MANUAL OF
PHYSICAL MEDICINE AND
REHABILITATION

Manual of

PHYSICAL MEDICINE AND REHABILITATION

Editor

Christopher M. Brammer, M.D.

Resident Physician
Department of Physical Medicine and Rehabilitation
University of Michigan Health System
Ann Arbor, Michigan

Associate Editor

M. Catherine Spires, M.D.

Clinical Assistant Professor
Associate Chair of Clinical Affairs
Chief of University Consult Services
Residency Program Director
Department of Physical Medicine and Rehabilitation
University of Michigan Health System
Ann Arbor, Michigan

HANLEY & BELFUS, INC. Philadelphia

Publisher: HANLEY & BELFUS, INC.
Medical Publishers
210 S. 13th Street
Philadelphia, PA 19107
800-962-1892; 215-546-7293
FAX (215) 790-9330
www.hanleyandbelfus.com

Note to the reader: Although the information in this book has been carefully reviewed for correctness of dosage and indications, neither the authors nor the editors nor the publisher can accept any legal responsibility for any errors or omissions that may be made. Neither the publisher nor the editors make any warranty, expressed or implied, with respect to the material contained herein. Before prescribing any drug, the reader must review the manufacturer's current product information (package inserts) for accepted indications, absolute dosage recommendations, and other information pertinent to the safe and effective use of the product described.

Library of Congress Cataloging-in-Publication Data

Manual of physical medicine and rehabilitation / edited by Christopher M. Brammer, M. Catherine Spires.
    p. ; cm.
  Includes bibliographical references and index.
  ISBN 1-56053-479-6 (alk. paper)
    1. Medical rehabilitation—Handbooks, manuals, etc. 2. Medicine, Physical—Handbooks, manuals, etc. I. Brammer, Christopher M., 1973- II. Spires, M. Catherine, 1947-
    [DNLM: 1. Physical Medicine—methods—Handbooks. 2. Physical Medicine—methods—Outlines. 3. Rehabilitation—methods—Handbooks. 4. Rehabilitation—methods—Outlines. WB 39 M2947 2002]
  RM930 .M36 2002
  617'.03—dc21
                                                                    2001051604

The publishers have made every effort to trace the copyright holders for borrowed material. If they have inadvertently overlooked any, they will be pleased to make the necessary arrangements at the first opportunity.

Manual of Physical Medicine and Rehabilitation   ISBN 1-56053-479-6

Last digit is the print number: 9 8 7 6 5 4 3 2 1

Dedication

To my wife Deanna—for her unconditional love and support

*To my children Trevor, Tori, and Cassidy—who show me
what things are really important in life*

*My parents and sister—for helping me build the foundation
on which I stand*

– C.M.B.

*To my friends and colleagues
For their support in all my endeavors:*

*Theodore M. Cole, M.D., Chair Emeritus, visionary of
life and the specialty of Physical Medicine and Rehabilitation*

*James A. Leonard, Jr., M.D., Chair,
outstanding clinician and teacher*

*Alice Cheesman, University of Michigan PM&R Residency
Training Coordinator, a tireless supporter of
the residents and training directors*

*Thurmond J. Johnson, M.D., resident and teacher,
for his commitment and dedication to
family and our profession*

*University of Michigan PM&R Department Graduates
and residents with whom I have had the privilege
of working*

–M.C.S.

Contents

III. THERAPEUTIC INTERVENTIONS

IV. APPENDIX

Contributors

Paula M. Anton, R.N., M.S.A.
Clinical Care Coordinator, Department of Nursing Administration, University of Michigan Health System, Ann Arbor, Michigan

Rita N. Ayyangar, M.D.
Clinical Assistant Professor, Division of Pediatric Rehabilitation, Department of Physical Medicine and Rehabilitation, University of Michigan Health System, Ann Arbor, Michigan

Anne Bradley, Ph.D.
Post-doctoral Fellow, Department of Physical Medicine and Rehabilitation, University of Michigan Health System, Ann Arbor, Michigan

Christopher M. Brammer, M.D.
Resident Physician, Department of Physical Medicine and Rehabilitation, University of Michigan Health System, Ann Arbor, Michigan

Andrew R. Briggeman, D.O.
Resident Physician, Department of Physical Medicine and Rehabilitation, University of Michigan Health System, Ann Arbor, Michigan

Lori L. Brinkey, M.P.T.
Physical Therapist, Division of Physical Therapy, Department of Physical Medicine and Rehabilitation, University of Michigan Health System, Ann Arbor, Michigan

Anthony Chiodo, M.D.
Clinical Assistant Professor, Department of Physical Medicine and Rehabilitation, University of Michigan Health System, Ann Arbor, Michigan

Anita S.W. Craig, D.O.
Clinical Instructor, Department of Physical Medicine and Rehabilitation, University of Michigan Health System, Ann Arbor, Michigan

Alicia J. Davis, C.P.O.
Senior Orthotist/Prosthetist, Orthotics and Prosthetics Center, Department of Physical Medicine and Rehabilitation, University of Michigan Health System, Ann Arbor, Michigan

Lisa A. DiPonio, M.D.
Clinical Instructor, Department of Physical Medicine and Rehabilitation, University of Michigan Health System, Ann Arbor, Michigan

Lynn E. Driver, M.S., C.C.C.
Speech-Language Pathologist, Division of Speech and Language Pathology, Department of Physical Medicine and Rehabilitation, University of Michigan Health System, Ann Arbor, Michigan

Jeffrey E. Evans, Ph.D.
Clinical Assistant Professor, Department of Physical Medicine and Rehabilitation, University of Michigan Health System, Ann Arbor, Michigan

Donald F. Green, M.D.
Resident Physician, Department of Physical Medicine and Rehabilitation, University of Michigan Health System, Ann Arbor, Michigan

Liza B. Green, M.D.
Resident Physician, Department of Physical Medicine and Rehabilitation, University of
Michigan Health System, Ann Arbor, Michigan

Bryan Grose, C.P.
Orthotics and Prosthetics Center, Department of Physical Medicine and Rehabilitation,
University of Michigan Health System, Ann Arbor, Michigan

Andrew J. Haig, M.D.
Associate Professor, Director, Spine Program, Department of Physical Medicine and Rehabilitation and Department of Surgery, University of Michigan Health System, Ann Arbor, Michigan

Anne Griffith Hartigan, M.D.
Resident Physician, Department of Physical Medicine and Rehabilitation, University of
Michigan Health System, Ann Arbor, Michigan

Gioia M. Herring, M.D.
Assistant Director, Adult Rehabilitation Inpatient Service, Clinical Instructor, Department
of Physical Medicine and Rehabilitation, University of Michigan Health System, Ann Arbor,
Michigan

Joyce L. Huerta, M.D.
Resident Physician, Department of Physical Medicine and Rehabilitation, University of
Michigan Health System, Ann Arbor, Michigan

Edward Albert Hurvitz, M.D.
Assistant Professor, Department of Physical Medicine and Rehabilitation, University of
Michigan Health System, Ann Arbor, Michigan

Mara M. Isser, D.O.
Resident Physician, Department of Physical Medicine and Rehabilitation, University of
Michigan Health System, Ann Arbor, Michigan

Sarah Clay Jamieson, M.D.
Lecturer, Department of Physical Medicine and Rehabilitation, University of Michigan
Health System, Ann Arbor, Michigan

David A. Klipp, M.D.
Resident Physician, Department of Physical Medicine and Rehabilitation, University of
Michigan Health System, Ann Arbor, Michigan

Benedict S. Konzen, M.D.
Assistant Professor, Department of Palliative Care and Rehabilitation Medicine, University
of Texas, M.D. Anderson Cancer Center, Houston, Texas

Karen B. Kurcz, M.A., C.C.C.
Speech and Language Pathologist, Division of Speech and Language Pathology, Depart-
ment of Physical Medicine and Rehabilitation, University of Michigan Health System, Ann
Arbor, Michigan

Ann T. Laidlaw, M.D.
Resident Physician, Department of Physical Medicine and Rehabilitation, University of
Michigan Health System, Ann Arbor, Michigan

Sharon K. McDowell, M.D.
Assistant Professor, Department of Physical Medicine and Rehabilitation, University of
Michigan Health System, Ann Arbor, Michigan

Karen L. Meyer, D.O.
Attending Physician, Munson Medical Center, Traverse City, Michigan

Sonya R. Miller, M.D.
Clinical Instructor, Associate Residency Director, Department of Physical Medicine and Rehabilitation, University of Michigan Health System, Ann Arbor, Michigan

Virginia S. Nelson, M.D., M.P.H.
Clinical Associate Professor, Department of Physical Medicine and Rehabilitation, University of Michigan Health System, Ann Arbor, Michigan

Austin I. Nobunaga, M.D., M.P.H.
Associate Clinical Professor, Department of Physical Medicine and Rehabilitation, University of Cincinnati, Drake Center, University Hospital, Cincinnati, Ohio

Jess W. Olson, M.D.
Resident Physician, Department of Physical Medicine and Rehabilitation, University of Michigan Health System, Ann Arbor, Michigan

Geeta Peethambaran, B.Sc., P.T.
Clinical Specialist, Division of Physical Therapy, Department of Physical Medicine and Rehabilitation, University of Michigan Health System, Ann Arbor, Michigan

William M. Scelza, M.D.
Resident Physician, Department of Physical Medicine and Rehabilitation, University of Michigan Health System, Ann Arbor, Michigan

Jennifer Shifferd, M.S., P.T.
Physical Therapist, Division of Physical Therapy, Department of Physical Medicine and Rehabilitation, University of Michigan Health System, Ann Arbor, Michigan

M. Catherine Spires, M.A., M.D.
Clinical Assistant Professor, Department of Physical Medicine and Rehabilitation, University of Michigan Health System, Ann Arbor, Michigan

Henry C. Tong, M.D.
Lecturer, Department of Physical Medicine and Rehabilitation, University of Michigan Health System, Ann Arbor, Michigan

Andrew G. Urquhart, M.D.
Assistant Professor, Department of Orthopaedic Surgery, University of Michigan Health System, Ann Arbor, Michigan

Seth Warschausky, Ph.D.
Associate Professor, Department of Physical Medicine and Rehabilitation, University of Michigan Health System, Ann Arbor, Michigan

Jacques S. Whitecloud, M.D.
Resident Physician, Department of Physical Medicine and Rehabilitation, University of Michigan Health System, Ann Arbor, Michigan

Mark J. Ziadeh, M.D.
Resident Physician, Department of Physical Medicine and Rehabilitation, University of Michigan Health System, Ann Arbor, Michigan

Foreword

The present is prologue to the future, and in our future we will find increasing numbers of people with disabilities, an increasing population of elderly persons, and an increasing need to enhance the productivity of our citizens. To meet these needs, medical rehabilitation has moved into the mainstream of health care.

The mainstream was a long time in coming. In 1947, The American Medical Association first recognized the American Board of Physical Medicine, and examination of candidates resulted in the issuance of 103 certificates for Physical Therapy Physicians. Within ten years, the Society of Physical Therapy Physicians (forerunner of the American Academy of Physical Medicine and Rehabilitation) boasted 300 members. In the 1970s, the AMA proposed standards of medical practice for physiatrists, and by the end of that decade their numbers had grown to 1200. Such growth was insufficient to meet national needs, and the Graduate Medical Education National Advisory Council recommended the specialty grow to 4000 members, which it did by 1992.

Growth brought with it changes beyond size. Electromyography and Pediatric Rehabilitation led the movement to subspecialize within physiatry. They soon were followed by other special interest groups such as spine physicians, sports medicine physicians, and spinal cord injury physicians. Around them grew a host of other medical and scientific scholars (including neurologists, orthopedists, internists, burn surgeons, pediatricians, pulmonologists, cardiologists, head injury technicians, physician assistants, and others) adding to the existing list of health care specialists who were already in the swim of medical rehabilitation: nurses, physical therapists, occupational therapists, orthotists and prosthetists, psychologists, speech and language pathologists, and many more. There are now more than 600,000 physicians in the United States. Only about 7000 are specialists in Physical Medicine and Rehabilitation, far too few to manage the nation's entire effort in medical rehabilitation.

As can be seen, the twentieth century was a time of confluence. Society and our system of medical care recognized that physical disability was one of the most important issues affecting the health of our nation. Physiatrists were key advocates for the evolution and they were greatly benefited by so many other professionals serving persons with chronic diseases and injuries in America. This group found support from policy makers and health care economists, and physical dysfunction took its place alongside organ pathology as a basis for extensive growth in research and technology to solve human problems related to injury and illness. Medical rehabilitation had moved into a place of recognition and respect.

Public Law 101.613, the Americans with Disabilities Act, enacted in July 1990, sets the civil rights expectation that people with disabilities should experience a life filled with more opportunity and compassion. Their future must include health professionals who have a full understanding of the issues regarding physical disabilities. In order for this to happen, the community of health practitioners whose priority is working with human disability will need ready reference to the information in this volume.

This big-little book, the *Manual of Physical Medicine and Rehabilitation*, is testimony to these changes, for its explicates how medical rehabilitation is practiced. The chapters are directed not only to physiatrists but also to the diverse work force of rehabilitation practitioners. They offer immediate and easy access to the essentials of medical rehabilitative care. The book is organized around the tried and true three-legged stool: the patient, the problem, and the therapy. Yet it flows out of the latest evidence-based interventions and evaluative tools. Chapters address the most frequently seen diagnoses and disabilities facing health practitioners of today. It spells out what to consider in a patient evaluation, how to approach problems, and what interventions to consider. It includes up-to-date medical information on both adult and pediatric populations as well as current disability issues that are comanaged by colleagues in the field. It is a book for both the student and the seasoned practitioner of medical rehabilitation. Its size makes it a ready reference for diagnostic dilemmas and therapeutic choices.

The *Manual of Physical Medicine and Rehabilitation* is written by residents in the field of PM&R at the University of Michigan and their faculty mentors. This group is keenly attuned to finding quick and understandable information that they found useful in their own development as specialists in medical rehabilitation. We hope it will help you, too.

Theodore M. Cole, MD
Professor Emeritus
Department of Physical Medicine
    and Rehabilitation
University of Michigan

Preface

We are pleased and humbled to witness the production of the *Manual of Physical Medicine and Rehabilitation*. It began as a vision to produce a practical guide of strategies and interventions that rehabilitation clinicians at varying levels of experience and training could use. The *Manual's* use is primarily focused toward the physiatric clinical management of patients. Its goal is to complement comprehensive textbooks and to provide a quick, mobile reference that one could carry in a lab coat.

Practical manuals play a vital role in clinical patient management and in medical student and resident training. Historic manuals such as the *Washington Manual of Medical Therapeutics* in internal medicine and the *Harriet Lane Handbook* in pediatrics are essential and standard tools for clinicians in those specialties. There is no reason to believe that such a manual focused on rehabilitation medicine should be any less useful to clinicians in this field.

Using University of Michigan clinicians with varying degrees of experience was a way to ensure that the diverse needs of the anticipated reading audience would be met. When available, resident physicians and fellows laid the foundation of the chapters. They attempted to provide the information that clinicians of their level of experience would need. Because of this aspect, the *Manual* is an invaluable resource and aid in the education of residents and fellows involved in rehabilitation medicine. For many training programs, it could be used as an integral part of didactic and clinical instruction. This work was further directed and enhanced by junior and senior faculty. Because of this relationship, we feel that this manual addresses the educational needs of the clinician ranging from the medical student to resident to seasoned attending physician, as well as allied health professionals.

The organization of the *Manual* mimics the natural presentation of the rehabilitation patient to inpatient services. The first unit encompasses the management of the rehabilitation patient by specific rehabilitation diagnosis. The etiology, clinical presentation, evaluation, and diagnosis of specific problems are outlined along with medical and rehabilitation interventions. The second unit discusses specific medical problems seen in the rehabilitation population, although not necessarily exclusive to one specific rehabilitation patient subset. The third unit describes the most common therapeutic interventions used in rehabilitation medicine. Appendices complement the chapters with additional topical information and provide resources, such as adult and pediatric emergency algorithms, that are essential to the practice of inpatient rehabilitation medicine.

Maintaining a concise form was a challenging task given the enormous amount of information that is seen in rehabilitation medicine. Thus, theory and basic science generally have been reduced with an emphasis on clinical presentation, evaluation, and treatment of the most common situations encountered. The outline format is used for easier organization and scanning. For quick reference, generous use of charts, tables, and illustrations provide great quantities of information in the most concise and organized form.

The *Manual* cannot act as a complete equation into which all patients can be inserted. The clinician must continue to use experience and judgment to understand which treatment interventions are indicated and appropriate. We also recognize that there are different practices in patient management across the United States, as well as internationally. Thus, we can summarize that the recommendations on patient management and care in the *Manual* are general guides that encompass common knowledge and practices, as well as clinical experiences from the University of Michigan.

We wish to thank many that have made important and essential contributions. We appreciate the support and guidance of James A. Leonard, Jr., M.D., Clinical Professor and Chair of the Department of Physical Medicine and Rehabilitation at the University of Michigan. Karen Hadwin, clinical administrator of the Department, contributed with suggestions and resources to improve the quality of the *Manual*. Administrative support and manuscript preparation from Ms. Alice Cheesman and Beth Benton were greatly appreciated. We certainly have benefitted from the inspiration and friendship of Thurmond Johnson, M.D. Bryan Grose, C.P., has produced outstanding illustrations that made concepts come to life. Drs. James Rae and Theodore Cole, former Department Chairmen, are to be thanked for establishing and building a strong, dedicated department from which the present generation of patients and clinicians are undoubtedly benefiting. Finally, and most importantly, thanks and appreciation go to the many contributors. Without their support and work, the *Manual* would simply have been a vision instead of a reality.

We are proud to present this work to our colleagues in the field of rehabilitation medicine, a field made of physicians in many specialties and health professionals in many disciplines. Whether a beginning resident or seasoned clinician, we hope that you find the *Manual* useful in the ultimate task of helping those patients who aim to improve their independence and return to life in their community.

Christopher M. Brammer, M.D.
M. Catherine Spires, M.D.

Chapter 1

AMPUTATION REHABILITATION

Joyce L. Huerta, M.D., and Sonya R. Miller, M.D.

I. Epidemiology

A. Lower extremity amputations

1. Peripheral obstructive disease accounts for 65–75% of all lower extremity (LE) amputations. The male-to-female ratio is 2.1:1.
2. Trauma accounts for 20–25% of LE amputations. Amputations due to trauma are more common in 17–55-year-old males. The male-to-female ratio is 7.2:1.
3. Malignancy accounts for 5% of LE amputations. Malignancy-related amputations are common in 10–20-year-olds.
4. Congenital limb deficiency is the cause of in 5–60% of all amputations in children. The male-to-female ratio is 1.5:1.
5. The prevalence is 1,230,000–1,546,000 major amputations; 80–85% of all amputations involve the LE.
6. Equal left and right occurrence.

B. Upper extremity amputations

1. The most common causes of upper extremity (UE) amputation are trauma and cancer.
2. The most common type of UE amputation is the transradial level, which accounts for 57% of all UE amputations.
3. Incidence of congenital UE deficiency is 4.1 per 10,000 live births. Left, terminal transverse radial limb deficiency is the most common congenital limb deficiency.
4. The right arm is more frequently involved in work-related injuries.

II. Types of Lower Extremity Amputations (Figs. 1 and 2)

A. **Transphalangeal:** excision of part of the toe(s).

B. **Toe disarticulation:** resection through the metatarsophalangeal (MTP) joint(s).

C. **Partial foot/ray:** resection of the metatarsal and digit.

D. **Transmetatarsal:** resection through all metatarsals.
1. Avoids equinovarus deformity.
2. Provides adequate lever arm.

E. **Lisfranc:** resection through the metatarsal and tarsal joint.
1. Transfer of the peroneus brevis to the cuboid and transfer of the anterior tibialis to the neck of the talus prevents equinovarus deformity.
2. Can be difficult to fit with orthosis or partial foot prosthesis.

F. **Chopart:** resection through the calcaneocuboid and talonavicular joints.
1. Transfer of the peroneus brevis to the cuboid and transfer of the anterior tibialis to the neck of the talus prevent equinovarus deformity.
2. Can be difficult to fit with orthosis or partial foot prosthesis.

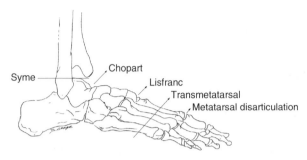

FIGURE 1. Types of lower extremity amputations (foot).

G. **Symes:** ankle disarticulation with or without removal of the medial/lateral malleoli and distal tibia/fibula flares.
   1. If the heel pad is not attached properly, there is the risk of heel-pad migration.
   2. 3% of all amputations.
H. **Transtibial:** below knee amputation (BKA).
   1. Ideal length is at the intersection between the middle and distal thirds of the limb.
   2. Ideal shape is cylindrical.
   3. Long BKA is > 5 0% of tibial length, medium BKA is 20–50% of tibial length; short BKA is < 20% of tibial length.
   4. 54% of all amputations.

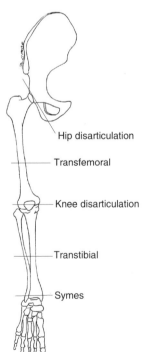

FIGURE 2. Types of lower extremity amputations (leg).

   I. **Knee disarticulation:** resection through the knee.
      1. Not an ideal length because it limits the amount of space available for components (the patient has to be fit with an above-knee prosthesis).
      2. 1% of all amputations.
   J. **Transfemoral:** above-knee amputation (AKA).
      1. Ideal length is just proximal to femoral condyles.
      2. Ideal shape is conical.
      3. Long AKA is > 60% of femoral length; medium AKA is 35–60% of femoral length; short AKA is < 35% of femoral length.
      4. 32% of all amputations.
   K. **Hip disarticulation:** resection through the hip; the pelvis is intact. (2% of all amputations).
   L. **End weight-bearing amputations**
      1. Transmetatarsal
      2. Chopart
      3. Lisfranc
      4. Symes
      5. Osetomyoplasty/Ertl procedure: an osteoperiosteal tube joins the ends of the bones, which ossify to form a sturdy weight-bearing bone bridge.
III. **Types of Upper Extremity Amputations** (Fig. 3)
   A. **Transphalangeal (partial finger):** resection may occur at distal interphalangeal (DIP), proximal interphalangeal (PIP), or metacarpophalangeal (MCP) levels.
   B. **Transmetacarpal:** resection through the metacarpals.

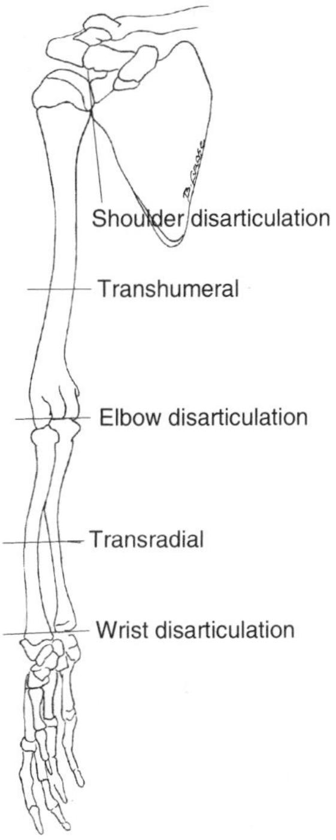

FIGURE 3. Types of upper extremity amputations.

Shoulder disarticulation

Transhumeral

Elbow disarticulation

Transradial

Wrist disarticulation

C. **Transcarpal:** transection through the carpal bones.
D. **Wrist disarticulation:** transection between the carpals and radius/ulna (1% of all amputations).
E. **Transradial (below elbow)**
   1. Long = > 80% of radial length; medium =55–80% of radial length; short = < 55% of radial length.
   2. 4% of all amputations.
F. **Elbow disarticulation:** transection through elbow joint (0.2% of all amputations).
G. **Transhumeral (above elbow)**
   1. Standard = 50–90% of humeral length; short = <50% of humeral length.
   2. 2% of all amputations.
H. **Shoulder disarticulation:** transection through shoulder joint (1% of all amputations).

IV. **Vascular Analysis**
   A. **Ankle brachial index (ABI)**
      1. ABI = lower extremity systolic blood pressure (BP)/brachial systolic BP.
      2. Normal = 1 or greater.
      3. Indicates normal blood flow and healing.
      4. Lowest ABI consistent with healing in a diabetic patient is 0.45; in a nondiabetic patient, 0.35. Healing is likely to be very slow.
   B. **Transcutaneous Doppler ultrasound**
      1. Triphasic waveform is normal; healing is normal.
      2. Biphasic waveform is normal; healing is normal.
      3. Monophasic waveform is abnormal and indicates impaired flow; poor healing potential.
   C. **Transcutaneous oxygen (TcO$_2$):** normal = 40 mmHg; healing will occur.

V. **Surgical Considerations**
   A. **Partial foot (transmetatarsal, Lisfranc, Chopart)**
      1. Bevel the inferior edges of the bones with a transmetarsal amputation to decrease pressure on plantar surface.
      2. Use only plantar skin for skin grafts on the plantar surface.
   B. **Transtibial**
      1. Bevel the ends of the tibia and fibula.
      2. The fibula should be 0.5–1.0 cm shorter than the tibia to promote a cylindrical shape.
      3. Avoid split-thickness skin grafts.
      4. Long posterior flap (Burgess procedure is preferred because the muscle padding facilitates total contact fitting).
      5. With a short BKA (at the level of the tibial tubercle), the fibular head should be removed. Otherwise, it may cause pain with prosthetic use.
      6. The nerves should be cut under tension to allow them to retract and decrease the risk of pain from neuroma formation.
      7. Myodesis should be performed, if possible. The posterior calf muscles are attached to the tibia. With a myodesis, the fascia and muscles are sutured directly to the bone. This technique creates the most structurally stable limb.
   C. **Transfemoral**
      1. Myodesis is the preferred method. It stabilizes the femur in adduction (via the adductor magnus), enhances hip flexion (via the rectus femoris), and enhances hip extension (via biceps femoris). Control of the limb in the socket is optimized.

2. Transect the nerves under tension to allow retraction and decrease risk of pain from neuroma development.
3. The fishmouth technique (equal anterior and posterior flaps) is preferred.
4. Avoid split-thickness skin grafts.

D. **Transradial**
   1. The long forearm residual limb is preferred for use of body-powered prosthesis.
   2. The medium forearm residual limb is preferred for externally powered prosthesis.
   3. Ideal shape of residual limb is cylindrical.

E. **Limb salvage vs. amputation**
   1. Amputation is indicated if one cannot reconstruct a vascular injury.
   2. Trauma often involves vascular or nerve injury, burn injury, cold injury, or nonhealing fractures. All may result in a limb that is less functional than a prosthesis.
   3. Limb should be salvaged only if it has sufficient sensation to be capable of productive feedback.
   4. Early amputation and prosthetic fitting are preferable to limb salvage that results in poor function.

F. **Guillotine amputation** (open amputation)
   1. Done in patients with infection to keep it from spreading.
   2. Usually revised to closed amputation.

VI. **Postoperative Management**
   A. **Rigid removal dressing (RRD)** is used for transtibial amputees (Fig. 4).
      1. Made of plaster of Paris or fiberglass and suspended by stockinette and supracondylar cuff.
      2. Benefits
         a. Controls edema
         b. Decreases pain
         c. Promotes wound healing
         d. Protects limb from trauma
         e. Desensitizes limb
         f. Allows daily inspection of limb
      3. Prosthetic socks may be added or omitted to maintain proper fit.
   B. **Immediate postoperative prosthesis (IPOP):** for transtibial amputees
      1. Rigid spica made of plaster of Paris and applied from distal limb to mid thigh.
      2. Benefits
         a. Prevents knee flexion contracture.
         b. Controls edema.
         c. Protects limb from trauma.
         d. Desensitizes limb.
         e. Can add pylon and foot to allow early ambulation.
         f. Usually worn for 3 weeks and changed weekly.
      3. The one disadvantage is that you cannot inspect the limb daily.
   C. **Soft dressing:** for transtibial and transfemoral amputees (Fig. 5).
      1. Elastic bandage (Ace wrap) or elastic shrinker.
      2. Should be worn 24 hours/day except for bathing.
      3. Elastic bandage should be applied in a figure-of-8 fashion.

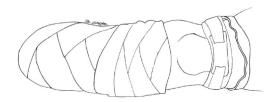

FIGURE 4. Rigid removable dressing.

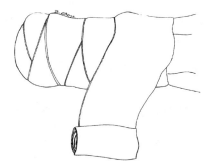

FIGURE 5. Figure-of-8 elastic bandage wrapping.

    4. Difficult to apply correct amount of compression with elastic bandage. If there is more compression proximally than distally, you create a tourniquet effect.

    5. Elastic bandage is the least effective method of edema control. It is best to use double-length, 4-inch bandage for BKAs and double-length, 6-inch bandage for AKAs.

    6. Shrinker sock provides even compression and is easy to don and doff.

    7. Patient can begin using stump shrinker 1–2 weeks after surgery if incision is healing well.

  D. **Semirigid postoperative dressing:** for transtibial amputees

    1. Unna paste applied over conventional soft dressing.

    2. Unna paste = zinc oxide, gelatin, glycerin, calamine

    3. Benefits

      a. Controls edema.

      b. Limits joint movement and prevents contracture formation.

  E. **Pain management**

    1. **Postoperative surgical pain** is best treated with narcotics. Consider patient-controlled analgesic (PCA) pump or epidural.

    2. **Phantom pain:** pain referred to the surgically removed limb or some area of the removed limb.

      a. Often described as cramping, squeezing, burning, sharp, or shooting.

      b. Up to 85% of amputees report phantom pain.

      c. Commonly develops in first month after amputation.

      d. More likely to develop in patients who had a lot of pain before amputation.

      e. Possible causes: peripheral nerve irritation, abnormal sympathetic function, and psychological factors.

      f. Treatment

     i. Transcutaneous electrical nerve stimulation (TENS) unit
    ii. Tricyclic antidepressants (TCAs): nortriptyline, amitriptyline (usually start with a low dose, 10–25 mg at bedtime).
   iii. Anticonvulsants: carbamazepine, gabapentin (usually necessary to titrate gabapentin to at least 300 mg 3 times/day; serum gabapentin levels can be monitored.).
    iv. Topical anesthetics—lidocaine gel, capsaicin
     v. Chemical sympathectomy
    vi. Beta blockers
   vii. Shrinker sock
  viii. Narcotics are not helpful.

3. **Phantom sensation:** awareness of missing limb.
   a. Not an unpleasant or painful sensation.
   b. Associated with subjective tingling sensation.
   c. Very common immediately after amputation.
   d. Usually felt in most distal aspect of limb.
4. **Tumor:** local recurrence of tumor can cause residual limb pain.
5. **Vascular disorders**
   a. Peripheral vascular disease can cause intermittent claudication in residual limb.
   b. Traumatic amputees may have damage to the vascular system that manifests as residual limb pain years after injury.

F. **Skin complications**
1. **Choke syndrome:** edema of the distal limb caused by lack of total contact between limb and prosthesis.
   a. Associated with proximal restriction of prosthesis around limb.
   b. Verrucous hyperplasia (Fig. 6) can develop if choke syndrome is not treated.
      i. Wart-like skin overgrowth on distal aspect of limb.
      ii. Caused by poor external compression and edema.
   c. Choke syndrome and verrucous hyperplasia are treated by improving total contact between limb and socket. This goal is achieved by adding a distal pad to socket, improving suspension, or making a new socket.
2. **Maceration**
   a. Caused by too much moisture next to skin.
   b. Treatment includes changing prosthetic socks frequently, using absorbent prosthetic socks, applying cornstarch or talc power to limb, and use of specially formulated antiperspirants.

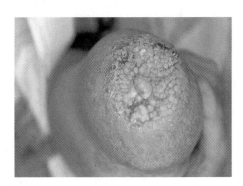

FIGURE   6. Verrucous hyperplasia in chronic choke syndrome.

3. **Contact dermatitis**
   a. Macular, papular erythematous rash; often pruritic.
   b. Treatment includes topical corticosteroids and removal of offending agent.
4. **Tinea corporis, tinea cruris** (fungal infections)
   a. Caused by excessive moisture with or without poor hygiene.
   b. Treatment includes use of antiseptic cleaner, oral antibiotics, and topical fungicides as well as decreasing excessive moisture.
5. **Folliculitis**
   a. Infection of hair follicles
   b. Caused by poor hygiene, sweating, poor socket fit, postioning of limb in socket.
   c. Treatment includes use of antiseptic cleaner, topical or oral antibiotics, incision and drainage, and avoiding high-pressure areas in socket.
6. **Epidermoid cyst**
   a. Sebaceous gland plugged with keratin.
   b. Treatment includes topical or oral antibiotics and incision and drainage.
7. **Skin adherence**
   a. Caused by scar tissue.
   b. Treatment includes friction scar massage, socket modification, and surgical revision.
8. **Skin grafts:** split-thickness skin grafts do not provide best residual limb coverage, especially on end-bearing surfaces.

G. **Other complications**
1. **Neuromas**
   a. Formation of scar tissue around distal end of a severed nerve.
   b. Potential source of stump and/or phantom pain.
   c. Often can be palpated on exam.
   d. Direct palpation of neuroma reproduces lancinating pain.
   e. Treatment includes modification of socket, local injection with anesthetic and corticosteroids, and surgical excision.
   f. May reoccur even when treated with surgery.
2. **Bone problems:** there are multiple sources of bone pain.
   a. Incorrectly stripped periosteum during surgery or from trauma.
   b. Hypermobile fibula that is longer than tibia.
   c. Unbalanced myodesis for transfemoral amputation can cause femur to extrude through muscle and skin.
   d. Severe hip or knee osteoarthritis.
3. **Contractures:** most common are hip and knee flexion contractures
   a. Knee flexion contracture of 10° or less can be treated conservatively (stretching with or without ultrasound and ambulating as much as possible).
   b. Knee flexion contracture of 25° or more may require hamstring lengthening with posterior knee capsule release or bent-knee prosthesis.
   c. Ability to accommodate a hip flexion contracture depends on limb length.
      i. 15° or more of hip flexion contracture in a long transfemoral residual limb results in a compensatory lumbar lordosis.
      ii. Short transfemoral residual limb can accommodate up to 25° of hip flexion contracture with accompanying loss of hip extension power.

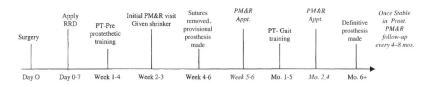

FIGURE 7.   Lower extremity amputee rehabilitation time line (vascular patient).

       iii. For transfemoral amputees, a hip flexion contracture contributes to knee instability and may result in use of a lockable knee.

   d. Knee or hip flexion contractures decrease cosmesis.

   e. Hip flexion contractures are prevented by avoiding prolonged sitting, using no pillows under the residual limb, and daily stretching.

   f. Knee flexion contractures are prevented by daily stretching and placing a board under the limb that promotes knee extension

VII. Therapy (Figs. 7 and 8)

  A. **Preprosthetic training:** period from hospital discharge to prosthetic fitting.

    1. **Goals for lower extremity**

      a. Maintain range of motion of the joints proximal to the level of amputation.

      b. Strengthen the gluteus medius and maximus for all levels of lower extremity amputation.

      c. Additional emphasis is placed on strengthening the hamstrings and quadriceps for Symes and transtibial amputees.

      d. Mobility training: wheelchair, walker, crutches

      e. Transfer training

      f. Activities of daily living training from seated/wheelchair level.

    2. **Goals for upper extremity**

      a. Maintain range of motion of the joints proximal to the level of amputation.

      b. Strengthen the scapular protractors, retractors, elevators and depressors.

      c. Activities of daily living training, especially if dominant upper extremity was amputated.

      d. If dominant upper extremity amputated, begin training patient to use other upper extremity as dominant arm.

  B. **Prosthetic Training**

    1. **Goals for lower extremity**

      a. All of the goals listed under preprosthetic training.

      b. Gait training with prosthesis on all surfaces.

      c. Improving balance on all surfaces.

      d. Ascending/descending stairs, curbs, ramps.

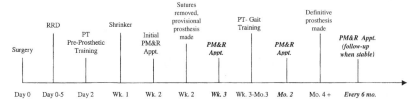

FIGURE 8.   Lower extremity amputee rehabilitation time line (traumatic patient).

  e. Prosthetic and skin care.
  f. Proper donning and doffing of prosthesis.
 2. **Goals for upper extremity**
  a. All of the goals listed under preprosthetic training.
  b. Prosthetic and skin care.
  c. Proper donning and doffing of prosthesis.
  d. Opening and closing of the terminal device.
  e. Grasping and releasing of objects.
  f. Prepositioning of the terminal device for activities.
  g. Training in activities of daily living, homemaking skills, occupational skills and recreational activities.

VIII. Energy Expenditure (Table 1)
IX. Pediatric Amputees
 A. **Etiology**
  1. In the first decade, about 68% of new pediatric amputees are due to congenital deformity, 27% to trauma, 3% to tumor, and 2% to disease.
  2. In the second decade, 63% of new pediatric amputations are due to trauma, 22% to tumor, 9% to disease, and 6% to late surgery for congenital deformity.
  3. Possible causes of congenital limb deficiency
   a. Exposure to teratogenic agents during limb development: thalidomide, excessive radiation.
   b. Congenital amniotic bands
   c. Certain genetically determined syndromes: Holt-Oram, Fanconi syndromes
 B. **Special considerations**
  1. **Bony overgrowth:** periosteal appositional growth
   a. Common in the skeletally immature, especially after a mid-shaft amputation.
   b. Risk is decreased if amputation is done through the joint, which preserves the epiphysis.
   c. Unlike adults, residual condyles tend to atrophy after amputation through the joint.
   d. Can be a source of pain.
   e. Transplanting an epiphysis over the bone end can limit occurrence and recurrence.

TABLE 1. Energy Expenditure of Amputees vs. Normal Subjects without Vascular Disease

Amputation Level	Percent Decrease in Gait Velocity	Percent Increase in Oxygen Consumption
Syme	32	13
Transtibial (vascular)	44	33
Transtibial (traumatic)	11	7
Knee disarticulation (traumatic)	24	53
Transfemoral (vascular)	55	87
Hip disarticulation	41	60
Transpelvic	50	93

2. **Leg length discrepancy**
    a. Can be caused by epiphyseal growth asymmetries in distal femoral plate, which contributes 70% to femoral growth lengthening.
    b. Proximal tibial plate contributes 56% to tibial growth lengthening.
3. **Skin**
    a. Split-thickness skin grafts, even on weight-bearing surfaces, are a good way to provide residual limb coverage, but full-thickness skin grafts are best.
    b. Surgical incisions tolerate more tension than in adults.
4. **Phantom pain:** uncommon in pediatric amputees.
5. **Timing of prosthetic fitting**
    a. UE prosthesis should be fitted when the child is learning to sit (about 6 months of age).
    b. LE prosthesis is fitted when the child is learning to stand (about 9–12 months of age).
    c. Transfemoral amputee scan be fitted at 6 months to promote symmetrical sitting.
C. **Prosthetic considerations**
    1. Initially, transfemoral amputation prostheses have a locked knee joint.
    2. Around age 3, a constant friction knee can be used for transfemoral amputees.
    3. Modifications and socket replacements are more common than with adults because of growth.
    4. Difference of 1 cm or more between sound and prosthetic limb is indication for new prosthesis.
    5. Children need a new LE prosthesis each year up to age 5, every 2 years from ages 5–12, and every 3–4 years to age 21.
D. **Common longitudinal deficiencies**
    1. **Fibular longitudinal deficiency:** fibular hemimelia
        a. Complete or partial absence of the fibula.
        b. Most common cause of congenital deficiency.
        c. Bilateral in 25% of cases.
        d. Leg length inequality can be severe.
    2. **Femoral longitudinal deficiency:** proximal femoral focal deficiency (PFFD)
        a. Partial deficiency of the femur with involvement of hip joint.
        b. Typical femur position is flexion, abduction, external rotation.
        c. Frequently associated with partial fibular absence and foot deformity.
        d. May be associated with tibial shortening, hip and knee flexion contractures.
        e. 10–15% are bilateral.
        f. Caused by failure of proximal femoral growth plate and chondrocytes to migrate proximally.
        g. Can be treated with van Ness rotation plasty and knee fusion.
    3. **Tibial longitudinal deficiency:** tibial hemimelia
        a. Complete or partial absence of the tibia.
        b. Associated with severe foot varus, leg shortening, knee and/or ankle instability.
        c. Can be associated with supernumerary digits, partial adactyly (floating thumb), central aphalangia of the hand (lobster claw).
        d. Can be part of an autosomal dominant syndrome.
        e. 30% of cases are bilateral.

X. Prosthetic Prescription
A. Lower extremity
1. Diagnosis
2. Socket
3. Liner
4. Suspension
5. Knee (for transfemoral)
6. Terminal device (foot)
7. Check/test socket

B. Upper extremity
1. Diagnosis
2. Socket
3. Terminal device
4. Suspension
5. Elbow (for transhumeral)
6. Control system
7. Body powered vs. externally powered
8. Check/test socket
9. Wrist unit

Bibliography
1. Barnes RW, Cox B: Amputations: An Illustrated Manual. Philadelphia, Hanley & Belfus, 2000.
2. Bowker JH, Michael JW (eds): Atlas of Limb Prosthetics: Surgical, Prosthetic, and Rehabilitation Principles, 2nd ed. St. Louis, Mosby, 1992.
3. Braddom RL: Physical Medicine and Rehabilitation, 2nd ed. Philadelphia, W.B. Saunders, 2000, pp 263–310.
4. DeLisa JA: Rehabilitation Medicine: Principles and Practice, 3rd ed. Philadelphia, Lippincott-Raven, 1998.
5. O'Young B, Young MA, Stiens SA (eds): PM&R Secrets, 2nd ed. Philadelphia, Hanley & Belfus, 2002.
6. Sanders G: Lower Limb Amputations: A Guide to Rehabilitation. Philadelphia, F.A. Davis, 1986.
7. Wilson AB Jr: Limb Prosthetics, 6th ed. New York, Demos Publications, 1989.

Chapter 2

BURN INJURY REHABILITATION

M. Catherine Spires, M.D., and Christopher M. Brammer, M.D.

I. Introduction

A. Burn injury is necrosis and damage of tissue secondary to exposure to an external agent such as flame, radiation or other agents of extreme temperature.

B. Burn injuries cause complex local and systemic responses involving the cardiovascular and pulmonary systems, microcirculation, metabolism, nutrition, endocrinology, and immunology.

C. Local and systemic reactions are time-dependent; the pathophysiologic responses of the acute period are distinct form those of a later period.

D. Burn injury has been a problem since the early use of fire by humans; Hippocrates and other ancients describe treatments for burn injuries.

E. Burn injury can result from thermal, electrical, frostbite, chemical, and radiation exposure.

F. The average person believes that a serious burn injury is the most devastating trauma that a person can sustain.

II. Epidemiology

A. The United State has the highest **incidence** of any industrialized nation.

1. Approximately 1.25 million people seek medical care for burn injuries each year.

2. Most burn injuries (approximately 90%) are thermal injuries, such as those due to direct flame.

3. Home-related accidents are responsible for one-third of burn injuries

4. 4% of people sustaining burn injury require hospitalization (50,000 per year).

5. Approximately 95% survive a major burn injury; in people whose burn is complicated by inhalation injury, the survival rate drops to 30%.

    a. Mortality is highest in very young and very old patients.

    b. Survival rate of severely burned people has dramatically increased over the past four decades.

B. **Children**

1. Account for 35% of burn injuries.

2. Scald injury is the most common type of childhood burn (72%).

3. Burn injury is the number-one cause of accidental death in children under age 2 years and the number-two cause of death in children under age 4.

4. 40% of patients admitted to hospitals for burns injuries are under age 10 or over age 50 years.

III. Costs

A. Mean length of hospital stay: 13.5 days.

B. Mean charges for hospitalization: $40,000; for the most severely injured: $200, 000.

    C. An estimated $2 billion is spent yearly in the U.S. for burn care; $30 million is spent each year for care of older women who sustain burn injuries related to ignition of clothing.

IV. Risk Factors

    A. **Male gender** (18–25-year-old group at greatest risk)

    B. **Premorbid conditions**

      1. Psychiatric disease

      2. Alcoholism and substance abuse

      3. Dementia

    C. **Risk factors for death**

      1. Age over 60 years or less than 2 years

      2. Burn size greater than 40%

      3. Inhalation injury

V. Etiology

    A. **Chemical burns**

      1. Alkali causes liquefaction necrosis.

      2. Acid causes coagulation necrosis.

    B. **Thermal Injuries:** protein denaturation occurs at 40°C.

    C. **Frostbite**

      1. Water in tissues crystallizes and causes tissue dehydration and damage.

      2. Due to exposure of tissue to temperature below freezing.

      3. Freezing temperatures may cause frostbite, depending on humidity, wind chill, altitude, duration of exposure, and other environmental factors.

      4. Frostnip or whitening of exposed area does not appear to cause damage but may increase the risk of frostbite in that area during future cold exposure.

    D. **Radiation**

      1. Primarily due to radiation treatment in civilian populations.

      2. Injury due to inhibition of cell proliferation.

      3. Delayed healing or chronic wounds may result from radiation therapy.

      4. Acute or chronic vascular changes may impair healing.

      5. After acute radiation, basal cells are damaged and tissue sloughs off, creating the wound; underlying tissue may be injured secondary to tissue hypoxia from obliterative endarteritis.

      6. Chronic wounds from radiation are difficult to manage.

    E. **Electrical burns**

      1. 3% of burns each year are secondary to electrical injury.

      2. Result in approximately 800 deaths per year; responsible for disproportionate amount of morbidity and mortality.

      3. Occur predominantly in young men ages 20–34, typically in the dominant arm while at work.

      4. Low-tension injuries occur at less than 500 volts; high-tension injuries occur above 1000 volts.

        a. The greater the amperage, the greater the injury; degree injury is related to current, resistance, and duration of exposure

        b. Cross-sectional area critical: as the area of exposure decreases, the current density increases, generating greater heat; therefore, fingers and toes are at greatest risk.

      5. Cutaneous injury does not necessarily reflect extent of injury because of "iceberg" effect. Deep tissue is more severely damaged than superficial or cutaneous inspection indicates.

6. Injury severity depends on voltage of source, amperage of current passing through tissues, resistance of tissues, duration of exposure, and pathway of current.
   a. Current traversing the most resistant tissue produces the greatest heat.
   b. Least conductive tissue is bone, followed by cartilage, tendon, skin, muscle, blood ,and nerve.
7. Complications include neurologic injuries and major limb amputation.

VI. Classification of Burns
A. **Etiology of injury** (see Section V. Etiology)
B. **Depth of injury**
   1. The skin is the largest organ of the body; total area ranges from 0.25– 1.9 m^2.
   2. Skin has multiple functions:
      a. Physical barrier against outside environment
      b. Immunologic function/infection
      c. Body temperature stabilization
      d. Facilitation of motion of body parts
      e. Appearance and personal identity
      f. Sensory organ
      g. Excretory organ
      h. Production of vitamin D
      i. Maintenance and prevention of loss of body fluids
   3. **Skin anatomy**
      a. **Epidermis** (external layer of skin; primary barrier to environment)
         i. Superficial layer is composed of nonviable cornified cells.
         ii. Keratinization occurs in epidermis; cells originate in basal layer and migrate outward, flatten, and break down, leaving keratin layer.
         iii. Cornified layer acts as barrier against environment.
      b. **Dermis**
         i. Prevents evaporative fluid loss.
         ii. Thermoregulation
         iii. Gives nutritional and mechanical support for epidermis.
         iv. Origin of skin appendages, such as hair follicles, sebaceous glands, and sweat glands.
         v. Collagen and elastic fibers give strength and flexibility to skin.
         vi. Vascular and cutaneous nervous tissues that mediate pain are found only in dermis.
      c. **Subcutaneous tissue**
         i. Supports dermis and epidermis.
         ii. Contains vascular plexuses and fat.
C. **Classification of injury depth** (Fig. 1)
   1. Depth is important determinant of healing.
   2. Traditional classification describes degree of injury, such as first , second, or third; the second common classification describes the injury in terms of partial or full thickness.
      a. **First-degree or superficial burn** (limited to epidermis)
         i. Mild swollen appearance of local tissue
         ii. No blistering
         iii. Erythematous and tender skin
         iv. Healing time of 2–3 days
         v. No scarring

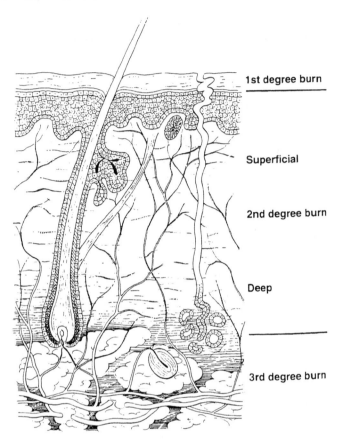

FIGURE 1. Normal skin histologic characteristics, with depth of burn injury indicated. (From Kucan JO: Burn and trauma. In Ruberg RL, Smith DJ Jr (eds): Plastic Surgery: A Core Curriculum. St. Louis, Mosby, 1994, p 212, with permission.)

      vi. Exfoliation of damaged epithelium in 5–10 days
     vii. Systemic effects are rare; patients typically do not need medical intervention.
   b. **Second-degree or partial-thickness burn** (entire epidermis and varying depths of dermis)
     i. Blistering; more painful than first-degree or superficial injury.
     ii. Superficial second-degree or superficial partial-thickness burn (limited to upper third of dermis)
      • Blistering
      • Very painful since cutaneous nerve endings are impaired but not totally damaged.
      • Heals in 7–14 days.
      • Epithelialization occurs by repopulation from cells that line skin appendages.
     iii. Deep second-degree or deep partial-thickness burn (more serious injury extending into deep dermis)

- Typically red and blanches with pressure.
- Less painful than superficial second-degree burn since most of the nerve endings are lost.
- Blistering is not typically seen.
- Fluid loss and metabolic effects are similar to those with third-degree burn.
- Marginal residual blood supply places wound at risk to convert to third-degree or full-thickness injury.
- Few epithelial cells survive; reservoir of epithelial cells is present in hair follicles and glands.
- Repopulation is very slow; although epithelial cells can regenerate and close the wound, healing can take several weeks or months, depending on wound dimensions.
- Typically skin grafting is required to expedite wound healing.
- Associated with significant scarring.

  c. **Third-degree, or full-thickness, burn** causes complete loss of epidermis and dermis. A deep partial-thickness burn and full-thickness burns are often difficult to distinguish clinically. When the depth of the wound is in question, the wound is treated as a full-thickness injury. Infection or inadequate circulation can convert a wound from a partial-thickness to a full-thickness wound.

    i. White, brown, or tan waxy appearance (may appear charred)
    ii. Dry, leathery texture
    iii. Thrombosed vessels
    iv. Insensitive to pain
    v. Re-epithelialization does not occur; no epithelial cells remain; granulation can occur.
    vi. Skin does not blanch or refill since the blood vessels are thrombosed.
    vii. Wound bed is avascular due to destruction of dermal blood vessels.
    viii. Require skin grafting unless the wound is small; in that case, healing can result from migration of skin from wound edges.
    ix. Dense, thick scarring results.

  d. **Fourth-degree burn**
    i. Extends to deep structures such as muscle, tendon, and bone.
    ii. May require amputation or extensive deep debridement.

C. **Total body surface area (TBSA).** Injured surface area refers to the extent of the burn expressed as a percent of body surface area. Surface area, like depth of injury, reflects severity of injury, prognosis, fluid resuscitation requirements, and type of treatment. It also determines which patients should be treated in a specialized burn center.

1. Average area of skin in adults is 1.8 m^2 (range = 1.2–1.9 m^2); in neonates, it is only 0.25 m^2.
2. Only partial-thickness or full-thickness burn sites are included in calculation of TBSA burned.
3. Surface area is determined most accurately by charts that are specific to the patient's age. Lund and Browden chart corrects for age-dependent differences (Fig. 2). Body surface determination is critical in children and adolescents.
4. In adults, surface area can be determined by using the rule of nines (Fig. 3), introduced by Pulasi and Tennison in the 1940s. It is a crude but time-honored estimation, particularly in emergency settings.

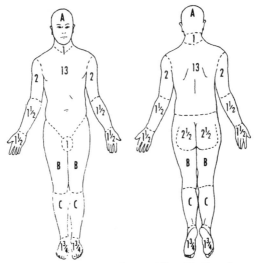

Relative Percentage of Areas Affected by Growth

	Age in Years					
	0	1	5	10	15	Adult
A—½ of head	9½	8½	6½	5½	4½	3½
B—½ of one thigh	2¾	3¼	4	4¼	4½	4¾
C—½ of one leg	2½	2½	2¾	3	3¼	3½

FIGURE 2.   Lund and Browder method of determining skin surface area; method corrects for differences in percentage of body surface areas by age. (From McManus WF: Immediate emergency department care. In Artz CP, Moncrief JA, Pruitt BA (eds): Burns: A Team Approach. Philadelphia, W.B. Saunders, 1979, p 154, with permission.)

     a. Unsatisfactory for children under age 15 since the surface area of the head is larger and the extremities are smaller than in adults.
     b. Based on the assumption that the body can be divided into 11 regions that represent 9% of the TBSA of the body with the perineum/genitalia equaling 1%
        i. Head and each upper extremity are 9%.
        ii. Anterior trunk, posterior trunk, and each lower extremity are 18%.
        iii. Palmar surface of hand equals approximately 1% of TBSA.
   5. Diagrams or computer-generated drawings are used to record specific sites of injury.
D. **Severity of injury**
   1. Severity of injury is determined by several factors, the most important of which are age and associated injuries or disease.
     a. Age: very young and very old people are the most vulnerable; minor and moderate injuries can be life-threatening in some instances.
     b. Among associated injuries, inhalation injury and head injury are particularly important.
     c. Premorbid disease or conditions (e.g., diabetes mellitus) can significantly affect morbidity and mortality.

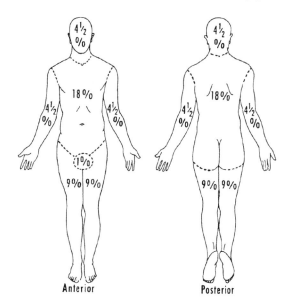

Anterior   Posterior

FIGURE 3.   Rule of nines used to determine body surface area injured. (From Moylan JA: First aid and transportation of burned patients. In Artz CP, Moncrief JA, Pruitt BA (eds): Burns: A Team Approach. Philadelphia, W.B. Saunders, 1979, p 153, with permission.)

      d. TBSA injured
      e. Depth of injury
      f. Body part injured (burn specialists are required for injuries to face, hands, genitalia, and feet)
    2. Major, moderate and minor burns (Table 1)
VII. Acute Evaluation and Treatment
   A. **Serious burn injury:** a pansystemic injury creating stress on entire body system.

TABLE 1.   Burn Injury Classification

Type of Injury	Major Burn	Moderate Burn	Minor Burn
Partial-thickness burns			
Children	> 20% TBSA	10–20% TBSA	< 10% TBSA
Adults	> 25% TBSA	15–25% TBSA	< 15% TBSA
Full-thickness burns	> 10% TBSA	2–10% TBSA	< 2% TBSA
Injury to face, eyes, ears, feet or perineum	+	–	–
Inhalation injury	+	–	–
Electrical injury	+	–	–
Comorbid factors of age, other trauma, or premorbid illness	+	–	–

Abbreviations: TBSA, total body surface area; +, presence of injury or comorbidity indicates a major burn requiring care at a burn center.
From American Burn Association: Hospital and pre-hospital resources for optimal care of patients with burn injury: Guidelines for development and operation of burn center. J Burn Care Rehabil 11:99–104, 1990.

1. Cascade of events is initiated with serious burn injury.
2. Local response to burn injury involves several factors.
   a. Local edema results from vasodilatation, increased extravascular osmotic activity, impaired cell membrane function, and microvascular permeability. If more than 30% TBSA is involved, edema is seen in nonburned regions.
   b. Heterogeneous reduction in perfusion creates local ischemia and necrosis with impaired microcirculation.
   c. Endothelial cells, platelets, and leukocytes migrate to injured area; platelets contribute to homeostasis and thrombosis.
3. Generalized response involves virtually every organ system.
   a. Hypovolemia is a major problem. Greatest fluid loss occurs in first 24 hours.
   b. Systemic hemodynamic changes include initial depression of cardiac output.
   c. Pulmonary function is near normal, but inhalation injury is the single most important cause of mortality, accounting for more than 50% of fire-related deaths. Inhalation injury is influenced by exposure time, concentration of fumes, composition of smoke, and extent of body burned.
   d. Thermoregulation is disrupted.
   e. Metabolic abnormalities include hypermetabolic state and negative nitrogen balance.
4. Initial goal of treatment is interruption of burning process and assessment of airway, breathing, and circulation (ABCs).
   a. Further assessment includes evaluation of TBSA involved, inhalation injury, and involvement of specialized body areas, such as face, perineum, hands, or feet.
   b. Patient's age, other injuries, and comorbid medical injuries are also considered.
B. **Specific goals of burn injury**
   1. **Restoration** of skin integrity, function, and appearance
   2. **Principles of wound care**
      a. Goals
         i. Prevent infection
         ii. Decrease pain
         iii. Prevent and suppress scarring
         iv. Prevent contracture
         v. Prepare wounds for grafting, if needed
   3. **Debridement** is removal of devitalized tissue to create a viable base for wound healing and grafting, if necessary; eschar favors infection and delays healing.
      a. Eschar is a coagulum of necrotic tissue composed of denatured collagen, elastin, and protein.
         i. Provides a medium for bacterial growth.
         ii. Promotes consumption of clotting factors
         iii. Has high degree of permeability and absorbs water from surrounding skin and tissue.
      b. Techniques of debridement
         i. Mechanical debridement
            • Wet-to-dry dressings
            • Hydrotherapy via water immersion or spraying

     ii. Debridement with enzymes
- Commercially available topical enzymes, such as sutilains, induce proteolysis, fibrinolysis, and collagenolysis.
- Specificity varies from agent to agent.
- May cause localized irritation, pain, cellulitis, and skin temperature elevation .

    iii. Surgical debridement
- Sequential debridement: thin slices of tissue are removed until a viable tissue bed is reached, indicated by brisk bleeding; less likely to lose viable tissue but blood loss can be significant.
- Fascial debridement: removes tissue down to fascia; ensures viable wound bed but leaves significant tissue defect.

4. **Escharotomy**
   a. Because burned skin is inelastic and unable to tolerate increasing interstitial edema, escharotomy is critical in circumferential burns. Tourniquet-like phenomenon may occur, creating necrosis, unless escharotomy is performed to release pressure.
   b. Escharotomy is excision through burned tissue at specified sites to relieve local pressure created by devitalized tissue.
      i. Done at specific sites of upper and lower extremities to relieve or prevent a compartment syndrome .
      ii. Done over chest wall if eschar prevents chest wall excursion.

5. **Wound dressings and skin grafts**
   a. Biologic dressings are biologic tissues used for wound closure.
      i. Allow early wound closure, which fosters pain relief, reduces infection, limits evaporative fluid loss, and reduces metabolic needs.
      ii. Dressings include cadaver tissue (homografts) and porcine grafts. Homografts are preferred, but supply is limited.
   b. Synthetic wound dressings
      i. Polyvinylchloride, polyurethanes, and other plastic membranes are water- and gas-permeable.
      ii. Nylon mesh embedded with silicon
      iii. Dressings impregnated with silver
   c. Autograft is surgical transfer of skin from one body site to another (Figs. 4 and 5).
      i. Applied once tissue bed is free of devitalized tissue and is not infected; a wound biopsy with a bacterial count less than 106 will accept a skin graft.
      ii. Split-thickness grafts may be applied in sheets or meshed.
      - Meshing involves creating small, staggered parallel slits in the sheet of skin for the purpose of expanding the size of the graft from 1.5 times to several times its normal surface area.
      - The greater the degree the mesh is expanded, the poorer the cosmetic outcome because the interstices epithelialize and the pattern of mesh persists after the wound is healed.

6. **Topical antibiotics** are applied to the open wounds to reduce bacterial proliferation and local infection.
   a. Sulfadiazine and mafenide acetate are the most commonly used. Sulfadiazine is broad-spectrum antibiotic but does not penetrate eschar.

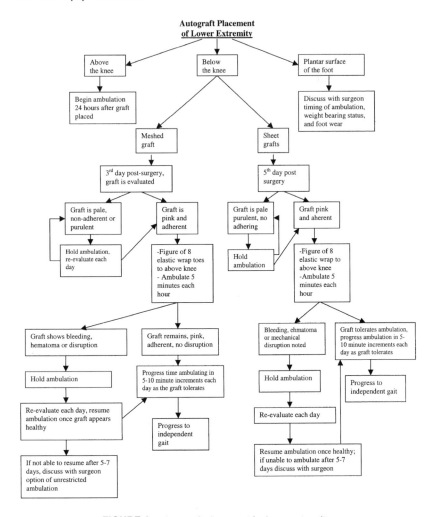

FIGURE 4. Autograft placement for lower extremity.

    b. Mafenide penetrates eschar but can induce acidosis and leukopenia.

    c. Dressings impregnated with silver are available; they can be left in place for several days, reducing pain and nursing needs.

7. **Wound healing** involves three processes that occur simultaneously:

    a. Immediately after injury, the inflammatory phase begin; it consists of initial vasoconstriction followed by vasodilatation, increased capillary permeability, and chemotaxis.

    b. Proliferative phase s marked by synthesis of collagen by fibroblasts and angiogenesis; this is the stage of scar formation.

    c. Contraction involves movement of scar edges toward the center of the wound; it reduces wound size and aids closure. Degree of contraction depends on looseness and redundancy of local tissue.

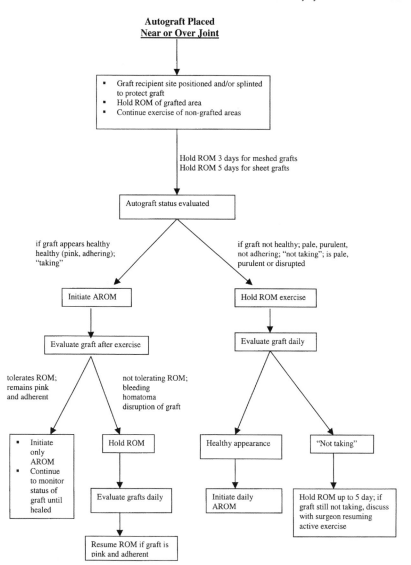

FIGURE 5. Autograft placement near or over joint

VIII. Acute Burn Rehabilitation (Table 2)
A. **Rehabilitation** is a multistage process.
   1. Requires months, even years of treatment.
   2. Ultimate goal is to assist patients in achieving optimal function.
B. **Goals** of acute burn rehabilitation
   1. Promote wound healing.
   2. Prevent complications of joint contracture, weakness, impaired endurance and loss of functional abilities.

TABLE 2.   Acute Burn Rehabilitation

Problem	Goal	Treatment
Burn injury extends across joint	Maintain normal range of motion	1. Active and passive range of motion (ROM) exercises 2. Splint involved joints 3. Position joints in anticontracture position
Loss of range of motion	Restore normal ROM	1. Prolonged stretching techniques 2. Active and active assistive ROM exercises 3. Position involved joint in a custom splint 4. Measure and monitor ROM
Loss of elbow, shoulder ROM	Restore motion	1. Classic sites for heterotopic ossification (HO): elbow and hip in children 2. Active exercise in available ROM 3. Begin work-up for HO
Exposed tendon	Prevent tendon destruction Prevent adhesions	1. Prevent desiccation by applying wet dressings 2. Splint in slack position 3. Exercise gently through limited ROM 4. Exercise adjacent joints avoiding stress on exposed tendon
Exposed extensor hood mechanism of hand	Prevent loss of extension mechanism	1. Splint in extension for 6 weeks 2. After 6 weeks begin active exercise
Joint capsule exposed but not open	Avoid drying of tissue	1. Wet dressings; irrigate 2. Gentle exercise through available ROM; splint otherwise
Open joint	Fusion; spontaneous ankylosis	1. Splint to protect wound or amputation inevitable; preserve length 2. Monitor for septic arthritis
Mobility and activities of daily living (ADLs)		
Gait abnormality; loss of mobility	Restore normal gait	1. Physical therapy for gait training; may require a gait aid 2. Monitor for gait deviations secondary to contracture, weakness, or pain
Impaired ADL skills	Independence in self-care	1. Occupational therapy 2. Assistive devices as needed
Hand burns	Restore normal function	1. Splinting hand in functional position 2. Elevate hand to decrease edema formation 3. Specific hand exercise program 4. Once wounds healed, they benefit from pressure glove
Other rehabilitation concerns		
Compression mononeuropathy	Prevention of nerve injury	1. Proper positioning 2. Avoid pressure over areas where peripheral nerves are superficial, e.g., fibular head 3. Monitor splints for proper fit and application
Inhalation injury	Restore pulmonary function	1. Percussion and postural drainage 2. Assisted cough techniques
Excessive secretions	Prevent pneumonia	

(Table continued on next page.)

TABLE 2.   Acute Burn Rehabilitation *(Continued)*

Problem	Goal	Treatment
Rehabilitation after skin grafts and joint release		
New skin grafts	Protect new graft from unwanted shear or stress	1. Splint until surgically cleared for motion 2. Elevate involved limb above level of heart 3. Avoid dependent position until cleared by the surgeon; 3–5 days typical except for lower extremities (see below) 4. Proper positioning 5. Resume exercise when surgeon clears
Resume ambulation after grafting to lower extremities	Independent gait and transfer	1. Begin weight bearing after cleared by surgeon; typically in 5–7 days 2. Use pressure wraps over newly grafted areas to prevent edema and sloughing 3. Begin with dangling legs in increasing increments of 5–10 minutes and monitor for edema
Release of contracture	Maintain ROM	1. Resume ROM when surgeon permits 2. Splint to maintain ROM 3. Monitor grafts

3. Individualized by burn location, depth of injury, percent of body surface injured, associated injuries, and complications.
4. Patient age as well as previous functional level and health are significant.
C. **Positioning:** Proper positioning is fundamental to prevent development of contractures and avoid compression neuropathies (see Fig. 6).
1. Underlying principle: keep tissues in an elongated state.
2. Patients assume positions of comfort, primarily flexion and adduction.
3. Typically positions of extension and abduction should be chosen, but positioning needs to be individualized according to specific injuries.
D. **Splinting** is used to prevent joint contractures, maintain proper positioning, and protect new skin grafts.
1. Joints that have overlying deep partial-thickness or full -thickness burns are at risk for developing contracture.
2. Splints are labor-intensive and add cost to patient care; the cost -benefit ratio must be favorable.

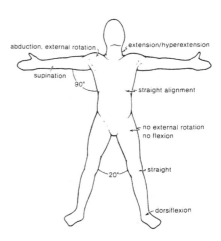

FIGURE 6. Suggested positioning guidelines for prevention of burn contractions. (From Helm PA, Kevorkian CG, Lushbaugh M, et al: Burn injury: Rehabilitation management in 1982. Arch Phys Med Rehabil 63:8, 1982, with permission.)

3. Splints must be user-friendly for patients and nursing staff. Poorly applied splints can cause nerve injury, loss of skin grafts, and worsening of burn wound.
4. Nonburn areas may require splinting; for example, to prevent ankle contractures during prolonged bed rest.
5. Custom splints can be designed for virtually all parts of the body.
    a. Commercially available designs can be used in selected cases.
    b. Type of splint depends on area of body injured.
    c. Splinting with functional goals in mind.
    d. Level of patient participation is important.
6. **Characteristics of a good splint**
    a. Easy to don and doff.
    b. Avoids pressure over bony prominence.
    c. Made of remoldable materials that can be modified as patient needs change.
    d. Compatible with wound dressings and topical medications.
7. Hand splints
    a. Resting hand splints position hand in wrist extension, 60–80° of metacarpophalangeal flexion, full interphalangeal extension, and thumb abduction.
    b. If injured hands are left unsplinted, the hands will contract with the metacarpophalangeal joints hyperextended, the proximal phalangeal joints flexed, and thumb in long abduction with loss of the palmar arches.
    c. Boutonnière deformity is common.
E. **Exercise**
1. Requires understanding of location, depth, and extent of burn.
2. Preexisting conditions affect the type of exercise that is appropriate (e.g., history of coronary artery disease).
3. **Initial goal of exercise** is to maintain normal ROM and strength.
    a. Active and active-assisted exercise is appropriate for alert patients.
    b. Slow passive exercise programs indicated for obtunded or critically ill.
    c. ROM exercises can be performed with the patient under anesthesia. This is a good choice to determine true ROM, especially for patient who cannot tolerate ROM because of pain.
4. **Stretching programs** are indicated when there is loss of normal ROM.
    a. Requires skin preconditioning.
    b. Preconditioning is moving a joint to the end of its ROM several times before applying a prolonged stretch.
    c. Stretching can be maintained until tissue blanching is observed; blanching indicates that capillary blood flow is impeded.
5. Once normal ROM is achieved, active exercise is preferred.
6. Strengthening should begin as tolerated.
    a. Strengthening programs should include progressive resistive exercise and other protocols to maximize recovery.
    b. Endurance training should also be included, with monitoring of cardiopulmonary response.
7. Post skin graft: see Figure 5.
E. **Early ambulation:**
1. Maintains independence, balance, and lower extremity ROM; decreases risk of deep venous thrombosis.
2. May begin as soon as patient's medical condition allows.
3. **Skin grafting** of lower extremities prevents patient from ambulating until stable circulation to graft sites is established (see Fig. 4).

a. Typically, patients cannot put their lower extremities in a dependent position for 5–7 days after grafting.
b. Begin with program of dangling lower extremities before initiating ambulation to determine if graft tolerates the dependent position.
c. Elastic wraps or other form of compression are indicated initially to avoid venous pooling, which results in graft sloughing.
d. Status of the graft should be checked before and after dangling or walking.
4. **Monitor for gait deviations.**
a. Gait deviations are common.
b. Gait abnormalities may be due to pain, focal or generalized weakness, contractures impaired sensation ,or central nervous system causes.
c. Some gait deviations resolve as wounds heal and pain resolves.

IX. **Postacute Rehabilitation (Table 3)**
A. Once wound care is no longer major priority; **primary focus** shifts to maximizing patient's potential for independence in work and community living.
B. **Wound and skin care**
1. Patients typically are discharged with a limited number of unhealed wounds.
2. Patients and family need to be educated about wound care and dressings.
3. Healed skin is fragile and easily abraded. Teach patients to monitor skin for breakdown due to splints, pressure garments, clothing, and other irritants.
4. Healed burn skin is sensitive to sun and chemicals. Educate patients and families about appropriate use of sun blocking agents and appropriate clothing.
5. Healed burn skin lacks natural lubricants.
a. Use moisturizers (e.g., cocoa butter, aloe) frequently.
b. Avoid prolonged submersion in water, especially hot water.
c. Avoid drying soaps and detergents.
d. Wash skin with mild soap and water.
e. Massage skin often.
C. **Scarring**
1. **First 3 months** after deep partial-thickness and full-thickness injury
a. Often, skin appearance is acceptable immediately after healing.
b. However, within 1–3 months, hypertrophic scarring occurs, creating irregular, raised, and red scars.
i. Hypertrophic scar and keloid are not synonymous terms.
ii. Hypertrophic scar remains within the confines of the original injury, whereas a keloid invades normal surrounding skin. Keloids are rare in children; dark-skinned adults are believed to be at greater risk.
2. **Scar suppression**
a. On histologic examination, hypertrophic scars show a random orientation of collagen, often in whorls and nodules.
b. Hypertrophic scars may take up to 2 years to mature, whereas nonhypertrophic scars demonstrate a parallel arrangement of collagen and mature in weeks to months.
c. **Pressure** facilitates parallel orientation of collagen during scar maturation, thereby smoothing the irregular appearance of hypertrophic scarring.
i. Application of continuous pressure improves appearance of scars.
ii. Methods of applying pressure include:
• Custom-fitted elastic garment that provides at least 25 mmHg of pressure and is worn at least 23 hours/day.
• Custom-fitted gloves and orthoses for the hands

TABLE 3. Postacute Burn Rehabilitation

Problem	Goal	Treatment
Joint contracture	Maintain normal ROM Restore normal ROM	1. Prolonged stretching techniques 2. Active and active assistive ROM exercises 3. Position involved joint in a custom splint 4. Measure and monitor ROM 5. Consider heterotopic ossification when ROM is lost despite appropriate exercise
Generalized weakness	Regain normal strength	1. Consider burn or critical care peripheral neuropathy or myopathy 2. Progressive strengthening; emphasize extension
Poor endurance	Normal cardiopulmonary function	General conditioning program
Scarring in healed partial- and full-thickness burns	Prevent or reduce scarring	1. Once wound is closed, apply pressure of at least 25 mmHg (capillary pressure) 24 hours/day until scars are no longer hyperemic and are soft and pliable (18–24 mo) 2. Custom-fitted garments 3. Elastic bandages 4. Elastic stockinet; molded inserts 5. Acrylic face masks 6. Splints 7. Local steroid injection for specific lesion of limited size
Pruritus	Reduce discomfort Prevent local trauma from scratching	1. Moisturize skin 2. Massage 3. Oral or topical diphenhydramine HCl 4. Oral hydroxyzine HCl 5. Wearing of pressure garments 6. Avoid overheating 7. Oatmeal baths; cool showers 8. Limited use of topical steroids or EMLA cream
Gait abnormality, abnormal posture	Normalize mobility and posture	1. Gait training 2. Assistive gait devices 3. Mirrors or other feedback regarding posture or gait 4. Evaluate for specific muscle weakness or contracture
Impaired ADLs	Restore functional independence	Occupation therapy for training and assistive devices
Impaired hand function	Restore fine motor and coordination	1. Occupational therapy (OT) for hand therapy 2. Fit with custom pressure gloves to maintain web spaces and reduce scarring 3. Sensory loss may be seen from inability of nerves to re-grow through scar tissue of loss from full-thickness burns 4. Gloves and protective hand garments 5. Patient education
Intolerance of heat and cold	Maintain normal body temperature	1. Appropriate clothing 2. Educate patient to avoid extreme temperatures

(Table continued on next page.)

TABLE 3. Postacute Burn Rehabilitation *(Continued)*

Problem	Goal	Treatment
Skin sensitivity and fragility	Prevent abrasions and local breakdown	1. Moisturizers to prevent dryness 2. Gloves and other protective garments 3. Avoid handling chemicals (e.g., gasoline, strong detergents) 4. Educate patient in skin care and protection
Sun sensitivity	Prevent sunburn	1. Use sun-blocking agents (UVA, UVB); SPF of at least 35 2. Specialized clothing with sun-blocking qualities 3. Hats, gloves
Inhalation injury	Increase pulmonary	1. Initiate pulmonary rehabilitation program 2. Energy conservation techniques

- Silicone sheeting is used to improve fit and contact over areas of irregular contour, such as the web spaces between fingers.
- Splints and orthoses
- Custom-made acrylic face masks preserve facial contours.
- Microstomia orthoses can be used to maintain the normal aperture of the mouth or to stretch local scarring about the mouth.

iii. **Pressure therapy** is continued until the scar is mature, (i.e., soft, nonindurated, and no longer hyperemic). Typically the scar matures in 18–24 months.

iv. **Problems caused by pressure therapy**
- Allergy to material used for garments or splints
- Monitor the influence of pressure on bone growth in children
- Dental occlusion should be followed in children or adolescents who wear a compression face mask, including custom acrylic face masks.

3. **Pigmentation**
   a. Burns that do not require skin grafting for closure typically repigment within 1–3 years.
   b. Relative hyperpigmentation may result, depending on native skin color, sun responsiveness, degree of UV light exposure, and body region.
   c. In the case of deeper partial-thickness burns or burns that require grafting, hypertrophy and hyperpigmentation may develop rapidly and intensely. The pigment changes appear to be influenced by a number of variables, including native skin color, depth of burn, and sun exposure.

D. **Joint function**
1. **Immobility and scarring lead to joint contractures**.
   a. Active exercise, proper positioning, and splinting are the best approach to joint contracture prevention; exercise should be done 3–4 times/day; patient and family teaching is important to re-enforce joint exercise.
   b. Stress functional activities to normalize joint use.
   c. Limited ROM of the joint can result from extrinsic factors, such as hypertrophic scarring or from intrinsic joint pathology.
   d. Careful examination of the tissues limiting function is crucial to prescribing the most effective therapy and achieving full function.
      i. Tautness of the skin that limits ROM indicates an extrinsic cause but does not eliminate the possibility of additional intrinsic joint disease, such as heterotopic ossification (HO).

        ii. When ROM becomes painful or is lost despite appropriate therapeutic exercise, HO must be ruled out.
- Bone scan is the most sensitive and earliest indicator.
- Radiographic changes are late.
- Elevated serum alkaline phosphatase is not highly specific.
- Develops primarily around major joints (the elbow is the most common site). In adults, calcification occurs in the medial fibers of the triceps; in children, along the brachialis muscle.

2. **Joint contracture that fails nonsurgical treatment**
   a. Surgery should be considered, especially if the contracture interferes with desired activities, mobility, or cosmesis.
   b. Surgery is indicated to release contracted skin and joints that do not respond to stretching exercise and modalities.
   c. Surgical procedures include simple releases, such as a Z plasty, or sophisticated reconstruction of facial and body contours
   d. For patients with sites of recurrent ulceration or skin breakdown, repeat skin grafting may be needed.

E. **Exercise**
   1. Exercise should continue in the postacute period.
   2. Goals include achieving or maintaining joint ROM, normal strength, normal cardiopulmonary function, and endurance.
   3. Resistive exercise programs are indicated.
   4. Keep in mind any premorbid or complicating conditions, such as diabetes mellitus and coronary artery disease (particularly important in the elderly)
   5. Children participate best in exercise programs that are activity-oriented and developmentally appropriate.
   6. Modalities can be used to help with stretching programs.
      a. Paraffin lubricates skin as well as provides warmth to make the skin more pliable for stretching. Position scar in stretched position and apply paraffin for 30 minutes.
      b. Ultrasound can be used to stretch specific, limited areas of scarring, such as a hypertrophic scar that creates band-limiting ROM.

F. **Gait and mobility**
   1. Ambulation should continue to focus on independence on all surfaces, progressing to gait without an assistive device.
   2. ROM of the trunk is critical to prevent abnormal gait patterns, such as the robotic motion seen with a stiff trunk.
   3. It is critical to get geriatric patients on their feet as soon as possible because they seem to show effects of immobility sooner than younger people.

G. **Adjustment**
   1. Psychological status before injury is a strong indicator of long-term psychological health after injury.
   2. Psychological and psychiatric disorders are likely to be exacerbated by a severe burn injury.
   3. Psychiatric disorders seen most commonly after injury include delirium, adjustment disorder, post-traumatic stress disorder, and major depression. Delirium is the most common disorder, followed by adjustment disorder.
   4. Patients surviving serious burns often do not receive the empathy from others that is typically seen with other disabilities. This finding may relate to the perception of burn scars as unattractive.

    a. Women and girls have lower self-esteem after burn injuries than men or boys with similar injuries.

    b. The more support patients believe they have from family and friends, the higher their self-esteem.

    c. Families and friends need to be educated about their key role in the emotional recovery of seriously injured people.

H. Cosmesis and appearance

1. Disfigurement, especially of the face, is a major concern to patients.
2. Special make-up is available to reduce the appearance of burn scar; it may be an acceptable option to some, depending on the extent and type of scarring.
3. Severe scarring is a frequent indication for surgery, as is correction of functional limitations, such as a contracture.
4. Plastic surgery may be used to reconstruct an ear, reduce scarring over the face, or allow adolescent female breast development.
5. Surgery requires a collaborative relationship with the surgeon as well as extensive discussion and education of the patient.
6. Often patients who have sustained a major burn injury are unwilling to pursue further surgery even if the physiatrist believes significant functional or cosmetic gains are possible. Many have undergone an extraordinary number of surgical procedures and are psychologically unable to tolerate additional surgery.

I. Return to school and work

1. Percent of deep partial thickness and full thickness injures correlates with the time needed to return to work or school (Table 4).
2. Postacute therapy programs must include focus on strength, endurance, power, and work-specific tasks. Work-hardening programs are typically indicated.
3. Hand burns, occupation, education, and age are important factors in determining return to work or school .
4. Burn sequelae that affect return to work or school include pruritus, cold and heat sensitivity, intolerance of sunlight, skin dryness and fragility, sensory loss, and intolerance of chemicals or other irritants.
5. Previous inhalation injuries often prevent return to work environments with dust, fumes, and other respiratory irritants.
6. Patients injured at work often find it difficult to resume work at the site of injury or to do similar tasks; many have to change occupations.

J. Outpatient rehabilitation

1. Discharge planning should begin as soon as the patient is admitted.

    a. Awareness of patient's social and financial resources

    b. Availability of burn care-specific treatment and therapy

    c. Home setting and social support system to which patient will return

TABLE 4.   Length of Stay in Acute Hospital

Percent TBSA Injured	Estimated Length of Stay (Days)
< 20	6–17
20–39	17–45
40–89	38–94
> 90	129–237

Modified from Ryan CM, Schoenfeld DA, Thorpe WP, et al: Objective estimates of the probability of death from burn injuries. N Engl J Med 338–366, 1998.

2. At discharge, patient should be independent in all aspects of care or have appropriate home or community services in place.
   a. Patients should know their exercise regimen, pressure suppression program, and wound care as well as the principles of skin protection and safety.
   b. Patients should be knowledgeable about goals and purpose of their treatment program and be able to direct others in their care, if necessary.
3. Regular and frequent follow-up medical care should be established, including the burn surgeon and physiatrist.
4. Outpatient physical and occupational therapy should be arranged with therapists experienced and knowledgeable in burn rehabilitation.

K. **Impairment**
1. The physiatrist is the most skilled provider for rating the patient's final level of impairment.
2. Burn patients have great difficulty in obtaining work disability.
3. Many impairment scales do not acknowledge intolerance of chemicals, heat and cold sensitivity, sensory impairment, or reduced endurance.
4. Mental health disorders, such as post-traumatic stress disorder and adjustment disorders related to returning to the site of injury or similar settings, are also often underrecognized.
5. Ultimately, it is the physiatrist's responsibility to determine when the patient is ready for school or work. The decision is complex and requires not only consideration of physical impairments and their sequelae. but also assessment of the patient's premorbid health, age, schooling, social situation, and mental health.

L. **Special notes about pediatric patients**
1. Approximately 40% of persons admitted to the hospital for burn care are children, and the number of children surviving severe burn injury is rising.
2. The major cause of death in children is respiratory insufficiency.
3. One outcome measure of efficacy of burn care is the rate of return to school. This measure includes documentation of the time from injury to return to the classroom as well as academic and behavioral performance after injury.
4. Although school reentry programs statistically have not shown improved adjustment to school in some studies, such programs are well received by teachers, parents, students, and school personnel.
   a. Staley et al. reported the results of their school reentry program and found that burn injury did not appear to have a negative impact on the child's functioning in school.
   b. Although students did not develop any new school performance problems on return to school, children with a history of school performance and behavioral problems continued to have problems at reentry. This finding was the same for very young children and adolescents.
5. Health care professional must maintain a low threshold for suspecting child abuse, which remains a major problem.
   a. Typically, nonaccidental pediatric burn injuries are not isolated events, but rather reflect a progression of abuse from minor injuries to more devastating injuries. At the time of evaluation for burn injury, abused children often have physical injuries from earlier abuse, which are in various stages of healing.
   b. Efforts have been made to construct the basic profile of the abused child. Studies show that the abused child is typically from a single-parent,

impoverished home that is welfare-dependent. Only 10% of abused children had parents who were employed, whereas 55% of parents of children who sustained accidental burns were employed.

c. Burns secondary to abuse tend to cover a larger surface area than accidental burns. Young found that burns of the hands, feet, or genitalia were involved in 100% of abuse cases. For cases of accidental burns, only 41% had burns in these areas.

d. Studies show no difference in gender distribution.

Bibliography

1. Achauer BM: Reconstructing the burned face. Clin Plastic Surg 19:623–636, 1992.
2. „American Burn Association: Hospital and prehospital resources for optimal care of patients with burn injury: Guidelines for development and operation of burn center. J Burn Care Rehabil 11: 98–104, 1990.
3. Barrow, RE, Herndon, DN: Incidence of mortality in boys and girls after severe thermal burns. Surg Gynecol Obstet 170:295–298, 1990.
4. Berstein N: Marital and sexual adjustment of severely burned patients: Medical aspects of human sexuality. Clin Plast Surg 9:337–346, 1982.
5. Blakeney P, Moore P, Meyer W, et al: Efficacy of school reentry programs. J Burn Care Rehabil 16: 469–472, 1995.
6. Bowden JL, Feller I, Tholen D, et al: Self esteem in severely burned patients. Arch Phys Med Rehabil 61:449–452, 1980.
7. Bringham PA, McLoughlin E: Burn incidence and medical care use in the United States: estimate, trends, and data sources. J Burn Care Rehabil 17:95–107, 1996.
8. de Chalain TM, Tang C, Thomson HG: Burn Area Color Changes after Superficial Burns in Childhood: Can They be Predicted? J Burn Care Rehabil 19:39–49. 1998
9. Helm PA, Kevorkian GC, Lusbaugh MS, et al: Burn injury: rehabilitation management. Arch Phys Med Rehabil 63:6–16, 1982
10. Helm, PA, Walker SC: Return to work after burn injury. J Burn Care Rehabil 13:53–55, 1992.
11. Helm PA, Walker SC, Peyton SA: Return to work following hand burns. Arch Phys Med Rehabil 67:297–299, 1986.
12. Knaysi GA, Crikelair GF, Cosman B: The rule of nines: Its history and accuracy. Plast Reconstr Surg 41:560–63, 1968.
13. Monafo WW: Initial management of burns. N Engl J Med 335:1581–1586, 1996.
14. Orr DA, Reznikoff M, Smith GM: Body image, self esteem and depression in burn injured adolescents and adults. J Burn Care Rehabil 10:454–461, 1989.
15. Questad KA, Patterson R, Boltwood MD, et al: Relating mental health and physical function at discharge to rehabilitation status at 3 months post burn. J Burn Care Rehabil 9:87–89, 1988.
16. Ryan CM, Thorpe WP, Mullin PA, et al: A persistent fire hazard for older adults: Cooking related clothing ignition. J Am Geriatr Soc 45:1283–1285, 1997.
17. Ryan CM, Schoenfeld DA, Thorpe WP et al: Objective estimates of the probability of death from burn injuries. N Engl J Med 338–366, 1998.
18. Saffle JR, Davis B, for the American Burn Association Registry Participant Group: Recent outcomes in the treatment of burn injury in the United States: A report from the American Burn Association Patient Registry. J Burn Care Rehabil 16:219–232, 1995.
19. Salisbury RE: Burn rehabilitation: Our unanswered challenge. J Burn Care Rehabil 13:495–497, 1992.
20. Sheridan RL, Hinson MI, Laing MH, et al: Long-term outcomes of children surviving massive burns. JAMA 83: 69–73, 2000.
21. Steiner H, Clark WJ Jr.: Psychiatric complications of burned adults: A classification. J Trauma 17:134–143, 1977.
22. Spires MC: Rehabilitation of patients with burns. In Braddom R, Dumitru D (eds): Physical Medicine and Rehabilitation. Philadelphia, W.B. Saunders , 2000.
23. Ward RS: Pressure therapy for the control of hypertrophic scar formation after burn injury: a history and review. J Burn Care Rehabil 12:257–262, 1991.
24. Watkins PN, Cook El, May SR, et al: The role of the psychiatrist in the team treatment of the adult patients with burns. J Burn Care Rehabil 13:19–27, 1992.

Chapter 3

CANCER REHABILITATION

Benedict S. Konzen, MD

I. General Principles

  A. Rehabilitation medicine aims to restore a person to the highest level of possible functioning after an illness or trauma. In general, the physiatrist assists the patient in maximizing function while maintaining or enhancing quality of life.

  B. Traditionally, a comprehensive interdisciplinary team approach involving therapies, nursing, and social services is used. In the care of patients with cancer, however, the focus expands to include the oncologist, surgeon, radiation oncologist, nutritionist, and often spiritual adviser.

  C. Cancer rehabilitation is a dynamic process. The patient's disease is often progressive, and medical interventions are typically ongoing. The physiatrist must recognize and make allowances for oncologic interventions. Life-sustaining chemoradiation therapy or surgical intervention may lead to fatigue, immunosuppression, or impairment of neuromuscular functioning. Potential secondary complications of treatment include peripheral neuropathy, lymphedema, and immobility. In addition, decubitus ulcers, deep venous thromboses, or pulmonary embolus may be seen after periods of immobility.

  D. Rehabilitation should occur throughout the course of any disease process. In advanced cancer, the goal should be to improve basic mobility, self-care and activities of daily living (ADLs). This goal often involves training family members in assisting the patient with basic needs, such as bowel/bladder management, skin care, and pain palliation.

  E. Although research studies are limited, the literature shows that despite tumor type, stage, or metastasis, rehabilitation improves endurance and performance of self-care, promotes safe ambulation, and limits pain.

II. Epidemiology

  A. After cardiovascular disease, cancer remains the second leading cause of death in the United States.

  B. In general, cancer incidence continues to trend upward, yet in recent years there has been a decline in specific tumor types-uterine, hematopoietic, and enterologic (oral, gastric and pancreatic).

  C. Tumor incidence is decreasing by age and demonstrates an upswing after the age of 55.

  D. Despite advances in treatment, certain tumor types still have marginal 5-year survival rates (< 30%), including tumors of the stomach, esophagus, liver, pancreas, lung/bronchus, and brain as well as multiple myeloma.

III. Tumor-induced Problems

  A. **Spinal cord involvement**

1. Up to 30% of all patients with cancer may experience metastatic involvement of the spinal cord. Of this group, 5% have associated spinal cord compression. Most metastatic tumors are extradural (95%); of these, up to 70% affect the thoracic cord, followed by lumbar and cervical levels in order of decreasing incidence.

2. Architecturally, the vertebral body is affected in 80% of cases, followed in frequency by the posterior elements.

3. Common presenting complaints include spinal pain when lying down, radiating pain, and radicular symptoms. Pain, however, may not be present. Key features to identify include:
   a. Weakness
   b. Sensory changes
   c. Gait abnormality (e.g., ataxia)
   d. Autonomic changes
   e. Impotence, bladder/bowel dysfunction (loss of sphincter control may be a late finding)

4. Treatment options vary. However, a thorough physical and neurologic examination comparing current findings with baseline is critical. Such findings should be promptly conveyed to the neurosurgeon and neurologist, and appropriate radiographic imaging and intervention should be determined. In general, however, back pain in the patients with cancer should prompt the physiatrist to obtain a bone scan or magnetic resonance imaging (MRI) scan.

5. **If there is high suspicion of spinal cord compromise:**
   a. Multilevel MRI should be obtained.
   b. Patient should be bolused with high-dose IV dexamethasone, 100 mg.
   c. Concurrently neurosurgical consultation should be undertaken.

6. Treatment may consist of surgery with resection, cord stabilization (either surgically or with bracing), and radiation therapy.
   a. Current interest lies in vertebroplasty/kyphoplasty using methylmethacrylate in patients with nonoperative vertebral compression fractures. The subsequent exothermic reaction may provide an antitumor effect.
   b. In **vertebroplasty**, methylmethacrylate is injected percutaneously via a needle under fluoroscopic guidance though the vertebral pedicle into the vertebral body. The goal is not so much the filling of the collapsed vertebral body as it is the fixing of the fractured superior plane of the wedge deformity. In effect, the anterior one-half to two-thirds of the vertebral body is filled in. There is, however, no restoration of vertebral height. Problems associated with vertebroplasty include cement extravasation (< 1% of cases).
   c. **Kyphoplasty** involves restoring height to the vertebral body while relieving pain and stabilizing the fractured plane. Kyphoplasty begins with the use of a needle inserted into the vertebral body. Much like angioplasty, an inflatable balloon is introduced through the trochar. The balloon is inflated in the collapse vertebra and subsequently removed. The void is filled with methylmethacrylate, and the vertebra "re-inflates." This procedure can reduce a 30° wedge deformity to 5°.
   d. Both procedures increase structural stability to the vertebral body and can markedly reduced pain without interfering with future palliative radiation to the site. As with any invasive neurosurgical procedure, relative

contraindications include sepsis, coagulopathy, vertebra plana deformity, or disruption in the posterior vertebral body wall.

B. **Additional neurologic complications**

1. **Spinal cord involvement by metastatic disease** is fairly common. Equally devastating are primary brain tumors-typically, gliomas—which account for 10% of all neurologic disease. Approximately 25% of common tumor primaries (lung, breast, gastrointestinal, and melanoma) metastasize to the brain.

2. **Tumor types of the brain** include glioblastomas (40%), astrocytomas (42%), oliogodendrogliomas (3.5%), medulloblastomas (3.6%), ependymomas (3%), and meningiomas (2%).

3. **Mental status changes** in patients with cancer patient have multiple causes.
   a. Reactive peritumoral edema
   b. Infection (commonly pneumonia, urinary tract infection)
   c. Intratumoral hemorrhage
   d. Obstructive hydrocephalus
   e. Hyponatremia
   f. Seizure activity
   g. Metabolic/endocrine disorders
   h. Hypoxemia (e.g., pulmonary embolus)
   i. Medications (e.g., corticosteroids, sedative-hypnotics, phenytoin)

4. A **thorough physical and neurologic examination** is critical. Findings should be correlated with aspiration risk, laboratory data (blood chemistries, blood and urine cultures, and evaluation of cerebrospinal fluid with chemistries and cytology) as well as neuroimaging (MRI/CT).

5. **Correction of sodium imbalance** should done cautiously.
   a. Rapid correction of sodium imbalance can lead to **central pontine myelinolysis**.
   b. Dramatic increases in edema can lead to a number of **central herniation syndromes**.
      i. Temporal (uncal) herniation beneath the tentorium is associated with pupillary dilatation, ptosis, homonymous hemianopsia, and hemiparesis/plegia secondary to cerebral peduncle herniation. Fixed and dilated pupil with concomitant bradycardia and hypertension are late findings in uncal herniation.
      ii. Tonsillar herniation through the foramen magnum is associated with nuchal rigidity with head flexion and increased extensor tone. Without intervention and posterior fossa decompression, coma and respiratory arrest will ensue.
      iii. Midbrain involvement may include Cheyne-Stokes respirations, stupor, and decerebrate rigidity and gaze paresis.

6. **Presenting deficits may also mimic those of patients with stroke.**
   a. Lesions of the frontal lobe affect voluntary motor control on the contralateral side.
   b. Disruption in Broca's area results in motor (expressive) language aphasia.
   c. Areas anterior to the motor areas are involved in complex behavioral and executive activities. Lesions here may impair judgement, abstract thought, tactfulness, and insight.
   d. Lesions of the parietal lobe will contralaterally affect light touch, proprioception, and pain input. There may be left-right discriminatory errors, spatial errors and disturbances of body image and apraxia.

e. Lesions of the temporal lobe result in an auditory aphasia-the patient hears but does not comprehend. The patient may be unable to read or write (alexia/agraphia).

f. Lesions of the occipital lobes may cause contralateral blindness or a visual agnosia.

7. **Multiple myeloma** has been associated with spinal cord/nerve root compression and entrapment neuropathies.

8. **Paraneoplastic syndromes**

a. Predominantly associated with small cell lung cancer, ovarian cancer, and lymphomas.

b. Occur in < 1% of all patients with cancer patients.

c. Include paraneoplastic peripheral neuropathies, cerebellar degeneration, and Lambert-Eaton myasthenic syndrome.

C. **Metastatic tumor to bone and risk of fracture**

1. The most frequent presenting complaint in metastatic bone disease is slowly progressive, localized, aching pain associated with weight-bearing and often worse at night. However, the presence or absence of pain does not directly correlate with degree of skeletal involvement.

2. **Primary bone tumors** are seen most often in children and are generally appendicular. In adults, the most common bony tumor is metastatic disease, generally in patients over the age of 40. The most common primary malignancies include breast, prostate, lung, and kidney. Metastatic bone disease, however, can affect both the axial and appendicular skeleton. Vertebrae (notably thoracic) are most commonly affected in metastatic disease, followed by the pelvis, ribs, femur, sternum, and skull. Specifically, metastatic breast carcinoma shows a predilection for the proximal femur. Prostate cancer commonly metastasizes to the pelvis.

3. **Pathologic fractures** are seen in 10–15% of patients with bone metastases (mets). Metastatic bone disease may also cause:

a. Early hypercalcemia may be characterized by fatigue, lethargy, nausea, and polyuria and may progress to mental status changes, pruritus, bradycardia, and coma. Treatment includes bisphosphonates, which inhibit bone resorption. A patient should be aggressively hydrated intravenously, and IV palmidronate is administered, 60–90 mg infused slowly over 2 hours and repeated every 48 hours as needed.

b. Intractable pain

c. Nerve impingement (at the cord, spinal root, peripherally, brachial plexus levels

IV. **Therapy-induced Problems**

A. The mainstay of cancer treatment is tumor-dependent and may include surgery and/or chemoradiation. Treatment may be curative or palliative. However, mainstream treatment protocols and aggressive life-sustaining measures are associated with secondary complications.

B. **Effects of chemotherapy**

1. Chemotherapy may affect both healthy and diseased tissues.

2. Its side effects can be profound and include:

a. **Peripheral neuropathy**

i. Most commonly implicated are vinca alkaloids (e.g., vincristine, vinblastine, navelbine), cisplatin, taxol, and procarbazine. On EMG, the vinca alkaloids demonstrate an axonal sensorimotor peripheral neuropathy. Cisplatin is associated primarily with an axonal sensory neuropathy. Clinically, patients report burning dysesthesias of the hands and feet.

    ii. Rehabilitation intervention focuses on desensitization techniques, splinting, adaptive equipment, proprioceptive/balance training, and pain management (neuropathic agents).

b. **Pancytopenia**

    i. Patients may demonstrate anemia, leukopenia, and/or thromobocytopenia. Functionally, patients may have reduced endurance, impaired immune function, and/or a bleeding dyscrasia.

    ii. Resistive or strenuous exercise is usually avoided in patients with hemoglobin under 8 gm/dl.

    iii. While most physical therapy protocols tend to discourage active mobilization of a patient with < 20,000 platelets, current ongoing investigation at MD Anderson Cancer Center tends to include patients with platelets > 7500. Rather than relying on platelet number, emphasis is placed on baseline stability, endurance, and evidence (or lack thereof) of an acute/active source of bleeding.

c. **Cognitive effects**

    i. Chemotherapeutic agents may have chronic, protracted effects.

    ii. Cytokines such as interferon-alpha, interleukin-2, and tumor necrosis factor have been linked with subacute frontal lobe dysfunction, subcortical dementia, and psychosis.

    iii. Treatment should include cognitive rehabilitation in conjunction with tricyclic antidepressants.

d. **Syndrome of inappropriate antidiuretic hormone (SIADH)** may result from use of vincristine or cyclophosphamide.

e. **Vocal cord paralysis.** Vinca alkaloids have been implicated in either unilateral or bilateral vocal cord paresis, which typically resolves with withdrawal of the drug.

C. **Effects of radiation therapy**

1. Radiation therapy remains a useful primary or adjuvant tool in both acute and chronic treatment and palliation of tumor and pain.

2. It may be associated with brachial plexopathy, peripheral nerve damage, radiation myelopathy, fibrosis/contractures, osteonecrosis, and cognitive impairments.

a. **Brachial plexopathy**

    i. Most radiation-induced brachial plexopathies are associated with tumors of the head/neck, breast, or lung. Generally they involve the upper trunk. Radiation-induced fibrosis entraps the nerve and constricts the vasa vasorum. These irreversible changes may occur anywhere from 1 month to 15 years after treatment.

    ii. As for any other plexopathy, treatment centers on edema and pain control, splinting, ranging, compensatory techniques, and adaptive equipment.

    iii. Imaging studies may not be able to differentiate between radiation- and tumor-induced plexopathy. EMG may demonstrate myokymic discharges in radiation plexitis. Although pathognomonic, myokymic discharges are not always present. Wertsch provides a useful table to differentiate between tumor and radiation plexopathy (Table 1).

TABLE 1. **Differentiation Between Tumor and Radiation Plexopathy**

Criteria	Tumor	Radiation
Pain at outset	Characteristic	Uncommon
Sensory symptoms as presenting complaint	Less common	More common
Weakness in upper plexus	Less common	More common
Lower trunk distribution	Characteristic	Rare
Latent interval		
Very early or very late		
< 6 mo	More common	Less common
< 5 yr	More common	Less common
Medium		
< 3 yr	Less common	More common
Rapid course	Characteristic	Uncommon
Radiation dose > 60 By	Less likely	More likely
Myokymic EMG	Not described	Characteristic

EMG = electromyogram.

   b. **Radiation-induced peripheral neuropathy.** As with plexitis, damage is the result of fibrosis and vascular insufficiency to the nerve.

   c. **Radiation-induced myelopathy**

      i. Occurring from 1 month to 3 years after treatment, radiation myelopathy is thought to result from demyelination of the posterior columns and lateral spinothalamic tracts.

      ii. Depending on dose, delayed radiation myelopathy may result in progressive and irreversible paraplegia or tetraplegia from 9 months to 3 years after treatment.

   d. **Cognitive effects**

      i. In a study by Meyer et al., 34% of patient undergoing chemoradiation demonstrated cognitive deficits.

      ii. Although acute effects of brain irradiation are rare, there may be subacute reversible demyelination.

      iii. Chronic effects may include focal necrosis, leukoencephalopathy, brain atrophy, and secondary radiation-induced tumors.

      iv. Radiation-induced reactions may include headache, nausea, vomiting, somnolence, and fever.

      v. Symptoms may be prevented with the use of corticosteroids (e.g., dexamethasone, 2 mg once or twice daily).

      vi. Subacute reaction (weeks to months after radiation) may be secondary to transient demyelination of oligodendroglia or changes in capillary permeability.

      vii. Transient neurologic deterioration, encephalopathy, or marked somnolence may mimic recurrent tumor.

        • MRI may be confusing, and subsequent positron emission tomography (PET) may be need to differentiate radiation necrosis from tumor recurrence.

        • Dexamethasone may be used to limit injury progression.

D. **Lymphedema**

   1. Common complication after surgical intervention and radiation therapy

   2. Associated most often with treatment of breast, uterine, ovarian, and prostate cancer

3. Postsurgical edema often resolves once lymphatic drainage is reestablished via anatomic channels. However, if lymph flow is blocked or remaining channels are insufficient, protein and fluid accumulate in the interstitium, leading to progressive stasis and fibrosis.
4. Node dissection, radiation therapy, infection, obesity, postsurgical trauma, and constriction of the affected site/limb exacerbate this condition.
5. Functionally, the patient with lymphedema may demonstrate impaired range of motion and functional use of the extremity, pain, and dermatolymphangitis. Pain must be fully-explored (neuropathic vs. mechanical) before initiating treatment for the lymphedema itself.
6. Often in patients with breast cancer undergoing mastectomy and lymph node dissection, paresthesias and dysesthesias of the posteromedial arm are encountered. They may be attributed to loss of the intercostobrachial nerve during the procedure.
7. The etiology of the lymphedema should be determined. Considerations include tumor recurrence, venous thrombosis, local inflammation, postradiation plexopathy, and/or trauma.
8. Left untreated, lymphedema may lead to loss of joint range of motion, pain, increased risk of infection, impaired limb functioning, and psychological features related to self-image and cosmesis. End-stage untreated lymphedema may progress to elephantiasis and, in rare instances, lymphangiosarcoma.
9. Gillis (2001) outlines a differential diagnosis for lymphedema (Table 2).
10. **Dermatolymphangitis** (DLA) refers to acute lymphedema with cellulitis and is often associated with postmastectomy lymphedema. Treatment options include dicloxacillin, 250–500 mg 4 times/day, or erythromycin, 250–500 mg 4 times/day.
11. The **goals of treatment** in secondary lymphedema are to improve lymphatic flow, reduce limb size, improve range of motion, and reduce the risk of infection. Treatment options may be either conservative (external compression) or invasive (surgery).
    a. Conservative management, also known as **complex decongestive therapy**, consists of manual lymphatic drainage, multilayered compression limb-wrapping, proper fitting of elastic compression garments, exercise, and skin emollients.
    b. Patient education involves instruction in self-massage, use of compression wraps and garments, and home exercises.
    c. External pneumatic compression pumps are rarely indicated and may indeed exacerbate damaged lymphatic vessels.
    d. Conservative measures should be attempted before surgery is considered.

TABLE 2. Differential Diagnosis for Lymphedema

	Lymphedema	Venous Insufficiency	DVT	Cellulitis
Color	Normal to pink	Normal/hemosiderin	Normal to red	Red
Heat	Minimal	Normal	Normal to warm	Hot
Pitting	+ early; – chronic	+	±	±
Symmetry	–	+	–	–
Doppler	Normal*	Normal	Abnormal	Normal

DVT = deep venous thrombosis.
* Bulky nodal disease can lead to DVT.

E. **Amputation and limb salvage** (see also Chapter 1: Amputation Rehabilitation)
  1. In a 30-year study of patients with cancer at the National Cancer Institute, 89% of all amputations were performed for sarcomas. In adults, most soft tissue sarcomas involve the extremities, whereas in children, the majority involve head/neck and genitourinary sites. Tumors are the leading cause of amputation in the 10–19-year-old group, and bone sarcomas cause 7% of all childhood cancers. Especially in children, limb-sparing techniques have gained increased popularity.
  2. **Standard treatment of sarcomas** involves wide resections. Since the 1970s with the advent of more efficacious chemotherapy, survival rates for patients with osteogenic sarcoma and Ewing's sarcoma have significantly improved.
     a. No statistical difference has been observed in local recurrence or long-term survival in patients who have undergone limb salvage vs. amputation.
     b. Salvage surgeries are usually undertaken in patients with upper extremity malignancies or proximal lower extremity involvement. This approach is largely due to marked functional deficits associated with amputation at these sites.
     c. In high-grade tumors of the leg and foot, wide resection with amputation is preferred. Usually such patients, who are future transtibial amputees, have an excellent functional prognosis.
  3. **Upper extremity limb-sparing procedures**
     a. **Scapulectomy with preservation of elbow and hand** may allow preservation of some shoulder flexion and abduction. Complications may include pain and forearm edema.
     b. In the **Tikhoff-Lindberg procedure**, the scapula, clavicle, and proximal humerus are removed en bloc. The result is loss of shoulder function but preservation of elbow and hand function.
     c. In **resection of the distal radius with wrist fusion and distal ulnar resection**, the key is that the more distal the resection, the greater the preservation of pronation and supination.
  4. **Lower extremity limb-sparing procedures**
     a. In **partial or total fibulectomy**, the knee remains stable, but peroneal nerve injury may lead to foot-drop.
     b. In **distal femur resection with knee arthrodesis**, the patient remains generally non-weight-bearing for weeks with the knee immobilized. Eventually the patient progresses to partial weight-bearing with posterior splinting.
     c. In patients with **knee joint resection, prosthetic replacement, and wide soft tissue resection**, function depends on the amount of muscle resected.
     d. In the **Van Ness rotational arthroplasty**, the knee joint and tumor are resected en bloc. The tibia is rotated 180°and fused to the residual femur. The reversed ankle acts as a knee joint for the below-knee prosthesis.
  5. In the **cancer-induced amputee**, treatment with chemotherapy and radiation may be associated with anemia, fatigue, impaired wound healing, or weight loss (which affects prosthetic fitting).

V. **Assessing Patients with Cancer for Inpatient Rehabilitation**
  A. As with any general rehabilitation candidates, patients with cancer may present initially as outpatients referred by a primary physician or, specifically in cancer, an oncologist or surgeon. More often, however, rehabilitation medicine

becomes aware of a patient through the hospital consultative service. Often a patient has already undergone surgical intervention, and a period of healing is anticipated before resumption of treatment, whether it be chemotherapy, radiation therapy, further surgical intervention, or palliation.

B. The postsurgical patient is often debilitated and demonstrates decreased endurance, impaired mobility, and impaired ability for self-care.
1. Depending on the severity of the intervention, the patient may have cognitive deficits; he or she may be immunocompromised or pancytopenic, nutritionally challenged, constipated, or not yet ambulating.
2. Secondary to immobility, the patient may have skin breakdown, pneumonia, or deep venous thrombosis.
3. Any future intervention by oncology specialists may be limited until patients have "sufficiently recovered." In the world of managed care, this approach equates to inpatient rehabilitation or subacute/long-term placement. However, unique to the treatment of patients with cancer is the final return home-whether with family or through hospice services.
4. **To start an effective rehabilitation program**, certain criteria must be met.
   a. **Is the patient a rehabilitation candidate?**
      i. Successful rehabilitation generally occurs when specific goals are identified before admission to the inpatient rehabilitation unit.
      ii. In cancer care, the physiatrist may be asked to teach family members how to care for a relative who is terminally ill and perhaps cognitively unable to respond.
      iii. In the vast number of cases, however, patients with cancer are no different from general rehabilitation patients. Their deficits may parallel the outcome of stroke, traumatic brain injury, spinal cord injury, or fracture with concomitant weight-bearing restrictions.
   b. **What is the discharge plan?**
      i. Rehabilitation is not a disposition plan. The goal of rehabilitation, especially in patients with cancer, is to restore the patient as close as possible to premorbid functioning while addressing quality-of-life issues.
      ii. Function is restored using a comprehensive team approach of therapists (physical, occupational, and psychological), nurses, nutritionists, social workers, and case managers.
      iii. Successful home or community reentry requires a mutual understanding and cooperative therapeutic interaction among patients, therapists, and future caregivers. The caregiver enables the patient either to proceed safely onward to the next therapeutic step or, in terminally ill patients, to come to terms with impending death.
      iv. Patients with cancer who are unable to undertake physically or emotionally acute inpatient rehabilitation and for whom further medical or interventional therapy is planned should be considered for subacute placement or, when necessary, skilled nursing placement.
      v. End-of-life issues are best addressed in a family conference with all medical specialists, family members, and the patient.
VI. **Commonly Faced Problems in the Care of Patients with Cancer**
   A. **Pain**
   1. Based on international studies, 60–90% of patients with cancer experience pain.

    a. Pain remains inadequately controlled in about 25%. Indeed, up to 40–50% of patients with cancer in the U.S. may fail to achieve adequate relief.

    b. Reasons for this discrepancy include inadequate assessment of pain and deficiencies in the practitioner's working knowledge of analgesic and opioid usage.

    c. Pain can be managed successfully by using a multifaceted approach, including surgery, radiation, chemotherapy, treatment of infection, use of pain medication, rehabilitation, and psychology services.

2. Pain may result directly from the tumor or from cancer therapy.

    a. Pain should be characterized as acute or chronic.

    b. It also should be determined whether the pain is somatic, visceral, or neuropathic.

3. In 1990, the World Health Organization devised a systematic approach to pain management that has demonstrated 90% efficacy in relieving cancer-based pain; it also relieves pain in 75% of terminally ill cancer patients.

    a. The first step is to use **aspirin, acetaminophen, or NSAIDs** for mild-to-moderate pain (Table 3).

       i. Adverse effects of NSAIDS, which may appear at any time, include renal failure, hepatic dysfunction, bleeding, and/or gastric ulceration.

      ii. No particular NSAID has demonstrated superiority over all others for pain relief.

     iii. Once the agent is selected, the dose should be titrated upward until either pain is relieved or the maximal dose has been reached.

     iv. Because NSAIDS have individual ceiling effects in terms of efficacy, another drug should be tried if a patient fails to respond to the first choice before NSAID therapy is discontinued altogether.

    b. If pain persists or increases, an opioid (codeine or hydrocodone) should be added to the NSAID regimen. However, combination products may be limited by their content of acetaminophen or NSAID.

    c. If pain persists and is moderate to severe at the outset, opioid potency or dosage should be increased.

    d. **Adjuvant analgesics** used in the treatment of cancer pain include:

       i. Tricyclic antidepressants, secondary amines (e.g., nortriptyline), or mexiletine, which have proven efficacy in dysesthesias associated with chemotherapy-induced neuropathies.

      ii. Carbamazepine has been used for lancinating pain, although its use may be limited in patients experiencing leukopenia.

     iii. Gabapentin has been used to treat lancinating and neuropathic pain. Indeed, it is a reasonable first- or second-line adjuvant medication. It has a benign side-effect profile and has few drug-drug interactions. Because gabapentin is excreted renally, doses should be monitored in patients with concomitant renal disease and patients on dialysis.

     iv. Topical adjuvants, such as capsaicin and lidocaine preparations, have been used in patients with cutaneous allodynia or hyperpathia.

    e. **Opioids** are analgesics used in the treatment of moderate-to-severe pain. Based on their specific receptor site, they may be classified as full agonist, partial agonists, or mixed agonist-antagonists.

       i. Full agonists, such as morphine, hydromorphone, codeine, oxycodone, hydrocodone, methadone, and fentanyl, have no ceiling effect to analgesic efficacy. In fact, large does of morphine (e.g., several

TABLE 3.   Dosing Data for Acetaminophen and NSAIDs

Drug	Usual Dose for Adults and Children ≥ 50 kg Body Weight	Usual Dose for Children and Adults ≤ 50 kg Body Weight
Acetaminophen and over-the-counter NSAIDs		
Acetaminophen	650 mg every 4 hr 975 mg every 6 hr	10–15 mg/kg every 4 hr 15–20 mg/kg every 4 hr (rectal)
Aspirin	650 mg every 4 hr 975 mg every 6 hr	10–15 mg/kg every 4 hr 15–20 mg/kg every 4 hr (rectal)
Ibuprofen (Motrin, others)	400–600 mg every 6 hr	10 mg/kg every 5–8 hr
Prescription NSAIDs		
Carpofen (Rimadyl)	100 mg 3 times/day	
Choline magnesium trisalicylate (Trilisate)	1000–1500 mg 3 times/day	25 mg/kg 3 times/day
Choline salicylate	870 mg every 3–4 hr	
Diflunisal (Dolobid)	500 mg every 12 hr	
Etodolac (Lodine)	200–400 mg every 6–8 hr	
Fenoprofen calcium (Nalfon)	300–600 mg every 6 hr	
Ketoprofen (Orudis)	25–60 mg every 6–8 hr	
Ketorolac tromethamine (Toradol)	10 mg every 4–6 hr to a maximum of 40 mg/day	
Magnesium salicylate (Doan's, Magan, Mobidin, others)	650 mg every 4 hr	
Meclofenamate sodium (Meclomen)	50–100 mg every 6 hr	
Mefenamic acid (Ponstel)	250 mg every 6 hr	
Naproxen (Naprosyn)	250–275 mg every 6–8 hr	
Naproxen sodium (Anaprox)	275 mg every 6–8 hr	
Sodium salicylate (Generic)	325–650 mg every 3–4 hr	
Parenteral NSAIDs		
Ketorolac tromethamine (Toradol)	60 mg initially, then 3 mg every 6 hr intramuscular dose not to exceed 5 days	

hundred milligrams every 4 hours) may be needed for severe pain. Morphine is the most commonly used opioid for moderate-to-severe pain.

ii. Morphine sulfate must be used with care in elderly patients and patients with renal disease. Morphine metabolites (morphine-3-glucuronide and morphine-6-glucuronide) have long half-lives and are renally excreted. Morphine also may impair cognitive functioning.

iii. Oxycodone and fentanyl preparations have benign metabolite profiles and are available in sustained-released formulations.

iv. Use of meperidine (Demerol) is discouraged because its metabolite, normeperidine, is toxic with chronic use.

v. In the initial evaluation of opioid-naïve patients with pain, the patient is provided with an immediate-release preparation, which is given liberally (at times hourly) as needed (Tables 4 and 5).

TABLE 4.   Dose Equivalents for Opioid Analgesics in Opioid-naive Adults and Children ≥ 50 kg Body Weight

Drug	Approximate Equianalgesic Dose		Usual Starting Dose for Moderate to Severe Pain	
	Oral	*Parenteral*	*Oral*	*Parenteral*
Opioid agonist				
Morphine	30 mg every 3–4 hr (repeat around-the-clock dosing)	10 mg every 3–4 hr	30 mg every 3–4 hr	10 mg every 3–4 hr
	60 mg every 3–4 hr (single dose or inter-mittent dosing)			
Morphine controlled-release (MS Contin, Oramorph)	90–120 mg every 12 hr	N/A	90–120 mg every 12 hr	N/A
Hydromorphone (Dilaudid)	7.5 mg every 3–4 hr	1.5 mg every 3–4 hr	6 mg every 3–4 hr	1.5 mg every 3–4 hr
Levorphanol (Levo-Dromoran)	4 mg every 6–8 hr	2 mg every 6–8 hr	4 mg every 6–8 hr	2 mg every 6–8 hr
Meperidine (Demerol)	300 mg every 2–3 hr	100 mg every 3 hr	N/R	100 mg every 3 hr
Methadone (Dolo-phine, other)	20 mg every 6–8 hr	10 mg every 6–8 hr	20 mg every 6–8 hr	10 mg every 6–8 hr
Oxymorphone (Numorphan)	N/A	1 mg every 3–4 hr	N/A	1 mg every 3–4 hr
Combination opioid/NSAID preparations				
Codeine (with aspirin or acetaminophen)	180–200 mg every 3–4 hr	130 mg every 3–4 hr	60 mg every 3–4 hr	60 mg every 2 hr (IM/SC)
Hydrocodone (in (Lorcet, Lortab, Vicodin, others)	30 mg every 3–4 hr	N/A	10 mg every 3–4 hr	N/A
Oxycodone (Roxi-codone, also in Percocet, Perco-dan, Tylox, others)	30 mg every 3–4 hr	N/A	10 mg every 3–4 hr	N/A

N/A = not available, IM = intramuscular, SC = subcutaneous.

- Once opiate use has stabilized, the amount used over a 24-hour period should be calculated. This amount is then divided in half and administered as morning and evening sustained-release doses.
- Breakthrough as-needed medication is often provided in an immediate-release preparation at 1–3-hour intervals. Rescue or breakthrough doses are typically 5–15% of the total daily dose.
- Ideally, one should use the same opioid as the sustained-release preparation. If the required amount of breakthrough pain medication increases, the sustained-released dose is increased accordingly.

f. At times, when pain remains under poor control despite increased amounts of the full agonist, additional analgesic techniques need to be explored.

TABLE 4.   Dose Equivalents for Opioid Analgesics in Opioid-naive Adults and Children < 50 kg Body Weight

Drug	Approximate Equianalgesic Dose		Usual Starting Dose for Moderate to Severe Pain	
	Oral	*Parenteral*	*Oral*	*Parenteral*
Opioid agonist				
Morphine	30 mg every 3–4 hr (repeat around-the-clock dosing)	10 mg every 3–4 hr	0.3 mg/kg every 3–4 hr	0.1 mg/kg every 3–4 hr
	60 mg every 3–4 hr (single dose or inter-mittent dosing)			
Morphine controlled-release (MS Contin, Oramorph)	90–120 mg every 12 hr	N/A	N/A	N/A
Hydromorphone (Dilaudid)	7.5 mg every 3–4 hr	1.5 mg every 3–4 hr	0.06 mg/kg every 3–4 hr	0.015 mg/kg every 3–4 hr
Levorphanol (Levo-Dromoran)	4 mg every 6–8 hr	2 mg every 6–8 hr	0.04 mg/kg every 6–8 hr	0.02 mg/kg every 6–8 hr
Meperidine (Demerol)	300 mg every 2–3 hr	100 mg every 3 hr	N/R	0.75 mg/kg every 2–3 hr
Methadone (Dolo-phine, others)	20 mg every 6–8 hr	10 mg every 6–8 hr	0.2 mg every 6–8 hr	0.1 mg/kg every 6–8 hr
Combination opioid/NSAID preparations				
Codeine (with aspirin or acetaminophen)	180–200 mg every 3–4 hr	130 mg every 3–4 hr	0.5–1 mg/kg every 3–4 hr	N/R
Hydrocodone (in (Lorcet, Lortab, Vicodin, others)	30 mg every 3–4 hr	N/A	0.2 mg/kg every 3–4 hr	N/A
Oxycodone (Roxi-codone, also in Percocet, Perco-dan, Tylox, others)	30 mg every 3–4 hr	N/A	0.2 mg/kg every 3–4 hr	N/A

N/A = not available, NR = not recommended.

   i. Intraspinal (epidural/intrathecal) administration
   ii. Intraventricular opioids
   iii. Regional local anesthetic blockade
   iv. Neurolysis of plexi (celiac, superior hypogastric
   v. Sympathetic blockade
   vi. In terminally ill patients, neuroablative techniques have been used, including rhizotomy, neurolysis of primary afferent nerves, cordotomy, and C1 midline myelotomy.
   vii. Periodically, pain is effectively eliminated by antineoplastic, neuroablative or neurolytic procedures.
      • Opioids may be weaned accordingly by providing half the prior daily dose for each of the first 2 days, then reducing the daily dose by 25% ever 2 days thereafter until the total dose in morphine equivalents is 30 mg/day.

- The drug may be discontinued after 2 days on the 30 mg/day dose.
- Transdermal clonidine (0.1–0.2 mg/day) may help reduce anxiety, tachycardia or other autonomic symptoms associated with opioid withdrawal.

4. **Nonpharmacologic modalities**
   a. Little human research exists in this field.
      i. In general, one should avoid heat and cold modalities over tumor or radiated sites.
         - Radiated skin has reduced sweat gland and circulation.
         - Heat should not be applied because temperatures below those cidal for cancer (44–45°C) may increase blood flow, accelerate tumor growth. and promote metastatic spread.
      ii. In the limited physiatric literature, use of ultrasound is contra-indicated over fields of possible tumor. The restriction in the use of ultrasound dates back to Hayashi's study in 1940.

B. **Bowel/bladder management**
   1. Patients with a lower motor neuron pattern of bowel, bladder and erectile impairment require ongoing management.
      a. Bladder management may consist of urinary monitoring (bladder scanning), establishment of an intermittent catheterization program, and subsequent urologic investigation.
      b. Bowel programs are designed to prevent incontinence and regulate colonic evacuation.
         i. Even in cases of intact neurologic functioning, the use of opiate pain medication delays colonic transit times.
         ii. A regulated bowel program of stool softener and colonic irritant (e.g., Senekot-S; suppository; digital stimulation; enemas with Theravac, milk, or molasses; saline, mineral oil, and glycerin [SMOG]) adds to good colonic health and reduces the risk of obstruction and nausea.

C. **Fatigue**
   1. One of the most frequent complaints of patients with cancer
      a. In one study fatigue affected up to 78% of patients and for the majority restricted daily routine.
      b. Diminished energy, motivation, or ability to attend may characterize fatigue. The patient can appear exhausted or present with generalized weakness.
      c. Patients may have an unusual desire for sleep and appear depressed or distressed.
   2. Treatment focuses on remediable factors, such as nutrition, infection, pain, hypercalcemia, hypothyroidism, or organ failure (cardiorespiratory/hepatic). In addition, principles of energy conservation in conjunction with graduated aerobic exercising have been shown to alleviate fatigue.

D. **Febrile neutropenia**
   1. Neutropenia is the major reason for hospitalization during or after chemotherapy; 48–60% of neutropenic patients have infection. In only 50% of such patients is the pathogenic organism identified; 60–70% of bacterial pathogens are gram-positive.
   2. Neutropenia is defined as a neutrophil count $< 500/mm^3$ or $< 1000/mm^3$ with anticipated decline to $500/mm^3$. In febrile neutropenia, a single oral temperature is $> 38.3°C$ (101°F) for at least 1 hour.

3. A **low-risk** neutropenic patient is one who will likely remain neutropenic for < 7–10 days. A patient at **high risk** will likely remain neutropenic for > 10 days.

4. **Risk factors** for infectious complications in neutropenic patients include:
   a. Degree and duration of neutropenia.
   b. Mucositis from chemotherapy
   c. Skin lesions arising after IV injection or bone marrow aspiration
   d. Local placement of tunneled or nontunneled IV catheters
   e. Immunosuppression secondary to cytotoxic or corticosteroid therapy
   f. Obstruction secondary to neoplastic disease
   g. Malnutrition
   h. Alteration of normal flora by antibiotics, prolonged hospitalization, or underlying disease

5. **Initial evaluation** includes blood cultures (from peripheral vessels and a catheter or port); culture of exudative lesions, urine, and stool; chest x-ray to rule out infiltrates; and basic blood chemistries and hematology (complete blood count with differential).

6. **Initial antibiotic therapy** consists of one of the following regimens:
   a. If vancomycin is needed, use vancomycin and ceftazidime.
   b. If vancomycin is not needed, proceed with either monotherapy or duotherapy.
   c. Monotherapeutic drugs include ceftazidime, cefepime, imipenem, or meropenem. Duotherapeutic drugs involve the use of an aminoglycoside and antipseudomonal beta-lactam.

7. **Antiviral drugs** are not routinely used unless herpetic or varicella-zoster lesions are present. Colony-stimulating factors are likewise not routinely used but may be considered in serious infection (pneumonia, sepsis); neutropenia lasting longer than 7 days; and neutropenia defined by < 100/mm^3.

8. Most importantly, **antibiotic prophylaxis** in afebrile neutropenic patients is not routinely done (with the exception of prophylaxis against *Pneumocystis carinii* pneumonitis) to avoid drug toxicity, antibiotic resistance, and/or fungal overgrowth.

9. In summary, initial antibiotic treatment in the febrile neutropenic patient may be mono- or duotherapeutic. Vancomycin is not routinely used as a first-line drug unless the patient has a documented indication for its use or a methicillin-resistant *Staphylococcus aureus* infection. The patient should be treated with broad antibiotic coverage for a minimum of 7 days. Empiric use of antiviral agents or the routine use of colony-stimulating factors is not recommended.

E. **End-of-life issues**
   1. The patient's initial focus is often "beating" the cancer and returning to his or her premorbid life.
   2. When this is not possible, rehabilitation services often provide the next step in improving function and quality of life. The physiatrist, along with the team of oncology specialists, is ask to discuss and assist with issues of future medical options.
   3. Ongoing appropriate care often requires involvement by social workers and case managers to discuss covered benefits, out-of- pocket costs, nursing and personal care needs, assistive equipment, and transportation needs. An involved staff with the assistance of chaplaincy or psychology may help

reduce stress and ease the difficulty of end-of-life decisions.

4. Hospice care is available to the patient who requires nursing care and has a prognosis of 6 months or less.
   a. While providing basic medical care, hospices emphasize supporting the patient emotionally, spiritually, and functionally.
   b. Hospice are may be offered in an inpatient or residential setting. In the residential setting, the services of hospice vary. The hospice benefit does not include around-the-clock nursing or home-health aides. The goal of hospice care is to involve and educate the family in the patient's final care.

Bibliography
1. Ahrar K: Vertebroplasty and kyphoplasty: Percutaneous management. Neurosurgical Grand Rounds, April 6, 2001. M.D. Anderson Cancer Center. Houston.
2. Brown GP: Febrile neutropenia. Phar 5825. Pathophysiology and Therapy Series. Infect Dis (Spring, 1999) [taken from websource http://www. courses.ahc.umn.edu].
3. Cheville AL: Pain management in cancer rehabilitation. Arch Phys Med Rehabil 82(Suppl 1):S84–387, 2001.
4. Cleeland CS, Gonin R, et al: Pain and its treatment in outpatients with metastatic cancer. N Engl J Med 330:592–596, 1994.
5. DeLisa J, et al: Rehabilitation for patients with cancer diagnoses. In DeLisa J (ed): Rehabilitation Medicine. Philadelphia, Lippincott-Raven, 1998 p 1294.
6. Foley KM: The treatment of cancer pain. N Engl J Med 313:84–95, 1985.
7. Francis K: Cancer Rehabilitation. Kessler Review 2000. Kessler Medical Rehabilitation Research and Education Corporation, March 10–19, 2000, section 11(1–18).
8. Gillis T: Oncology rehabilitation. Baylor College of Medicine. 35th Comprehensive Review Course in Physical Medicine and Rehabilitation, March 13, 2001, Houston.
9. Gillis T, Cheville A, et al: Oncologic rehabilitation. Arch Phys Med Rehabil 82(Suppl 1):S63–S68, 2001.
10. Gokaslan Z: Metastatic disease of the spine: Conventional treatment. Neurosurgical Grand Rounds, April 6, 2001. M.D. Anderson Cancer Center, Houston.
11. Hayashi S: Der einfluss der ultraschallwellen und ultrakurtzwellen auf den maligen Tumor. J Med Sci Biophys Jpn 6(138):182, 1940.
12. King, JC; Williams RP; McAnelly RD; Leonard, EI. Rehabilitation of tumor amputees and limb salvage patients, Phys Med Rehabil State Art Rev 8:297–320, 1994.
13. Kottke F, Lehmann J, Delateur B: Diathermy and superficial heat, laser and cold therapy. In Krusen's Handbook of Physical Medicine and Rehabilitation, 4th ed. Philadelphia, W.B. Saunders, 1990, pp 283–367.
14. Marciniak CM, Sliwa JA, Spill G, Heinemann AW: Functional outcome following rehabilitation of the cancer patient. Arch Phys Med Rehabil 77:54–57, 1996.
15. Meyers CA: Neuropsychological aspects of cancer and cancer treatment. Phys Med Rehabil State Art Revi 8:229–242, 1994.
16. O'Young B, Young M, Stiens Sl (eds): PM&R Secrets, 2nd ed. Philadelphia, Hanley & Belfus, 2002.
17. Polednak AP, Flannery JT: Brain, other central nervous system, and eye cancer. Cancer 75(Suppl 1):330–337, 1995.
18. U.S. Department of Health and Human Services: Management of Cancer Pain. Clinical Practice Guideline 9. Washington, DC, U.S. Department of Health and Human Services, AHCPR Publication Number 94-0592, 1994.
19. Wertsch J: Differentiating between tumor and radiation plexopathy. Baylor College of Medicine. 35th Comprehensive Review Course in Physical Medicine and Rehabilitation, March 11, 2001, Houston.

Chapter 4

MULTIPLE SCLEROSIS REHABILITATION

Mara M. Isser, D.O., and Anthony Chiodo, M.D.

I. General Principles

A. Multiple sclerosis (MS) is an inflammatory disease of the central nervous system distinguished by discrete areas of demyelination, frequently causing functional and cognitive disabilities.

B. These disabilities are secondary to weakness, bowel and bladder dysfunction, spasticity, gait abnormalities, emotional and cognitive impairment, and sexual dysfunction.

C. Recognition of the resulting impairments determines the interventions that will improve in the patient's quality of life.

II. Epidemiology

A. Multiple sclerosis is the third most common cause of disability in people between the ages of 15 and 50 years.

B. MS affects 200,000–500,000 persons in the United States.

C. Average age at onset is 28 years.

D. 73% of affected people are women.

E. Prevalence rate is < 1/100,000 in equatorial areas compared with 6–14/100,000 in Southern Europe and Southern U.S. In Northern U.S. and Canada, the prevalence is 30–80/100,000.

F. Incidence rates determined by where a person lives before age 15.

G. Risk of MS after age 60 is minimal.

III. Etiology

A. Unknown; many hypotheses exist.

B. Current research points to an autoimmune process in genetically predisposed people after exposure to an environmental stimulus.

C. Hypotheses

1. **Genetic:** Certain HLA (HLA DR2) antigens are more prevalent in patients with MS and in children of patients with MS.

2. **Autoimmune:** Response is triggered by an infectious agent, as noted by an increase in IgG oligoclonal bands in cerebral spinal fluid

3. **Viral:** Direct infection from a slow virus, possibly herpes simplex, measles, or rubella; however, no specific virus has been consistently identified in MS.

4. **Geography:** Increased incidence in northern climates as long as person lived there for the first 15 years of life.

5. **Race:** Northern Europeans and their descendants have a higher incidence than Asians, Africans, and Eskimos.

IV. Pathophysiology

A. **Inflammation and gliosis** (disappearance of oligodendrocytes) in the central nervous system cause formation of plaques.

    1. Plaques occur in the white matter, frequently in the periventricular area of the cerebrum, spinal cord, brainstem, optic nerve, and perivenous areas.

    2. Initiating event is thought to be an autoimmune reaction against normal myelin by T lymphocytes when they recognize certain antigens bound to human lymphocyte antigen molecules (HLA). Cytokines such as tumor necrosis factor (TNF) and interferon cause more T cells to mount an inflammatory response.

  B. With recurrent attacks, further gliosis occurs. Extension and coalescence of plaques cause larger areas of demyelination and eventual secondary axonal damage.

  C. Cytokines cause a breakdown of the blood-brain barrier.

  D. T cells cross the blood-brain barrier, attach to certain HLA molecules, and release lymphotoxin, interferon gamma, and TNF, which increase the inflammatory response and attack myelin.

  E. Cytokines also cause B cells to produce antibodies that combine with complement to attack oligodendrocytes and myelin.

V. Clinical Presentation and Diagnosis

  A. **Differential diagnosis**

    1. Cervical spondylotic myelopathy: usually affects the older population; associated with more pain and fewer bladder disturbances.

    2. Vestibular neuronitis: vestibular tests may be abnormal but indiscernible from MS.

    3. Systemic lupus erythematosus (SLE): antinuclear antibody test is positive in 25% of MS patients; 37–42% of patients with SLE have neurologic symptoms.

    4. AIDS: usually associated with spastic paraparesis and sensory ataxia.

    5. Sjögren's syndrome: patients can also present with a relapsing-remitting course, internuclear ophthalmoplegia, or cerebellar symptoms.

    6. Lyme disease: patients may have relapsing-remitting course, oligoclonal bands in CSF. Possible to distinguish by serologic testing.

    7. Sarcoidosis: CNS involved in 5% of patients.

    8. Tropical spastic paresis: sensory changes with pain in lower extremities and neurogenic bladder caused by HTLV-1.

    9. Diseases with single lesions and a relapsing course: arteriovenous malformation, glioma, and meningioma.

    10. Carcinoma: associated with peripheral neuropathy; usually presents in older people with rapidly progressively course.

    11. Cerebrovascular disease: scattered lesions secondary to emboli may appear similar to MS lesions on imaging studies.

  B. **Symptoms at onset**

    1. Weakness

    2. Paresthesias (most common symptom)

    3. Gait abnormalities

    4. Optic neuritis (associated with pain in eye or forehead and scotomas)

    5. Diplopia

    6. Vertigo

    7. Ataxia

    8. Disturbed nutrition

  C. **Signs and symptoms during course of MS**, in decreasing order of occurrence (Table 1)

TABLE 1.   Signs and Symptoms During the Course of Multiple Sclerosis

Signs and Symptoms	Percent	Signs and Symptoms	Percent
Paresthesias	100	Impotence	40
Weakness	100	Lhermitte's sign	40
Abnormal reflexes	80	Pain	30
Cerebellar signs	80	Depression	30
Spasticity	75	Muscle wasting	20
Fatigue	75	Dementia	10
Decreased alternating	70	Facial weakness	3
movements		Unilateral hearing loss	3
Heat intolerance	60	Epilepsy	2
Nystagmus	50	Visual failure	1
Intellectual loss	40	Trigeminal neuralgia	1

From Taylor RS: Rehabilitation of persons with multiple sclerosis. In Braddon RL (ed): Physical Medicine and Rehabilitation. Philadelphia, W.B. Saunders, 2000, with permission.

D. **Physical findings**
   1. Spasticity
   2. Weakness
   3. Ataxia
   4. Loss of sensation
   5. Increased muscle stretch reflexes
   6. Pathologic reflexes (e.g., Babinski's sign)
   7. Optic disk pallor
   8. Abnormal papillary responses
   9. Nystagmus
   10. Ophthalmoparesis
   11. Visual field deficits
   12. Cranial nerve abnormalities
   13. Cognitive impairments
E. **Diagnostic studies**
   1. **Magnetic resonance imaging (MRI)**
      a. Positive findings seen in 95% of patients with MS.
      b. Multiple white matter lesions appear as bright areas on T2-weighted images, usually in the brainstem, optic nerve, periventricular region, cerebellum, corpus callosum, and spinal cord.
      c. Gadolinium aids in diagnosis because it crosses the blood-brain barrier and shows areas of acute inflammatory changes and reactivated chronic plaques.
      d. Approximately 75% of lesions detected on MRI do not correlate with clinical findings.
      e. Negative MRI nearly rules out MS.
   2. **Evoked potential recordings**
      a. Measures varied conduction time through myelinated pathways and helps to identify demyelination detected clinically.
      b. Can measure somatosensory-evoked potentials, brainstem auditory-evoked potentials, or visual-evoked potentials
   3. **Cerebrospinal fluid (CSF) analysis**
      a. No CSF findings are diagnostic, although they can be consistent with MS.
      b. CSF protein is elevated in one-fourth of patients with exacerbations.
      c. 60–70% of patients have an increase in IgG.

TABLE 2. Diagnosis of Multiple Sclerosis

Possible MS
- History of relapsing and remitting neurologic symptoms.
- Only one site of involvement noted by clinical symptoms, imaging or laboratory studies.
- No other diagnostic explanation of symptoms.

Probable MS
- Two documented attacks with at least one lesion being diagnosed with imaging, clinical, or laboratory studies.
- One documented attack with at least two separate lesions shown with imaging, clinical, or laboratory studies.

Definite MS
- Two attacks separated by at least 1 month with evidence of two lesions based on clinical symptoms, laboratory, or imaging studies.

Note: An attack is considered symptoms lasting longer than 24 hours.
From Taylor RS: Rehabilitation of persons with multiple sclerosis. In Braddon RL (ed): Physical Medicine and Rehabilitation. Philadelphia, W.B. Saunders, 2000, with permission.

     d. The IgG index is the ratio of CSF IgG to albumin divided by the ratio of serum IgG to albumin; abnormalities are found in 90% of cases.

     e. Normal CSF shows polyclonal IgG. IgG is oligoclonal in 85–95% of patients with MS.

F. **Criteria for diagnosis** (Table 2)
1. Remains a clinical diagnosis but must satisfy at least three criteria: (1) neurologic deficits that (2) occur in different areas of the CNS at different times and (3) do not result from another disease process.
2. Quantitative definition, provided by Schumacher, describes neurologic deficits involving at least two sites at two or more points in time, lasting longer than 24 hours, at least 1 month apart, or worsening symptoms for longer than 6 months.

VI. Natural History and Prognosis
A. **Clinical classification:** based on clinical course and neurologic deficits (Fig. 1).
1. **Relapsing-remitting**
   a. Accounts for majority of cases.
   b. Most attacks occur in first 5–10 years.
   c. Episodes of acute worsening with recovery and stable course between relapses.
   d. Responds best to treatment; progressive courses respond the least.
2. **Secondary progressive**
   a. Begins as relapsing-remitting
   b. Later develops into gradually worsening course with increasing neurologic deterioration.
3. **Primary progressive**
   a. Most likely to occur with onset of disease after 40 years of age.
   b. Gradual worsening of neurologic function from onset.
   c. 15% of patients present with this course.
4. **Progressive relapsing:** gradual worsening of neurologic function with superimposed acute relapses.
5. **Plateau:** disease appears clinically inactive from initial presentation.
6. **Benign:** 10 years after initial diagnosis of relapsing-remitting MS, the patient has few or no neurologic deficits.
7. **Malignant**
   a. Primary progressive MS with a consistently progressive course.
   b. Can lead to death 5 years from onset.

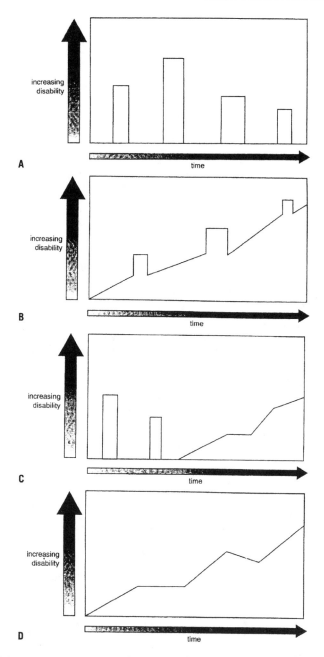

FIGURE 1.   Clinical course definitions of multiple sclerosis. A, Relapsing-remitting: relapses with full or partial recovery. B, Progressive-relapsing progressive disease with acute relapses. C, Secondary-progressive: initially relapsing-remitting followed by progression with, or without, relapses. D, Primary progressive: disease progression. (From Saffir M, Rosenblum D: Multiple sclerosis. In Grabois M, et al: Physical Medicine and Rehabilitation. The Complete Approach. Malden, MA, Blackwell Science, Inc.., 2000, with permission.)

B. **Functional classification scales**
  1. Kurtzke Disability Status Scale (DSS) measures 10 levels of impairment.
  2. Kurtzke Expanded Disability Status Scale (EDSS) consists of DSS with assessment of eight additional areas (Table 3).

TABLE 3.   Kurtzke Expanded Disability Status Scale (EDSS)

0	Normal neurologic examination (all grade 0 in FS*)
1.0	No disability, minimal signs in one FS (i.e., grade 1)
1.5	No disability, minimal signs in more than one FS* (more than one FS grade 1)
2.0	Minimal disability in one FS (one FS grade 2, others 0 or 1)
2.5	Minimal disability in two FS (two FS grade 2, others 0 or 1)
3.0	Moderate disability but with moderate disability in one FS (one grade 3) and one or two FS grade 2; or two FS grade 3; or five FS grade 2 (others 0 or 1)
3.5	Fully ambulatory but with moderate disability in one FS (one grade 3) and one or two FS grade 2; or five FS grade 2 (others 0 or 1)
4.0	Fully ambulatory without aid, self-sufficient, up and about some 12 hr a day despite relatively severe disability consisting of one FS grade 4 (others 0 or 1), or combinations of lesser grades exceeding limits of previous steps; able to walk without aid or rest some 500 m
4.5	Fully ambulatory without aid, up and about much of the day, able to work a full day, may otherwise have some limitation of full activity or require minimal assistance; characterized by relatively severe disability usually consisting of one FS grade 4 (others 0 or 1) or combinations of lesser grades exceeding limits of previous steps; able to walk without aid or rest some 300 m
5.0	Ambulatory without aid or rest for about 200 m; disability severe enough to impair full daily activities (e.g., to work a full day without special provisions) (usual FS equivalents are one grade 5 alone, others 0 or 1; or combinations of lesser grades usually exceeding specifications for step 4.0)
5.5	Ambulatory without aid or rest for about 100 m; disability severe enough to preclude full daily activities; (usual FS equivalents are one grade 5 alone, others 0 or 1; or combination of lesser grades usually exceeding those for step 4.0)
6.0	Intermittent or unilateral constant assistance (cane, crutch, brace) required to walk about 100 m with or without resting (usual FS equivalents are combinations with more than two FS grade 3+)
6.5	Constant bilateral assistance (canes, crutches, braces) required to walk about 20 m without resting (usual FS equivalents are combinations with more than two FS grade 3+)
7.0	Unable to walk beyond approximately 5 m even with aid, essentially restricted to wheelchair and transfers alone; up and about in wheelchair some 12 hr a day (usual FS equivalents are combinations with more than one FS grade 4+; very rarely pyramidal grade 5 alone)
7.5	Unable to take more than a few steps; restricted to wheelchair; may need aid in transfer; wheels self but cannot carry on in standard wheelchair a full day; may require motorized wheelchair (usual FS equivalents are combinations with more than one FS grade 4+)
8.0	Essentially restricted to bed or chair or perambulated in wheelchair, but may be out of bed itself much of the day; retains many self-care functions; generally has effective use of arms (usual FS equivalents are combinations, generally grade 4+ in several systems)
8.5	Essentially restricted to bed much of day; has some effective use of arm(s); retains some self-care functions (usual FS equivalents are combinations generally 4+ in several systems)
9.0	Helpless bed patient; unable to communicate effectively or eat/swallow (usual FS equivalents are combinations, almost all grade 4+)
10.0	Death due to multiple sclerosis

* Excludes functional system (FS) grade 1.
From Kurtzke JF: Rating neurologic impairment in multiple sclerosis: An Expanded Disabilities Status Scale (EDSS). Neurology 33:1444–1453, 1983, with permission.

a. The eight functional areas assessed are pyramidal, cerebellar, brainstem, sensory, bowel and bladder, visual, cerebral (or mental) and other (Table 4).

b. 10-point scale assesses maximal function and limitations.

c. Most commonly used.

3. Minimal Record of Disability: measures impairment, disability, and handicap.

4. Incapacity Status Scale assesses functional disability

5. Environmental Status Scale classifies social handicap in areas of work, financial status, home management, transportation, social life, and amount of personal assistance needed.

C. **Factors associated with poor prognosis**

1. Progressive disease at onset

2. Male sex

3. Age at onset > 40 years

4. Involvement of multiple systems at onset

5. Short interval between first two relapses

6. Poor recovery from relapse

7. Multiple cranial lesions on T2-weighted MRI at onset

D. **Factors associated with increasing number of exacerbations**

1. Infection

2. Pregnancy

3. Emotional stress

4. Heat and fatigue (causes transient weakness)

5. Trauma

VII. Medical Treatment

A. Goal: to arrest disease progression and prevent relapses.

B. Begin disease-modifying treatment before neurologic deficits have persisted longer than 6 months, especially in patients with poor prognostic factors.

C. Treatment by clinical subtype

1. **Relapsing-remitting MS**

   a. **For exacerbation**

      i. Steroids

      ii. Decrease length as well as severity of exacerbation by decreasing either CNS edema or immune response.

      iii. Does not alter course of disease.

      iv. Be certain to treat all infections before initiating therapy.

      v. For mild-to-moderate exacerbation, initially use oral prednisone, 60–100 mg/day tapered over 1–3 weeks.

      vi. For moderate-to-severe exacerbations use methylprednisilone, 1000 mg IV, over 2–3 hours/day for 3–7 days.

   b. **To alter disease course**

      i. Interferon is treatment of choice. Subtypes include beta-1a (Avonex), which may cause flulike side effects (treat with NSAIDs or prednisone) and beta-1b (Betaseron).

         • Studies with beta-1b have shown 33% decrease in number of exacerbations, 50% decrease in severity, and 60% decrease in plaques seen on MRI; however, there was no decrease in disability.

         • Injection site reactions can be prevented by using different sites, sterile technique, and smaller gauge needles.

Table 4. Kurtzke Functional Systems

Pyramidal functions

0. Normal
1. Abnormal signs without disability
2. Minimal disability
3. Mild or moderate paraperesis or hemi-paresis; severe monoparesis
4. Marked paraparesis or hemiparesis; moderate quadriparesis; or monoplegia
5. Paraplegia, hemiplegia, or marked quadriparesis
6. Quadriplegia
V. Unknown

Cerebellar functions

0. Normal
1. Abnormal signs without disability
2. Mild ataxia
3. Moderate truncal or limb ataxia
4. Severe ataxia, all limbs
5. Unable to perform coordinated movements because of ataxia
V. Unknown
X. Is used throughout after each number when weakness (grade 3 or more on pyramidal) interferes with testing

Brainstem functions

0. Normal
1. Signs only
2. Moderate nystagmus or other mild disability
3. Severe nystagmus, marked extraocular weakness, or moderate disability of of other cranial nerves
4. Marked dysarthria or other marked disability
5. Inability to speak or swallow
V. Unknown

Sensory functions (revised 1982)

0. Normal
1. Vibration or figure-writing decrease only, in one or two limbs
2. Mild decrease in touch or pain or position sense and/or moderate decrease in vibration in one or two limbs; or vibratory (c/s figure writing) decrease alone in three or four limbs
3. Moderate decrease in touch or pain or or position sense, and/or essentially lost vibration in one or two limbs; or mild de-crease in touch or pain and/or moderate decrease in all proprioceptive tests in three or four limbs
4. Marked decrease in touch or pain or loss of proprioception, alone or combined, in one or two limbs; or moderate decrease in touch or pain and/or severe proprio-ceptive decrease in more than two limbs
5. Loss (essentially) of sensation in one or two limbs; or moderate decrease in touch or pain and/or loss of proprioceptive for most of the body below the head
6. Sensation essentially lost below the head
V. Unknown

Bowel and bladder functions (revised 1982)

0. Normal
1. Mild urinary hesitancy, urgency, or retention
2. Moderate hesitancy, urgency, retention of bowel or bladder, or rare urinary incontinence
3. Frequent urinary incontinence
4. In need for almost constant catheterization
5. Loss of bladder function
6. Loss of bowel and bladder function
V. Unknown

Visual (or optic) functions

0. Normal
1. Scotoma with visual acuity (corrected) better than 20/30
2. Worse eye with scotoma with maximal visual acuity (corrected) of 20/30 to 20/59
3. Worse eye with large scotoma, or moderate decrease in fields, but with maximal visual acuity (corrected) of 20/60 to 20/99
4. Worse eye with marked decrease of fields and maximal visual acuity (corrected) of 20/100 to 20/200; grade 3 plus maximal acuity of better eye of 20/60 or less
5. Worse eye with maximal visual acuity (corrected) less than 20/200; grade 4 plus maximal acuity of better eye of 20/60 or less
6. Grade 5 plus maximal visual acuity of better eye of 20/60 or less
V. Unknown
X. Is added to grades 0 to 6 for presence of temporal pallor

Cerebral (or mental) functions

0. Normal
1. Mood alterations only (does not affect DSS score)
2. Mild decrease in mentation
3. Moderate decrease in mentation
4. Marked decrease in mentation (chronic brain syndrome, moderate)
5. Dementia or chronic brain syndrome—severe or incompetent
V. Unknown

Other functions

0. None
1. Any other neurologic fundings attributed to MS (specify)
V. Unknown

From Delisa JA, Gans BM (eds): Rehabilitation Medicine: Principles and Practice. Philadelphia, Lippincott-Raven, 1998.

- May see slight increases in liver enzymes, leukopenia, anemia, or depression.
- Monitor liver transaminases and complete blood counts.
- Indications to discontinue interferon include worsening disability over 6 months, treatment with 3 courses of steroids in 1 year, and detection of serum interferon beta-neutralizing antibodies.

  ii. Glatiramer acetate (Copaxone)
- Autoantigen in MS
- Studies show 29% decrease in number of exacerbations and improvement on Expanded Disability Scale, but MRI studies show little change.
- Side effects include mild injection site reactions as well as short periods of flushing, chest tightness, shortness of breath, and anxiety.
- May be most effective in patients who have developed neutralizing activity to interferon.

  iii. Immunosuppressive agents
- Because of high toxicity, periodic laboratory monitoring of hematologic, hepatic, renal, and infectious disorders is recommended.
- Research into the benefits of immunosuppressive agents, including azathioprine, cyclosporine A, methotrexate, and cyclophosphamide, is ongoing.
- Azathioprine, a purine analog that decreases cell- and humeral-mediated immunity, reduces relapse rate. It may be useful in patients who do not improve with glatiramer acetate or interferon.

2. **Progressive MS**
  a. Methotrexate
    i. Inhibits dihydrofolate reductase as well as cell- and humeral-mediated immunity and has anti-inflammatory effects.
    ii. Patients with secondary progressive MS benefited most.
  b. Cyclophosphamide
    i. Alkylating agent with many toxic effects, including alopecia, nausea, vomiting, hemorrhagic cystitis, leukopenia, myocarditis, infertility, and pulmonary interstitial fibrosis.
    ii. Used in nonresponders to methotrexate who have rapidly progressive disease.

D. Future treatment options may include remyelination strategies and inhibition of myelin-reactive T cells.

VIII. Treatment and Rehabilitation of Specific Problems

A. **Fatigue**
1. Common symptom that worsens with heat, stress, and activity; it can occur daily and drastically affect function.
2. Treatment
  a. Amantadine: antiviral agent that increases dopaminergic activity in peripheral and central nervous systems, thus improving energy level and function.
  b. Pemoline: central stimulant, often prescribed for attention-deficit hypeactivity disorder, that improved fatigue in one study.
  c. Psychosocial treatment includes helping patients maintain environmental control by teaching energy conservation techniques, time management, and work simplification.

    d. Depression may be associated with fatigue; treating depression may improve fatigue.

B. **Weakness and sensory dysfunction**

  1. Assess range of motion, muscle tone, skin integrity, sensation, postural control, balance, muscle tone, strength, and endurance.

  2. Studies have shown that, although autonomic response to exercise has been impaired, exercise does increase strength and endurance.

  3. Patients with greater neurologic impairment do not reach the same intensity or endurance level during therapies.

  4. Treatment goals of physical therapy

    a. Relapsing-remitting course: achieve prior level of function.

    b. Chronic progressive course: maintain current level of function.

  5. Treatment goals of occupational therapy: functional abilities and activities of daily living (ADLs) should be assessed.

  6. Treatment strategies

    a. Providing assistive devices as indicated

    b. Compensatory strategies, especially for energy conservation

    c. Hand function

    d. Fine motor control

C. **Spasticity** (see chapter on Spasticity)

  1. Increased tone can either help patient with transfers and standing or impaired mobility, transfers, self-care, and sexual activity.

  2. Treat the patient only if it causes pain or decreases function.

  3. Treatment strategies

    a. Avoidance of noxious stimuli.

    b. Daily stretching program.

    c. Casting or splinting.

    d. Medications

D. **Ataxia, dysmetria, and other movement disorders**

  1. Symptoms

    a. Can range from mild to severe.

    b. Affect function significantly, including balance, sitting, standing, and walking; wide-based gait is required for support.

    c. Fine motor skills are affected; patients require help with ADLs.

  2. Treatment strategies

    a. Medications: A small number of studies have showed decreases in tremor with isoniazid, primidone, clonidine, and inderal.

    b. Physical interventions

      i. Strengthening of stabilizing muscles, with improved balance and endurance

      ii. Use of arm weights to decrease tremor

      iii. Adaptive equipment, including weighted utensils, canes, walkers, and supportive seating systems for truncal instability

E. **Paresthesias**

  1. Pain can be severe and result in disability.

  2. Management

    a. Acute pain: carbamazepine, baclofen, or phenytoin.

    b. Chronic pain: tricyclic antidepressants or transcutaneous electrical nerve stimulation.

F. **Depression**

1. Incidence: 27–54%.
2. Occurrence does not correlate with severity of disease or physical or cognitive status.
3. Secondary to combination of organic and psychological factors.
4. Treatment includes pharmacotherapy, psychotherapy, stress management, exercise program, and vocational counseling.

G. **Speech and language disorders:** see chapter on Speech and Language Pathology.
   1. 40% of patients have problems with voice, articulation, and swallowing.
   2. 50% have cognitive defects.
   3. Voice pathology
      a. Includes impaired loudness control, voice harshness, defective articulation, impaired emphasis, and pitch control. Dysarthria can be ataxic, spastic, or both.
      b. Management depends on type of resulting dysarthria but may include palate exercises and working on speech rate, voice strength, and phrasing.
   4. Cognitive disorders
      a. Include short-term memory impairment (most common) and slowed mental processing.
      b. Management includes verbal cueing and memory strategies.

H. **Dysphagia**
   1. Secondary to cranial nerve involvement.
   2. Occurs in 10–33% of patients as result of decreased pharyngeal peristalsis and delayed swallowing reflex.
   3. Assessed with three-phase video swallow study.
   4. Treatment includes diet modification, swallowing precautions, oral-motor therapy, and alternative feeding regimens such as feedings through gastrostomy tube.

I. **Sexual dysfunction**
   1. Affects 75% of men and 50% of women.
   2. Symptoms
      a. Men report difficulty in achieving and maintaining an erection, decreased sensation, fatigue, and decreased libido.
      b. Women report decreases in sensation and libido, fatigue, difficulty in achieving orgasm, and decreased arousal and lubrication.
   3. Neurogenic bladder, spasticity, contractures, and weakness also cause sexual dysfunction.
   4. Treatment strategies
      a. Decrease fatigue with pacing.
      b. Manage spasticity with medical intervention (see chapter on Spasticity).
      c. Control bowel and bladder dysfunction with medical interventions as well as timed voiding programs and pelvic floor strengthening exercises. (see Chapters 15 and 16 on Neurogenic Bladder and Bowel Management).
      d. Prostaglandin injections, mechanical devices, or vasodilating medications may aid erectile dysfunction in men.
      e. Vaginal lubricants may benefit women.

J. **Bladder dysfunction** (see Chapter 15, Neurogenic Bladder Management)
   1. 79% of patients develop urologic symptoms, including urgency, frequency, and urge incontinence.

    2. Other symptoms include postvoid dribble, nocturia, increased frequency, dysuria, hesitancy, and decreased force and stream.

K. **Bowel dysfunction** (see chapter on Bowel Dysfunction)

    1. Occurs is two-thirds of patients.

    2. Symptoms include constipation, bowel incontinence, and fecal urgency.

Bibliography

1. Braddom RL (ed): Physical Medicine and Rehabilitation. Philadelphia, W.B. Saunders, 2000.
2. Cohen JA, Kinkel RP, Ransohoff RM, et al: Management of multiple sclerosis. N Engl J Med 337:1604–1611, 1997.
3. Delisa JA, Gans BM (eds): Rehabilitation Medicine: Principles and Practice. Philadelphia, Lipincott-Raven, 1998.
4. Garrison SJ, Grabois M, Hart KA, Lehmkuhl LD (eds): Physical Medicine and Rehabilitation: The Complete Approach. Malden, MA, Blackwell Science, 2000.
5. Kraft GH: Rehabilitation still the only way to improve function in multiple sclerosis. Lancet 354:2016, 1999.
6. Kraft GH, Taylor RS (eds): Multiple Sclerosis: A Rehabilitative Approach. Philadelphia, W.B. Saunders, 1998.
7. Lisak RP, Tselis AC: Multiple sclerosis: Therapeutic update. Arch Neurol 56:277–280, 1999.

Chapter 5

REHABILITATION FOLLOWING TOTAL HIP AND TOTAL KNEE ARTHROPLASTY

Mark J. Ziadeh, M.D., Lisa A. DiPonio, M.D., and Andrew Urquhart, M.D.

I. General Principles

A. **Arthroplasty** is the replacement of a joint to relieve pain and improve range of motion, thereby improving the patient's functional status.
   1. Arthroplasty in various forms was first attempted more than 100 years ago but was not routinely successful until the past 40 years.
   2. Currently, total hip arthroplasty (THA) and total knee arthroplasty (TKA) are two of the most common orthopedic surgical procedures performed.
B. **Incidence:** Approximately 300,000 total joint arthroplasties are done annually in the United States.
C. **Indications for arthroplasty**
   1. Severe disabling pain
      a. Generally in the groin, thigh, or buttocks for hip disease or in the knee.
      b. Pain can be secondary to many conditions, including osteoarthritis (most common), rheumatoid arthritis, avascular necrosis, developmental dysplasia, and posttraumatic arthritis.
   2. Failed nonoperative management of pain
      a. Medications: nonsteroidal anti-inflammatory drugs (NSAIDs), acetaminophen, intra-articular steroid injections.
      b. Physical therapy
      c. Use of assistive devices for ambulation
      d. Activity modifications
   3. Decreased range of motion and function
   4. Impaired activities of daily living
   5. Fractures that cannot be repaired with standard reduction or fixation
D. **Contraindications**
   1. Absolute: active sepsis, local infection, quadricep muscle deficiency for TKA
   2. Relative
      a. Muscle weakness or paralysis around the joint
      b. Traditionally, being young or very active was a relative contraindication, but THA and TKA are now done in these patients with good early results.
E. **Possible indications for acute inpatient rehabilitation**
   1. Medical complications

2. Preexisting functional impairment
3. Arthroplasty revision
4. Bilateral arthroplasty
5. Persistent pain
6. Press-fit fixation of THA requiring non-weight-bearing
7. Decreased range of motion (generally with TKA)
8. Comorbidity: cerebrovascular accidents, amputations, congestive heart failure

II. Total Hip Arthroplasty (THA)

A. THA is replacement of both the acetabulum and femoral head components of the joint.
B. **Hemiarthroplasty** replaces only the femoral head component; performed primarily for displaced femoral neck fractures in the elderly.
C. **Surgical concerns**
   1. **Surgical approaches**
      a. Posterolateral (most common approach; gluteus maximus is split, gluteus medius is preserved)
      b. Anterolateral (second most common approach; both gluteus maximus and gluteus medius are split)
      c. Anterior
      d. Lateral
   2. **Materials:** generally metal alloy components articulating with ultrahigh-molecular-weight polyethylene.
   3. **Methods of fixation**
      a. **Polymethylmethacrylate** (PMMA)
         i. Also called bone cement
         ii. No adhesive qualities
         iii. Interdigitates with the endosteal surface of the bone to provide a mechanical bond
         iv. Peak stability achieved in 24 hours
         v. Generally allows full weight-bearing as tolerated immediately postoperatively but determined by surgeon
         vi. Poor mechanical properties can lead to fatigue and possibly aseptic loosening.
      b. **Press-fit stabilization**
         i. Reaming of the bone and machining of the implant ensure a stable fit.
         ii. Generally non-weight-bearing or toe-touch weight-bearing for 6 weeks after surgery but determined by surgeon.
      c. **Bioactive ceramics**
         i. Most common are hydroxyapatite and tricalcium phosphate.
         ii. Initial press-fit stabilization is needed.
         iii. Goal of biologic fixation between the bone and the implant.
         iv. Generally two types of implant surfaces are used:
            (a) **Porous surface for bone ingrowth**
               • Beads or mesh on the surface of the implant provides a porous metal matrix with a pore size of 100–400 microns, allowing bony ingrowth.
               • Minimal motion allowed at the bone-implant surface (< 50 microns) postoperatively; therefore, usually toe-touch weight-bearing or partial weight-bearing for 6 weeks is required, but determined by surgeon.

(b) **Roughened surface for bone ongrowth**
- Corundum-blasted roughed surface of the implant allows for bony ongrowth.
- This surface can also be used without a bioactive ceramic.
- Usually toe-touch weight-bearing or partial weight-bearing for six weeks, but determined by surgeon.

D. **Hip precautions**
1. Generally observed for 8–12 weeks, allowing time for pseudocapsule to form.
2. Maintained to avoid hip dislocations (usually occur shortly after surgery).
3. Instructed and reinforced by occupational and physical therapy.
   a. **Posterior hip precautions** (of greater concern with posterolateral surgical approach)
      i. No internal rotation past neutral while hip is in flexion
      ii. No adduction across the midline
      iii. No hip flexion > 70–90°
      iv. A hip abductor pillow can be used to assist patients in maintaining precautions.
      v. After a THA revision, the surgeon may elect to use an abductor brace with hip hinge to maintain strict posterior hip precautions.
   b. **Anterior hip precautions** (of greater concern with anterior or lateral surgical approach): avoid hyperextension, external rotation, and adduction.
   c. **Conditions predisposed to hip instability and dislocations**
      i. Abductor insufficiency: seen in surgical approaches in which gluteus medius is split or with previous surgery.
      ii. Soft tissue or bony impingement: caused by scars from previous surgeries or heterotopic ossification.
      iii. Inadequate soft tissue tension: caused by short leg, short femoral component, or previous surgery.
      iv. Historically, use of a posterior surgical approach without capsule repair resulted in a higher incidence of dislocations (5%).

E. **Weight-bearing restrictions**
1. Cemented prostheses: usually weight-bearing as tolerated immediately postoperatively.
2. Uncemented prostheses: toe-touch weight-bearing usually for 6 weeks, progressing to full weight-bearing by 12 weeks.

F. **Muscle strengthening principles**
1. Limited isometric contractions of the quadriceps and hip extensor muscles, initially leading to strengthening of the hip flexion and knee extension with increased resistance as tolerated.
2. Limit unsupported straight-leg raises or hip flexion if non-weight-bearing or toe-touch weight-bearing restrictions are in place to avoid torsional forces at the implant-bone interface.
3. Isometric exercise of the ankle dorsiflexors and plantar flexors promote lower extremity venous blood flow and may aid in preventing deep venous thrombosis (DVT).
3. Strengthening of upper extremities is important for transfers and ambulating with an assistive device
4. May be started in a preoperative exercise program.

G. **Range of motion (ROM)**
1 Important to maintain full active ROM in the nonoperated joints.

2. Must maintain specified hip ROM precautions with THA to avoid dislocation.

H. Suggested post-THA rehabilitation protocol

1. **Postoperative day 1**

   a. Patient may be limited by pain and lack of endurance.

   b. Instruct patient on supine bed exercises.

      i. Quadriceps sets (isometric tightening quadriceps muscles)

      ii. Gluteal sets (isometric tightening buttock muscles)

      iii. Ankle pumps (active ankle dorsiflexion and plantarflexion)

      iv. Hip and knee flexion (heel slides—"slide" heel of operated leg toward buttock and back toward foot of bed)

   c. Initial teaching about hip precautions (provide written instructions)

   d. Stand patient at bedside, using toe-touch weight-bearing (TTWB) for all THA revisions and uncemented primary THA and weight-bearing as tolerated (WBAT) for all cemented or hybrid THA, unless otherwise indicated by orthopedic surgeon.

   e. Begin occupational therapy training in use of assistive devices (AD) for activities of daily living (ADLs) and for maintaining hip precautions.

2. **Postoperative day 2**

   a. Patient instructed in further supine bed exercises.

      i. Quadriceps sets with rolled towel under knee

      ii. Straight leg raises—hip flexor and quadricep strengthening with unoperated leg bent and foot flat; lift operated leg with straight knee to lift foot is 12 inches off bed.

      iii. Supine hip abduction sets with no adduction past midline. (No abduction exercises if anterior approach was used or if THA included trochanteric osteotomy.)

   b. Review hip precautions again with patient and family member, if available.

   c. Begin teaching bed and chair transfers.

   d. Ambulate with AD (may need to start in parallel bars) and TTWB or WBAT on level surfaces.

   e. Continue occupational therapy, ADLs.

3. **Postoperative day 3 through discharge**

   a. Continue practicing supine bed exercises.

   b. Begin standing exercise program. (Exclude this program if anterior approach was used.)

      i. Standing gluteal strengthening: lift operated leg straight back, with kneecap pointing straight ahead and toes pointing toward floor; no rotation of leg.

      ii. Standing hip abduction strengthening: lift operated leg out to the side, one hand on counter or chair back; no leaning toward one side. (No abduction exercises if anterior approach was used or if THA included trochanteric osteotomy.)

   c. Continue transfer skills and ambulation on level surfaces; add higher level transfer training (e.g., toilet, car).

   d. Ambulate up and down 4 steps with AD using TTWB or WBAT, as appropriate.

   e. Continue occupational therapy, ADLs; train caregivers if appropriate.

I. Discharge criteria/rehabilitation goals

1. Patient and family should demonstrate clear understanding of dislocation precautions.

2. Patient should be safe and independent in ambulation on level surfaces and in ascending and descending 4 steps with appropriate AD.
3. Patient should be independent with bed, chair, toilet, and car transfers.
4. Patient should be able to demonstrate both supine and standing THA exercises.
5. Patient should be modified independent with ADLs or trained caregiver support.
6. Outpatient physical therapy, if appropriate, should be arranged before discharge.
7. Equipment, such as bedside commode, should be ordered if appropriate.

J. **Postdischarge issues**
   1. Maintain hip precautions until cleared by orthopedic surgeon (generally 8–12 weeks).
   2. Maintain AD use until weight-bearing restrictions change.
   3. No driving until reaction time returns.
      a. More important for right-sided arthroplasties.
      b. Consider driving safety evaluation.
   4. Educate patient in avoiding high-impact activities and vigorous sports.
   5. Prognosis: THAs now have 90% success rate at 10 years.

K. **Complications**
   1. **Dislocation**
      a. Most common complication after THA.
      b. Occurs in about 1% of THAs with anterior surgical approach and 5% with posterolateral surgical approach without capsule repair, and 1% with capsule repair.
      c. Increased incidence after revisions.
      d. Signs and symptoms: pain with weight-bearing, difficulty ambulating, or a malrotated leg.
      e. Diagnosis: clinical exam and radiographic evidence.
      f. Treatment: evaluation by surgeon for correction.
   2. **Infection**
      a. **Superficial wound infection/cellulitis**
         i. Decreased incidence with use of prophylactic antibiotics before and 24 hours after surgery.
         ii. Signs and symptoms: pain, redness, and warmth around the incision.
         iii. Diagnosis: clinical exam.
         iv. Treatment: generally responds well to cephalexin, 500 mg orally every 6 hours for 10 days, but discuss with surgeon before treatment because a superficial wound infection can be the first sign of a deep infection.
      b. **Deep infection**
         i. Can occur early (< 3 months after surgery) or late (> 3 months after surgery).
         ii. Signs and symptoms: pain with weight-bearing, fever, prolonged drainage from the surgical incision; laboratory tests may be normal.
         iii. Diagnosis: clinical exam, possible joint aspiration, laboratory tests. (C-reactive protein generally returns to normal within 3 weeks, and erythrocyte sedimentation rate generally returns to normal within 6 months after surgery if there is no infection).
         iv. Treatment
            • Early infection: assessment by surgeon for possible incision and debridement, and intravenous antibiotic therapy.

- Late infection: assessment by surgeon for incision and debridement and possible prosthetic replacement or chronic suppressive antibiotic therapy.
3. **Nerve injury** (increased incidence with revisions or prior surgery)
   a. **Sciatic nerve** (most common)
      i. Peroneal fibers more affected than tibial fibers.
      ii. Seen in posterolateral surgical approach.
      iii. Signs and symptoms: impaired sensation of the foot, weakness of the ankle dorsiflexors or ankle plantar flexors.
      iv. Diagnosis: clinical exam, x-ray to check for leg length discrepancy, ultrasound to check for possible hematoma.
      v. Treatment: early recognition and treatment of reversible causes (correct any leg length discrepancy or remove hematoma). If there is no identifiable cause, treatment is usually supportive in patients with axonal continuity and no source of ongoing compression.
   b. **Femoral nerve** (less common)
      i. Seen with anterior or lateral surgical approach.
      ii. Signs and symptoms: weakness of the quadricep muscles.
      iii. Diagnosis: clinical exam, x-ray, and ultrasound.
      iv. Treatment: similar to sciatic nerve injuriers; usually supportive in patients with axonal continuity and no source of ongoing compression.
   c. **Obturator nerve** (less common)
      i. Seen with anterior or lateral surgical approach.
      ii. Signs and symptoms: weakness of hip abductor muscles.
      iii. Diagnosis: clinical exam, x-ray, and ultrasound.
      iv. Treatment: similar to sciatic nerve injuries; usually supportive in patients with axonal continuity and no source of ongoing compression.
4. **Aseptic loosening**
   a. Signs and symptoms: pain in the groin or buttocks region, increased with weight-bearing. Patients with a loose femoral component may complain of start-up pain, which lessens with further activity.
   b. Diagnosis: clinical exam, radiographic evidence.
   c. Treatment: evaluation by surgeon for correction, possible revision.
5. **Deep venous thrombosis (DVT)**
   a. Refer to Chapter 13, Deep Venous Thrombosis for details.
   b. Patients are at high risk for DVT after total joint arthroplasty.
      i. Affects up to 50% of patients who do not receive prophylaxis.
      ii. Incidence of about 25% with aspirin prophylaxis.
      iii. Incidence drops to approximately 5% with warfarin or low-molecular-weight heparin prophylaxis.
   c. Signs and symptoms: pain, redness, or swelling.
   d. Diagnosis: clinical diagnosis is unreliable; therefore, diagnostic studies are needed if DVT is suspected.
   e. Treatment: refer to Chapter 13, Deep Venous Thrombosis.
6. **Heterotopic ossification**
   a. Risk factors include prior surgery or revision, prior heterotopic ossification, male gender, and ankylosing spondylitis.
   b. May be prevented by low-dose radiation (local, one-time dose of 600 rads), indomethacin (started within 48 hours of surgery), or etidronate.
   c. Signs and symptoms: decreased ROM, pain with ROM.

    c. Diagnosis: clinical exam, radiographic evidence, or bone scan.

    d. Treatment: evaluation by surgeon. Usually must wait until the ossification matures (> 1 year) and then correct surgically.

  7. **Limb-length discrepancy**

    a. Usually secondary to contractures around the hip or to an increase or decrease in the size of the components.

    b. A perceived leg length discrepancy can be due to abductor weakness.

    c. Signs and symptoms: gait abnormality.

    c. Diagnosis: clinical exam, radiographic evidence.

    d. Treatment: physical therapy, muscle strengthening, or orthotics.

III. Total Knee Arthroplasty (TKA)

A. Total replacement: both the femorotibial and patellofemoral articulating surfaces are replaced with prosthetic components.

B. The patella may or may not be resurfaced.

C. **Surgical concerns**

  1. **Surgical approach:** anterior midline incision is the most common.

  2. TKA may be posterior cruciate ligament-preserving or posterior stabilized.

  3. Deep dissection is usually a medial arthrotomy with splitting of the quadriceps rectus tendon, splitting of the vastus medialis oblique, or elevation of the vastus medialis oblique from the medial septum.

  4. **Materials**

    a. Tricompartmental replacements: most common; can be a fixed-bearing prosthesis or a mobile-bearing prosthesis.

    b. Unicompartmental replacements: only the abnormal side of the knee (usually the medial) is replaced.

  3. **Methods of fixation**

    a. PMMA is the most common method of fixation.

    b. Press-fit fixation, which is similar in principle to THA, can be used.

D. **Weight-bearing restrictions**

  1. Usually WBAT with cemented prosthesis

  2. Partial weight-bearing for grafting or tendon or muscle repairs

E. **Range of motion** (ROM)

  1. Time course depends on surgeon's preference.

  2. Generally, passive, active assisted, and active ROM should begin as soon as possible postoperatively to maximize function.

  3. Passive ROM may be accomplished by continuous passive motion (CPM) machine.

    a. Begin on postopertaive day 1; set machine at 0–40°, if tolerated, and advance according to patient tolerance.

    b. Generally, advance by no more than 40° per day as tolerated, to achieve 0–90° range.

F. **Suggested post-TKA rehabilitation protocol**

  1. **Postoperative day 1**

    a. Pain and lack of endurance may limit patient.

    b. Patient instructed in supine bed exercises.

      i. Quadriceps strengthening (isometric tightening of quadriceps muscles with knee straight)

      ii. Gluteal strengthening (isometric tightening of buttock muscles)

      iii. Ankle pumps (active ankle dorsiflexion and plantarflexion)

iv. Straight leg raises—hip flexor and quadriceps strengthening (unoperated leg bent with foot flat; lift operated leg with straight knee to lift foot 12 inches off bed)

c. Begin active and passive ROM exercises to the operated knee within the patient's pain tolerance, unless contraindicated.

    i. Stress full extension.

    ii. Patients who are unable to reach full extension should be placed in a knee immobilizer for 1 hour in the morning and 1 hour in the afternoon/evening to avoid knee flexion contracture.

d. Stand patient at bedside with knee immobilizer and WBAT, unless otherwise indicated.

e. Begin ADL therapies with occupational therapist.

2. **Postoperative day 2**

a. Instruct patient in further bed exercises.

    i. With 6-inch towel rolled under operated knee, lift heel off bed until operated knee is fully straight; hold 10 seconds; repeat.

    ii. Hip and knee flexion (heel slides—slide heel of operated leg toward buttock and back toward foot of bed).

b. Continue active and passive ROM exercises to the operated knee within the patient's pain tolerance, unless contraindicated; emphasize complete straightening of the operated knee.

c. Begin transfer training.

d. Continue ADL therapies with occupational therapist.

e. Begin ambulation.

    i. Use AD.

    ii. WBAT (unless otherwise indicated).

    iii. Begin on level surfaces (begin in parallel bars if needed).

    iv. Surgeon may elect to have patient wear knee immobilizer when ambulating until he or she can independently do a straight leg raise.

3. **Postoperative day 3 through discharge**

a. Continue bed exercises.

b. Continue active and passive ROM.

c. Continue ADL therapies.

d. Teach bed, chair, toilet, and car transfers.

e. Begin seated exercise program (sitting on a straight-backed chair).

    i. Sitting with thighs supported on chair, bend operated knee as far back as possible; hold 10 seconds; straighten operated knee completely; and hold 10 seconds).

    ii. Sitting far back in chair, place foot of operated leg flat on floor, then scoot forward in chair, increasing the angle of knee flexion; hold 60 seconds, and then scoot back. Repeat, each time scooting farther forward until knee is bent 90°.

    iii. Sitting back in chair, place foot of operated leg onto the seat of a second chair; tighten thigh muscles to push the operated leg down into full extension.

f. Teach prone exercise: lying prone, bend operated knee, trying to touch heel to buttocks. Hold 10 seconds. Lower foot back down and repeat.

g. Continue ambulation training with AD; begin stair training.

G. **Discharge criteria/rehabilitation goals**

1. Patient should be safe and independent in ambulation on level surfaces and in ascending and descending 4 steps with an appropriate AD.
2. Patient should be modified independent with bed, chair, toilet, and car transfers.
3. Patient and family should be trained in TKA exercise program, and patient should be able to continue exercises at home.
4. Patient should have achieved as close to 95° of knee flexion as possible.
5. Functional ROM needed at knee (may affect discharge disposition)
   a. Normal gait: 0–67°
   b. Climbing stairs: 0–83°
   c. Descending stairs: 0–90°
   d. Getting up from a chair: 0–93°
6. Patient should be modified independent with ADLs or trained caregiver support.
7. Outpatient physical therapy, if appropriate, should be arranged before discharge.

H. **Postdischarge issues**
   1. Continue exercise program.
   2. No driving until reaction time returns.
      a. More important for right-sided arthroplasties.
      b. Consider driving safety evaluation.
   3. Prognosis: TKAs now have > 95% success rate at 10 years.

I. **Complications** (similar to those associated with THA)
   1. **Infection**
      a. Most common complication after TKA.
      b. Signs and symptoms: similar to THA, as well as increase in pain or progressive loss of limb motion.
      c. Diagnosis: similar to THA.
      d. Treatment: similar to THA.
   2. **Aseptic loosening**
      a. Seen with tibial and patellar components.
      b. Signs and symptoms: knee pain with weight-bearing.
      c. Diagnosis: radiograph demonstrating a radiolucent line around the prosthesis.
      d. Treatment: evaluation by surgeon for possible revision.
   3. **Peroneal nerve palsy**
      a. Uncommon but may be seen after correction of valgus deformity.
      b. May also be secondary to nerve compression.
      c. Signs and symptoms: foot drop, ankle eversion weakness, sensory loss on lateral foot and/or web space between first and second toes.
      d. Diagnosis: clinical exam; electrodiagnostic study may be helpful.
      e. Treatment: usually supportive unless ongoing nerve entrapment or compression is present.
   4. **Patellar instability:** may be due to patellar tendon rupture.
   5. **Decreased ROM of knee**
      a. May be avoided by aggressive, early ROM and use of CPM.
      b. Signs and symptoms: difficulty in advancing in rehabilitation program
      c. Diagnosis: clinical exam, x-ray.
      d. Treatment: evaluation by surgeon, possible knee manipulation if ROM is not functional.

6. **DVT**
   a. High incidence after lower extremity arthroplasty (5–40%).
   b. Incidence can be decreased to about 5% with the use of warfarin or low-molecular-weight heparin.
   c. Early ROM or CPM may also decrease the incidence.
   d. Refer to Chapter 13, Deep Venous Thrombosis.

Bibliography
1. Braddom RL (ed): Physical Medicine and Rehabilitation, 2nd ed. Philadelphia, W.B. Saunders, 2000.
2. Brander VA (ed): Rehabilitation following hip and knee arthroplasty. Phys Med Rehabil Clin North Am 5(4), 1994 [entire issue].
3. Canale ST (ed): Campbell's Operative Orthopaedics, 9th ed. St. Louis, Mosby, 1998.
4. DeLisa JA (ed): Rehabilitation Medicine: Principles and Practice, 3rd ed. Philadelphia, Lippincott-Raven, 1998.
5. Grabois M: Physical Medicine and Rehabilitation. The Complete Approach. Oxford, Blackwell Science, 2000.
6. Kottke FJ (ed): Krusen's Handbook of Physical Medicine and Rehabilitation, 4th ed. Philadelphia, W.B. Saunders, 1990.
7. Ruddy S (ed): Kelley's Textbook of Rheumatology, 6th ed. Philadelphia, W.B. Saunders, 2001.

Chapter 6

PARKINSON'S DISEASE REHABILITATION

Jess W. Olson, M.D., and Anita S. W. Craig, M.D.

I. **General Principles**
   A. **Definition:** Parkinson's disease (PD) is a chronic progressive disease characterized by the presence of tremor, rigidity, postural instability, and bradykinesia. It was first described by James Parkinson over 180 years ago, allthough descriptions of patients with tremor and akinesia are found in ancient Indian literature from 4500–1000 BC.
   B. **Epidemiology**
      1. PD occurs throughout the world in all ethnic groups with a slight predominance of males over females and of Caucasians over Asians and African Americans.
      2. Affects 0.3% of total population (1% of population older than 55 years).
      3. 5–10% of patients who eventually develop PD have symptoms before age 40.
      4. More than 1 million people in the U.S. have PD, and 50,000 new cases are diagnosed annually.
      5. Mortality rate is 2–5 times higher in patients with PD than in age-matched controls.
      6. Studies demonstrate little concordance among monzygotic vs. dizygotic twins, although recent studies have shown increased concordance among monzygotic twins if one twin has early-onset PD.
   C. **Risk factors**
      1. Age: Incidence increases sharply after age 50.
      2. Family history: Persons with a first-degree relative with PD have 3-fold greater risk.
      3. Sex: Men have slightly higher incidence rates than women.
      4. Race: Caucasians are at slightly greater risk than African Americans or Asians.
      5. Smoking: Nonsmokers have higher risk than smokers.
   D. **Etiology:** The cause of PD is unknown. Four prominent hypotheses are accelerated aging, toxin exposure, genetic predisposition, and oxidative stress.
   E. **Pathophysiology**
      1. Associated with the degeneration of dopaminergic neurons in the substantia nigra pars compacta (SNPC), which sends axons to the striatum (caudate nucleus and putamen).
      2. It is estimated that 80% of neurons are lost before the disease becomes clinically evident.
      3. The SNPC and striatum, along with the globus pallidus and subthalmic nucleus, make up the basal ganglia. The basal ganglia plays a major role in voluntary movements and postural adjustments.

    4. During neurodegeneration neurons develop characteristic cytoplasmic inclusion bodies called Lewy bodies.

II. Diagnosis

A. Diagnosis of Parkinsonian syndrome is based on presence of **bradykinesia and at least one of following:**

1. Muscular rigidity
2. 4–6 hz resting tremor
3. Postural instability not caused by primary visual vestibular, cerebellar, or proprioceptive dysfunction.

B. **Exclusion criteria**

1. Parkinsonism due to identifiable causes (e.g., stroke, traumatic brain injury, brain tumor)
2. Oculogyric crisis
3. Sustained remissions
4. Supranuclear gaze palsy
5. Cerebellar signs
6. Early severe autonomic insufficiency
7. Early severe dementia
8. Poor response to large doses of levodopa

C. **Supportive criteria:** Three or more of the following are required for diagnosis of definite PD:

1. Unilateral onset
2. Resting tremor
3. Progressive signs and symptoms
4. Persistent asymmetry
5. Excellent early response to levodopa
6. Clinical course > 5 years

D. **Ancillary tests**

1. No single test or procedure can verify the diagnosis of PD.
2. Magnetic resonance imaging (MRI) scans are usually normal, with variable amounts of atrophy.
3. F-dopa positron emission tomography (PET) may show decreased tracer uptake in putamen.
4. Single-photon emission computed tomography (SPECT) may show decrease in dopamine transporters.

E. **Differential diagnosis**

1. **Drug-induced disease:** Most commonly neuroleptics such as haloperidol, but also metoclopramide, prochlorperazine, methyldopa, reserpine, amiodarone, lithium, and several anticonvulsants.
2. **Toxin-induced disease:** MPTP (byproduct of meperidine synthesis), manganese poisoning, and herbicides; uncommon causes: cyanide and carbon monoxide poisoning.
3. **Vascular PD**
4. **Structural lesions** (tumors)
5. **Normal-pressure hydrocephalus**
6. **Infections:** sequelae of encephalopathy and Creutzfeldt-Jakob disease (associated with rapid dementia)
7. **Trauma**
8. **Metabolic disorders** (hypothyroidism and hypoparathyroidism)
9. **Neurogenerative disorders**

   a. Progressive supranuclear palsy (early postural instability and inability to look down)
   b. Multisystem atrophy
   c. Alzheimer's disease
   d. Diffuse Lewy-body disease
   e. Corticobasal degeneration
10. **Hereditary disorders**
   a. Wilson's disease
   b. Huntington's disease
   c. Machado-Joseph disease
   d. Shy-Drager syndrome (early and profound autonomic failure)
   e. Fahr's disease
11. **Essential tremor** (usually stable with action and resolves with rest)
12. **Psychogenic PD**

III. Common Features

A. **Tremor** (most common presenting feature)
   1. Resting tremor of 4–6 cycles/sec in 75% of patients at some point in PD.
   2. Usually begins unilaterally in the upper extremity.
B. **Rigidity:** resistance to passive movement in flexors and extensors that is velocity-independent and usually occurs proximally before distally.
C. **Dyskinesia:** impaired voluntary movements, often during peak effect times of levodopa.
D. **Bradykinesia** (slowness of movement): leads to decrease in automatic movements and difficulty in maintaining movement.
E. **Postural instability**: usually a late sign; extensor muscles are weaker than flexor muscles, leading to stooped posture.
F. **Akinesia:** advanced stage of bradykinesia characterized by difficulty with initiating movement and "freezing."
G. **Masked facies**
H. **On-off phenomenon**
   1. Patients taking levodopa go from a relatively mobile state to a relatively immobile state with increased tremor, rigidity, and bradykinesia.
   2. Occurs in 50% of patients after 5 years when effects of levodopa wear off at unpredictable times.
   3. "Off" stage can last from minutes to hours.
I. **Sleep disturbance**
   1. Affects 75–95% of patients.
   2. May be due to parkinsonian symptoms, medications, depression, dementia, or urologic problems.
J. **Urinary dysfunction**
   1. Occurs in 58–71% of patients and often manifests as nocturia.
   2. Most often due to detrusor hyperreflexia with poorly sustained contractions and incomplete emptying, although it can also be related to anticholinergic drugs.
K. **Dermatologic findings:** patients often develop seborrheic dermatitis.
L. **Visual disturbances:** patients can develop blurry vision, decreased blinking, and impaired conjugate gaze and smooth pursuit.
M. **Psychiatric symptoms**
   1. Depression and anxiety in about 40% of patients each.
   2. Psychosis can occur with high doses of dopaminergic drugs.

N. **Autonomic dysfunction**
1. Patients often develop orthostatic hypotension that may be exacerbated by dopaminergic therapy, sometimes leading to syncopal episodes.
2. Many patients require decreases in blood pressure medications.

O. **Sexual dysfunction:** may result from decreased interest, depression, bradykinesia, autonomic dysfunction, and medications (anticholinergics, antidepressants, antihypertensives).

P. **Gastrointenstinal (GI) dysfunction:** constipation occurs in about 50% of patients secondary to bradykinesia of the GI tract and antiparkinson medications.

Q. **Dysphagia**
1. Occurs in about 50% of patients.
2. Affects all three phases of swallowing: voluntary oral preparation phase, involuntary pharyngeal phase, and esophageal phase.
3. Due to impaired motor movements throughout swallowing sequence.
4. Often worsens in later stages of PD.

R. **Cognitive dysfunction**
1. Subcortical dementia is slightly more common than in people without PD, but it is a late finding.
2. Patients with PD also have deficits with visuospatial discrimination, frontal lobe executive function, memory retrieval, and bradyphrenia.

S. **Olfactory dysfunction:** frequently occurs before motor symptoms and does not improve with medications.

T. **Speech dysfunction:** speech becomes rapid, monotonous, and of low volume.

U. **Hyperhidrosis:** paroxysms of drenching sweats occur as levodopa effects wear off.

IV. **Classification of Disability** (Hoehn and Yahr)
A. **Stage I:** unilateral involvement only, usually with minimal or no functional impairment.
B. **Stage II:** bilateral or midline involvement without impairment of balance.
C. **Stage III:** bilateral disease with impaired postural reflexes but preserved ability to ambulate independently. Patients are physically able to live independently and continue some forms of employment with mild-to-moderate disability.
D. **Stage IV:** severe disease requiring considerable assistance, but patients are still able to walk and stand unassisted.
E. **Stage V:** end-stage disease; patients are confined to bed or chair.

V. **Medical Therapy**
A. **General principles**
1. No medications have been proved to act as neuroprotectants. Despite some initial enthusiasm, further testing has shown that both selegiline and vitamin E are ineffective neuroprotectants.
2. Drugs used to treat various stages of PD are summarized in Table 1.
   a. **Therapy for mild PD:** amantidine, which has some beneficial effects and fewer side effects than dopamine agonists or levodopa. It is also convenient to take.
   b. **Therapy for moderate PD**
      i. Levodopa
      - Used in mild, moderate, and severe PD.
      - Almost always accompanied by carbidopa, a peripheral decarboxylase inhibitor.

TABLE 1.   **Common Parkinson's Disease Medications**

Class	Indication	Important Adverse Effects
Anticholinergic (benztropine, trihexyphenidyl)	Therapy in moderate PD; improves tremor and rigidity	Peripheral: dry mouth, blurred vision, constipation, difficulty with urination Central: confusion, memory problems; particularly problematic in elderly
Dopamine releaser (amantadine)	Early PD or in conjunction with levodopa in late PD	Confusion, visual hallucinations, leg edema, livedo reticularis
Dopamine precursor (levodopa)	Main treatment for PD along with dopamine agonist	Peripheral: nausea, vomiting, hypotension; helped by addition of carbidopa Central: dyskinesias, psychiatric disturbances At higher doses, variable plasma levels lead to on-off phenomenon
Dopamine agonist: ergot-derived (bromocriptine, pergolide; gabergoline, lisuride)	Main treatment for PD along with levodopa	Peripheral and central dopaminergic side effects, pedal edema, pleuropulmonary reaction, retroperitoneal fibrosis, erythromelalgia At high doses, brings about cortical side effects such as confusion or hallucinations
Dopamine agonist: non–ergot-derived (ropinirole, pramipexole, apomorphine)	Monotherapy or used with levodopa to potentiate its effects	Peripheral and central dopaminergic side effects with no pleuropulmonary reaction, retroperitoneal fibrosis, or erythromelalgia At high doses, brings about cortical side effects such as confusion or hallucinations
Monoamine oxidase-B inhibitor (selegiline)	Sometimes used in early PD, but usually in later PD to potentiate levodopa	Increased dopaminergic effects of other drugs, insomnia, and confusion; may cause hypertensive reactions
Catechol O-methyl-transferase inhibitor (tolcapone, entacapone)	Potentiates levodopa	Increased effects of dopaminergic drugs and diarrhea Liver tests liver needed every 6 months
Antihistamine: diphenhydramine	Used instead of anticholinergics for tremor control	Similar to anticholinergic, but decreased side effects

- More selective than dopamine agonists but has less predictable pharmacokinetics, leading to on-off phenomenon at high doses.
  ii. Dopamine agonists
  - Used in mild, moderate, and severe PD.
  - Provides smoother pharmacokinetics than levodopa but can cause cortical side effects at increased dosages.
c. **Therapy for severe PD**
  i. Combination of levodopa and dopamine agonists allows smaller doses of each and thus leads to fewer side effects.
  ii. Adjuvants to levodopa
  - Sustained-release levodopa
  - Monoamine oxidase-B (MAO-B) inhibitors
  - Catechol-O-methyltransferase (COMT) inhibitors

    iii. Anticholinergics
- Used in late stages of PD to decrease cholinergic activity of basal ganglia.
- Particularly effective in decreasing tremors, rigidity, and dystonia but have less effect on bradykinesia and gait disorders

B. **Treatment for PD signs and symptoms** (Table 2)

TABLE 2. Treatment for Signs and Symptoms of PD

Problem	Therapy/Treatment
Gait and posture difficulties: flexed posture, difficulty with initiating gate, shuffling steps, poor base of support, poor gate adjustment, "freezing"	Often not helped with pharmacologic treatment Therapy should emphasize trunk mobility, weight shifting, and balance; cadence can be used to initiate and maintain gait Patient's home should be evaluated to remove objects that may cause tripping and to add adaptive equipment
On-off phenomenon: late-stage levodopa-resistant motor disturbances	Increase dose of levodopa or use controlled-release levodopa; may also use dopamine agonist or MAO-B inhibitor to potentiate the effect of levodopa Provide liquid carbidopa-levodopa mix to be taken when episode comes on
Tremor	Often helped with anticholinergic medications and relaxation techniques
Bradykinesia and hypokinesia	Daily range of motion and stretching exercises Constant repetition of tasks to improve ability to complete them
Dyskinesia (involuntary motor movements): occurs after about 5 years of levodopa use, often at peak levels	Often must change to controlled-release or more frequent smaller doses to keep lesser, more consistent level of levodopa May want to start COMT inhibitor
Speech (hypokinetic dysarthria)	Improved with levodopa Intensive speech therapy involving breath and rate control, articulation, and increased volume
Constipation	Small frequent meals with increased fiber, fluid, stool softeners, and/or laxatives Decrease anticholinergics Increase exercise
Dysphagia	Avoid foods with mixed consistencies; eat thickened foods Use aspiration precautions Assess patient with swallow study Take medications 30 min before meal
Delayed gastric emptying	Start with domperidone, 10 mg 3 times/day
Cognition difficulties	Rule out other causes such as medications, infections, alcohol, Alzheimer's disease, hypothyroidism, B_{12} deficiency, stroke, depression, tumor, or hemorrhage Refer for evaluation by neuropsychologist Assess ability to live and work independently in early disease
Orthostatic hypotension	Teach patient methods to rise slowly from bed Decrease blood pressure medications Wear compression stockings Increase salt and fluid intake Eat smaller meals and decrease alcohol intake Try fludrocortisone, 0.1 mg/day; increase up to 1 mg/day If fludrocortisone does not increase blood pressure enough, add milodrine, 2 mg 3 times/day up to 10 mg 3 times/day

Table continued on following page

TABLE 2.   Treatment for Signs and Symptoms of PD *(Continued)*

Problem	Therapy/Treatment
Urinary problems: urgency, frequency, nocturia	Watch for frequent urinary tract infections Initially check urinalysis, post-void residuals, kidney function May need to work up neurogenic bladder with cystography, cystometrography, and/or cystoscopy Hyperactive detrusor may respond to oxybutinin, 5 mg 3 times/day; propantheline, 30 mg 4 times/day; or toltero-dine, 2 mg twice daily
Sexual dysfunction	Check prolactin, testosterone, luteinizing hormone, and thyroid-stimulating hormone for correctable problem Consider decreasing antihypertensives (particularly beta blockers) and antidepressants (particularly selective sero-tonin reuptake inhibitors [SSRIs]); both can cause impotence Consider sildenafil or yohimbine for impotence
Sleep problems	Difficulty with initiation may be treated with tricyclic anti-depressants, benzodiazepines, diphenhydramine, or chloral hydrate Evaluate for depression For daytime sleepiness, try selegiline, caffeine, or methyl-phenidate Sometimes insomnia is helped with bedtime dose of con-trolled-release levodopa
Hyperhidrosis	Treat similarly to on-off phenomenon with adjunctive agents such as dopamine agonists, COMT inhibitors, or MAO-B inhibitors, to potentiate effects of levodopa
Psychiatric disorders	For psychosis, first decrease anticholinergic medications, then direct dopaminergic agents If problem persists, slightly decrease levodopa and/or start clozapine or olanzapine (watch for agranulocytosis with clozapine) Treat depression with SSRIs

C. **Alternative treatments**
 1. **Surgerical targeting**
   a. Motor thalamus: interrupting the ventrointermediate thalamic nucleus provides about 80% improvement in tremor.
   b. Internal segment of globus pallidus: pallidotomoy leads to 80% im-provement in dyskinesias and some improvement in motor abilities.
   c. Subthalmic nucleus
 2. **Other research**
   a. Implanted deep brain electrodes
   b. Transplanting fetal dopaminergic neurons
   c. Gene therapy to slow or reverse progression of PD
D. **Occupational and physical therapy** (Table 3)
 1. Studies involving physical and occupational therapy (PT/OT) have varying results: some show significant improvement, some slight improvement, and some no improvement.
 2. **General consensus:** PT/OT has a small and somewhat short-term effect on PD symptoms. Patients often make small gains in function during therapy, then lose them as disease progresses or when they stop therapy. Still unclear which specific therapies result in improvement and which, if any, provide long-term benefit.

TABLE 3. Physical Therapy for Symptoms of PD

Symptom	Therapy
Truncal instability	Range of motion trunk exercises Strengthen low back and hip extensors Have patients use mirrors to correct posture
Slowed gait and decreased stride length	Various walking cadence exercises Use rhythmic acoustic stimlui from stereo or metronome Use visual cues on floor, such as white lines, to practice increased stride length Increase arm swing
Tremor	Slow stretching exercises
Slowness of simultaneous movement	Complete frequent repetition of each functional activity patient is trying to improve
Speech impairment	Prosodic exercises Breathing exercises
Standing up	Go through mental rehearsal of sequence before activity
Complicated tasks	Break down all tasks into component parts, and execute each task separately
Micrographia	Use lined paper Encourage large strokes
Rigidity	Do relaxational exercises involving stretching and slow rhythmic movements

3. **General rehabilitation concepts**
    a. Patients should concentrate on one task at a time.
    b. Patients should break down complex tasks into separate parts and do each part separately.
    c. Patients should participate in active aerobic and range-of-motion exercises as much as possible.
    d. Patients need to keep participating in therapy, or gains will be lost.

Bibliography
1. Adler C, Ahlskog J (eds): Parkinson's Disease and Movement Disorders: Diagnosis and Treatment Guidelines for the Practicing Physician. Totowa, NJ, Humana Press, 2000.
2. Braddom R (ed): Physical Medicine & Rehabilitation, 2nd ed. Philadelphia, W.B. Saunders, 2000.
3. Carr J, Shepard R: Neurological Rehabilitation: Optimizing Motor Performance. Oxford, Butterworth Heinemann, 1998.
4. Cohen A, Weiner W (eds): The Comprehensive Management of Parkinson's Disease. New York, Demos Publications, 1994.
5. DeLisa J, Gans B (eds): Rehabilitation Medicine: Principles and Practice, 3rd ed. Philadelphia, Lippincott-Raven , 1998.
6. Lang A, Lozano A: Medical progress: Parkinson's disease. Part I. N Engl J Med 339:1044–1053, 1998.
7. Lang A, Lozano A: Medical progress: Parkinson's disease: Part II. N Engl J Med 339:1130– 1143, 1998.
8. Lewitt P, Oertel W (eds): Parkinsonís Disease: The Treatment Options. London, Martin Dunitz 1999.
9. Morris M: Movement disorders in people with Parkinson disease: A model for physical therapy. Phys Ther 80:578–596, 2000.
10. O'Sullivan S, Schmitz T: Physical Rehabilitation: Assessment and Treatment, 4th ed. Philadelphia, F.A. Davis, 2001.
11. Schenkman M, et al: Management of individuals with Parkinson's disease: Rationale and case studies. Phys Ther 69:944–954, 1989.
12. Stern G (ed): Advances in Neurology: Parkinson's Disease, vol. 80. Philadelphia, Lippincott Williams & Wilkins, 1999.
13. Stern M, Hurtig H (eds): Parkinson'sdisease and parkinsonian syndromes. Med Clin North Am 83(2), 1999 [entire issue].

Chapter 7

PEDIATRIC REHABILITATION

Karen L. Meyer, D.O., and Virginia S. Nelson, M.D., MPH

I. History

A. Patient's name, name and relationship of caregivers present

B. Reason for referral and source of referral

C. **Birth history:** where born, complications, term, birth weight, Apgar scores, feeding history, age at discharge, intensive care admissions, ventilator dependence, hospitalizations

D. **Maternal history:** prenatal care, unusual weight gain or loss, hypertension, infection (e.g., rubella), induction, mode and duration of delivery, use of anesthesia, intrapartum complications, expected and actual date of birth, alcoholism, diabetes, use of anticonvulsants, history of spontaneous abortion and other births, complications with other pregnancies, use of street drugs

E. **Developmental history** (see Appendix D for developmental milestones)
   1. Gross motor: rolling, sitting, crawling, walking
   2. Fine motor: pincer, drawing, stacking
   3. Social: play, dressing, helping,
   4. Speech: words, sentences

F. **Medical history:** especially surgeries, interventions related to presenting problem, medications (especially related to seizures), bowel, bladder, behavior

G. **Therapy history:** where, what kind, how much

H. **School history:** school district, type of classroom (see Appendix D for different educational settings and referral plan for special education), plans for future, knowledge of system, level of education, success in school

I. **Functional history**
   1. Eating: orally? with utensils? what kind of treatment? weight gain? gastrostomy tube problems? choking while eating?
   2. Dressing: upper limbs, lower limbs, buttons and snaps, braces, ability to tie shoes
   3. Bathing: safety and accessibility in tub, tub seat
   4. Hygiene: who does it? what kinds of problems?
   5. Mobility: how does child get around the house? school? mall? How does child travel in car?
   6. Adaptive equipment: braces, wheelchair, walker, cane , adaptive car seat (ask type, when and where obtained, reason for use)
   7. Communication: age-appropriate? augmentative communication device?

J. **Social history:** family, vocation if out of school, source of income, type of home and accessibility

K. **Allergies**

L. **Family history:** history of diagnosis or problem same as or related to patient's

    M. **Review of systems:** focus on swallowing difficulties, appetite, how long it takes to eat a meal, breathing difficulty, constitutional symptoms (weight gain or loss, fever, chills), nausea or vomiting, sleeping habits, seizures, pain, bowel and bladder control, constipation or loose stool, change in range of motion, change in strength or sensation

    N. **Vital signs** (Table 1)

II. Physical Examination

    A. For younger children, do as much as you can by watching, playing, and having parents do things.

    B. Observe mobility, hand function, language, cognition, functional strength, and range of motion.

    C. Have toys available, and avoid wearing the white coat.

    D. Assess weight, height, head circumference (see Appendix D for recording charts and normal values).

TABLE 1. Selected Physiologic Guidelines in Childhood

1. Carorie and fluid requirements

Age	Cal/kg	Protein (gm/kg)	Water (ml/kg)
Infancy	120	2.2	120–150
1 yr	110	2.0–2.2	120–135
2–3 yr	100	1.8–2.0	100–125
4–6 yr	85–90	1.5–1.6	90–100
7–10 yr	80–85	1.5	75–100
11–14 yr	60–70	1.2	50–70
15–18 yr	50–60	0.8–1.0	40–60

2. Blood pressure and heart rate

Age	In Seated Position		At Rest
	Systolic	Diastolic	Heart Rate/Min
Infancy	80	55	125
1 yr	90	55	120
2–5 yr	90–94	55	100–110
6–9 yr	95–98	55–60	90–100
10–13 yr	98–109	60–65	85–90
14–18 yr	110–115	63–68	70–80

3. Vital capacity

Newborn	5 Years	10 Years	15 Years
100 cc	1300 cc	2300 cc	4000 cc

4. Urinary output: 2 ml/kg/hr in infants and young children

5. Maximal bladder volumes

Age	Volume
0–1 yr	25–75 cc
1–5 yr	100–150 cc
6–9 yr	200–250 cc
9 plus yr	300–350 cc

From Molnar GE, Alexander MA: Pediatric Rehabilitation. Philadelphia, Hanley & Belfus, 1999, with permission.

E. Head, ears, eyes, nose, throat: assess gum care, thrush in more severely impaired and immunocompromised patients, oral hygiene.
F. Cardiopulmonary assessment is specially important with patients with swallowing or pulmonary concerns and patients at risk for aspiration.
G. Abdominal assessment is especially important with patients with bowel programs, gastrostomy tubes, or other abdominal concerns.
H. Rectal assessment is rarely necessary except for suspected impaction or questions about spinal cord function.
I. Skin: look for erythema under braces, decubitus ulcers.
J. Assess extremities for active and passive range of motion, including test for hip dysplasia in infants and children with impaired mobility (see Section IX, Congenital Disorders). Document tone, condition of skin, edema, and fit of braces.
K. Assess neurologic function, including mental status, head and trunk control, cranial nerves, strength, sensation, balance, gait, cerebellar, tone, reflexes (see Appendix D for reflex development).

III. Approach to Pediatric Patients
A. **Communication with parent**
1. Treat the patient as a person, not a diagnosis.
2. Recognize that parents are experts on their child.
3. Explain what you are looking for and what you find.
4. Be sensitive to the parents' need for information. If you don't know, say so.
5. Acknowledge their sense of urgency, and call back promptly.
6. Be sensitive to how and what you write in the progress notes. Parents often read them, and they should match the tone and information that you conveyed at the visit.
7. Be knowledgeable about free services and resources, such as early intervention and school programs (authorized by federal law with funds passed from federal to state and local education agencies).

B. **Functions of physical therapist (PT)**
1. To position child for function: alignment, skin protection, cardiovascular status, nutrition, assessment of developmental level by caregiving and play.
2. To prevent deformity: influence muscle length, manage tone, preserve joint integrity, prevent/reduce pain.
3. To make suggestions about mobility and adaptive devices based on level of function.
4. To design task and manage environment: give choices, incorporate repetition, change as necessary.

C. **Functions of occupational therapist (OT)**
1. To position child for function: alignment, skin protection, nutrition, assessment of developmental level by caregiving and play.
2. To make suggestions for self-care, life roles/relationships, developmental and adaptive devices.
3. To teach manipulative and perceptual skills.

D. **Task design and environmental management:** design tasks and manage environment by giving choices; incorporate repetition, and change as needed.

E. **Function of speech and language pathologist**
1. To aid in recognition of speech and language disorders.
2. To aid in developing or restoring communication and oral motor function.
3. To make suggestions about adaptive communication devices.

4. To assess dysphagia, to improve swallowing in children with dysphagia, and to make suggestions about adaptive feeding devices (also may be done by OT).

F. **Function of neuropsychologist**
   1. To recognize and aid in confronting maladaptive issues relating to disability.
   2. To perform and analyze psychological assessment through testing, including tests for cognitive and intellectual function, adaptive behavior, psychosocial function, and neuropsychological testing (often used in brain injury).

G. **Functional measurement:** WeeFIM is used most commonly (see Appendix D).
   1. Domains: self-care, mobility, cognition (18 items total)
   2. Scores based on child's ability: documentation on a circular graph at 7 levels of performance.

IV. Cerebral Palsy (CP)

A. **Description**
   1. CP is a symptom complex (not a disease) that has multiple etiologies; diagnosis usually is made (at earliest) at 9–12 months of age.
   2. CP is the leading cause of childhood disability.
   3. CP is a disorder of tone, posture, or movement due to a lesion in the developing brain.
   4. CP is static, but symptoms may change with maturation.
   5. Lesions result in paralysis, weakness, incoordination, or abnormal movement.
   6. There is no cure, but CP is not contagious.
   7. Motor development is slowed.
   8. Some children may "outgrow" the diagnosis.
   9. The two major types of CP are determined by location of lesion: **pyramidal** and **extrapyramidal**. Pyramidal type is more common (about 75% of cases). Symptoms and anatomic lesions may overlap (Table 2).

B. **Epidemiology**
   1. Prevalence of CP has remained constant despite improved prenatal care.
   2. Constant prevalence is likely due to increased survival of premature infants with low birth weight.
   3. Prevalence of one subtype (choreoathetoid CP, which is due to kernicterus related to hyperbilirubinemia) has decreased.
   4. Overall incidence: 2.0-3.0/1000 live births.

C. **Etiology**
   1. CP has multiple etiologies, many still unknown; often no specific cause is found.
   2. 70–80% of causes are prenatal; **prematurity** is most common precursor to CP.

TABLE 2. Comparison of Symptoms of Pyramidal and Extrapyramidal CP

	Pyramidal (Spastic)	Extrapyramidal (Dyskinetic)
Involuntary movements	Rare	Often
Tone	Increased	Alternating
Type of tone	Spastic (clasped knife)	Rigid (lead pipe)
Deep tendon reflexes	Increased	Normal to increased
Clonus	Present	Present occasionally
Contractures	Early	Late
Primitive reflexes	Delayed	Persistent

TABLE 3. Risk Factors

Prenatal	Perinatal	Postnatal
Congenital malformations	Prematurity (< 32 weeks)	Trauma
Socioeconomic factors	Birth weight < 2500 gm	Infection
Intrauterine infections	Growth retardation	Intracranial hemorrhage
Teratogenic agents	Abnormal presentations	Coagulopathies
Maternal mental retardation	Intracranial hemorrhage	
Maternal seizures	Trauma	
Maternal hyperthyroidism	Infection	
Placental complications	Bradycardia and hypoxia	
Additional trauma	Seizures	
Multiple gestation	Hyperbilirubinemia	

From Molnar GE, Alexander MA: Pediatric Rehabilitation. Philadelphia, Hanley & Belfus, 1999, with permission.

3. **Risk factors** (Table 3)
4. **Hypoxic-ischemic encephalopathy** (HIE) is a clinical entity described in 1976 and sometimes equated with neonatal encephalopathy. It may cause CP and differs from asphyxia (low Apgar score and acidosis), which refers to the first minutes after birth and rarely causes CP. Symptoms of HIE persists for hours and days after birth. HIE has five major subtypes (Table 4).

D. **Diagnostic testing** is used to categorize and predict clinical course.
  1. Head ultrasound: useful in the first 2 weeks of life
  2. Magnetic resonance imaging (MRI): best after 2–3 weeks of age or older
  3. Computed tomography
  4. Magnetic resonance spectroscopy (MRS): still in research stage
  5. Metabolic studies to rule out mitochondrial and storage diseases
  6. Chromosomes (when dysmorphic features are present)

E. **Classification/syndromes**
  1. **Pyramidal (spastic) lesions:** motor cortex, internal capsule, and/or corticospinal tract; most common (75% of cases)
    a. **Spastic quadriplegia**
      i. Involves all four extremities.
      ii. Can be associated with diffuse HIE.
      iii. Often affects cognitive region as well as motor areas of brain.
      iv. Swallowing/feeding often a problem.
      v. About 50% have seizures.
      vi. Visual impairment common.
      vii. Children with moderate to severe quadriplegia have poor walking prognosis.
      viii. Highest incidence of mental retardation, proportional to severity.
      ix. Significant oromotor dysfunction
    b. **Spastic triplegia**
      i. Involves three extremities, classically bilateral lower and one upper extremity.
      ii. Features similar to those of spastic quadriplegia.
    c. **Spastic hemiplegia**
      i. Involves one side of the body; usually arm is more affected than leg.

TABLE 4. Hypoxic-Ischemic Encephalopathy Subtypes

	Ischemic/Hemorrhagic Periventricular Leukomalacia	Parasagittal Cerebral Injury	Focal and Multifocal Neuronal Necrosis	Selective Neuronal Necrosis	Status Marmoratus
Infant affected	Typically premature	Typically term	Both premature and term	Both premature and term (most common)	Both premature and term (rarest)
Injury location	Within bilateral white matter adjacent to lateral ventricles, motor cortex	Within bilateral cortical and adjacent sub-cortical white matter, motor cortex	Within vascular distribution, most commonly left middle cerebral artery distribution	Within hippocampus, thalamus, basal ganglia, pons	Within basal ganglia
Sequelae	Spastic diplegia Spastic quadriplegia Visual defects in more severe injury Mental retardation in more severe injury	Spastic quadriplegia	Spastic hemiplegia Spastic quadriplegia Seizures	Seizures Mental retardation	Choreoathetosis
Other			Associated with porencephaly	Coexists with other subtypes	Coexists with other subtypes

      ii. Most cases are congenital (70–90%).

      iii. Usually due to unilateral vascular lesion of middle cerebral artery.

      iv. Associated with porencephaly and visual, sensory, and perceptual deficits.

      vii. Seizures are common (about 50% of cases).

      viii. Growth retardation of affected limbs is common.

  d. **Spastic diplegia**

      i. Involves legs more than arms.

      ii. Motor cortex primarily affected.

      iii. Affects 80% of patients with CP who were preterm.

      iv. Associated with intraventricular hemorrhages in 28-32-week infant and with periventricular leukomalacia or porencephaly.

      v. Associated with seizures (20–25%), visual deficits (63%), strabismus (50%), and cognitive impairment (30%).

  f. **Spastic monoplegia** involves one extremity; rare, usually very mild.

2. **Extrapyramidal (dyskinetic) lesions**

  a. Involves basal ganglia, thalamus, subthalamic nucleus, and cerebellum.

  b. Infants generally are hypotonic at birth.

  c. Associated with oromotor difficulties, including dysarthria, swallowing difficulties, drooling

  d. Associated with hyperbilirubinemia and Rh incompatibility; therefore, incidence reduced because of adequate treatment.

  e. May also be due to incomplete resuscitation (rare in U.S.).

  f. Normal intelligence in approximately 78% of cases.

  g. **Athetosis**

      i. Slow, writhing movements and involuntary movements, especially in distal extremities.

      ii. Antagonist and agonist muscles are active.

  h. **Chorea:** quick, jerky-like movements, irregular.

  i. **Choreoathetoid:** both athetosis and choreiform movements.

  j. **Ataxia**

      i. Large-amplitude, involuntary movements.

      ii. Generally athetoid movement dominates.

      iii. Pure ataxic CP is rare.

  k. **Dystonia**

      i. Tremor and wide-based, drunken-like gait with uncoordinated movements.

      iii. Associated with nystagmus and dysmetria.

      iv. May be associated with cerebellar lesion.

      v. Slow, rhythmic movements with tone changes, generally in trunk and extremities.

      vi. Abnormal postures.

3. **Mixed types:** features from both classifications (e.g., spastic-athetoid type, in which child may have predominantly dyskinetic movements with underlying component of spasticity).

F. **Associated problems**

  1. **Orthopedic**

    a. **Scoliosis**

      i. Affects 25% of ambulatory children and virtually all nonambulatory children.

    ii. Surgery indicated in angles > 40°, bracing for angles of 25–40°, usually with thoracolumbosacral orthosis.

  b. **Hip dislocation**

    i. Imbalance of muscle strength (i.e., strong adductor muscles vs. weak abductor muscles) pulls hip out of socket, causing pain, decreased leg movement at the hip, deformity, and pelvic obliquity.

    ii. Surgery may be needed to lengthen tight medial muscles; sometimes the bone must be cut (osteotomy) and the head of the femur directed inward more acutely so that it will stay in the acetabulum.

  c. **Contractures**

    i. Spasticity and imbalance of muscle strength causes shortening of muscles and immobility of certain joints, especially hips, knees, ankles, elbows, and wrists.

    ii. Treatments include PT, OT, braces, posterior rhizotomy, botulinum toxin injections in tight muscles, antispasticity medications, intrathecal baclofen, and orthopedic surgery. (See Chapter 19, Spasticity.)

    iii. Special adaptive equipment can assist in preventing contractures and facilitate normal movements patterns: orthoses, side lyer, bolster chair, prone stander, standing parapodium, corner chair, scooter board, walkers, and bath chairs.

2. **Spasticity** (See Chapter 19, Spasticity.)
3. **Mental retardation**
  a. Most important factor influencing rehabilitation.
  b. Seen in 50% of children with CP.
  c. Most common in spastic quadriplegia.
  d. Common error is to underestimate cognition in persons with dysarthria or anarthria.
4. **Communication disorders**
  a. Occurs in 40% of children with CP (especially quadriplegia and extrapyramidal types).
  b. Due to oral motor problems.
  c. Sometimes causes misdiagnosis of mental retardation and great frustration in children with CP and normal intelligence.
  d. Critical that every child with CP be given a chance to communicate.
    i. Encourage oral speech constantly.
    ii. Begin speech therapy early and continue throughout childhood.
    ii. Communication system can be developed.
5. **Neurobehavioral problems**
  a. Entire spectrum from attentional problems to autism may be seen.
  b. Prevalence rates may reach 50%.
6. **Seizures**
  a. Seen in 50% of children with CP.
  b. Associated with spastic (pyramidal) CP, most frequently in spastic hemiplegia and quadriplegia.
  c. All types of seizures are seen, but incidence of generalized focal and multifocal seizures is increased.
  d. Child needs appropriate antiseizure medications.
7. **Cortical sensory deficit**
  a. Spastic hemiplegia

b. Child needs to be aware of risks related to lack of sensation (e.g., burns).

c. Adaptation to deficit, such as visual input, should be stressed.

8. **Visual deficits**

   a. 50–92% of children with CP have refractive errors and/or strabismus.

   b. Homonymous hemianopsia is associated with spastic hemiplegia.

   c. Cortical vision impairment is associated with spastic diplegia, hemiplegia.

9. **Sensorineural hearing loss**

   a. Affects 10% of children with CP.

   b. Associated with hyperbilirubinemia.

   c. May require hearing aids.

10. **Nutrition problems**

    a. Affect 50-70% of children with CP.

    b. Due to oral motor problems related to swallowing.

    c. Most common in spastic quadriplegia and extrapyramidal (dyskinetic) types.

    d. May require tube feeding or special diet.

    e. Referral to speech language pathologist is recommended.

    f. May require video-fluoroscopically guided swallowing study.

11. **Drooling**

    a. Due to oral motor problems.

    b. Treatment includes oral medications (cetirizine, glycopyrrolate) or scopolamine patch as well as surgery to excise salivary glands, redirect parotid ducts, and/or sever chorda tympani nerves.

12. **Dentition**

    a. Caries may be less frequent in younger children with CP than age-matched controls, possibly due to delayed eruption.

    b. Caries more prevalent later in life. Saliva is protective.

    c. Other problems include enamel dysgenesis, malocclusion, and gingival hyperplasia due to poor oral hygiene and medications (especially phenytoin).

    d. Problems with dentition are associated with oral motor dysfunction and are more common in children who do not eat orally.

    e. Adequate oral hygiene may require aid from caregiver.

13. **Neurogenic bladder:** may be due to incoordination and lack of voluntary control over hypertonic pelvic floor (also see Chapter 15, Neurogenic Bladder Management).

14. **Vasomotor problems:** in pyramidal (spastic) types, with coolness/edema of affected limbs.

15. **Temperature instability:** especially in severely affected child with spastic quadriplegic CP; environment should be regulated.

16. **Gastrointestinal problems:** reflux (H_2 blockers or proton pump inhibitors), constipation (See Chapter 16, Neurogenic Bowel Management).

17. **Pulmonary problems**

    a. Deficient ventilation

    b. Bronchopulmonary dysplasia in premature infants

    c. Aspiration in children with oral motor dysfunction, who require aspiration precautions.

    d. Some may require tracheostomy, mechanical ventilation.

    e. Sleep apnea may be central or obstructive

G. **Prognosis in CP**
 1. Best prognosis with ataxic CP and diplegic CP in terms of mobility, communication, and cognition.
 2. Extrapyramidal group has lowest rate of mental retardation. Overall mental retardation rate is 30–50%, with the highest rate in children with rigid, atonic, and severe spastic quadraplegic CP.
 3. Walking prognosis
    a. Almost all children with hemiplegia walk. Upper limb weakness and deformity are usually the chief concerns.
    b. Most children with diplegia walk (at least with aids).
    c. Sitting independently before age 2 is a good sign for independent walking; most children who do not sit by 4 years will *not* walk.
    d. Most children with moderate to severe quadriplegia do not walk.
    e. Persistence of primitive reflexes and absence of protective reflexes by 1 year of age are poor prognostic signs.
 4. 90% of children with CP survive to adulthood.
V. **Neural Tube Defects (NTD) and Myelomeningocele**
 A. **Definition:** failure of neuralization of primitive neural tube between third and fourth weeks in utero; neural tube is closed by 28 days in utero.
 B. **Annual incidence**
    1. 0.7–1.0/1000 in U.S. or 4000 total (< 1 birth/hour).
    2. Incidence is declining at a rate of 3–7%/year.
    3. Geographic variation
 C. **Etiology:** unknown, yet many theories
    1. Genetic factors: increased familial incidence and recurrence rate of 2.4–5% after birth of one affected child; rate doubles after birth of two affected children.
    2. Maternal factors: increased age, lower socioeconomic status, folate or zinc deficiency, hyperthermia, ethnic background, previous miscarriage.
    3. Environmental factors: teratogens such as agent orange, aminopterin, valproic acid, alcohol abuse; possible increased incidence in spring conceptions.
 D. **Spectrum of NTD**
    1. **Spina bifida:** general term describing bony defect resulting from failure of mesodermal closure around the neural canal.
       a. **Spina bifida occulta**
          i. Least severe, with no neurologic damage.
          ii. Radiographs demonstrate defective closure of posterior vertebral arches, typically at L5 and S1.
          iii. No associated hydrocephalus.
       b. **Spina bifida aperta**
          i. **Meningocele**
             • Opening in back with direct exposure of meninges.
             • Patient is neurologically normal with no associated hydrocephalus.
          ii. **Myelomeningocele**
             • Spinal cord, nerves, and meninges are exposed
             • Neurologic compromise and Arnold-Chiari type II malformation are seen in nearly all cases.
             • Hydrocephalus is found in 80%.
             • 75% are located in lumbosacral region.

2. **Encephalocele/ cranial meningocele:** defect of skull in which brain tissue and/or meninges herniate through cranial fissure.
3. **Anencephaly:** absence of the brain and cranial vault, with cerebral hemispheres completely missing or reduced to small masses; generally incompatible with life.
4. **Lipomeningocele:** fatty mass (lipoma) entangled with nerve roots.

E. **Prenatal diagnosis**
   1. Fetal ultrasound: look for hydrocephalus, Arnold-Chiari malformation (ACM; banana sign), leg movement, determination of gestational age, obliteration of cysterna magna.
   2. Amniocentesis (16-18 weeks) reveals elevations in alpha-fetoprotein (AFP), and acetylcholinesterase.
   3. Maternal serum AFP is elevated, but elevation may be due to other causes.

F. **Prenatal considerations**
   1. Counseling and preparation
   2. Delivery at tertiary center so appropriate specialists are available.
   3. Vaginal delivery vs. cesarean section: cesarean section before labor improves motor outcome.
   4. Intrauterine decompression of hydrocephalus has extremely poor outcome.

G. **Initial physical exam focus**
   1. Lesion (anatomic level, intactness of skin, associated problems)
   2. Head (hydrocephalus, fontanelles, sutures, encephaloceles)
   3. Lower extremity function (reflex versus voluntary movements)
   4. Sphincter function (bladder size, reflexes)
   5. Associated anomalies (club feet, omphalocele, cardiac)

H. **Initial diagnostic study options** to assess associated malformations
   1. Ultrasound (head, spinal cord, kidneys, associated heart defects)
   2. Vesicoureterogram/intravenous pyelogram (to assess kidneys)
   3. Renal scan (for kidney malformation)
   4. Urodynamics (for neurogenic bladder)
   5. MRI of head and spine (to assess central nervous system)
   6. Electrocardiogram/echocardiogram (cardiac assessment)
   7. Skeletal x-rays (vertebral)

I. **Medical complications**
   1. **Neurologic problems**
      a. **Hydrocephalus**
         i. Due to the ACM-II deformity or aqueductal stenosis.
         ii. Overall incidence: 80%.
         iii. I.Q. is not associated with degree of hydrocephalus or number of shunt revisions.
         iv. Intelligence is correlated with history of ventriculitis.
         v. Prophylactic antibiotics are given for delayed closure (> 48 hr); improve outcomes by decreasing incidence of ventriculitis.
         vi. Neuroimaging should be done in all cases of suspected shunt malfunction (Table 5).
         vii. No change in ventricular size is seen in 3–5% of documented shunt malfunctions.
      b. **Arnold-Chiari malformation** (ACM-II, ACM-II)
         i. Caudal displacement and elongation of the medulla, pons, cerebellar tonsils.

TABLE 5.   Possible Symptoms of Shunt Malfunction

Infants	Toddlers	School-age Children	Adults
Bulging fontanelle	Vomiting	Headaches	Headaches
Vomiting	Lethargy	Vomiting	Vomiting
Irritability	Irritability	Lethargy	Lethargy
Change in appetite	Seizures	Seizures	Seizures
Lethargy	Headaches	Irritability	Redness or swelling
Sunsetting eyes (CN VI palsy with abduction paralysis	Swelling along shunt tract	Swelling along shunt tract	along shunt
Seizures	Redness along shunt tract	Redness along shunt tract	
Vocal cord paralysis with stridor		Decreased school performance	
Swelling or redness along shunt track			

From Johnson C: Developmental Disabilities Review Course Syllabus. San Antonio, Children's Association for Maximum Potential, with permission.

    ii. Causes obstruction of outflow of fourth ventricle.

   iii. Present in most children with myelomeningocele and hydrocephalus, but symptomatic in only 20%.

   iv. Stridor and difficulty in swallowing may be the first presenting symptoms.

    v. Other symptoms include apneic spells, aspiration, motor weakness, and opisthotonus and sleep problems.

   vi. Upper respiratory symptoms in a child with ACM-II are more likely due to CNS causes than pulmonary causes.

  vii. **Central ventilatory dysfunction** (CVD) in children with ACM-II
- Incidence: about 6-30% of children with ACM-II.
- Now the major cause of mortality in myelomeningocele.
- Mortality rate of 20–75%; death may be sudden.
- Pulmonary signs are stridor and difficulty in swallowing, as above.
- Treatment is neurosurgical, including decompression of high intracranial pressure by shunt revision, posterior fossa craniotomy, and cervical laminectomy.

 viii. **Tethered cord**
- Term for abnormal attachment of spinal cord at its distal end, with traction of conus medullaris and cauda equina. Traction causes decreased metabolism of nerve tissue.
- Most children with myelomeningocele have tethered cord, but the vast majority are asymptomatic.
- Signs include deterioration of lower limb strength, decreasing upper limb strength and coordination, rapidly progressive scoliosis, changing reflex level, spasticity, change in bowel/bladder function, and paresthesias.
- Detect with MRI.
- Asymptomatic tethered cord should not be released.

   ix. **Hydrosyringomyelia** (HSM)
- Tubular cavitation in spinal cord likely due to increased cerebrospinal fluid pressure.
- 5–40% incidence.

- Symptoms include loss of upper limb function, upper limb paresthesias and weakness, loss of pain and temperature sensation, changing upper limb reflexes, and progressive scoliosis.
- Neuroimaging of head as well as cord is required; MRI is best option.

x. **Diastematomyelia:** sagittal cleavage of the spinal cord.

xi. **Neurogenic bowel and bladder**
- Continence for both is now possible in 70–90% of cases if one establishes consistent routine.
- Independent toileting may not be developed until age 10–15 years in children with myelomeningocele.
- Frequent urodynamic studies and prophylactic clean intermittent catheterizations can prevent renal deterioration, previously the main cause of mortality.
- Treat only symptomatic bacteriuria with antibiotics.

2. **Skeletal problems**
   a. Vertebral anomalies
   b. Cleft lip/palate
   c. Club feet
   d. Hip dislocation (not all need relocation)
   e. Scoliosis, kyphosis, lordosis

3. **Skin problems**
   a. Decubitus ulcers can be prevented by specialized cushions, pressure relief, and skin care (see Chapter 18: Pressure Ulcers).
   b. Latex allergy
      i. Common: estimated to affect 59% with myelomeningocele.
      ii. Current standard of care is to avoid latex in all children with NTD.
      iii. May cause intraoperative anaphylactic reaction and cardiovascular collapse; nonlatex materials should be used during surgery.
      iv. Swelling after blowing up or handling balloons is early clue.
      v. Cross-reactions may occur when child eats bananas, avocados, or water chestnuts.

4. **Learning disability**
   a. Affects two-thirds of children with myelomeningocele.
   b. Examples include problems with math (> reading), attention deficit hyperactivity disorder, visual-motor disturbances, and/or central auditory processing disorder (normal hearing, yet inability to make sense out of words or to process language adequately).

5. **Associated aging problems**
   a. Growth: because basal metabolic rate is less in myelomeningocele, fewer calories are needed.
   b. Increased risk of cardiovascular disease due to increased prevalence of obesity, inactivity, and renal disease.
   c. Sexuality
      i. Females are usually fertile and at increased risk of having child with myelomeningocele; folate should be started preconceptually.
      ii. Males usually demonstrate sexual dysfunction, but several assistive devices and surgeries are available.
      iii. Girls and boys have been reported to experience precocious puberty.

J. **Prognosis in myelomeningocele** (Table 6)
K. **Prevention:** prenatal vitamins and folic acid before conception

TABLE 6.   Prognosis in Myelomeningocele

Motor Level Spinal Cord Segment	Critical Motor Function Present	Mobility-Activity Range		
		Schol Age	Adolescent	Adult
T12	Totally paralyzed lower limbs	Standing brace Wheelchair	Wheelchair	Wheelchair No ambulation
L1–L2	Hip flexor muscles	Crutches Braces Wheelchair	Wheelchair Household ambulation	Wheelchair Nonfunctional ambulation
L3–L4	Quadriceps muscles	Crutches Braces Household ambulation Wheelchair	Crutches Household ambulation Wheelchair	50% wheelchair Household ambulation with crutches
L5	Medial hamstrings Anterior tibial muscles	Crutches Braces Community ambulation	Crutches Community ambulation	Community ambulation with crutches
S1	Lateral hamstring and peroneal muscles	Community ambulation	Community ambulation	Community ambulation, 50% with crutch or cane
S2–S3	Mild loss of intrinsic foot muscles possible	Normal	Normal	Limited endurance due to late foot deformities

From Johnson C: Developmental Disabilities Review Course Syllabus. San Antonio, Children's Association for Maximum Potential, with permission.

VI. Special Considerations in Children with Spinal Cord Injury (SCI)

A. Also see Chapter 8, Spinal Cord Injury Rehabilitation.

B. **Statistics**

1. Approximately 10,000 SCIs occur each year in the United States; 3–5% occur in children under age 15 years and 20% in people under age 20.

2. Boys are four times more likely to have SCIs than girls overall; in children under 9 years old, male-to-female ratio = 1.5:1.

3. In younger children, there is no statistically significant racial trend, whereas in those over 15 years the percentage of African-Americans is higher than their representation in the general population (from specialized hospital data).

4. Younger children more commonly have high cervical lesions, whereas older children are more likely to have lower cervical lesions, probably because of relatively large size of head in younger children.

5. Due to motor vehicle collisions in 39% (overall leading cause.)

6. Pedestrian-automobile collisions are the cause in 11% overall.

7. Hadley et al. found falls to be the second leading cause in children under 10 years, whereas sports were the second leading cause at ages 15 and 16. Vogel et al. found violence to be the second leading cause in children under age 9 and sports the second leading cause in children aged 9 years and older.

C. **SCI without obvious radiologic abnormality (SCIWORA)**

1. Additional classification in children; thought to result from elasticity of pediatric spine, which allows transient displacement of structures with injury to the spinal cord during subsequent self-reduction.

2. Can present with normal plain radiographs, but abnormalities may be seen on MRI.
3. In children under age 10, SCIWORA is present in 20–40% of SCIs. Younger children are more likely to have SCIWORA than older children.
4. Lesions are often complete with poor prognosis for recovery of function.

D. **Medical issues in children with SCI**

   1. **Immobilization hypercalcemia**
      a. Affects 10–23% of patients with SCI, with highest risk in adolescent boys with tetraplegia and complete lesions, usually in acute phase.
      b. Presentation: anorexia, nausea, vomiting, malaise, and behavioral changes.
      c. Obtain calcium and phosphorus levels.
      d. Treatment
         i. Hydration (at least 150% of maintenance needs)
            • 0.9 normal saline can be used.
            • If patient is able to drink, encourage oral hydration as well.
         ii. Furosemide (1mg/kg per dose) assists in excretion of calcium and extra fluid if needed.
         iii. In refractory cases, calcitonin (100 mg subcutaneously once or twice daily) may be used.
         iv. Etidronate may be used in older adolescents, but should not be used in growing children because of risk of rachitic syndrome.

   2. **Deep venous thrombosis** (DVT; also see Chapter 13, Deep Venous Thrombosis)
      a. Less common in prepubertal children, although it still occurs.
      b. Occurs most commonly during first few weeks after SCI.
      c. Recommended prophylaxis against DVT in pubertal children includes minidose heparin or low-molecular-weight heparin or calf compression.
      d. Treatment: heparinization, then warfarin for 3–6 months or low-molecular-weight heparin.

   3. **Latex allergy** (also see Section V, Neural Tube Defects and Myelomeningocele) has incidence of 6–18% in children with SCI.

   4. **Spasticity** affects approximately 50% of children with SCI , especially those with incomplete lesions (see Chapter 19, Spasticity).

   5. **Musculoskeletal effects**
      a. Most common complication is contracture during periods of rapid growth.
      b. Hip subluxation affects 90% of patients with SCI in early childhood.
      c. Scoliosis affects 90% of patients with SCI before puberty.
      d. Pathologic long bone fractures affect 14% (not necessarily related to growth).

   6. **Syringomyelia**
      a. Affects up to 50% of children with SCI.
      b. Development of cavitation and cystic lesion within spinal cord, with progressive neurologic compromise.
      c. Symptoms may include pain, sensory loss, motor weakness, severe spasticity, excessive sweating, orthostatic hypotension, Horner's syndrome.

   7. **Respiration and airway**
      a. All children with high tetraplegia (C1–C4 levels) have some type of partial or complete respiratory dysfunction requiring full-time or part-time mechanical ventilation (Table 7).
      b. Types of mechanical ventilation are outlined in Table 8.

TABLE 7. Muscles of Respiration

Muscle	Nerve	Innervation
Diaphragm	Phrenic	C3–C5
Intercostal muscles	Intercostal	T1–T12
Abdominal muscles		
External oblique	Intercostal	T6–T12
Internal oblique	Intercostal	T10–T12
	Ilioinguinal	L1
Transversus	Thoracic	L1–T12
Rectus	Thoracic	T7–T12
Cervical muscles		
Trapezius	Accessory	Cranial nerve XI and C3–C4
Sternocleidomastoid	Accessory	Cranial nerve XI and C2–C3

From Apple D (ed): Top Spinal Cord Inj Rehabil 2000; 6(Suppl):13, with permission.

TABLE 8. Types of Mechanical Ventilation

Type	Indications	Limitations	Advantages
BiPAP-trach	Respiratory support for child who can initiate breath Transition between trach-IPPV and mask-BIPAP Improve functional residual capacity Augment tidal breathing with pressure support Stabilize airways Improve pulmonary hygiene Rest respiratory muscles Intolerance of mask	Not usable for child who has no respiratory effort Trach imposes changes in lifestyle (e.g., swimming) Requires external battery and alarms Inability to trigger in small babies	Direct access to trachea for suctioning Smaller machine than *traditional* ventilator Shorter learning curve than traditional IPPV Leak compensation in children with uncuffed trachs
BIPAP-mask	Respiratory support for child who can initiate breath Improve tidal breathing with pressure support Augment tidal breathing with pressure support Stabilize airway Improve pulmonary hygiene Rest respiratory muscles	Portable with external battery Skin irritation on face may limit use Not usable with severe oral motor dysfunction No direct trachea access for suctioning Not useable for child who has no respiratory effort Not practical for 24-hr use	No trach (noninvasive) Less costly than IPPV Shorter learning curve Better humidification than passover humidifier and trach
Trach-IPPV	Full respiratory support	Trach imposes changes in lifestyle (e.g., swimming)	Ventilator is portable and can be transported on wheelchair
Cuirass	Respiratory support for child who can initiate breath independently but needs some support	Must be custom-made for small children and those with chest deformities (e.g., scoliosis) Does not work well with decreased lung compliance No internal battery; electrically powered	No trach No face mask
Iron lung	Respiratory support for child who can initiate breath independently but needs some support Rest respiratory muscles	Large size; does not fit well in most homes Does not work well with decreased lung compliance Use requires assistance Positioning is difficult Portable unit (Porta-lung) weight about 100 lbs	Machinery is simple to service No face mask, sometimes no trach May be used with or without trach

From Molnar GE, Alexander MA (eds): Pediatric Rehabilitation, 3rd ed. Philadelphia, Hanley & Belfus, 1999, with permission.

c. **Emergency tracheotomy tube change**
- Remain calm and work quickly, but do not rush.
- Check size of tracheostomy tube. Try to insert tube of same size; if you cannot, insert tube that is one size smaller.
- Position the child on a flat surface with a roll under the shoulders (if available) and extend the child's neck.
- Hold the tracheostomy tube in place.
- Cut ties and take out tube.
- Insert new tube.
- Remove obturator.

D. **Rehabilitation issues**
1. **Wheelchairs** (See Chapter 21, Mobility Aids)
   a. Should be obtained as soon as possible after injury and frequently re-assessed as child grows.
   b. Children as young as 2 years can use power chairs; all children should be fitted by age 3 or 4 years.
   c. Electric riding toys are available commercially.
   d. If child is transported by van or school bus in wheelchair, it should meet local and state transportation standards.
   e. Safety is important part of both manual and power chair training.
2. **Orthotics** for standing and ambulation (Tables 9 and 10)

TABLE 9. Comparison of Orthotic Options at C7, T5, and T12–L1

	C7	T5	T12–L1
Primary mobility	Wheelchair	Wheelchair and RGO/ HKAFO	Wheelchair and RGO/ HKAFO
Standers/ parapodium	Full body support Exercise, household, classroom use	Full body support Functional indoor use May pivot walk with parapodium/walker	May be initial means of upright mobility for early standing
RGO	Not generally recommended Limited exercise use on level surfaces only Requires modified walker Requires physical assistance	Household and classroom ambulator Limited outdoor use Walker or forearm crutches Assistance required, depending on age	Short community ambulator Walker or crutches, depending on age Midthoracic uprights to control lordosis
HKAFO	Not recommended	Same as above for RGO Walker or crutches with swing to/through gait	Same as above for RGO Crutches with swing-through gait
KAFO	Not recommended	Not recommended	Household ambulation Watch for development of lordosis Energy-consuming
AFO	Positioning use only	Positoning use only	Positioning use only
TLSO	Recommended for trunk support and postural alignment	Recommended for trunk support and postural alignment	May be used for postural alignment

RGO, reciprocating gait orthosis; HKAFO, hip-knee-ankle-foot orthosis; KAFO, knee-ankle-foot orthosis; AFO, ankle-foot orthosis; TLSO, thoracolumbosacral orthosis.
Adapted from Creitz LL, Nelson VS, Haubenstricker L, Backer G: Orthotic prescriptions. In Betz RR, Mulcahey MJ (eds): The Child with a Spinal Cord Injury. Rosemont, IL, American Academy of Orthopedic Surgeons, 1996, p 552.

TABLE 10. Comparison of Orthotic Options at L3 and L5

	L3	L5
Primary mobility	RGO/KAFO and wheelchair	AFO/GRAFO
Standers/ parapodium	May be initial means of upright mobility for early standing	Not applicable
RGO	Independent community ambulation Independent functional activities May be able to unlock knees	Generally not used at this level Consider use if hip extensors/ abductors are weak
HKAFO	Same as above for RGO	Same as above for RGO
KAFO	Same as above for RGO Watch for development of lordosis	May use to control genu valgum or varum Watch for development of lordosis
AFO	Positioning use If quadricps are strong, may be able to use for standing and/or walking	Watch for knee deformity May not need crutches
TLSO	Not required for ambulation	Not required for ambulation

RGO, reciprocating gait orthosis; HKAFO, hip-knee-ankle-foot orthosis; KAFO, knee-ankle-foot orthosis; AFO, ankle-foot orthosis; TLSO, thoracolumbosacral orthosis; GRAFO, ground reaction ankle-foot orthosis.
Adapted from Creitz LL, Nelson VS, Haubenstricker L, Backer G: Orthotic prescriptions. In Betz RR, Mulcahey MJ (eds): The Child with a Spinal Cord Injury. Rosemont, IL, American Academy of Orthopedic Surgeons, 1996, p 552.

3. **Education and vocation**
   a. Necessary adaptations include architectural barriers, attitudinal barriers, and how to function with different physical skills (e.g., new ways to access computers or two sets of books—one at home and one at school).
   b. School staff needs education about SCI; helpful if members of rehab team can visit school to discuss SCI.
4. Training of patient and family (Table 11)

VII. Special Considerations in Children with Traumatic Brain Injury (TBI)
   A. **Epidemiology and statistics**
      1. TBI is leading cause of death in U.S. in children older than 1 year.
      2. Approximately 10/100,000 children die each year from brain injury.
      3. Annual incidence for children is approximately 185/100,000/yr. Boys have higher incidence than girls (4:1 ratio for adolescents).
      4. Leading causes of TBI for children are transportation-related (39%), falls (28%), sports and recreational activities (17%), and assault (7%).
   B. **Mechanisms of injury**
      1. **Primary injury** caused by direct impact
         a. Cerebral contusion
         b. Epidural hematoma
         c. Skull fracture
         d. Penetration wound to brain
         e. Deceleration and shearing forces (contrecoup)
      2. **Secondary injury**
         a. Hypotension
         b. Hypoxia
         c. Hydrocephalus
         d. Mass lesion
         e. Midline shift or herniation leading to infarction
         f. Cerebral edema, particularly in children

TABLE 11. Teaching List for Care of a Ventilator-dependent Child with Tetraplegia

Respiratory care
Respiratory assessment
  Signs of respiratory distress
  Signs of respiratory infection
  Listening to breath sounds
  Use of pulse oximeter
Tracheostomy care
  Anatomy and purpose of tracheostomy
  Stoma care
  Trach tie changes
  Trach changes
  Safety issues
Suctioning
Percussion and postural drainage
Use of manual resuscitation bag
Nebulizer treatments
Vent training
  Mechanics
  Circuits
  Alarms
  Troubleshooting
Nutrition
Tube feedings
  Orientation to feeding pump
  Information about formula
  Setting up feeding
  Administrastion of feeding
  Flushes
  Checking for residuals
  Venting tube
  Cleaning of feeding equipment
  Storage of formula
How to check child's weight
Oral motor stimulation techniques
Other methods of feeding
Development
Assessment of developmental level
Appropriate stimulation and activities
Home speech therapy program
Rest patterns
Use of computer
Use of environmental control unit
Interaction of hospital team
Orientation as member of interdiscipli-
  nary team
Participation in discharge planning
Interactions of community-care providers
Orientation to home-care providers
Access to services
Participation as member of community-based
  care team
Developing independence in care routine

Emergency care
Cardiopulmonary, trach resuscitation
Emergency resources
How to access emergency medical services
Identify closest emergency department
How to transport patient
Equipment
Go-bag
Musculoskeletal system
Learning about spinal cord injury
Transfers (e.g., lift, sliding board)
Assessment of function
Range-of-motion exercises
Therapy interventions
  Home physical therapy program
  Home occupational therapy program
  Use of splints
Mobility equipment (e.g., power or manual
  wheelchair)
Neurologic system
Physiology of spinal cord injury
Autonomic dysreflexia
Body temperature regulation
Safety issues
Skin care
Review care of trach and GT stoma
Assessment of skin
  Potential for irritation at stomas
  Potential for pressure sores
  Potential for burns due to lack of sensation
Wound care
Positioning and pressure relief
GI care
Anatomy and purpose of tube
  Assessing stoma
  Skin care
Bowel program
Genitourinary system
Signs and symptoms of infection
Intermittent catheterization
Bladder/urethral spasms
Medications
Actions
Side effects
Administration

Travel independently with patient on unit; independently take patient off nursing unit, take patient outside hospital on day pass, perform 12-hr care from early morning to bedtime, perform 12-hr care from bedtime to morning, leave on pass from hospital or home simulation in hospital for 24 hr.

TABLE 12.   Rating of Severity of Brain Injury

	Mild	Moderate	Severe	Profound
Initial Glasgow Coma Scale	13–15 with no deterioration	9–12 with no deterioration	3–8	
Posttraumatic amnesia	< 1 hr	1–24 hr	> 24 hr	
Duration of unconsciousness	< 15–30 min	15 min–24 hr	1–90 days	> 90 days

3. **Growing skull fracture** may develop in children who are very young at time of trauma. Arachnoid protrudes through dural tear, resulting in cyst that can contribute to a widening skull deficit that may require operative repair.

C. **Classification and evaluation**
 1. Classification (Table 12)
 2. Glasgow Coma Scale modified for young children (Table 13)
 3. COAT assessment of posttraumatic amnesia in children (Appendix D)
 4. Ranchos Los Amigos Scale (see Chapter 10, Traumatic Brain Injury)

D. **Associated complications**
 1. **Motor deficits**
  a. Focal deficits, hemiparesis
  b. Diffuse damage (balance, coordination, speed of response)
  c. Balance deficits (may be due to cochlear or vestibular dysfunction or true vertigo)
  d. Tremor
  e. Dystonia
   i. Rare motor impairment, more common with childhood injuries.
   ii. Characterized by rhythmic, twisting motion of trunk, head, and extremities.
  f. Spasticity and rigidity (See Chapter 19, Spasticity)
 2. **Common sensory deficits**
  a. Anosmia
  b. Hearing impairment
   i. May result from central processing deficit, peripheral nerve damage, cochlear injury, middle ear disruption, or sensorineural hearing loss.
   ii. Common with basilar skull fractures.

TABLE 13. Glasgow Coma Scale for Young Children: Modification of Scoring of Verbal Responses*

Verbal Score	Adult and Older Child	Young Child
5	Oriented	Smiles, oriented to sound, follows objects, interacts
4	Confused, disorderd	Cries but consolable, interacts inappropriately
3	Inappropriate words	Cries but is inconsistently consolable, moaning
2	Incomprehensible sounds	Inconsolable crying, irritable
1	No response	No response

* Scoring of eye opening and motor responses same as for adults.
Modified from Simpson CA, Cockington RA, Hanien A, et al: Head injuries in infants and young children: The value of the paediatric coma scale. Childs Nerv Syst 7:183, 1991

c. Vision impairment
   i. May result from injury to cranial nerves, eyes, optic chiasm, optic tracts, radiations, or cortical structures.
   ii. Prisms are used for homonymous hemianopsia, patching for diplopia.
3. **Common cognitive deficits**
   a. Impairment of arousal and attention
      i. May be treated with amantadine, Ritalin.
      ii. Ritalin is not to be used in children under age 4 or 5.
      iii. Neurostimulants should be used with hesitation in children under age 2 years (also see Chapter 10, Traumatic Brain Injury, and Chapter 23, Pharmacology).
   b. Agitation (also see Chapter 10, Traumatic Brain Injury): all medications should be used with hesitation in children under age 2 years.
   c. Memory impairment
   d. Altered IQ performance correlates with severity of injury.
   e. Impairment of communication (see Chapter 20, Speech, Language, and Swallowing Concerns).
   f. Behavioral sequelae
      i. Children who sustain TBI during preschool years have increased risk of later behavioral problems that interfere with school performance.
      ii. Often manifested as lack of impulse control.
   g. Abnormal emotional expression
   h. Abstract reasoning impairment
   i. Social isolation
E. **Associated medical conditions** (also see Chapter 10, Traumatic Brain Injury)
   1. **Neuroendocrine dysfunction** (due to compression of pituitary and hypothalamus by edema, fractures, hemorrhage, increased intracranial pressure, ischemic necrosis)
      a. **Diabetes insipidus**
         i. Caused by deficiency of antidiuretic hormone (ADH), which is produced in posterior pituitary.
         ii. Symptoms include hypernatremic dehydration, polyuria, and polydipsia.
         iii. Treated with restriction of oral fluid intake and 1-deamino-8-arginine vasopressin (DDAVP) if indicated. Carbamazepine may also be helpful.
      b. **Syndrome of inappropriate antidiuretic hormone secretion** (SIADH)
         i. Characterized by decreased urine output, hyponatremia, and decreased serum osmolarity.
         ii. Treated with fluid restriction and demeclocyline (if fluid restriction is not possible).
      c. **Cerebral salt-wasting**
         i. Characterized by hyponatremia with signs of dehydration due to direct neural effects and renal tubular dysfunction.
         ii. Patients are volume-depleted; therefore, fluid restriction is contraindicated.
      d. **Precocious puberty**
         i. Initial signs occur 2–17 months after severe brain injury.
         ii. Girls at greater risk with 54.5% incidence; incidence in boys, 4.5%.
         iii. Often results in short bone stature.
         iv. Consider treatment with luteinizing hormone-releasing hormone (LHRH).

2. **Respiratory dysfunction**
   a. Usually late complication; may result from prolonged intubation.
   b. Associated problems may include stenosis of trachea in glottic or sub-glottic areas, tracheomalacia, and vocal cord injury or paralysis; acquired central hypoventilation during sleep also may develop.
3. **Gastrointestinal concerns**
   a. Patients may need parenteral nutrition.
   b. Increased risk of GI hemorrhage
      i. Due to factors such as stress and steroid treatment.
      ii. Prevention includes H_2 receptor blockers or proton pump inhibitors.
      iii. Neurogenic bowel (see Chapter 16, Neurogenic Bowel Management)
4. **Bladder concerns** (see Chapter 15, Neurogenic Bladder Management)
   a. Neurogenic bladder or cognitive-based problems may require timed voiding program.
   b. In contrast to adults, diapers are often used for children.
   c. Intermittent catheterization used less commonly in children.
5. **Central autonomic dysfunction**
   a. Presumed to be caused by hypothalamic or brainstem dysfunction.
   b. More common in patients with hypoxic injury.
   c. Starts early after acquired brain injury. Episodes can last for several hours and may occur many months after injury.
   d. Characterized by unexplained elevated temperatures not treated with antipyretics (e.g., acetaminophen), systemic hypertension, tachycardia, sweating, generalized rigidity, decerebrate posturing, and rapid breathing.
   e. May be related to poorer prognosis and correlated with worse cognitive and motor outcomes 1 year or more after injury.
   f. Treat hyperthermia with cooling blankets and sponge baths.
   g. Hypertension often treated with propranolol.
      i. Pediatric dose initiated at 1.0 mg/kg/day, divided into 2 doses.
      ii. May be titrated upward to 2–4 mg/kg/day, divided into 2 oral doses.
      iii. Maximum = 640 mg/day or 8 mg/kg/day.
      iv. Intravenous dosing not indicated for children.
6. **Heterotopic ossification** (see Chapter 14, Heterotopic Ossification)
   a. Ectopic bone formation occurs in 14-23% of children with TBI.
   b. More common in children over age 11 years, children with more severe injury, and children with two or more extremity fractures.
   c. Most commonly affects the hips and knees.
   d. Rarely results in functional impairment or requires surgical intervention in children.
7. **Posttraumatic epilepsy**
   a. Related to severity of the brain injury.
   b. When treatment of ongoing seizures is needed, switch from phenytoin to carbamazepine, which interferes less with brain recovery.
8. **Cerebral atrophy** (hydrocephalus ex vacuo) and true **hydrocephalus**
   a. Commonly seen in severe TBI.
   b. Hydrocephalus associated with clinical deterioration due to enlarged ventricles as result of obstruction of cerebrospinal fluid (CSF) flow or absorption with increased CSF pressure and volume.
   c. In hydrocephalus ex vacuo, ventricular system is enlarged to fill the vacuum resulting from loss of brain volume (cerebral atrophy).

F. **Community reintegration**
 1. **Transition to school**
    a. If child requires inpatient rehabilitation, early contact with school is essential to facilitate transition.
    b. Children require an individual education plan (IEP), which varies from state to state.
       i. By law all children are entitled to a free and appropriate education.
       ii. As children with TBI improve in function, they need more frequent IEP reviews.
    c. Children with TBI are more likely than the general population to require special education services.
 2. **Discharge**
    a. Most children are discharged home from inpatient rehabilitation with in-home services or care from family members.
    b. Other settings include day treatment centers, medical foster placement, group homes, or skilled nursing facilities; options depend on state of residence and funding.
 3. **Return to sports and recreational activities**
    a. Children with severe brain injury should not participate in contact sports, especially football, ice hockey, and soccer, or risky activities such as horseback riding and driving all-terrain vehicles, motorcycles, or snowmobiles.
    b. Children should wear helmets when riding a bike and be properly restrained with seat belts and car seats in motor vehicles.
    c. Each year up to 20% of high school football players sustain a concussion.
    d. Second-impact syndrome is defined as fatal outcome from repetitive minor head injuries within a short period. Caution must be taken in returning a child to sports activity.
G. **Outcomes**
 1. More than two-thirds of deaths from brain injury occur at the scene or en route to hospital.
 2. Children with acquired brain injury who have survived the initial stabilization period and become enrolled in a rehabilitation program generally live for many years.
 3. Children in vegetative states usually live for years, dramatically longer than adults with similar function. One-half of children still in vegetative states at 1 year after injury were still living 7–8 years later.
VIII. **Anoxic Encephalopathy**
 A. **Epidemiology and statistics**
 1. Drowning is the third leading cause of death in children aged 1–14 years.
 2. Death rate of 3/100,000 in 1–14-year-olds in U.S.
 3. Male-to-female ratio = 3.3:1.
 4. Morbidity rates: 1/300 for boys, 1/913 for girls hospitalized for near-drowning by age 19.
 5. Young children may drown in any water, including toilets, bathtubs, and pails. Freshwater drownings predominate (98% of cases).
 6. Increased risk with seizure disorders, alcohol use, and lapse of supervision of young children.
 B. **Pathophysiology**
 1. Pulmonary: hypoxia, pulmonary edema, aspiration and pneumonia, acute respiratory distress syndrome.

2. Neurologic: anoxic/hypoxic injury with brain cell damage and death, cerebral edema, increased intracranial pressure.
3. Cardiovascular: low cardiac output, high systemic vascular resistance, arrhythmias.
4. Electrolyte disorders (rare): hemodilution, hypervolemia, metabolic acidosis due to anoxia.

C. **Prognosis**
1. Poor outcome usual in patients who arrive at emergency department (ED) with flaccidity.
2. Any movement in ED, even posturing, is predictive of better neurologic outcome.
3. Glasgow Coma Scale score of 3 in ED is usually predictive of poor neurologic outcome or death.
4. Sustained intracranial pressure (ICP) > 20 mmHg predicts poorer prognosis
5. Children who still require CPR in the ED have a poorer neurologic outcome or death.
6. All-or-nothing phenomenon: good outcome or death/vegetative state.

D. **Associated complications**
1. **Motor deficits**
   a. Severe hypertonicity and opisthotonic posturing (may decrease with time).
   b. Contractures frequently develop, even with best of care.
   c. Early hip subluxation/dislocation may occur.
   d. Dyskinesia may be present in less severely involved patients.
2. **Cognitive deficits**
   a. Vegetative state or severe cognitive dysfunction is more common than in traumatic brain injuries.
   b. Goals are frequently maintenance rather than progression of skills.

E. **Associated medical conditions** (see Section VII, Traumatic Brain Injury)

F. **Rehabilitative management:** similar to TBI, except overall poorer prognosis and less progress of skills in children with anoxic encephalopathy.

G. **Prevention**
1. At least 5-foot fencing of swimming pools
2. "Child-proof" home: protection from open water (e.g., close toilets)
3. Safety education and legislation
4. Alcohol and drug abuse prevention
5. CPR training
6. Enforcement of life jacket use
7. Teaching children to swim at an early age.

IX. Rheumatologic Disorders
A. **Juvenile rheumatoid arthritis** (JRA)
1. **Statistics**
   a. Incidence: 13.9/100,000/year.
   b. Most common connective tissue disorder in children.
   c. Childhood cases account for about 5% of rheumatoid arthritis cases
2. **Classification**
   a. Defined by American Rheumatism Association as presence of arthritis lasting 6 weeks or longer and starting under the age of 16 years.
   b. Onset is classified in first 6 months as oligoarthritis (< 5 joints), polyarthritis (≥ 5 joints), or systemic arthritis.

TABLE 14. Juvenile Rheumatoid Arthritis

Onset	Median Age at Onset	Sex	Joints Involved	Serology	HLA	Outcome
Polyarticular			≥ 5			
RF-negative	1–3 yr	Girls	Large joints; knee, wrist, elbow, ankle, often symmetric	Sometimes ANA-positive	—	Variable
RF-positive	12 yr	Girls	Similar to adult-onset RA	ANA-positive	DR4	Severe arthritis in > 50%
Pauciarticular			≤ 4			
Type I	1–3 yr	Girls	Large joints:knee, ankle, elbow	ANA-positive RF-negative	DR5 DR6 DR 8	Chronic iritis: risk for loss of vision, good outcome for arthritis
Type II	10 yr	Boys	Large joints: hip, sacroiliac	ANA-negative RF-negative	B27	Acute iritis, may progress to spondylo-arthropathy
Systemic	Any	Boys or girls	Varied	ANA-negative RF-negative	—	Poor outcome with poly-articular involvement

RF = rheumatoid factor, ANA = antinuclear antibody. From Molnar GE, Alexander MA (ed): Pediatric Rehabilitation. Philadelphia, Hanley & Belfus, 1999, with permission.

 c. Five types are summarized in Table 14.
  i. Polyarticular: RF-negative in 90%, RF-positive in 10%.
  ii. Pauciarticular: 50% of total; accounts for largest percentage of children with JRA.
 3. **Etiology:** unknown (perhaps involves genetic predisposition, immunologic abnormalities, infection, and trauma)
 4. **Pathophysiology**
  a. Stimulation of B cells and T cells with infiltration in the synovial tissues → inflammation and hypertrophy of synovial tissues increases synovial fluid → increased joint pressure and swelling of the joint → chronic synovitis and effusion, erosion of cartilage and bone → enzymes cause destructive changes in articular cartilage, bone, and other surrounding structures.
  b. This process takes longer in children.
 5. **Differences between children and adults with rheumatoid arthritis**
  a. Systemic features more common in children.
  b. Adults have joint destruction earlier.
  c. Children may develop atrophy and contracture earlier due to disuse of joint, even if asymptomatic.
  d. Children have large -joint involvement more frequently than adults.
  e. Hand deviation: children have ulnar deviation at the wrist with loss of extension, radial deviation of fingers at metacarpophalangeal (MCP) joint with finger flexion.
  f. Tenosynovitis is more common in children than bursitis.
  g. Rheumatoid nodules occur less frequently in children.
  h. Children have cervical spine and temporomandibular joint involvement more often than adults.

    i. Children tend to be ANA-positive, RF-negative, whereas adult RA is generally RF-positive.

    j. Disturbance in growth and development is major issue in children.

    k. 30% of children with JRA develop osteopenia; calcium supplements are recommended.

6. **Diagnostic testing**
   a. 20% of children and 80% of adults with rheumatoid arthritis are RF-positive.
   b. Erythrocyte sedimentation rate (ESR) may be elevated.
   c. Platelet count is elevated.
   d. White blood cell count is elevated.
   e. Anemia of chronic disease may be present.
   f. Joint fluid shows increased protein, low glucose, and low to normal complement and cell count, (5000–80,000 cell/mm^3).

7. **Radiographic findings**
   a. Early: few findings except for soft tissue swelling.
   b. Periarticular bone demineralization seen on x-ray once 50% demineralization is present.
   c. Later: subchondral erosions and loss of joint space.

8. **Medical issues** depend on joint involvement.
   a. **Cervical spine**
      i. More commonly involved in children than adults.
      ii. Symptoms include decreased range of motion, pain, and muscle spasm.
      iii. Neutral position encouraged to decrease flexion contracture risk.
      iv. Subluxation of atlantoaxial joints can lead to erosion of transverse ligament.
      v. Excessive flexion can cause neurologic sequelae,
      vi. Firm collar should be worn with automobile travel.
      vii. Affected children should not participate in contact sports.
      viii. Caution required during intubation for anesthesia.
      ix. Treatment may require surgical fusion.
   b. **Temporomandibular joint**
      i. Involved in 50% of children with JRA.
      ii. Associated with micrognathia and facial asymmetry.
   c. **Shoulder** (involved in 8% of cases)
   d. **Elbow**
   e. **Wrist**
      i. Flexion contracture common in children.
      ii. Ulnar deviation also may be seen.
   f. **Hands**
      i. Loss of flexion and extension range
      ii. Swan neck deformity: hyperextension of proximal interphalangeal (PIP) joints
      iii. Boutonnière deformity: flexion of PIP joint with hyperextension of distal interphalangeal (DIP) joints; MCP hyperextension may occur.
      iv. Ring splints may be useful.
   g. **Hip**
      i. Children have flexion contractures with internal rotation and adduction vs. external rotation and abduction in adults.

      ii. Lumbar lordosis is common.

      iii. Lateral subluxation can occur.

  h. **Knee**

      i. Flexion contracture

        • Flexed position maintained for comfort to decrease intrarticular pressure and pain induced by hamstring spasm.

        • Eventually leads to quadriceps atrophy and weakness.

      ii. Valgus tendency secondary to:

        • Muscle weakness

        • Hamstring spasm, which pulls the tibia laterally

        • Overgrowth of medial femoral condyle

        • External tibial torsion

        • Internal rotation at the hip

        • Vastus medialis atrophy

  i. **Ankle and foot**

      i. Flat-footed gait: metatarsophalangeal (MTP) joint has decreased push-off.

      ii. Clawtoe deformity: spasm of long toe flexors leads to hyperextension at MTP, which leads to flexion of interphalangeal joints.

      iii. Varus hindfoot: weight-bearing over lateral foot border.

      iv. Valgus deformity

      v. Plantarflexion contracture: toe-walking, pain in heel

      vi. Treated with molded foot-orthotics, University of California Berkeley Laboratory foot orthosis (UCBL), ankle-foot orthosis, lift for leg length discrepancy.

9. **Treatment**

  a. **Drug therapy** (Table 15): general guidelines

      i. First-line agents: nonsteroidal anti-inflammatory drugs (NSAIDs) with patient/family education, family support, rehabilitation, and nutrition.

      ii. Second–line agents: safer disease-modifying antirheumatic drugs (DMARDs; also also called slow-acting antirheumatic drugs [SAARDs]). The safer DMARDs are in bold print, the moderately toxic in regular print, and the highly toxic in italics.

Auranofin	Azathioprine	Methotrexate
Chloroquine	*Chlorambucil*	Cyclosporine
Hydroxychloroquine	D-Penicillamine	*Cyclophosphamide*
Sulfasalazine	Gold	

      iii. Third-line agents: corticosteroids.

      iv. Fourth-line agents: the moderately toxic SAARDS, which are immunosuppressive (e.g., methotrexate, cyclosporine).

      v. Final resort: experimental therapy

  b. **Rehabilitation**

      i. Posture: in hip and knee flexion, lumbar lordosis, internal rotation of the femur, genu valgum of the knee, with tibial external rotation and decreased knee extension.

      ii. Strengthen with isometric exercises plus recreational activities such as throwing a ball, riding a bike, and swimming.

      iii. Rest

      iv. Passive range-of-motion exercises

TABLE 15. Drug Therapy in Juvenile Rheumatoid Arthritis

Drug	Dosage	Usage/Length of Treatment	Side Effects
Aspirin	80–100 mg/kg/d qid up to 25 kg; otherwise, 650 mg qid	At least 6–8 wk	Drowsiness, tinnitus, hyperventilation, concern of Reye's syndrome if used during varicella or influenza, reduced platelet function, GI irritation
Naproxen	10–20 mg/kg/d bid, suspension available	At least 6–8 wk	GI irritation, cutaneous pseudoporphyria, cutanea tarda
Ibuprofen	35–45 mg/kg/d qid 45 mg/kg/d if using suspension	At least 6–8 wk	GI irritation, rash, aseptic meningitis
Tolmetin	25–30 mg/kg/d tid		GI irritation
Indomethacin*	1–2 mg/kg/d tid	For fever and pericarditis in systemic in systemic JRA	Headache, epigastric pain, difficulty paying attention
Diclofenac*	2–3 mg/kg/d qid		Mild GI effects
Piroxicam*	0.3–0.6 mg/kg/d	Advantage of once-a-day dosing	
Gold salts	0.75–1 mg/kg/wk max 50 mg/wk	At least 6 mo use early for polyarthritis	Mucosal ulcers, rash, proteinuria, nephropathy, leukopenia, thrombocytopenia, anemia
Auranofin*	0.1–0.2 mg/kg/d qd or bid; max 9 mg/d		GI effects, rash
Hydroxychloroquine	5–7 mg/kg/d; max 400 mg/d	8–12 wk	Macular degeneration
D-Penicillamine	3 mg/kg/d; max 250 mg/d	3 mo	Bone marrow suppression, renal effects, rash, autoimmune effects, proteinuria
	6 gm/kg/d; max 500 mg/d	3 mo	
	10 gm/kg/d; max 750 mg/d	1–3 yr For polyarthritis, not systemic or pauciarticular	
Sulfasalazine*	40–60 mg/kg/d divided 3–6 doses	6–8 wk	GI effects, rash, hypersensitivity, renal toxicity, headache
Methotrexate*	0.25 mg/kg/wk orally; increase at 2–4 wk intervals to 1.0 mg/kg/wk; can be given SQ		Avoid use with NSAID because it may potentiate bone marrow suppression, GI effects, hepatotoxicity
Azathioprine*	0.5–2.0 mg/kg/d	Take for 1 yr or more; monitor every 1–2 mo	GI effects, liver effects, dose-related leukopenia
Cyclophosphamide*	0.5–1gm/m^2 IV monthly		Alopecia, nausea, vomiting, bladder effects, pulmonary fibrosis, leukopenia, thrombocytopenia
Cyclosporine	3–5 mg/kg/d		Immunosuppression, hypertension, renal insufficiency

Table continued on following page

TABLE 15. Drug Therapy in Juvenile Rheumatoid Arthritis *(Continued)*

Drug	Dosage	Usage/Length of Treatment	Side Effects

Corticosteroids
  Prednisone
	0.1–1.0 mg/kg/d orally;
	  max 40 mg
		Most potent anti-
		  inflammatory agent
			Growth failure, adrenal
			  suppression, osteopenia,
			  cushingoid appearance,

Pulse steroid
  methylpred-
  nisolone
	10–30 mg/kg/dose;
	  max 1 gm
			avascular necrosis,
			  weight gain, cataracts,
			  psychosis, myopathy

qid = 4 times/day, tid = 3 times/day, bid = 2 times/day, qd = once daily; NSAID = nonsteroidal anti-in-
flammatory drug, IV = intravenously, SQ = subcutaneously, GI = gastrointestinal.
* Not approved for use in children.
From Molnar GE, Alexander MA (eds): Pediatric Rehabilitation, 3rd ed. Philadelphia, Hanley &
Belfus, 1999, with permission.

  v. Adequate nutrition
  vi. Adaptive equipment
  vii. Training in activities of daily living (ADLs) and ambulation to im-
       prove function
  viii. Prevention of contractures with splinting
  ix. Treatment of contractures with serial casting for 48–72 hours, then
      repeat; dynamic splinting; surgery
c. **Surgical management**
  i. Soft tissue release
  ii. Posterior capsulotomy
  iii. Tendon lengthening
  iv. Synovectomy
  v. Joint replacement once growth completed
10. **Outcomes**
a. **Classes** according to American College of Rheumatology
  i. Class I: completely able to perform usual ADLs as well as voca-
     tional, and avocational activities.
  ii. Class II: able to perform usual self-care and vocational activities but
      limited in avocational activities.
  iii. Class III: able to perform usual self-care activities but limited in vo-
       cational and avocational activities.
  iv. Class IV: limited in ability to perform usual self-care, vocational,
      and avocational activities.
b. **Poor outcome factors**
  i. Delay in treatment
  ii. Later age at onset
  iii. Longer duration of disease, lack of remission
  iv. RF positivity
  v. Unremitting course
  vi. Multiple small joint involvement
  vii. Early erosion on x-ray
  viii. Hip involvement
c. Death rate: 2–4% in children; death rate in North America alone is < 1%.
B. **Juvenile-onset spondyloarthropathy**
1. HLA-B27–associated clinical syndrome in children under age 16 with related arthritis, enthesitis (pain at the insertion of tendon to bone), and
   tenosynovitis involving joints of lower limbs, spine, and sacroiliac (SI) joint.

2. Patients are seronegative.
3. More common in boys than girls.
4. Cases with SI joint involvement are termed **seronegative enthesopathy and arthropathy** (SEA) syndrome.
   a. Defined by age of onset before 17 years, seronegativity, enthesitis (usually at heel or knee), and pauciarticular arthritis (usually of lower limbs).
   b. Usually progresses to ankylosing spondylitis or other spondyloarthropathy.

C. **Ankylosing spondylitis** (AS)
   1. Incidence: 2.0/100,000 in U.S.
   2. Male-to-female ratio: 6.1–2.6:1.
   3. 90% of white patients are HLA-B27-positive vs. only 9% in general population.
   4. Etiology unknown, possible genetic susceptibility.
   5. Tarsal involvement and enthesopathy at onset are more common in AS vs. JRA.
   6. Later < 50% have upper limb involvement.
   7. Development of axial symptoms and radiographic sacroiliitis leads to pain and decreased range of motion.
   8. Arthritis is asymmetric.
   9. Outcome is poorer with hip involvement.
   10. Compared with adults, children are more likely to have peripheral joint involvement (82%), most commonly in lower limbs and hip joint, although shoulder, costoclavicular joint, and sternoclavicular joint can be affected.
   11. Enthesitis occurs more commonly in children at onset (patella, tibial tuberosity, Achilles tendon)
   12. Up to 27% have uveitis (treated with ophthalmic steroids).
   13. **Treatment**
      a. Drug therapy: NSAIDs and glucocorticoid injection.
      b. Rehabilitation includes maintaining range of motion, prevention of hip contracture, strengthening of hip extensors and quadriceps, trunk extension, and swimming.

D. **Reiter's syndrome**
   1. Not common in children, yet more frequent in boys over age 8 years.
   2. Symptoms include conjunctivitis, urethritis, and symmetric arthritis.
   3. Occurs after infection with *Chlamydia trachomatis, C. pneumoniae, Salmonella* sp., *Shigella flexneri*, and *Yersinia enterocolitica*.
   4. **Treatment**
      a. Drug therapy: NSAIDs are primary agents; if course is aggressive and unremitting, immunosuppressive agents can be used.
      b. Rehabilitation includes range-of-motion exercises, isometric exercises (goal is to maintain erect posture with trunk extension), and breathing exercises for chest expansion.

E. **Arthritis associated with inflammatory bowel disease**
   1. Affects 10–20% of children with ulcerative colitis and Crohn's disease.
   2. Arthritis is usually pauciarticular; spondylitis may be present.
   3. **Treatment:** management of bowel disease, NSAIDS, physical therapy

F. **Psoriatic arthritis**
   1. Inflammatory arthritis in children under 16 years associated with psoriasis that either precedes onset or occurs within 15 years.

2. Higher incidence in girls ,with peak age of onset of arthritis at 7–11 yr and psoriasis at 9–13 yr.
3. 50% present with monoarticular arthritis; eventually most cases involve > 5 joints in asymmetric pattern.
4. Small joints of hands/feet may be involved.
5. Anterior uveitis is common.
6. Lab results: elevated ESR; RF-negative; antinuclear antibodies (ANA) may be positive; synovial fluid mostly polymorphonuclear neutrophils.
7. **Treatment**
   a. Drug therapy: NSAIDs, SAARDS, intra-articular steroid injections, topical agents for psoriasis.
   b. Rehabilitation: PT and OT to maintain joint range of motion and function.

G. **Systemic lupus erythematosus (SLE)**
   1. Multisystem autoimmune disease with episodic inflammation and vasculitis associated with positive ANA and widespread immune complex deposits.
   2. Incidence: 0.6/100,000 population.
   3. 20% of cases begin in childhood, with female-to-male ratio of 4.5:1.
   4. Etiology unknown; may be immunologic, genetic, environmental, infectious.
   5. Children more likely to present with systemic disease.
   6. Symptoms involve malaise, fatigue, weight loss, anorexia (Table 16).
   7. **Diagnostic tests**
      a. Positive ANA
      b. Anti-DNA antibody
      c. Low complement
      d. Anemia (complete blood count [CBC])
      e. Leukopenia (CBC)
   8. **Treatment**
      a. Drug therapy
         i. NSAIDs
         ii. Prednisone
         iii. Hydroxychloroquine
         iv. Immunosuppressive agents
         v. Intravenous immunoglobulin (IVIG)
         vi. IV cyclophosphamide
      b. Rehabilitation
         i. Adequate nutrition must be ensured.
         ii. Physical activity should be maintained.

TABLE 16. Diagnostic Criteria in Systemic Lupus Erythematosus*

Malar rash	Cytopenia
Discoid lupus rash	Positive immunoserology
Photosensitivity	Lupus erythematosus cells
Oral or nasal mucocutaneous ulceration	Anti-native DNA antibodies
Nonerosive arthritis	Anti-Sm antibodies
Nephritis	False-positive test for syphilis
Encephalitis	Positive antinuclear antibody
Pleuritis or pericarditis	

• Four or more of the 11 criteria are required for clinical diagnosis.
Adapted from Tan EM, Cohen AS, Fries JF, et al: The 1982 revised criteria for the classification of systemic lupus erythematosus. Arthritis Rheum 25:1271, 1982.

   iii. Physical therapy: range-of-motion exercise, strengthening, functional training with ambulation.
   iv. Occupational therapy: functional training in ADLs.
9. **Outcome**
   a. Poor with hematuria, proteinuria, persistent hypertension, pulmonary hypertension, chronic active disease, or diffuse proliferative glomerulonephritis.
   b. Ten-year survival rate > 80%

H. **Dermatomyositis**
   1. Multisystem inflammatory disease (mainly muscle and skin)
   2. Incidence: 0.22–0.55/100,000 population.
   3. Peak age of onset is between 5 and 9 years of age; ratio of girls to boys increases with age.
   4. Associated with coxsackie B virus and *Toxoplasma gondii.*
   5. May be immune-mediated process related to genetic predisposition secondary to association with HLA-B8 in 72% and DR3.
   6. Can occur in blood vessels of dermal connective tissue, GI tract, and nerves.
   7. Clinical picture: deep tendon reflexes may be preserved until later in course; progressive symmetric weakness proximally (greater in lower than upper limbs), skin rash, and arthralgias.
   8. Involvement of respiratory muscles (pharyngeal and palatine) with dysphagia.
   9. Calcium deposits in up to 70% of cases (most commonly in knee and elbow).
   10. Vasculitis may involve GI tract.
   11. Myocarditis develops in some patients.
   12. **Diagnostic tests**
       a. Elevated creatine phosphokinase (CPK)
       b. Elevated aspartate aminotransferase (AST)
       c. Elevated alanine aminotransferase (ALT)
       d. Elevated ANA titer
       e. Normal ESR
       f. Elelctromyography: normal nerve conductions; low-amplitude, short-duration polyphasic motor units with early recruitment; positive sharp waves; fibrillations; and complex repetitive discharges.
       g. Muscle biopsy: inflammatory myopathy with focal degeneration and regeneration, fibrosis, and variation in fiber size.
   13. **Treatment**
       a. Drug therapy
          i. Corticosteroids, immunosuppressive agents
          ii. Follow lung function.
          iii. Follow swallowing.
          iv. Limit calcinosis.
       b. Rehabilitation
          i. PT started in acute phase to prevent contracture with passive range-of-motion exercises and splinting.
          ii. Unnecessary immobilization should be avoided.
          iii. When inflammation has subsided, initiate strengthening of muscles and endurance training, hydrotherapy (if available) for range of motion and decreased muscle pain.
   14. **Outcome:** approximately 20% have chronic course; prognosis related to degree of vasculitis.

TABLE 17. Types of Scleroderma

Morphea	Systemic sclerosis
Localized	Diffuse cutaneous sclerosis
Generalized	Limited cutaneous sclerosis
Guttate morphea	Mixed connective tissue disease
Liver scleroderma	CREST syndrome (calcinosis, Raynaud's phenomenon,
En coup de sabre	esophageal dysfunction, sclerodactyly, telangiectasia)

I. **Scleroderma**
   1. Types are summarized in Table 17; disease presents with linear or focal cutaneous involvement.
   2. Greater incidence in girls than boys.
   3. Average age at onset: 8–10 years, with duration of 7–9 years.
   4. Etiology may be immunologic, metabolic, and vascular.
   5. Morphea: circumscribed area of hardened skin; self-limiting over 2–3 yr.
   6. **Linear scleroderma**
      a. Atrophic, erythematous area becomes fibrotic, binding skin to underlying tissue.
      b. Results include soft tissue atrophy, facial or other areas of asymmetry.
      c. Children account for nearly half of cases of linear scleroderma.
   7. **Systemic form**
      a. Uncommon in children.
      b. Characterized by stiffness, skin tightness, loss of range of motion, GI involvement with dysphagia and malabsorption, pulmonary and renal complications (causes of death).
   8. **Treatment** is nonspecific.
      a. Drug therapy
         i. Topical corticosteroids or D-penicillamine for skin disease
         ii. Systemic corticosteroids for progressive linear disease
         iii. Methotrexate
         iv. Nifedipine for Raynaud's phenomenon
         v. Captopril for hypertension
         vi. H_2 blockers or proton pump inhibitors for esophageal dysmotility
      b. Rehabilitation
         i. PT includes range-of-motion exercises, prevention of contractures, soft tissue massage, stretching exercises (moist heat can be applied in advance), and range of motion of mouth and face to maintain oral opening.
         ii. OT includes adaptive equipment and work with functional ADLs.
         iii. Serial casting
         iv. Splinting
      c. Surgery for severe facial involvement, joint contractures
   J. **CREST syndrome** (**c**alcinosis, **R**aynaud's phenomenon, **e**sophageal dysfunction, **s**clerodactyly, **t**elangiectasia): unclear if it is separate entity from systemic sclerosis (scleroderma).
   K. **Mixed connective tissue disorder**
      1. Diagnostic criteria
         a. Raynaud's phenomenon or swollen hands
         b. Positive tests for anti-ENA (extractable nuclear antigen) and anti-RNP (ribonucleoprotein)

      c. Mixed findings of two connective tissue disorders from following list: SLE, scleroderma, and polymyositis/dermatomyositis

   2. More common in girls > 6 years old

L. **Lyme disease**

   1. Incidence: 5.2/100,000.

   2. Etiology: spirochete *Borrelia burgdorferi*, transmitted by deer tick *Ixodes dammini.*

   3. Appears 1–30 days after a tick bite and disappear within 4 weeks of onset.

      a. Initial phase: fever, fatigue, headache, arthralgia, myalgia, stiff neck, erythema migrans

      b. Late disease: arthritis (knee most common), cardiac disease, neurologic disease including meningitis, radiculitis, cranial nerves (Bell's palsy)

   4. Lab results

      a. Antibody detection

      b. Up to 30% of patients are ANA-positive, RF-negative.

   5. **Treatment**

      a. Antibiotics for 21 days (doxycycline, amoxicillin, erythromycin).

      b. Early Lyme arthritis: 30-day course of oral antibiotics.

      c. Late disease: IV antibiotics (ceftriaxone).

M. **Rheumatic fever** (rare in U.S.)

   1. Affects boys and girls equally, occurring in children older than 4 yr.

   2. Most commonly affected joints: knees, elbow, ankles, and wrists .

   3. Diagnosed by Jones criteria (Table 18).

N. **Septic arthritis:** viral vs. bacterial

   1. Viral: parvovirus 19, rubella, hepatitis B, Epstein-Barr, varicella.

   2. Bacterial: *Neisseria gonorrhoeae, Hemophilus influenzae, Staphylococcus aureus.*

O. **Reactive arthritis:** after infection with *S. aureus, Yersinia enterocolitica, Salmonella* sp., *Shigella* sp, or *Campylobacter* sp.

P. **Other causes of arthritis in children**

   1. Hemophilia: hemarthrosis.

   2. Kawasaki disease: acute phase, self-limited.

   3. Sickle cell disease: septic arthritis, noninflammatory joint effusion, chronic synovitis.

X. **Congenital Disorders**

  A. **Congenital limb deficiences**

    1. **Definitions**

TABLE 18. Jones Criteria for the Diagnosis of Rheumatic Fever*

Major	Minor	Preceding Group A Streptococcal Infection
Carditis	Fever	Throat culture
Polyarthritis	Arthralgia	Rapid streptococcal antigen
Chorea	Elevated ESR or CRP	Elevated streptococcal antibody
Erythema marginatum	Prolonger PR interval	
Subcutaneous nodules		

ESR = erthrocyte sedimentation rate, CRP = C-reactive protein.
* Two of the major criteria or one major with two minor criteria are required for diagnosis with evidence of preceding streptococcal infection.
Adapted from Dajani AS, Avoub E, Bierman Z, et al: Guidelines for the diagnosis of rheumatic fever: Jones criteria, updated. JAMA 268:2069, 1992.

     a. **Amelia:** absence of a limb.

     b. **Hemimelia:** absence of half of a limb.

     c. **Phocomelia:** flipper-like appendages.

     d. **Acheiria:** missing hand.

     e. **Adactyly:** absent metacarpal or metatarsal.

     f. **Aphalangia:** absent finger or toe.

2. **Upper limb deficiencies** (absence)

     a. Incidence: 4.1/10/000 live births.

     b. Most common deficiency is left arm transradial deficiency.

     c. Associated upper limb syndromes are seen with radial deficiency.

         i. **TAR syndrome** (thrombocytopenia with absence of radius)

         ii. **Fanconi syndrome** with associated anemia and leukopenia

         iii. **Holt-Oram syndrome** with associated congenital heart defects

         iv. **Baller-Gerold syndrome** with associated craniosynostosis

         v. **VACTERL syndrome** with vertebral involvement, anal atresia, cardiac involvement, tracheoesophageal fistula, renal involvement, and limb involvement.

     d. Mostly without hereditary implication, except for hand deficiencies such as central ray deficiencies, adactyly, or lobster claw deformities.

     e. Craniofacial anomalies often associated.

3. **Lower limb deficiency**

     a. Fibular longitudinal deficiency (fibular hemimelia) is most common congenital lower limb deficiency; occurs bilaterally in 25% of cases.

     b. Transtibial deficiency: more common than transfemoral or transverse deficiency of the thigh/amelia.

     c. Longitudinal deficiency of tibia occurs in 1 in 1 million births.

         i. Manifests clinically as varus foot, short leg, unstable knee, and or unstable ankle.

         ii. Treatment of choice is disarticulation at knee.

     d. Longitudinal deficiency of femur or partial proximal femoral focal deficiency (PFFD): congenital defect of shaft of femur.

         i. Incidence: 1 in 50,000 births.

         ii. 10-15% of cases are bilateral.

4. **Treatment**

     a. Surgical: depends on type of deformity, whether unilateral or bilateral, presence of hip joint, amount of coxa vara, presence of pseudarthrosis, and limb length discrepancy.

     b. Prosthesis (See Chapter 26, Prosthetics)

         i. First fitting of upper limb prosthesis when child is able to sit (6 months). Elbow joint should not be added until age 3–5 years.

         ii. First fitting of lower limb prosthesis when child is able to pull up to stand (9–10 months). Knee joint should not be added until age 3–5 years.

B. **Congenital anomalies (deformities)**

1. **Upper limb anomalies/conditions**

     a. **Syndactyly**

         i. Incidence: 1 in 2200 births.

         ii. Most common between third and fourth fingers, second and third toes, where digital rays fail to separate during eighth postconceptional week.

     b. Simple dominant or simple recessive

     c. **Polydactyly:** supernumary digits

    d. **Brachydactyly:** shortness of digits
    e. **Scapula:** bipartite coracoid, duplication of acromial process, dysplasia of glenoid and scapular clefts
    f. **Sprengel's deformity:** congenitally high scapula, failure of scapula to descend from the cervical region overlying first through fifth ribs.
    g. **Congenital brachial plexopathy**
       i. Incidence: 0.5–2.6/1000 live births.
      ii. Affects males and females equally.
     iii. Usually unilateral, can be bilateral.
     iv. Most common etiologies are large baby and shoulder dystocia.
      v. Caused by injury to brachial plexus by excessive lateral traction to fetal head or neck and/or intrauterine propulsion due to force of contractions.
     vi. Classifications (Table 19).
     vii. Evaluate with physical examination, electromyography, MRI, myelography.
    viii. Treat with range-of-motion exercises, strengthening, splinting; encourage use of affected arm.
     ix. Rarely is surgery needed.
      x. Surgical procedures, if warranted, include neurolysis, nerve graft reconstruction, and nerve transfers.
     xi. **Prognosis:** overall 80–90% favorable prognosis with most improvement in first 3 months; poor prognosis with avulsion.

2. **Spine anomalies/conditions**
    a. **Klippel-Feil syndrome:** brevicollis or short neck, low hairline, restricted neck movement with number of cervical vertebra usually decreased; several elements in cervical spine may be lacking, with smaller nerve roots and intervertebral foramina.
    b. **Cleft vertebral column (raschischisis):** vertebral abnormalities that affect axial structure of spine.
    c. **Congenital scoliosis**
       i. < 20°, observe; > 40°, consider surgery.
      ii. Bracing between 20–40°, generally with thoracolumbosacral orthosis for apices at T8 or below and Milwaukee Brace for apices above T8.
     iii. Associated with cardiac abnormalities in 10% of cases as well as GI abnormalities.
     iv. Associated with renal abnormalities in 25% of cases.
      v. Family history positive in 5–10% of siblings, offspring.
     vi. Any progressive curvature warrants immediate surgical referral.

TABLE 19. Classification of Congenital Brachial Plexopathy

Plexopathy	Level (Nerve Roots/Trunk)	Clinical Findings (Related Weakness)
Duchenne-Erb's palsy (most common)	C5–C6 ± C7 Upper trunk	Weakness of shoulder abduction, external rotation, elbow flexion, supination, wrist extension, finger extension
Klumpke's plexopathy	C8–T1 Lower trunk	Weakness of elbow extension, pronation, wrist flexion, hand weakness, associated with Horner's syndrome
Pan plexopathy	C5–T1 Arm, entire plexus	Weakness of all motions listed above, flail chest

  d. **Neuromuscular spinal deformities:** common in Friedreich's ataxia (up to 80%), spinal muscular atrophy (up to 65%), Duchenne muscular dystrophy (up to 90%), cerebral palsy with spastic quadriplegia (up to 70%), and myelodysplasia (up to 60%).
  e. **Congenital cervical stenosis:** transient quadriplegia.
  f. **Congenital torticollis** (wryneck deformity; infant with head tilt).
    i. Relatively common
    ii. Most commonly associated with breech delivery and sternocleidomastoid fibroma.
    iii. More common if infant sleeps on back.
    iv. Neck motion is limited by contracture of sternocleidomastoid.
    v. Resolves spontaneously in 90% of cases; 10% require operative correction.
    vi. Treatment includes range-of-motion exercises, correct posture, possible botulinum toxin injection.
    vii. Assess for coexistent hip dysplasia, which also is associated with breech delivery.
3. **Lower limb anomalies/conditions**
  a. **Congenital dislocation of knee/patella** (rare)
  b. **Multipartite patellae** (fractioned knee)
    i. Fragment may attach to main body of patella,,
    ii. Usual presentation is in older child or athlete with knee pain and patellofemoral-type symptoms.
4. **Hip dysplasia** (ranges from instability to displacement)
  a. Two basic types
    i. **Congenital:** develops in utero, perinatally, or postnatally; early in utero, associated with other severe malformations, such as arthrogryposis and myelomeningocele.
    ii. **Developmental:** usually develops within first 2 weeks after birth with subluxation or dislocation; higher incidence with breech deliveries.
  b. Diagnosis
    i. Ortolani's sign: palpable click with flexing and abduction, causing reduction.
    ii. Barlow's sign: slowly moving hip into adduction causes dislocation.
    iii. Galeazzi's sign: femoral shortening with asymmetric knee levels with infant supine and heels together, hip and knees flexed.
    iv. Ultrasound is imaging technique of choice.
  c. **Treatment** with reduction, Pavlik harness, or alternative orthoses.
    i. If conservative treatment not successful, open reduction may be needed.
    ii. Other surgery for stabilization may be necessary (i.e., osteotomies).
  d. Avascular necrosis is uncommon but may occur. If ossification of femoral head is not seen by 1 year of age, avascular necrosis is suspected.
5. **Anteversion of femoral head/neck:** coxa valga and coxa vara.
6. **Femoral retroversion**: more common in patients with Down syndrome or Ehlers-Danlos syndrome.
7. **Tibial torsion**
8. **Infantile tibia vara** (Blount's disease)
9. **Genu varum:** associated with Blount's disease, hypophosphatemic rickets, metaphyseal chondrodysplasia, focal fibrocartilaginous dysplasia.

10. **Genu valgum**
11. **Talipes equinus** (clubfoot): foot in equinus with forefoot and hindfoot varus and severe adduction.
    a. Incidence: 1 in 400 live births with 1 in 10 chance of inheritance if parent is affected.
    b. Can result from intrauterine crowding.
    c. Also associated with myelodysplasia, arthrogryposis, and hip dislocation.
12. **Pes planus:** failure of tarsal bones to separate; rigid form is associated with other anomalies in 50% of cases.
13. **Talocalcaneal coalition** (48% of coalitions)
14. **Calcaneonavicular coalition** (43% of coalitions)
15. **Rigid cavus foot:** may be related to metatarsalgia, clawing, and intrinsic muscle atrophy; atrophy may be caused by an underlying neurologic condition.
16. **Arthrogryposis multiplex congenita:** multiple joint contractures present at birth.
17. **Treatment** of conditions 4–15 includes casting, orthotics, physical therapy for gait training, range-of-motion exercises, compensatory strengthening, and surgery (if necessary).
18. **Constitutional conditions of bone:** five categories
    a. Category 1: defects of tubular bone or spinal growth, either present at birth or manifested late in life; includes achondroplasia and various types of dwarfism, chondrodysplasias, epiphyseal and spondyloepiphyseal dysplasias.
    b. Category 2: disorganized cartilage and fibrous components; includes fibrodysplasia and multiple cartilaginous exostoses.
    c. Category 3: abnormal bone density or structure; includes osteopetrosis and osteogenesis imperfecta.
    d. Category 4: metabolic conditions generally affecting calcium or phosphorous metabolism; includes types of rickets and mucopolysaccharidoses.
    e. Category 5: extraskeletal disorders; includes sickle cell anemia, renal osteodystrophy, and hyperparathyroidism.

Bibliography
1. Betz RR: The Child with a Spinal Cord Injury. Rosemont, IL, American Academy of Orthopaedic Surgeons, 1996.
2. Campbell SK: Physical Therapy for Children. Philadelphia, W.B. Saunders, 1994.
3. Dubowitz V: Muscle Disorders in Childhood, 2nd ed. Philadelphia, W.B. Saunders, 1995.
4. Molnar GE: Pediatric Rehabilitation, 3rd ed. Philadelphia, Hanley & Belfus, 1999.
5. Staheli LT: Fundamentals of Pediatric Orthopedics. Philadelphia, Lippincott-Raven, 1998.

Chapter 8

SPINAL CORD INJURY REHABILITATION

William M. Scelza, M.D., and Austin I. Nobunaga, M.D., M.P.H.

I. **General Principles**
   A. Traumatic spinal cord injury (SCI) can be a devastating event, and rehabilitation is the first step in renewing a sense of independence.
   B. Physiatrists need to be able to coordinate a team of health care professionals as well as manage the medical concerns of patients.
   C. Rehabilitation of patients with SCI lasts long beyond their stay on an acute rehabilitation unit; both short- and long-term goals should be set as soon as possible to help ease the transition.

II. **Epidemiology and Statistics**
   A. **Incidence:** approximately 10,000 new cases per year (30–40 per million).
   B. **Prevalence:** currently estimated at > 200,000 persons in U.S.
   C. **Gender:** approximately 4:1 male-to-female ratio.
   D. **Average age** = 32.3 years old (54.1% of new injuries affect people 16–30 years old); average age continues to increase.
   E. **Causes of traumatic SCI** (Table 1)

TABLE 1.   Causes of Traumatic Spinal Cord Injury by Gender and Year

Gender/Cause	Year of Injury					Total
	1973–1977	*1978–1982*	*1983–1988*	*1989–1993*	*1994–1998*	
Males						
Auto accidents	34.0	34.7	32.0	28.5	29.7	31.4
Falls	17.2	15.7	19.2	19.7	21.7	19.0
Gunshot	12.7	13.0	15.7	24.1	22.4	18.3
Diving	10.6	10.6	9.3	6.0	4.8	8.0
Motorcycle	6.9	7.9	6.6	5.2	4.6	6.1
Falling objects	6.7	4.4	3.5	3.1	2.9	3.8
Medical/surgical	0.7	1.3	1.6	2.0	2.5	1.7
Pedestrian	1.5	1.3	1.7	1.7	1.7	1.6
All others	10.4	12.4	12.0	11.7	12.2	11.8
Females						
Auto accidents	49.9	53.7	51.9	50.6	49.1	51.0
Falls	15.7	16.1	19.0	17.7	19.8	18.0
Gunshot	13.6	11.1	9.3	12.6	11.1	11.3
Medical/surgical	1.8	2.0	4.2	5.1	5.7	4.1
Diving	5.1	4.2	3.3	2.3	2.5	3.2
Pedestrian	1.6	2.6	2.4	2.5	2.2	2.3
Motorcycle	3.3	2.4	1.4	0.5	2.0	1.7
Falling objects	0.8	0.5	0.5	1.0	1.0	0.8
All others	8.4	7.4	8.0	7.7	6.6	7.5

Data reported are percentages. Data from Nobunaga AI, Go BK, Karunas RB: Recent demographic and injury trends in people served by the Model Spinal Cord Injury Core Systems. Arch Phys Med Rehabil 80:1372–1382, 1999, with permission.

F. **Trends**
    1. Increase in violence from 13.9% in 1973–1977 to 21.8% in 1994–1998.
    2. Violence and motor vehicle accidents much more likely in persons < 30 years old.
    3. Falls are more common in persons > 45 years.
    4. Incidence higher in summer than winter months and on weekends vs. week days.
G. **Level and extent**
    1. Paraplegia (incomplete): 19.7%
    2. Paraplegia (complete): 26.1%
    3. Tetraplegia (incomplete): 30.2%
    4. Tetraplegia (complete): 23.3%
III. **Anatomy of the Spine and Spinal Cord**
    A. **Spine and nerve roots** (Fig. 1)

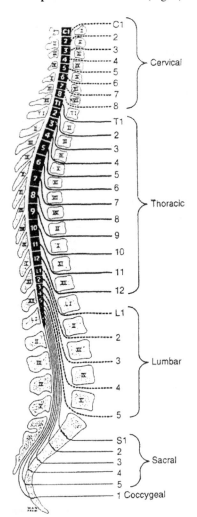

FIGURE 1.   Anatomy of spine and nerve roots. The conus medullaris lies in the L1–L2 interspace. The dural cul-de-sac ends at S2. (From Haymaker W, Woodhall B: Peripheral Nerve Injuries, 2nd ed. Philadelphia, W.B. Saunders, 1952, p 32, with permission.)

TABLE 2.   Reflexes

Level	Reflex
C5	Biceps
C6	Brachioradialis
C7	Triceps
T6–T12 (abdominal)	Superficial abdoinal reflex*
L1—L2	Cremasteric
L4	Patella
S1	Achilles
S3–S4	Bulbocavernosus
S3–S5	Anal wink

* With the patient supine, gently stroke a blunt object toward the umbilicus. The normal response is a brief and brisk movement of the umbilicus toward the stimulus.

1. Vertebrae: 7 cervical, 12 thoracic, 5 lumbar, 5 sacral (fused).
2. Nerve roots: 8 cervical, 12 thoracic, 5 lumbar, 5 sacral.
3. Dorsal root: afferent (sensory) messages from body.
4. Ventral root: efferent (motor) from anterior horn cells.
5. Dermatomes (see p. 125 for dermatomal distributions)
6. Reflexes (Table 2)
7. Blood supply
   a. Anterior spinal artery supplies anterior two-thirds of spinal cord.
   b. Paired posterior spinal arteries supply posterior third of spinal cord.
   c. Both are supplied via radicular arteries, the largest of which is the artery of Adamkiewicz, which enters the spinal canal in the lower thoracic segments but sends branches as high as the T4 level.
B. **Major long tracts and organization of the spinal cord** (Fig. 2)
   1. Dorsal columns = ascending tracts that relay proprioception.
   2. Anterior spinothalamic tract = ascending tracts that relay pain and temperature sensation.

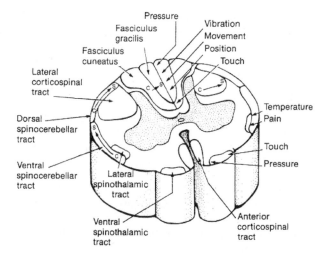

FIGURE 2.   Cross-sectional organization of spinal cord, indicating ascending and descending spinal cord tracts. C → S = cervical to sacral in direction of arrow. (From Burke DC, Murray DC: Handbook of Spinal Cord Medicine. New York, Raven Press, 1975, p 7.)

   3. Corticospinal tracts = descending tracts from brain (upper motor neurons) that relay motor information to anterior horn cells.
   4. Anterior horn cells = cell bodies that arise from anterior horn of spinal cord are primary efferent fibers that innervate muscle (lower motor neurons).
   5. Somatotropic organization = how the specific segments (i.e., cervical, thoracic, lumbar, and sacral) are organized within the individual tracts of the spinal cord.

IV. Acute Management
   A. Recognize trauma and **suspect SCI**.
   B. **ABCs: a**irway, **b**reathing, **c**irculation.
   C. **Always immobilize spine** with backboard and cervical precautions to prevent or minimize neurologic compromise.
   D. Appropriate resuscitation and treatment of **other injuries**.
   E. **High-dose steroids** (30 mg/kg methylprednisolone IV loading dose for 15 minutes followed by 5.4 mg/kg/hour IV over next 23 hours) may be of benefit, if administered within 8 hours of injury. Much debate still surrounds the benefit of steroids.
   F. Be aware of **spinal shock**, defined as initial flaccid paralysis below the level of injury after an upper motor neuron lesion.
      1. Increased tone and spasticity begin to develop hours to weeks afterward.
      2. Spinal shock can initially present with hypotension.
      3. Differentiate between cardiogenic shock, acute blood loss, and other conditions.
      4. Return of the bulbocavernosus reflex heralds the end of spinal shock.
   G. **Further spine stabilization with orthosis or surgery**, as indicated.

V. Spinal Cord Syndromes
   A. **Brown-Sequard syndrome**
      1. **Pathophysiology:** hemisection of spinal cord due to trauma, tumor, and the like.
      2. **Clinical features**
         a. Produces ipsilateral paralysis and loss of proprioception due to the crossing of the corticospinal tracts and dorsal columns in the brainstem.
         b. Produces contralateral loss of pain and temperature sensation due to local crossing of the spinothalamic tracts in the spinal cord.
   B. **Central cord syndrome**
      1. **Pathophysiology**
         a. Primarily a lesion in the central gray matter and medial white matter tracts in the cervical spinal cord due to compression/ischemia.
         b. Lesion affects the local gray matter and medial laminations of the corticospinal and spinothalamic tracts, which supply the upper extremities, with relative sparing of the lateral laminations, which supply the lumbar and sacral lesions.
         c. Usually seen in hyperextension injuries to the cervical spine, particularly in older persons with degenerative arthritis in the cervical spine.
      2. **Clinical features**
         a. Produces greater weakness in upper extremities than lower extremities with sacral sparing.
         b. Sometimes referred to as the "walking quad" because most patients have sufficient lower extremity strength for ambulation but more significant upper extremity involvement and weakness.

C. **Anterior cord syndrome**
   1. **Pathophysiology**
      a. Typically involves disruption in blood flow to the anterior spinal artery (trauma, embolus, hypotension).
      b. Causes ischemia/infarction of the anterior two-thirds of the spinal cord, corresponding to the distribution of the anterior spinal artery.
   2. **Clinical features:** absence of motor function and pain sensation, with preserved proprioception.
D. **Conus medullaris syndrome**
   1. **Pathophysiology:** injury to the sacral spinal cord at the level of the conus medullaris.
   2. **Clinical features**
      a. Similar to cauda equina syndrome, but sacral reflexes may be preserved.
      b. "True" spinal cord injury with upper motor neuron findings.
E. **Cauda equina syndrome**
   1. **Pathophysiology:** lesion of the lumbosacral nerve roots within the neural canal.
   2. **Clinical features**
      a. Results in flaccid paralysis and sensory loss to the lower extremities because lesion involves the peripheral nerves.
      b. Areflexia of the bowel and bladder.
      c. Lower motor neuron findings.
F. **Syringomyelia (syrinx)**
   1. **Pathophysiology**
      a. Gradual enlargement of a fluid filled cyst within the central canal of the spinal cord, usually beginning at the zone of injury.
      b. Asymptomatic cysts may be present in up to 50% of patients and can cause neurologic decline in up to 5% of patients.
   2. **Clinical features**
      a. Expands rostrally and caudally and may cause neurologic decline (weakness, loss of reflexes, numbness, respiratory decline) as it causes more spinal cord damage.
      b. Incomplete injuries may sustain further neurologic decline below the neurological level of injury as well with caudal migration.
      c. MRI is diagnostic tool of choice in absence of contraindication (e.g., metal fragments, surgical hardware); then CT myelogram may be necessary.
      d. Often difficult to treat. Diuresis and avoidance of certain positions is usually first-line treatment.
      e. Percutaneous tap may be dangerous because of position of syrinx and is usually of only transient benefit.
      f. Syringoperitoneal shunts may be considered to prevent the progression of neurologic deficits. Shunt obstruction may be problematic.
V. **Clinical Evaluation and Examination**
   A. **Definitions**
      1. **Neurologic level:** most caudal segment with normal sensory and motor function on both sides of the body.
      2. **Sensory level:** most caudal segment with normal sensory function (both pin-prick and light touch); recorded bilaterally.
      3. **Motor level:** most caudal key muscle that is at least grade 3, provided that all key muscle groups above are judged to be normal (for those levels

not represented by key muscle groups, the sensory level is used); recorded bilaterally.

4. **Skeletal level:** level at which radiographic abnormality is seen.
5. **Incomplete injury:** partial preservation of sensory and/or motor function below the neurologic level; includes the lowest sacral segment.
6. **Motor incomplete:** partial preservation of sensory and/or motor function in the sacral segments S4–S5. The patient also must have *either* voluntary anal sphincter contraction *or* sparing of motor function more than three levels below the motor level.
7. **Complete injury:** no sensory and motor function below the level of injury.
8. **Zone of partial preservation:** used only in complete injuries. It is the most caudal segment below the neurologic level of injury with some sensory and/or motor function; recorded as sensory and motor levels bilaterally.

B. **Neurologic examination** (Figs. 3 and 4)
1. **Sensory exam:** pin-prick and light touch tested in the 28 dermatomes on the right and left sides. (Pin-prick is intact only if sensation is normal and sharp-dull discrimination is accurate).
2. **Motor exam:** testing motor strength in 10 defined myotomes on the right and left sides.
3. **Rectal exam:** assess sensation to anal mucocutaneous junction. Motor function defined as presence or absence of voluntary contraction of external anal sphincter.
4. Determine **motor and sensory levels** on the right and left sides.
5. Assign level on **ASIA Impairment Scale** (Fig. 5).
6. Determine **zone of partial preservation** if injury is complete.
7. **Add motor and sensory scores**.

VII. **Medical Complications**
A. **Cardiovascular**
1. **Deep venous thrombosis** (DVT) (See chapter 13, Deep Venous Thrombosis)
   a. **Pathophysiology:** risk factors include paralysis, associated trauma/fractures, transient hypercoaguble state, surgical procedures, and previous DVT.
   b. **Clinical features**
      i. May be present as early as 3 days after injury; risk is increased up to 1 year (highest in first 2 weeks).
      ii. Pulmonary embolism is most severe complication.
      iii. Signs and symptoms include unilateral swelling, pain, erythema, and low-grade temperature.
   c. **Diagnosis and treatment**
      i. Diagnosis via Doppler ultrasound. Venogram is gold standard test.
      ii. Full anticoagulation with heparin and warfarin for 3–6 months or as long as clinically warranted. Vena caval filter should be placed if anticoagulation is contraindicated and/or pulmonary reserve is decreased.
   d. Clinical practice guidelines for **DVT prophylaxis** (See chapter 13, Deep Venous Thrombosis)
      i. Anticoagulant prophylaxis with low-molecular-weight or unfractionated heparin within 72 hours of injury (if no contraindication is present).

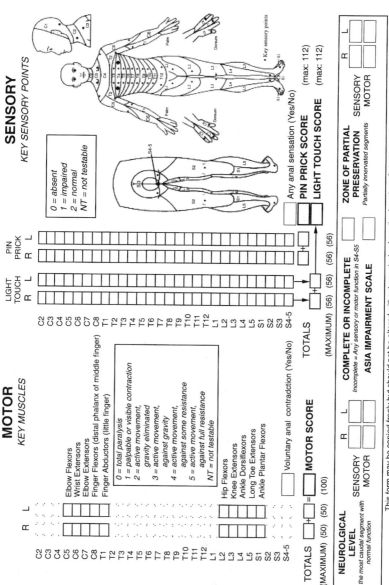

FIGURE 3. Standard neurologic classification of spinal cord injury. (Courtesy of American Spinal Injury Association.)

L	7 Complete Independence (Timely, Safely) 6 Modified Independence (Device)	No Helper
E V E L S	**Modified Dependence** 5 Supervision 4 Minimal Assist (Subject = 75%+) 3 Moderate Assist (Subject = 50%+) **Complete Dependence** 2 Maximal Assist (Subject = 25%+) 1 Total Assist (Subject = 0%+)	Helper

ADMIT   DISCH

Self Care
A. Eating
B. Grooming
C. Bathing
D. Dressing-Upper Body
E. Dressing- Lower Body
F. Toileting

Sphincter Control
G. Bladder Management
H. Bowel Management

Mobility
Transfer:
I. Bed, Chair, Wheelchair
J. Toilet
K. Tub, Shower

Locomotion
L. Walk/Wheelchair   W ☐   W ☐
                       C ☐   C ☐
M. Stairs

Communication
N. Comprehension   A ☐   A ☐
O. Expression   V ☐   V ☐
                       V ☐   V ☐
                       N ☐   N ☐
Social Cognition
P. Social Interaction
Q. Problem Solving
R. Memory

Total FIM

Leave no blanks; enter 1 if patient not
testable due to risk.

FIGURE 4. Functional Independence Measure (FIM). (Courtesy of American Spinal Injury Association).

ii. Recommended prophylaxis course is 8 weeks for uncomplicated motor complete injuries, 12 weeks (or until discharge) for motor complete injuries and other risk factors. However, course may be individualized depending on condition and needs of patient.

iii. Vena caval filter should be considered if anticoagulant prophylaxis is contraindicated, prophylaxis fails, or patient has high cervical lesion or limited pulmonary reserve.

iv. If DVT is present, exercise and mobilization of the patient should be withheld for 48–72 hours.

2. **Autonomic dysreflexia (AD)**

a. **Definition:** an acute syndrome of uninhibited sympathetic discharge as a result of noxious stimuli.

b. **Pathophysiology**

i. Patients typically have SCI at the level of T6 and above. Noxious stimuli below the lesion stimulate splanchnic sympathetic response

☐ **A = Complete:** No motor or sensory function is preserved in the sacral segments S4-S5.

☐ **B = Incomplete:** Sensory but not motor function is preserved below the neurological level and includes the sacral segements S4-S5

☐ **C = Incomplete:** Motor function is preserved below the neurological level, and more than half of key muscles below the newurological level have a muscle grade less than 3.

☐ **D = Incomplete:** Motor function is preserved below the neurological level, and at least half of key muscles below the neurological level have a muscle grade of 3 or more.

☐ **E = Normal:** motor and sensory function is normal

FIGURE 5. American Spinal Injury Association (ASIA) scale for assessment of impairment.

CLINICAL SYNDROMES

☐ Central Cord
☐ Brown-Sequard
☐ Anterior Cord
☐ Conus Medullaris
☐ Cauda Equina

(splanchnic outflow between T6 and L2) that cannot be inhibited because of SCI.

  ii. This can cause severe vasoconstriction and elevated blood pressure (BP). Elevated BP may be sensed by carotid baroreceptors and may cause reflex bradycardia due to increased parasympathetic output. Secondary inhibition of sympathetic outflow from higher centers is unable to pass below the lesion.

  iii. Common causes include bladder distention, urinary tract infection, impacted bowel, pressure ulcers, ingrown toenails, fracture, or anything that can be considered noxious stimuli.

c. **Clinical features**

  i. The major sign is paroxysmal hypertension (20–40 mmHg increase above baseline). Recall that normal systolic BP in patients with SCI can run 90–100 mmHg, especially in tetraplegia. Other signs and symptoms include bradycardia/tachycardia and headache. Flushing and sweating may be present above the level of the lesion.

d. **Treatment**

  i. If left untreated, AD can result in hypertensive crisis, seizures, arrhythmia, stroke, or even death.

  ii. The first and most important step is to decrease BP. Sit the patient upright and remove support hose/abdominal binder. Now identify the noxious stimuli. Catheterize the patient (use lidocaine jelly because irritation may exacerbate problem), disimpact the bowel, remove tight clothing, and check the skin. In most cases, this protocol identifies the cause of AD and reverses the symptoms.

   iii. If primary measures result in no improvement, consider a short acting antihypertensive medication with rapid onset while continuing to investigate causes. Also watch for symptomatic hypotension. Monitoring in an intensive care unit may be necessary.

   iv. **Antihypertensive agents:** no specific "best agents" have been identified. Below is a list of medications commonly used in the management of AD:

- Nifedipine, 10 mg orally, is a calcium-channel blocker and arterial vasodilator commonly used as a first-line agent. Dose may be repeated in 30–60 minutes.
- Nitropaste: $\frac{1}{2}$ to 2 inches applied directly to skin. Nitrates are venous dilators and are easily applied and may be wiped off. Watch for hypotension.
- Hydralazine, 10–20 mg IV or orally, is a potent arterial dilator usually reserved for more severe cases.
- Clonidine is started at 0.1 mg orally. This alpha$_2$ agonist decreases central sympathetic outflow and acts quickly. A patch form may be used as a prophylactic agent.
- Alpha$_1$ antagonists sometimes are used as prophylactic agents to suppress hypertensive episodes. Be careful in patients with underlying systolic blood pressure < 100 mmHg.
- Nitroprusside is a potent intravenous agent used for hypertensive emergencies. Patients must be in an intensive care setting when this medication is used.

   v. Medications should be used reluctantly. Once the noxious stimuli is identified and removed, BP will fall. After giving an antihypertensive agent, one may have to treat hypotension with IV fluids and/or Trendelenburg position, thus increasing the risk of bladder distention and another episode of AD.

B. **Metabolic/bone**

  1. **Heterotopic ossification** (see chapter14, Heterotopic Ossification)

   a. **Definition:** deposition of new bone around a joint. It is actual bone and not merely calcification of soft tissues.

   b. **Clinical features**

    i. Particularly found below the level of the spinal cord lesion. It may severely limit ROM, fuse joints, alter seating, or predispose patient to a pressure ulcer.

    ii. Poorly understood onset is usually within first 6 months of injury.

    iii. Signs include swelling, redness and warmth of the extremity (often confused with DVT or fracture) and decreased ROM about a joint.

   c. **Diagnosis:** plain x-rays, triple-phase bone scan (usually shows changes 7–10 days before plain X-ray), elevated alkaline phosphotase levels.

   d. **Treatment**

    i. Disodium etidronate (20 mg/kg/day for 2 weeks, then 10 mg/kg/day for ~12 weeks). Bisphosphonate limits extent of ossification but does not reverse it. Also has been used for prophylaxis.

    ii. Important for physical therapist to maintain range of motion without pushing to extremes and causing more damage.

      iii. Surgery to remove HO may be indicated only after bone matures (stable exam, stable x-rays, normal alkaline phosphatase levels, decreased uptake of triple phase bone scan), or reoccurrence is likely.

      iv. Radiation and indomethacin has also been taken prevent HO.

2. **Immobilization hypercalcemia**

  a. **Pathophysiology**

      i. Immobilization after SCI causes an increase in bone resorption.

      ii. Sometimes bone resorption exceeds ability of kidneys to excrete calcium, leading to hypercalcemia.

      iii. Bone mass and calcium metabolism eventually reach a steady state 6 or more months after injury, and patient is left with decreased bone mass below the level of the lesion.

  b. **Clinical features**

      i. Onset usually 2 weeks to 6 months after injury, most frequently in adolescent males.

      ii. Symptoms of hypercalcemia include lethargy, fatigue, nausea, anorexia, cramping, polydipsia, and polyuria.

      iii. Hypercalciuria develops first, followed by hypercalcemia and onset of clinical symptoms.

      iv. Also consider other causes (e.g., hypercalcemia of malignancy).

  c. **Treatment**

      i. Treat initially with aggressive intravenous fluids with normal saline for mild to moderate hypercalcemia (10.4–12.0 mg/dl).

      ii. May also add furosemide to prevent fluid overload and inhibit calcium reabsorption from the kidneys.

      iii. IV bisphosphonates may be required for severe hypercalcemia.

      iv. Bisphosphonates, calcitonin, weight bearing (if possible) also used for long-term treatment.

C. **Pulmonary**

1. **Muscles of respiration**

  a. Diaphragm: innervated by cervical roots C3–C5 (phrenic nerve).

  b. Intercostal muscles: innervated by thoracic spinal segments. Some cervical and shoulder girdle muscles also may contribute during strong inspiration.

  c. Abdominal muscles: innervated by thoracic spinal segments; primarily muscles of expiration. Contraction squeezes abdominal contents superiorly and elevates diaphragm, particularly in strong expiration and cough.

2. **Changes with SCI**

  a. Patients with high cervical spinal cord injuries (C3 and above) are usually ventilator-dependent because of loss of phrenic nerve function to the diaphragm.

  b. Patients with thoracic spinal cord injuries lose intercostal and abdominal muscles that aid in inspiration and expiration. The higher the level, the more severe the dysfunction. Cough is also impaired.

  c. Expiration is primarily due to elastic recoil of rib cage and is a passive process.

  d. Patients with tetraplegia may lose expiratory reserve; thus, inspiratory capacity usually equals vital capacity.

  e. Effects of positioning in tertaplegic persons: Vital capacity improves with supine position. The relative displacement of the diaphragm into the chest in the supine position aids in diaphragmatic function (paradoxical pattern of respiration).

f. Abdominal binder aids in respiration while patient is in upright position because of displacement of abdominal contents and diaphragmatic position.

3. **Other concerns**
    a. Aggressive pulmonary toilet and assisted cough maneuvers important to maintain good pulmonary hygiene.
    b. Effective diagnosis of swallowing dysfunction and implementation of compensatory strategies to minimize risks of aspiration and other complications.
    c. Attempt to minimize environmental risks (e.g., smoking cessation, pneumococcal/influenza vaccinations, and regular medical follow-up).

4. **Tracheostomy management**
    a. Tracheostomy indicated for all patients who require long-term ventilatory support.
    b. Cuffed tracheostomy for patients who have poor pulmonary reserve and/or difficulty with clearing secretions. Avoid over inflating cuff (> 25 cmH_2O) to prevent subglottic stenosis.
    c. Cuffless tracheostomy may be used in stable ventilator-dependent patients to aid with communication.
    d. Implement appropriate tracheostomy care.

5. **Basic ventilator concerns**
    a. Long-term mechanical ventilation usually needed for patients with spinal cord injuries at C3 and above.
    b. Most common mode is positive pressure mechanical ventilation.
    c. Tidal volumes maintained at 10–15 ml/kg are recommended.
    f. Positive end-expiratory pressure (PEEP) of up to 5 cm may be used without significant risk of barotrauma.
    g. Adjust FiO_2 to maintain arterial oxygen saturation > 92%.

6. **Ventilator weaning**
    a. **General considerations**
        i. All patients with C2 tetraplegia need some form of ventilatory assistance.
        ii. Most C3 and C4 tetraplegics should be able to wean completely from ventilatory assistance.
        iii. Virtually all C5 tetraplegics should be able to wean completely from ventilator if their medical condition permits.
    b. **Requirements for weaning**
        i. Patients must be willing to begin weaning and be free from any medical conditions (e.g., pneumonia, atelectasis, pulmonary effusions).
        ii. Secretions must be minimal.
        iii. Vital capacity must be sufficient (> 1000 cc or 15cc/kg).
        iv. Negative inspiratory force (NIF) > 20 ccH_2O.
        v. Patients must be closely supervised by certified respiratory therapist.
    c. **Monitoring of weaning**
        i. Patient must advance slowly through wean protocol.
        ii. Monitor vital signs and respiratory parameters (forced vital capacity, NIF, and oxygen saturation) very closely.
        iii. Follow arterial blood gases when indicated.

iv. **Discontinue wean** in presence of any of following:
- Tachycardia.
- Tachypnea.
- Hypertension or hypotension
- Cyanosis
- Significant increase in FiO_2 requirements.
- Mental status changes.

D. Gastrointestinal concerns

1. **Neurogenic bowel** (See chapter 16, Neurogenic Bowel Management)
   a. Major medical and social concern for persons with SCI.
   b. Innervation from sacral segments (parasympathetic/sympathetic) and enteric nervous system (within the bowel).
   c. Because of impaired somatic innervation at external anal sphincter, sensation of fullness and urge to defecate also are impaired.
   d. Lower motor neuron bowel (as may be seen in cauda equina syndrome) has characteristics of slowed stool propulsion and little or no tone of sphincter mechanisms.
   e. Upper motor neuron bowel (as seen in lesions above the conus medullaris) may be associated with longer mouth-to-cecum transit times. Hyperactive/hypoactive peristalsis may be present, and increased sphincter tone may lead to colonic distention and need for mechanical/chemical trigger to defecate.

2. **Ileus**
   a. Altered neurologic input, metabolic, pneumonia, or dietary changes may contribute to development of ileus, especially in the acute stages of SCI.
   b. Signs and symptoms: abdominal pain and distention, absent bowel sounds. Serial X-rays exams aid in diagnosis and following progress.
   c. Treat with decompression and supportive care. Surgical consultation should be considered if symptoms do not improve in timely matter with decompression.

3. **Diarrhea**
   a. Be suspicious of *Clostridium difficile* colitis, especially in patients with history of antibiotic use. Evaluate for other potential infectious causes as well.
   b. High-level stool compaction can sometimes present with diarrhea as liquid stool passes around the obstruction. Abdominal X-rays may help aid in diagnosis.
   c. Review all medications. Excessive use of laxatives, stool softeners, or antibiotics may also cause diarrhea.

4. **Acute abdomen**
   a. Index of suspicion must be high because altered abdominal sensation and muscle function may not provide typical symptoms that normally direct examiner to intra-abdominal process.
   b. Autonomic dysreflexia may be presenting symptom.
   c. Low threshold for surgical consulatation because of poor localization of abdominal complaints.
   d. Consider use of ulcer prophylaxis with H_2 antagonists or proton pump inhibitors, especially if patient is in acute stress from injury, takes steroids, or has other risk factors.

E. **Neurogenic bladder** (see chapter 16, Neurogenic Bladder Management)
   1. Innervation from sympathetic/parasympathetic sacral micturation center. Higher cortical and pontine centers provide volitional and coordinated sphincter control, respectively.
   2. Lower motor neuron bladder (as with cauda equina syndrome) is a high-volume bladder without presence of detrusor sphincter dyssynergia. Little or no contractile force from detrusor muscle.
   3. Upper motor neuron bladder (as with spinal lesions above the conus medullaris) is a low-volume spastic bladder. Detrusor sphincter dyssynergia is present and puts patients at risk for upper urinary tract complications.
   4. Major medical and social implications for persons with SCI.
F. **Spasticity** (see chapter 19, Spasticity)
   1. **Pathophysiology:** after acute SCI and a phase of spinal shock, development of reflexes and tone gradually begins to increase. This process often coincides with motor recovery.
   2. **Clinical features: phasic and tonic patterns**
      a. Phasic stretch reflex characterized by presence of velocity dependent hypertonicity, clonus, and extensor pattern.
      b. Tonic stretch reflex often elicited by noxious stimulus (i.e., pressure ulcer) and tends to be flexor in nature.
   3. **Treatment**
      a. Depends on whether spasticity interferes with such functions as transfers, ADLs, sleep, perineal care, or seating posture of patient.
      b. Spasticity can be of benefit to patients in such activities as standing and transfers. Thus, many factors must be taken into consideration before treatment is initiated.
G. **Skin care** (see chapter 18, Skin Care).
   1. Many factors can contribute to the formation of pressure ulcers in patients with SCI, incuding:
      a. Insensate skin
      b. Decreased muscle mass/poor nutrition
      c. Pressure over bony protuberances
      d. Excessive sitting/lying
      e. Spasticity or contractures
      f. Improper fitting garments
      g. Burns from hot water
   2. It is important to recognize and address these potential hazards with appropriate preventive measures and care.
H. **Pain in SCI**. Pain in persons with SCI has been difficult to classify. It may be due to various types of repetitive trauma above the neurologic level, or it may be neuropathic pain below the level of injury. For specific treatment, see chapters 11, Acute and Chronic Pain, and 23, Pharmacology.
   1. **Pain above neurologic level of injury**
      a. **Nocireceptive**
         i. May result from trauma or previous surgery.
         ii. Overuse injuries (e.g., rotator cuff tendinopathy in chronic wheelchair users) are common. Weakness due to prolonged immobilization also may contribute to such musculoskeletal conditions.
         iv. Headache associated with autonomic dysreflexia.

b. **Neuropathic**

　i. Compressive neuropathies (e.g., carpal tunnel syndrome), especially in users of wheelchair and other assistive devices.

　ii. Central causes, such as nerve root irritation or syringomyelia.

2. **Pain at or below neurologic level of injury**

a. **Nociceptive**

　i. Often in the zone of partial preservation and may be much different from similar conditions above neurologic level.

　ii. Be aware of previous injuries, spinal instability, and infections.

　iii. Acute abdomen should always be considered.

b. **Neuropathic**

　i. Radicular pain and paresthesias, particularly in the zone of partial preservation, may be present with nerve root irritation.

　ii. Hyperesthesia and allodynia are common.

　iii. Neuropathic pain below complete injuries, often described as burning/cold or "pins and needles" in nondermatomal patterns, is very common.

　iv. Complex regional pain syndrome also may be observed.

VIII. **Goals for Rehabilitation**

　A. Educate patient and family about SCI.

　B. Maximize proficiency with mobility and self-care and/or learning to direct care as necessary.

　C. Teach appropriate bowel and bladder routines.

　D. Prevent comorbidities (e.g., contractures, skin break down, pulmonary care) associated with SCI.

　E. Assess psychological well-being and initiate community/vocational reintegration.

　F. Define long-term goals based on severity of injury and family/community resources.

　G. **Strive for maximal independence.**

IX. **Outcomes**

　A. **Expected motor outcomes**

　　1. Perform ASIA exam within 72 hours after injury.

　　2. Repeat ASIA exam 3–7 days after injury.

　　3. Repeat after any surgical intervention or complaint of changing neurologic status.

　　4. Monitor periodically until plateau achieved.

　　5. Monitor periodically throughout lifetime.

　　6. Majority of recovery occurs in first 2 months and slows over next 3–6 months. Recovery has been noted as long as 2 years after injury.

　B. **Motor recovery**

　　1. In complete tetraplegia, key muscles with grade 1 or 2 strength that are one level below muscles with grade 3 strength or better (motor level) have 90% chance of reaching antigravity at 1 year.

　　2. Key muscles with grade 0 strength have 45% chance of reaching antigravity in 1 year and may continue to improve.

　　3. In tetraplegics, one level may drastically increase functional outcomes.

　　4. Not relevant for paraplegics because there are no key muscles for recovery in thoracic region.

　C. **Prognosis for ambulation**

　　1. ASIA A: 3–6% recover functional strength in lower extremities.

TABLE 3. Typical Functional Outcomes in Patients with Complete Spinal Cord Injury

Location of Injury	Pressure Relief	Wheelchair Transfers	Wheelchair Propulsion	Ambulation	Orthotic Devices	Transportation	Communication
C3–C4	Independent in power recliner wheelchair; dependent in bed or manual wheelchair	Total dependence	Independent in pneumatic or chin control-driven power wheelchair with power recliner	Not applicable	Upper extremity externally powered orthosis, dorsal cock-up splint, BFOs	Dependent on others in accessible van with lift; unable to drive	Independent with adapted equipment for phone or typing
C5	Most require assistance	Assistance of one person with or without transfer board	Independent in powered wheelchair indoors and outdoors; short distances in manual wheelchair with adapted handrims indoors	Not applicable	As above	Independent driving in specially adapted van	As above
C6	Independent	Potentially independent with with transfer board	Independent moderate distances in manual wheelchair with plastic rims or lugs indoors; assistance needed outdoors; independent in hand-driven wheelchair	Not applicable	Wrist-driven orthosis, universal cuff, writing devices, built-up handles	Independent driving in specially adapted van	Independent with adapted equipment for phone, typing, and writing; independent in turning pages
C7	Independent	Independent with or without transfer board, including car, except to or floor with assistance	Independent in manual wheelchair indoors and outdoors, except stairs	Not applicable	None	Independent driving in car with hand controls or specially adapted van; independent placement of wheelchair into car	As above
C8–T1	Independent	Independent, including to and from floor and car	Independent in manual wheelchair indoors and outdoors; with curb escalators; assistance on stairs	Exercise only (not functional with	None	As above	Independent

Table continued on following page

TABLE 3. Typical Functional Outcomes in Patients with Complete Spinal Cord Injury *(Continued)*

Location of Injury	Pressure Relief	Wheelchair Transfers	Wheelchair Propulsion	Ambulation	Orthotic Devices	Transportation	Communication
T2–T10	Independent	Independent	Independent	Exercise only (not functional with orthoses); may not require assistance	Knee-ankle-foot orthoses with forearm crutches or walker	As above	Independent
T11–T12	Independent	Independent	Independent	Functional ambulation indoors with orthoses; stairs using railing	Knee-ankle-foot orthoses or ankle-foot orthoses with forearm crutches	As above	Independent
L3–S3	Independent	Independent	Independent	Community ambulation; independent indoors and outdoors with orthoses	Ankle-foot orthoses with forearm crutches or canes	As above	Independent

Location of Injury	Pulmonary Hygiene	Feeding	Grooming	Bathing	Dressing	Bowel and Bladder Routine	Bed Mobility
C3–C4	Totally assisted cough	May be unable to feed self; use of BFOs with universal cuff and adapted utensils indicated; drinks with long straw after set-up	Total dependence	Total dependence	Total dependence	Total dependence	Total dependence
C5	Assisted cough	Independent with specially adapted equipment for feeding after set-up	Independent with adapted equipment	Total dependence	Assistance with upper extremity dressing; dependent for lower extremity dressing	Total dependence	Assisted by others and by equipment

Table continued on following page

TABLE 3.   Typical Functional Outcomes in Patients with Complete Spinal Cord Injury *(Continued)*

Location of Injury	Pulmonary Hygiene	Feeding	Grooming	Dressing	Bathing	Bowel and Bladder Routine	Bed Mobility
C6	Some assistance required in supine position; independent in sitting position	Independent with equipment; drinks from glass	Independent with equipment	Independent with upper extremity dressing; assistance needed for lower extremity dressing	Independent in upper and lower extremity bathing with equipment	Independent for bowel routine; assistance needed with bladder routine	Independent with equipment
C8–T1	As above	Independent	Independent	Independent	Independent	Independent	Independent
T2–T10	T2–T6 as above; T6–T10, independent	Independent	Independent	Independent	Independent	Independent	Independent
T11–L2	Not applicable	Independent	Independent	Independent	Independent	Independent	Independent
L3–S3	Not applicable	Independent	Independent	Independent	Independent	Independent	Independent

BFO = balanced forearm orthosis.

From Staas WE, Formal CS, Freedman MK, et al: Spinal cord injury and spinal cord injury medicine. In DeLisa JA (ed): Rehabilitation Medicine, Principles and Practice, 3rd ed. Philadelphia, Lippincott Williams & Wilkins, 1998, pp 1276–1277, with permission.

2. ASIA B: 50% become ambulatory (prognosis better for patients with intact sacral pin sensation).
3. ASIA C: 75% become ambulatory in the community.
4. ASIA D: 95% become ambulatory in the community.
5. Prognosis worse with age > 50 years.

D. **Expected functional outcome**
   1. Table 3 (on previous three pages) offers guide to expected outcomes for persons who are motor-complete at 1 year after injury.
   2. Obviously patient's medical condition, social supports, cognitive abilities, and access to other resources have profound impact on outcomes.
   3. Guideline used for setting of goals and objective comparison of outcomes from different institutions.

Bibliography

1. American Spinal Injury Association: International Standards for Neurological Classification of Spinal Cord Injury, Revised. Chicago, American Spinal Injury Association, 2000.
2. Bryce TN. Ragnarsson KT: Pain after spinal cord injury. Phys Med Rehabil Clin North Am 11:157–168, 2000.
3. Bracken MB, Shepard MJ, et. al: Methylprednisolone or tirilazad mesylate administration after acute spinal cord injury: 1-year follow up. Results of the third National Acute Spinal Cord Injury randomized controlled trial. J Neurosurg 89:699–706, 1998.
4. Braddom RL. Rocco JF: Autonomic dysreflexia: A survey of current treatment. Am J Phys Med Rehabil 70(5):234–241, 1991.
5. Consortium for Spinal Cord Medicine: Clinical practice guidlines: Acute management of autonomic dysreflexia: Adults with spinal cord injury presenting to health-care facilities. Washington, DC: Paralyzed Veterans of America, 1997.
6. Consortium for Spinal Cord Medicine: Clinical practice guidlines: Outcomes following traumatic spinal cord injury: Clinical practice guidelines for health-care professionals. Washington, DC: Paralyzed Veterans of America, 1999.
7. Consortium for Spinal Cord Medicine: Clinical practice guidlines: Prevention of thromboembolism in spinal cord injury. Washington, DC: Paralyzed Veterans of America, 1999.
8. Lanig IS, Peterson P: The respiratory system in spinal cord injury. Phys Med Rehabil Clin North Am 11:29–43, 2000.
9. Little JW, Burns S,. James JJ, Stiens SA: Neurologic recovery and neurologic decline after spinal cord injury. Phys Med Rehabil Clin North Am 11:73–89, 2000.
10. Massagli TL, Cardenas DD: Immobilization hypercalcemia treatment with pamidronate disodium after spinal cord injury. Arch Phys Med Rehabil 80:998–1000, 1999.
11. Nobunaga AI, Go BK, Karunas RB: Recent demographic and injury trends in people served by the Model Spinal Cord Injury Care Systems. Arch Phys Med Rehabil 80:1372–1382, 1999.
12. Staas WE, Formal CS, Freedman MK, et al: Spinal cord injury and spinal cord injury medicine. In Delisa JA (ed): Rehabilitation Medicine Principles and Practice. 3rd ed. Philadelphia, Lippincott-Raven, 1998, pp 1259–1291.
13. Stiens SA, Bergman SB, Goetz LL: Neurogenic bowel dysfunction after spinal cord injury: Clinical evaluation and rehabilitative management. Arch Phys Med Rehabil 78(3 Suppl):S86–102, 1997.
14. Wagner R, Jagoda A: Spinal cord syndromes. Emerg Med Clin North Am 15(3):699–711, 1997.
15. Weingarden SI: The gastrointestinal system and spinal cord injury. Phys Med Rehabil Clin North Am 3:765–781, 1992.

Chapter 9

STROKE REHABILITATION

Christopher M. Brammer, M.D., and Gioia M. Herring, M.D.

I. General Principles

A. Stroke is a common problem that leaves many people with life-altering functional and neurologic deficits.

B. Timely recognition and treatment in the acute phase are important to minimize the permanent damage caused by various destructive factors.

C. Continued rehabilitation from the acute phase throughout the patient's medical course and beyond is essential to maximize recovery and restore function.

D. Understanding the management of patients with stroke throughout their acute presentation until discharge is essential so that the rehabilitation specialist can design an appropriate rehabilitation plan.

E. **Epidemiology**
1. 4,400,000 stroke survivors (2.2 million males, 2.3 million females).
2. Third leading cause of death (1 of every 14.5 deaths) after heart disease and cancer.
3. 600,000 strokes per year (500,000 new; 100,000 recurrent).
4. New stroke occurs every 53 seconds; death from stroke, every 3.3 minutes.
5. 29% of patients with strokes die within the first year (increased risk patients > 65 years), according to the Framingham Heart Study.
6. 72% of strokes occur in patients > 65 years of age.
7. After age 55, risk of stroke more than doubles in each successive decade.
8. 14 % of patients have a recurrent stroke or transient ischemic attack (TIA) within 1 year.
9. 50–70% of stroke survivors regain functional independence, whereas 15–30% are permanently disabled.

F. **Costs:** $4940 per hospitalization for TIA; $11,010 per hospitalization for cerebrovascular accident (CVA); $3.8 billion paid by Medicare for stroke care in 1996.

G. **Risk factors** (Table 1)

H. **Guidelines for primary prevention** (Table 2)

I. **Etiology and classification**
1. **Temporal**
   a. TIA: temporary neurologic deficit lasting < 24 hours and resolving completely.
   b. Reversible ischemic neurologic deficit (RIND): temporary neurologic deficit lasting > 24 hours but with eventual resolution.
   c. Stroke: neurologic deficit lasting > 24 hours with lasting neurologic deficits.
2. **Disease mechanism** (Table 3)

TABLE 1.   Risk Factors for Stroke

Nonmodifiable	Modifiable	Potentially Modifiable
Age	Hypertension	Obesity
Gender	Cardiac disease (e.g.,	Physical inactivity
Genetic predisposition	atrial fibrillation)	Heavy alcohol use
Race/ethnicity	Diabetes	Hyperhomocysteinemia
	Lipids	Drug abuse
	Cigarette smoking	Hypercoagulability states
	Asymptomatic carotid	Antiphospholipid antibody
	stenosis	Factor V Leiden
	Sickle cell disease	Prothrombin 20210 mutation
		Protein C deficiency
		Protein S deficiency
		Antithrombin III deficiency
		Hormone replacement therapy
		Oral contraceptive use
		Inflammatory processes

From Goldstein LB, et al: Primary prevention of ischemic stroke: A statement for healthcare professionals from the Stroke Council of the American Heart Association. Circulation 103:163–182, 2001, with permission.

II. Acute Evaluation and Treatment of Stroke

A. **Immediate goals:** localize deficit, stabilize patient, and salvage ischemic penumbra

B. **Evaluation:** ischemic vs. hemorrhagic stroke

1. Airway, breathing, circulation

2. **Differential diagnosis** of stroke: traumatic brain injury, hypertensive encephalopathy, intracranial mass, seizure with persistent symptoms, complex migraine, metabolic disturbances, hyper or hypoglycemia, poison or medication induced, uremia, psychiatric disorders, and shock.

3. **Differentiating stroke by mechanism**

   a. **Ischemic**

      i. **Thrombotic**
         - Symptoms progress over hours to days.
         - Classic patient awakes with minimal deficits that progress in a stepwise pattern.
         - History of prior TIA or stroke is common.

      ii. **Embolic**
         - Symptoms occur very rapidly, usually in seconds.
         - Typically the patient is awake and involved in an activity.
         - Patients often have no history of TIA or stroke.

   b. **Hemorrhagic**

      i. Headache and insidious loss of consciousness more common than in ischemic stroke. Other symptoms include nausea, vomiting, and elevated blood pressure.

      ii. Symptoms may not fit the anatomic distribution of a specific blood vessel.

      iii. Nuchal rigidity and retinal hemorrhages may be present; however, nuchal rigidity is not exclusive to hemorrhage (also seen in meningitis and inflammatory cause of ischemic stroke).

      iv. Many intracranial hemorrhages are lobar.
         - Occipital: ipsilateral eye pain and hemianopsia.

TABLE 2.   Guidelines for Primary Prevention of Stroke

Factor	Goal	Recommendations
Hypertension	SBP < 140 mmHg DBP < 90 mmHg	Measure BP in all adults at least every 2 years. Promote lifestyle modification: weight control, physical activity, moderation of alcohol intake, moderate sodium intake. If BP > 140/90 mmHg after 3 months of life habit modification or if initial BP > 180/100 mmHg, add antihypertensive medication; individualize therapy to patient's other requirements and characteristics.
Smoking	Cessation	Strongly encourage patient and family to stop smoking. Provide counseling, nicotine replacement, and formal programs as available.
Diabetes	Improved glucose control; treatment of hypertension	Diet, oral hypoglycemics, insulin.
Asymptomatic carotid stenosis		Endarterectomy may be considered in selected patients with > 60% and < 100% carotid stenosis, performed by surgeon with < 3% morbidity/mortality rates. Careful patient selection guided by comorbid conditions, life expectancy, patient preference, and other individual factors. Patients with asymptomatic stenosis should be fully evaluated for other treatable causes of stroke.
Atrial fibrillation		
Age < 65 y, no risk factors[†]		Aspirin
Age < 65 y, with risk factors[†]		Warfarin (target INR: 2.5; range: 2.0–3.0)
Age 65–75 y, no risk factors[†]		Aspirin or warfarin
Age 65–75 y, with risk factors[†]		Warfarin (target INR: 2.5; range: 2.0–3.0)
Age > 75 y, with or without risk factors[†]		Warfarin (target INR: 2.5; range: 2.0–3.0)
Lipids		
Initial evaluation (no CHD)		
TC < 200 mg/dl and HDL ≥ 35 mg/dl	General education	Repeat TC and HDL within 5 years or with physical examination
TC < 200 mg/dl and HDL < 35 mg/dl		Lipoprotein analysis
TC 200–300 mg/dl and HDL ≥ 35 mg/dl and < 2 CHD risk factors*		Dietary modification, reevaluation in 1–2 years
TC 200–239 mg/dl and HDL < 35 mg/dl or < 2 CHD risk factors•		Lipoprotein analysis
TC ≥ 240 mg/dl		Lipoprotein analysis
LDL evaluation		
No CHD and < 2 CHD risk factors*	LDL < 160 mg/dl	6-month trial of diet modification. Drug therapy if LDL remains ≥ 190 mg/dl.
No CHD but ≥ 2 CHD risk factors	LDL < 130 mg/dl	6-month trial of diet modification. Drug therapy if LDL remains ≥ 160 mg/dl.
Definite CHD or other atherosclerotic disease	LDL < 100 mg/dl	6- to 12-week trial of Step II diet. Drug therapy if LDL remains ≥ 130 mg/dl.
Physical inactivity	≥ 30 min of moderate intensity activity daily	Moderate exercise (e.g., brisk walking, jogging, cycling, or other aerobic activity) Medically supervised programs for high-risk patients (e.g., cardiac disease) and adaptive programs depending on physical/neurologic deficits

Table continued on following page

TABLE 2.   Guidelines for Primary Prevention of Stroke *(Continued)*

Factor	Goal	Recommendations
Poor diet/nutrition		Diet containing at least 5 servings of fruits and vegetables per day may reduce risk of stroke.
Alcohol	Moderation	No more than 2 drinks/day for men and 1 drink/day for nonpregnant women
Drug abuse	Cessation	In-depth history of substance abuse should be included as part of complete health evaluation for all patients

SBP = systolic blood pressure, DBP = diastolic blood pressure, INR =international normalized ratio, CHD = coronary heart disease, TC = total cholesterol, HDL = high-density lipoprotein, LDL = low-density lipoprotein.
* CHD risk factors: men ≥ 45 years, women ≥ 55 years or early menopause without hormone replacement therapy, family history of premature CHD, smoking, hypertension, HDL > 35 mg/dl, diabetes mellitus.
† Atrial fibrillation risk factors: hypertension, diabetes mellitus, poor left ventricular function, rheumatic mitral valve disease, prior TIA/stroke, systemic embolism or stroke, prosthetic heart valve (may require higher target INR).
From Goldstein LB, Adams R, Becker K, et al: Primary prevention of ischemic stroke: A statement for healthcare professionals from the Stroke Council of the American Heart Association. Circulation 103:162, 2001, with permission.

- Parietal: anterotemporal headaches, contralateral sensory loss, mild hemiparesis.
- Frontal: bifrontal headaches and contralateral arm weakness.
- Temporal: dysphasia and pain around the ear.
- Other common locations include putamen, thalamus, brainstem, and cerebellum.
   v. Seizures common in lobar rather than deep hemorrhage.
4. **Clinical syndromes**
   a. **Left- vs. right-sided** (also see Chapter 20, Speech, Language, and Swallowing Dysfunctions)
      i. Right hemisphere mediates learned behaviors in initiation, planning, general intellectual function, visual-spatial and visual-motor judgment (right parietal lobe). Emotional disorders such as flat affect, impulsivity, and emotional lability also may be seen. Patients are generally slower in relearning activities of daily living (ADLs).
      ii. Left hemisphere controls language in 97% of the population.
   b. **Vascular distribution and clinical deficits** (see Appendix E, Figs. 1 and 2).

Table 3.   Mechanisms of Acute Stroke

Ischemic	**85%**
Thrombotic	60%
Large vessel extracranial	
Small vessel intercranial	
Embolic	20%
Cardiac	
Intra-arterial	
Aortic	
Paradoxical	
Other	5%
Hypertension	
Vasculitis	
Hemorrhagic	**15%**
Intracerebral	10%
Subarachnoid	5%

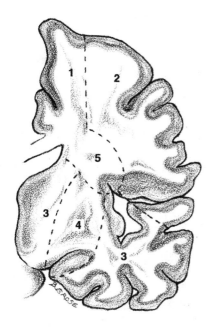

FIGURE   1. Vascular   supply   and distribution of cerebral arteries. Areas: 1, anterior cerebral artery, including the callosomarginal and pericallosal arteries; 2, middle cerebral artery; 3, posterior cerebral artery to the diencephalon and inferior temporal lobe; 4, medial striate arteries to the internal capsule, globus pallidus, and amygdala; 5, lateral striate arteries to the caudate nucleus, putamen, and internal capsule.

5. **Determining clinical severity** (see Appendix E)
   a. NIH Stroke Scale: determines neurologic severity of stroke based on 15 items.
   b. Hunt and Hess Scale: classifies subarachnoid hemorrhage on a scale of 1–5 based on the severity of clinical symptoms

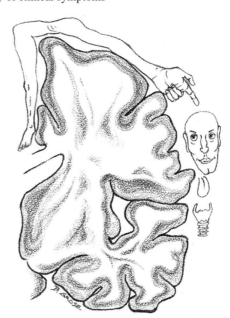

FIGURE 2.   Motor area of the brain.

    c. Mini-Mental Status Examination: widely used assessment that screens 7 domains related to mental status; must take into account education level and normal aging.

6. **Laboratory evaluation:** glucose, electrolytes, creatinine, blood urea nitrogen, complete blood count with differential and platelets, prothrombin time, partial thromboplastin time, and erythrocyte sedimentation rate should be performed.

7. **Radiologic imaging**

    a. **Head computed tomography (HCT)** (Table 4)

       i. HCT has many diagnostic applications during acute and subacute periods.

         • Used to rule out hemorrhagic process, neoplasm, infectious source, vascular aneurysm or malformation before use of anticoagulation or antithrombotic therapy for acute stroke.

         • Can be used to evaluate brain tissue, cerebrospinal fluid space, skull, and brain tissue perfusion.

         • Used when symptoms cannot be explained by one cerebrovascular lesion.

         • Can be used to provide serial evaluations of anticoagulated patients.

         • Can be used to look for edema, hemorrhagic conversion, mass effect, or hydrocephalus in patients who have deteriorated or remain comatose. This application is of particular concern for patients receiving anticoagulation.

      ii. HCT is limited in viewing the posterior fossa, specifically the brainstem, because of artifact production by surrounding bony structures.

     iii. In general, noncontrast-enhanced CT is standard of care. Section cuts < 5 mm are used for the posterior fossa to the base of the cerebral hemispheres; 8-mm sections are used for remainder of the brain.

TABLE 4.   **Computed Tomography Imaging in Stroke**

Time	Findings
Hemorrhagic process	
0–3 days	Hematomas appear as hyperdense areas due to increased hemoglobin in red blood cells (RBCs).
4–21 days	Progresses to isodense character similar to cerebrospinal fluid as hemoglobin from lysed RBCs is reabsorbed.
> 21 days	Hypodense areas similar to cerebrospinal fluid. Hemosiderin deposits around the periphery may show ring enhancement.
Ischemic process	
< 12 hours	Mass effect without mild gyral flattening or poorly demarcated areas are seen.
12–24 hours	Areas of decreased density that are poorly defined.
3–5 days	Well-defined hypodense areas. Edema may be seen as hypodensity involving white and gray matter.
6–13 days	Sharper demarcation of hypodense area is seen.
14–21 days	Infarcted area may become isodense compared with normal surrounding brain tissue. Contrast-enhanced studies may detect hypodense zone.
> 21 days	Sharper demarcation with cystic lesion appears. Ipsilateral ventricle may enlarge later.

TABLE 5.   Magnetic Resonance Imaging in Stroke

| Type/Time | Blood Product | MRI Signal Compared with Brain Parenchyma | |
		T1-Weighted Image	T2-Weighted Image
Hemorrhagic			
< 24 hr	Oxyhemoglobin	Isodense	Hyperdense
1–3 days	Deoxyhemoblogin	Isodense	Hyper-hypodense
3–7 days	Intracellular methemoglobin	Iso- to hyperdense	Hypodense
7–21 days	Extracullular methemoglobin	Hyperdense	Hyperdense
> 21 days	Hemosiderin	Hypodense	Hypodense
Ischemic		Hypodense	Hyperdense

   b. **Magnetic resonance imaging (MRI) of the head** (Table 5)
      i. Superior to HCT for imaging vessels, blood flow, and smaller lesions (e.g. lacunar strokes).
      ii. Performed in following situations
         • If HCT is negative and clinical suspicion remains high.
         • When a superior view of the vertebrobasilar area is needed.
         • Immediately after acute infarctions (within first 24 hours).
         • When dissection is suspected.
   c. **Magnetic resonance arteriography**
      i. May be used as screening tool to explain vascular mechanisms of stroke for later consideration of cerebral arteriography.
      ii. Less accurate than cerebral angiography; may miss small aneurysms and vascular malformations.
      iii. Safer than conventional angiography; requires no radiation or IV dye.
      iv. Superior to angiography and HCT in detecting cavernous malformations; may provide more important information about time course of hemorrhage.
   d. **Cerebral angiography**
      i. Should be considered for patients without known cause of bleeding who are clinically stable surgical candidates. Timing is based on clinical stability.
      ii. Not indicated when HCT imaging shows no definitive structural lesion.
8. **Other diagnostic tests**
   a. Electrocardiogram and cardiac monitoring: used to rule out cardiac arrhythmias (e.g., atrial fibrillation).
   b. Echocardiography
      i. Transthoracic echocardiography (TTE) is recommended for screening for embolization source.
      ii. Transesophageal echocardiography (TEE), although more sensitive than TTE in detecting cardioemboli, is an uncomfortable and expensive procedure reserved for patients with unidentified source of emboli.
   c. Carotid ultrasound: used to evaluate degree of stenosis in carotid arteries when the anterior circulation is suspect. .
   d. Transcranial Doppler: evaluates flow characteristics of intracranial vessels as well as determines degree of cerebral vasospasm.
   e. Lumbar puncture: should be considered if encephalitis or subarachnoid hemorrhage is suspected in light of negative imaging.

C. **Acute management of ischemic stroke**
1. **Anticoagulation**
   a. Considered only after hemorrhagic source (cerebral or elsewhere) is ruled out and no other bleeding contraindications are present.
   b. Indications
      i. Suspected embolic source
      ii. Potentially reversible event after acute stroke
      iii. DVT prophylaxis (if no contraindications) (see Section 6 below).
   c. Tissue plasminogen activator (tPA)
      i. Proven to be beneficial within 3 hours of initial onset of symptoms.
      ii. Dosing: 0.9 mg/kg (maximum of 90 mg), 10% as bolus and remainder in 60-minute infusion.
      iii. Risk of bleeding is approximately 6.4%.
      iv. Blood pressure must be lowered below 180 mmHg with no other risk factors present. Refer to Adams et al. for specific protocols.
      v. Management takes place predominantly in regional tertiary care centers with dedicated acute stroke care teams to evaluate eligibility for anticoagulation.
   d. Intravenous heparin
      i. Not proven to be efficacious or detrimental in management of acute ischemic events other than strokes caused by embolic or hypercoagulable state.
      ii. Initiation is based on preference of clinician caring for patient. Its use may place patient at risk for bleeding, with the potential for producing large hemorrhagic transformations.
   e. Aspirin may produce modest benefit in preventing recurrent thrombotic events at dosages of 80–325 mg.
2. **Blood pressure management**
   a. Blood pressure lowering is contraindicated unless a hypertensive crisis exists, resulting in end-organ damage (e.g., hypertensive encephalopathy, nephropathy, or retinopathy). Other medical complications that may require blood pressure reduction include acute myocardial infarction, heart failure, and arterial dissection.
   b. Maintenance below systolic level of 220 mmHg or calculated mean arterial blood pressure (MAP) of 130 mmHg or below 180/105 mmHg if the patient is receiving thrombolytic therapy. MAP = sum of systolic pressure plus 2 times diastolic pressure divided by 3.
   c. Blood pressure reduction may cause further ischemic injury secondary to inadequate autoregulation of cerebral vasculature, which results in decreased blood flow to damaged cerebral tissue and surrounding ischemic penumbra. MAP should not be lowered > 20 mmHg.
   d. If blood pressure reduction is warranted, calcium channel antagonists should be avoided because they can relax cerebral vasculature. Medications not affecting the cerebral vasculature include oral and intravenous alpha/beta antagonists (labetalol), alpha$_2$ antagonists (clonidine), and angiotensin-converting enzyme (ACE) inhibitors (enalapril).
   e. Many acute stroke patients have elevated blood pressures for first 48 hours after injury.
3. **Fever**
   a. Full fever workup should be done to rule out treatable infectious causes.

b. Antipyretic drugs should be given to lower metabolic requirements and prevent further cerebral injury. If necessary, cooling blankets can also be used.

c. Many studies have found that hyperthermia worsens prognosis. Reith found that a 1° increase in temperature was associated with a 2.2 greater risk of poor outcome independent of other risk factors.

4. **Seizures**: may occur in approximately 5% of patients with ischemic stroke. (See Appendix A for acute treatment algorithm).

5. **Electrolyte management, fluid balance, and nutrition**

a. **Hyponatremia** (plasma sodium concentration < 134 mEq/L) may be present in up to 30–35% of patients with subarachnoid hemorrhage.

   i. Usually develops 2–10 days after subarachnoid hemorrhage.

   ii. Early clinical changes may include confusion and mental status deterioration, muscle cramps, lethargy, anorexia, and nausea. Later signs with progressive hyponatremia may include further mental status deterioration, seizures, asterixis, and coma (generally seen when sodium levels fall below 120 mEq/L).

   iii. Determine cause and classification by determining whether hyponatremia occurs in setting of hypo-, iso-, or hypertonic fluid balance. Rule out other numerous causes of hyponatremia before implementing treatment.

   iv. **Fluid overhydration:** most common cause of hyponatremia; decreasing fluid therapy usually corrects the situation.

   v. **Salt-wasting syndrome**
   - Hyponatremic patients tend to have negative fluid balance, low central venous and pulmonary wedge pressures, declining weight, negative sodium balance, and excessive natriuresis.
   - Administering isotonic saline or Ringer's lactate can aid in restoring blood volume. Fludrocortisone acetate (1 mg orally 2 times/day) can be used with or without sodium chloride tablets to minimize or eliminate negative sodium balance.

   vi. **Syndrome of inappropriate antidiuretic hormone** (SIADH)
   - Hyponatremic patients tend to have stable fluid balance (hypotonic isovolemic). Pulmonary and capillary wedge pressures are normal or elevated along with stable or elevating body weight.
   - Laboratory evaluation reveals increased urine sodium > 30 mEq/L and urine osmolarity levels greater than serum osmolarity.
   - Treatment includes fluid restriction to < 1 L/day. Loop diuretics such as furosemide, 40–80 mg/day, can be used to decrease positive fluid balance. Demeclocycline, 300–600 mg 2 times/day, as well as others can be used to inhibit ability of antidiuretic hormone to increase water absorption.

   vii. Regardless of cause, correct sodium level slowly (0.5–1.0 mEq/L/hr); only half of deficit should be corrected in first 24 hours. A slower correction of 10 mEq/L/24 hr is indicated in patients with chronic hyponatremia. Correction too quickly can cause **cerebral edema** and **central pontine myelinosis** (CPM). CPM evolves several days after sodium correction with disorders of upper motor neurons, spastic quadriparesis, pseudobulbar palsy, and mental status changes.

    viii. Severe cases may warrant hypertonic saline administration with or without a loop diuretic in a monitored environment such as an intensive care unit.

    ix. Morbidity and mortality rates can exceed 40% when serum sodium concentration is < 110 mEq/L.

  b. Avoidance of hypotonic fluids is essential to prevent potential worsening of cerebral edema.

  c. Aggressive management of hyperglycemia is indicated. Worsening of ischemic areas occurs with worsening hyperglycemia. Jorgensen et al. found that elevated blood glucose on admission was related to poorer outcome.

6. **Acute-setting DVT prophylaxis** (see Chapter 13, Deep Venous Thrombosis)

  a. Incidence of DVTs among acute stroke survivors who have not received any type of prophylaxis is approximately 42%.

  b. Prophylaxis is recommended for patients not receiving any other type of anticoagulation (i.e., IV heparin or warfarin) with risk factors for DVT formation such as limited mobility, malignancy, age > 40 years, or recent fractures. Patients with limited mobility include those unable to ambulate >150 feet/day, although 50 feet has been reported by some to be sufficient.

  c. McGuire and Harvey recommend weight-based treatment protocol for DVT prophylaxis:

    i. Heparin, 5000 units subcutaneously every 12 hr for patients < 70kg

    ii. Heparin, 5000 units 8 hours for patients 70–100kg

    iii. Low-molecular-weight heparin (Lovenox), 30 mg subcutaneously 2 times/day for patients > 100 kg

    iv. Low-molecular-weight heparins (e.g., Lovenox, Fragmin) have increased bioavailability in subcutaneous fat because of their small size.

  d. Anticoagulation is contraindicated in patients with active bleeding source. Alternatives for such patients include aspirin, sequential compression devices, elastic support stockings, and/or inferior vena cava (IVC) filter placement.

  e. Inadequate evidence supports duration of treatment beyond 14 days. The assumption is that the risk of DVT decreases over time, but no data describe the time course of risk reduction. It is likely that the risk of DVT varies according to presence of other risk factors, such as severe paresis and immobility.

D. **Acute management of hemorrhagic stroke**

1. **Blood pressure management**

  a. Goal is to decrease bleeding from ruptured cerebral arteries and arterioles.

  b. Recommendations for pressure parameters

    i. MAP of 130 mmHg

    ii. Cerebral perfusion pressure > 70 mmHg

    iii. Systolic blood pressure > 90 mmHg and < 180 mmHg

2. **Intracranial pressure** (ICP)

  a. Elevated ICP defined as ≥ 20 mmHg for > 5 minutes.

  b. Presentation 48–72 hours after insult with peak edema at 3–5 days.

  c. Contributing factors include hypercarbia, hypoxia, hyperthermia, acidosis, hypotension, and hypovolemia.

d. May present clinically with decline in level of consciousness, changes in breathing pattern, enlargement of pupil ipsilateral to infarcted hemisphere, loss of venous pulsations or papilledema on ophthalmoscopic exam, progression of focal neurologic deficit, and contralateral signs of weakness and hyperreflexia.

e. **Treatment** may include:
   i. Correction of exacerbating factors
   ii. Elevating head of bed
   iii. Fluid restriction (< 2 L/24 hr)
   iv. Osmotherapy with 20% mannitol (0.25–0.5 g/kg every 4 hr with maximum of 2 gm/24 hr) with or without furosemide (40–80 mg every 2–8 hours) to obtain serum osmolality of 300–320 mOsm/L.
   v. Hyperventilation producing hypocarbia-induced cerebral vasoconstriction. Goal is PCO_2 of 25–30 mmHg.
   vi. Medical/surgical interventions, such as ventricular drains and intracranial pressure monitors, may be required.
   vii. Barbiturates, which can lower ICP, may be considered if above approach fails, but systemic effects, such as, hypotension may limit their use.
   vii. Steroids are generally avoided because of unproven effectiveness and side effects. They may be of some benefit in patients with vasogenic strokes (i.e., tumor).

3. **Seizures**
   a. Seen in 6–7% of patients with intracranial hemorrhage.
   b. More prevalent in lobar than deep hemorrhages.
   c. See Appendix A for acute seizure management.

4. **Vasospasm**
   a. Approximately 70% of patients have vasospasm in first 2 weeks after bleeding of vascular origin.
   b. Signs and symptoms include increase or change in headache, decreased consciousness, and waxing and waning appearance of focal neurologic deficits.
   c. Transcranial Doppler may aid in diagnosis.
   d. Nimodipine lessens likelihood of ischemic stroke from vasospasm, particularly after subarachnoid hemorrhage. Dose is 60 mg every 4 hours for up to 21 days. Hypervolemic hemodilution and induced hypertension are also used to lower viscosity and increase perfusion pressure with persistent vasospasm.

5. **Surgical intervention and hematoma removal**
   a. May be considered based on etiology of ICP, age, size of hemorrhage, area of hemorrhage, and patient's current clinical status.
   b. Ventricular peritoneal shunting can be effective in decreasing ICP.
   c. Evacuation should be considered, especially for hematomas > 2.5 cm.

III. Medical Problems of Patients with Stroke

A. Cardiovascular

1. Because of strong association between thrombotic strokes and pre-existing arteriosclerotic heart disease, cardiovascular screen/examination should be performed to evaluate modifiable risk factors (see Table 2). Precautions should be implemented when appropriate (Table 6).

TABLE 6. Cardiac Precautions for Inpatient Rehabilitation

Contraindictions to exercise/activities
1. Recent significant change in electrocardiogram (i.e., ST-segment changes)
2. Recent complicated myocardial infarction (≤ 3 weeks)
3. Unstable angina pectoris
4. Resting heart rate < 50 or > 140 beats per minute (bpm)
5. Cardiac rate and/or rhythm that causes acute drop in blood pressure, angina, and/or dizziness to near-syncope
6. Uncontrolled heart failure
7. Extreme dyspnea at rest
8. Acute infections (e.g., myocarditis, pericarditis, acute febrile state)
9. Untreated thrombophlebitis
10. Recent systemic or pulmonary emboli

Relative contraindications to exercise/activity
1. Aortic stenosis
2. Resting systolic blood pressure < 90 or > 200 mmHg
3. Resting diastolic blood pressure > 110 mmHg
4. Heart rate < 50 or > 120 bpm
5. Frequent or complex ventricular ectopy
6. Cardiomyopathy
7. Severe left ventricular dysfunction (ejection fraction < 30%)
8. Dyspnea on exertion

Activity should be terminated if any of the following occurs:
1. New onset of cardiopulmonary symptoms
2. Heart rate decreases > 20% or increases > 50% of baseline resting heart rate
3. Systolic blood pressure increases to > 240 mmHg
4. Disatolic blood pressure increases to > 120 mmHg
5. Systolic blood pressure decreases ≥ 30 mmHg from baseline or to < 90 mmHg

From Fletcher BJ, Dunbar S, Coleman J, et al: Cardiac precautions for nonacute patient settings. Am J Phys Med Rehabil 72:140–143, 1993.

2. **Generalized deconditioning** (see Chapter 12, Deconditioning and Bed Rest)
3. **DVT** (see Chapter 13, Deep Venous Thrombosis)
   a. Up to 42% of patients who have not received prophylaxis develop DVT after first week.
   b. Incidence: 55% in the paretic limb.
   c. Prospective studies have demonstrated no increased risk of intracranial bleeding in patients on DVT prophylaxis (low-dose unfractionated heparin) started on second day after spontaneous intracerebral hemorrhage compared with regimens started on day 4 or 10.
   d. Alternatives to anticoagulation include sequential compression devices (which should be worn constantly to be maximally effective), antithrombotic compression stockings, and IVC filter placement.
   e. Sixth American Council of Chest Physicians' (ACCP) Consensus Conference on Antithrombotic Therapy makes following recommendations for DVT prophylaxis in stroke patients:
      i. **Ischemic stroke**
         • When indicated, routine use of low-dose unfractionated heparin (LDUH) or low-molecular-weight heparin (LWMH); LMWH is more efficacious in reduction than LDUH, though more costly.
         • When heparin is contraindicated, mechanical prophylaxis with elastic stockings and intermittent pneumatic compression (IPC) should be used.

    ii. **Hemorrhagic stroke**
- No studies have focused on DVT prophylaxis in patients with hemorrhagic stroke to date.
- Neurosurgical patients (including elective cranial and spine surgery) should use IPC devices with or without elastic stockings
- Postoperative LDUH or LMWH is acceptable alternative, although risk of bleeding is increased.
- Combining physical and pharmacologic intervention in patients at high risk for DVT may provide more protection than either modality alone.

B. **Pulmonary**
1. **Pulmonary embolism** (PE) (see Chapter 13, Deep Venous Thrombosis)
   a. Incidence of 10–20% among patients with acute stroke.
   b. Accounts for approximately 5–25% of deaths 1 week after stroke.
   c. 90% originate from lower extremity DVTs; therefore, prophylaxis is essential.
2. **Pneumonia**
   a. Occurs in approximately 30% of stroke patients.
   b. Often secondary to clinical or subclinical aspiration.
   c. Aspiration is defined as penetration of contrast material below level of true vocal cords. It is a consequence of dysphagia (difficulty in swallowing).
   d. Aspiration is missed in 40% of patients on bedside exam. However, a videofluoroscopic swallow study (VFSS) usually identifies aspiration.
   e. Subclinical or silent aspiration has been reported in 8–40% of stroke patients.
   f. Not all patients who aspirate develop pneumonia.
   g. Risk factors for aspiration pneumonia include brainstem stroke, tracheostomy, gastric reflux, emesis, nasogastric tubes, compromised immune system, chronic lung disease, difficulty in handling secretions, and recurrent pulmonary infections. Bedside dysphagia exam reveals wet-sounding voice, weak voice, and cough.
   h. Prevention includes early mobilization, aggressive pulmonary toilet, incentive spirometry, deep-breathing exercises, reflux and emesis prevention, and tube feedings or diet modification strategies in patients with dysphagia.
   i. Any patient suspected of having impaired swallowing mechanism should avoid oral ingestion until a formal assessment can be performed.

C. **Gastrointestinal** (also refer to Chapter 16, Neurogenic Bowel Management)
1. Common complaints may include nausea and constipation.
2. **Neurogenic bowel** results from interrupted cerebral input between cerebral cortex, pons, and spinal defecation center, causing uninhibited reflex emptying.
3. **GI motility** is normal, although it may be altered by certain medications.
4. Using the gastrocolic reflex may be necessary in conjunction with a **bowel medication regimen** and timed voiding program (see Chapter 16, Neurogenic Bowel Management).
5. **Dysphagia** (see Chapter 20, Speech, Language, and Swallowing Disorder)
   a. Incidence: 30–65% among stroke patients.
   b. Can be diagnosed by bedside swallowing evaluation, though VFSS is more accurate.

    c. Positive gag reflex does not rule out dysphagia.

    d. Dysphagia may be secondary to delayed pharyngeal phase, although altered control of lips and tongue is seen in strokes affecting the cranial nerves.

    e. Dysphagia may be present in brainstem, unilateral, and bilateral hemispheric strokes.

    f. Risk factors include impaired cognition and location (e.g., brainstem).

    g. Treatment includes dietary modification for minimal aspiration and enteral supplementation (e.g., nasogastric or nasoduodenal tubes) for severe aspiration. Semipermanent enteral tube should be placed if > 75% of nutritional needs cannot be met by diet modification alone. Gastrojejunal tube placement, as opposed to gastric tube placement, theoretically reduces the risk of gastroesophageal reflux because of protection by pyloric sphincter.

  6. **Nutrition** (Table 7)

    a. Complicated problem related to severity of dysphagia as well as premorbid condition.

    b. In acute period after stroke, the patient is in a hypermetabolic state, which increases nutritional needs.

    c. Malnourished patients consistently scored lower on the Barthel Index.

    d. Visceral protein stores, including albumin, prealbumin, and transferrin, can be measured via serum analysis.

    e. Prealbumin may give better estimate of short-term nutritional variability; albumin estimates nutritional health over longer period.

    f. Nutritional supplementation may be necessary. See Appendix C for detailed description of formulas and adverse reactions to tube feeding.

  7. **Language and communication** (see Chapter 20, Speech, Language, and Swallow Dysfunction)

    a. Approximately 30% of stroke survivors have some type of language or communication dysfunction.

    b. Full testing of fluency, expression, comprehension, naming, reading, writing, and repetition should become part of the initial evaluation. The American Speech-Language-Hearing Association Functional Assessment of Communication Skills for Adults and Boston Diagnostic Aphasia Examination can be used to document deficits.

  8. **Cognition**

    a. Approximately 15–25% of stroke survivors have a cognitive deficit.

    b. Mini-Mental State Examination can be used to screen for such deficits, although there may be a high correlation between results and educational level.

    c. Neurobehavioral Cognitive Status Examination can be used to assess dementia severity in multiple areas, including consciousness, orientation, memory, language, and reasoning.

F. **Genitourinary** (refer to Chapter 15, Neurogenic Bladder Management)

  1. Incidence of urinary incontinence: approximately 44–60% in patients with acute stroke.

  2. In absence of ischemic insult to pontine micturition center, normal synchronous destrusor-sphincter synergy is preserved.

  3. Over time bladder function can evolve from flaccid, atonic bladder (early) to spastic, hyperreflexic bladder within a few weeks.

TABLE 7.   Interventions for Secondary Medical Complictions Affecting Food Intake in Patients with Stroke

Upper extremity hemiparesis or paralysis	Teach patient to use unaffected hand, even if paralyzed hand has been dominant.
	Consult occupational therapist, use assistive devices to assist in eating skills, when appropriate.
	Provide opportunities for feeding rehabilitation for as long as progress is noted.
	Encourage self-feeding; provide finger foods.
	Prevent fatigue.
	Maintain human dignity.
Disorientation	Give clear, repeated, slow-paced instruction and demonstrations.
Altered level of consciouness	Encourage participation of family.
	Review medications (antipsychotic and sedative anticholinergics can impair mental status)
	Be nonjudgmental about changes in personality.
Altered emotional behavior (e.g., depression, iras-cibility, lability, indifference)	Reassure with word or touch.
	Medications (e.g., antidepressants such as methylphenidate) have side effect of appetite suppression
	Oral supplements may be helpful.
	Tube feedings may be helpful in patients who refuse to eat.
	Lability may not reflect actual emotion.
Dysphagia	Dysphagia evaluation, consultation with speech-language pathologist, clinical dietitian.
	Implement dysphagia diet and/or tube feedings.
Apraxia	Break down tasks into familir set of small steps.
	Monitor quantity eaten.
	Continually encourate eating.
Visuospatial perceptual deficits	Give directions and discussion on unaffected side.
	Depending on level of cognition, present food within visual field or train patient to rotate tray to previously "hidden food" and purposefully look to side of "blind spot."
	Remediation and computer-controlled audiovisual-based rehabilitation programs can be useful for improving feeding skills.
Denture ill fit due to facial paralysis or gum shrinkage during denture removal	Dental consultation.
	New set of dentures, if necessary.
	In meantime, use liquid complete nutritional formula and/or soft, pureed diet.
Obesity	Reduced-energy diet, because excessive weight can interfere with mobility and long-term outcome.
Decubitus ulcers	Adequate energy and protein.

From Finestone HM, Green-Fienstone LS: Nutrition and diet in neurological rehabilitation. In Lazar RB (ed): Principles of Neurologic Rehabilitation. New York, McGraw-Hill, 1998, with permission

4. Risk factors for incontinence include impaired cognitive status, neglect, premorbid benign prostatic hypertrophy, and diabetes-induced parasympathetic autonomic neuropathy.

5. **Treatment plan**

   a. Determine cause of incontinence (i.e., spastic vs. flaccid bladder). Evaluation includes accurate fluid intake and output amounts, frequency and timing of voids, postvoid residuals, and assessment of current medication that may contribute to incontinence.

   b. Discontinue indwelling (Foley) catheters, which may lead to infections and anatomic and functional changes. Urinary incontinence should be managed with clean intermittent catheterizations, timed voiding schedule, or external (condom) catheters.

    c. Eliminate moisture and chemical irritation of perineal area to prevent skin breakdown.

    d. Slowly advance bladder management medications, such as ditropan, urecholine, or hytrin, to minimize potential side effects.

    e. Other treatment options for incontinence include Kegel exercises and biofeedback.

G. **Skin** (see Chapter 18, Pressure Ulcers: Prevention and Care)

    1. Approximately 15% of stroke patients develop decubitus ulcers.

    2. Early prevention is best management. Risk assessment for decubitus ulcer formation should be performed on admission to hospital.

    3. Other methods of decubitus ulcer prophylaxis include proper body positioning, pressure relief orthotics (e.g., L'nard boots, heel/elbow protectors), specialty mattresses and overlays, and wheelchair cushions.

H. **Depression**

    1. Prevalence among acute stroke survivors ranges from 25% to 79%. One-third of affected patients develop major depression.

    2. Possible causes include medication side effects, disruption of catecholaminergic system (decreased serotonin and noradrenaline), grief reaction to loss, hypothyroidism, infection, or pre-existing/underlying psychiatric condition.

    3. Clinical signs and symptoms include decreased energy, insomnia, agitation, loss of interest, decreased sexual desire, feeling of worthlessness, impaired concentration, behavior changes, suicidal thoughts, decreased or increased appetite.

    4. Diagnosis may be difficult, particularly in aphasic or cognitively impaired patients. A combination of methods should be used, such as clinical observation by the rehabilitation team, family, and rehabilitation psychologist; observation of the family or caregiver; and depression screening scales (e.g., Geriatric Depression Scale [GDS], Center for Epidemiologic Studies of Depression [CES-D], Beck Depression scale).

    5. Pharmacologic treatment includes selective serotonin reuptake inhibitors (SSRIs), tricyclic antidepressants (TCAs), and psychostimulants (e.g., methylphenidate) (see Chapter 23, Pharmacology). Electroconvulsive therapy may be considered in severe cases of depression that are resistant to medical management.

    6. Psychotherapy should be used in combination with medications.

    7. Depression can negatively affect rehabilitation program, causing longer length of stay, greater ADL disability, greater cognitive deficits, and higher 10-year mortality rate.

I. **Neurologic**

    1. **Spasticity** (refer to Chapter 19, Spasticity)

        a. Can begin days to weeks after stroke.

        b. Mass contraction of multiple muscle groups is seen in flexor and extensor patterns (Table 8).

        c. Medications, such as tizanidine, dantrium, clonidine, and baclofen, can be effective alone or in combination for systemic spasticity. Local spasticity can be managed with chemical neurolysis (phenol injections) or chemical deinnervation (botulinum toxin injections).

TABLE 8.   Basic Limb Synergy Patterns

	Flexion Synergy	Extensor Synergy
Upper extremity	Shoulder retraction	Shoulder protraction
	Arm abduction	Arm adduction
	Arm external rotation	Arm internal rotation
	Elbow flexion	Elbow extension
	Forearm supination	Forearm pronation
	Wrist flexion	Wrist extension
	Wrist radial deviation	Wrist ulnar deviation
	Digit extension	Digit flexion
Lower extremity	Hip flexion	Hip extension
	Thigh abduction	Thigh adduction
	Thigh external rotation	Thigh internal rotation
	Knee flexion	Knee extension
	Ankle dorsiflexion	Ankle plantarflexion
	Ankle supination	Ankle pronation
	Digit extension	Digit flexion

    d. Adjuncts therapies include stretching, therapeutic modalities, serial casting, and range-of-motion (ROM) exercises.

2. **Seizures**

    a. Approximate risk at onset is 5–10% after stroke, with a higher incidence of 24% in patients with subarachnoid hemorrhage (SAH). These seizures occur mostly in the first 2 weeks after stroke.

    b. Seizure prophylaxis should be considered in higher-risk patients (i.e. SAH) and then discontinued after 1 week if no seizures occur.

    c. Transition from more sedating anticonvulsants (e.g., phenytoin) to less sedating (e.g., carbamazepine) can help increase alertness in cognitively impaired patients without compromising efficacy.

    d. See Appendix A for acute seizure management.

3. **Hydrocephalus**

    a. Communicating hydrocephalus, secondary to impaired absorption of cerebrospinal fluid, is more common than the noncommunicating subtype.

    b. Clinical signs and symptoms include incontinence, gait impairment, behavior changes (e.g. confusion), or lack of neurologic and/or functional improvement.

    c. Most easily diagnosed by HCT to evaluate ventricular size.

    d. If present, neurosurgical consultation should be obtained for possible ventricular shunt placement.

J. **Pain** (also see Chapter 11, Acute and Chronic Pain)

1. **Central post-stroke pain**

    a. Occurs in 2% of patients.

    b. Peripheral causes should be ruled out before treatment.

    c. May be treated with gabapentin and/or tricyclic antidepressants, therapeutic modalities, and desensitization techniques.

2. **Shoulder pain**

    a. Possible causes include spasticity, bursitis, shoulder subluxation, tendinitis, traction neuropathies of the brachial plexus, regional complex pain syndrome, and rotator cuff tears/impingements.

    b. Pain often arises during periods of increased spasticity as opposed to periods when the limb is flaccid.

    c. Treatment, although variable according to cause, is aimed at supporting and strengthening muscles around the shoulder. Support and proper positioning can be accomplished with a sling, lapboard, or tray. The therapeutic program should focus on ROM and strengthening of the trapezius and other shoulder stabilizers.

    d. Pain can be treated with local modalities, systemic pain medications, anesthetic/corticosteroid injections, or topical analgesics (e.g. capsaicin cream), if appropriate to specific etiology.

    e. Functional electrical stimulation may be of benefit in shoulder subluxation.

K. **Falls**

  1. One-third of stroke patients fall during course of rehabilitation, most often during transfers or when they are reaching and/or bending from wheelchair.

  2. Serious injury occurs in 2–4% of falls, resulting in fractures, abrasions, lacerations, and subdural hematomas.

  3. Risk factors include right hemispheric stroke, urinary incontinence, polypharmacy, neglect and visuospatial deficits, impulsivity, confusion, male gender, and poor ADL performance.

  4. Prevention strategies include adequate supervision, fall prevention education for patient and family, minimizing of sedative and diuretics, and strengthening and balance programs.

  5. Restraints should be last resort.

IV. Neurological and Functional Recovery

A. **General considerations**

  1. To develop realistic rehabilitation program for stroke survivors, it is important to have a clear understanding of the natural history of both neurologic and functional recovery.

  2. This information helps to estimate expected improvement of any given underlying deficit with rehabilitation as well as provides information to patient/family about the prognosis of the deficit.

  3. Regardless of the rehabilitation program, no studies indicate that one program is superior to another for accelerating or extending a patient's recovery.

B. **Neurologic recovery phases**

  1. **Early stage** (0–3 months after stroke) includes recovery of ischemic penumbra from metabolic toxins, edema, pressure, and hemorrhage due to initial insult.

  2. **Late stage** (> 3 months after stroke) involves neuroplastic reorganization that affects structure and function. This includes repair of damaged pathways and incorporation of other neurons to perform new functional tasks.

C. **Motor recovery patterns**

  1. Large motor strokes affecting the extremities (i.e., main branch of the middle cerebral artery) recover in a proximal-to-distal pattern. Extremities are initially flaccid and then develop spasticity with large synergy patterns (Table 9). Coordinated movements and decreased spasticity usually follow.

  2. Recovery of lower extremity is generally greater than recovery of upper extremity because of need for more complex control recovery in upper extremities.

D. **Language recovery patterns**

  1. Language recovery is generally more unpredictable than motor recovery.

  2. Most recovery occurs in the first 3–6 months after stroke but can occur up to 2 years after stroke.

TABLE 9. Brunstrom Stages of Motor Recovery After Stroke

Stage	Clinical Characteristics	Spasticity
1	Flaccid. No activation of limb. No passive or active resistance.	None
2	Flexor and extensor synergies appear with weak initiated movements.	Developing
3	Voluntary movements are present, but activation is in synergy patterns.	Prominent
4	Selective activation of muscles outside synergy patterns patterns occurs.	Decreasing
5	Motor activation is selective and independent of limb synergies	Continued decrease
6	Purposeful, isolated movements are coordinated and smooth	Occasional with fast movements

    3. Fluent aphasics generally have better recovery than nonfluent aphasics.

    4. Receptive aphasia generally recovers earlier than expressive aphasia.

E. **Stroke and impairment scales**

    1. Impairment scales, such as the National Institutes of Health Stroke Scale (NIHSS) (Appendix E), Scandinavian Neurological Stroke Scale (SSS), and Mathew Scale, have been used extensively for evaluation of treatment outcomes in numerous randomized, controlled trials.

    2. Clinically the scales have been used to monitor neurologic deficits within first 24 hours after acute stroke as well as neurologic deterioration and improvement during acute hospitalization and to provide gross prognostic information.

    3. Trial of Org 10172 in Acute Stroke Treatment (TOAST) found that the NIHSS correlated well with poor outcome at 3 months using a score of > 16, whereas a score < 6 was indicative of a good prognosis.

    4. Unlike the other impairment scales, the SSS also has a prognostic section that can be used for long-term follow-up.

F. **Disability scales**

    1. Disability scales evaluate the functional consequence of a neurologic deficit.

    2. More commonly used scales evaluate limitations of the capacity to perform specific ADLs. At the most basic level, ADLs are skills needed to live independently.

    3. Scales dedicated to the evaluation of ADLs generally assess independence in self-care (e.g., eating, grooming, dressing), transfers, and ambulation.

    4. Barthel Index (BI) and Functional Independence Measure (FIM) are the most widely used disability scales in acute stroke trials and clinical assessments. The Modified Rankin Scale is also used. (See Appendix E).

G. **Overall neurologic and functional recovery**

    1. Tremendous amount of research into post-stroke neurologic and functional recovery has originated from the **Copenhagen Stroke Study**, a prospective, consecutive, and community-based study of 1197 unselected stroke patients, all of whom were treated on a distinct stroke unit from the time of acute hospitalization to completion of rehabilitation. Stroke severity was measured by the SSS and functional deficits by the BI.

    2. **Results of the study**

a. 21% of patients died during hospitalization; 15% went to nursing homes; 64% were discharged to their own home.
b. Best neurologic function was reached in 80% of survivors at 4.5 weeks and in 95% by 11weeks from the time of stroke onset.
c. Best ADL function was reached in 80% and 95% of stroke survivors at 6 and 12.5 weeks, respectively.
d. Neurologic recovery preceded functional recovery by about 2 weeks on average.
e. Initial stroke severity is one of the most important factors determining neurologic and functional recovery, mortality, and discharge disposition. As expected, patients with more severe neurologic deficits had a higher mortality rate, longer course of recovery, and lower rate of discharge to home (Tables 10 and 11).
f. Discharge rates to home varied with stroke severity: very severe, 14%; severe, 34%; moderate, 74%; mild, 93%.
g. Independent rates of function varied with stroke severity: very severe, 4%; severe, 13%; moderate, 37%; mild, 68%.

3. **Determinants of poorer prognosis:** increased body temperature and/or elevated blood glucose at time of admission; diabetes; stroke progression; atrial fibrillation; treatment on general neurologic and medical wards.
   i. Treatment on a dedicated stroke unit from the time of acute admission to end of rehabilitation improved overall outcome.
   ii. Relative risk of dying was reduced by 50%, discharge to nursing home by 40% and length of stay by 30%.

H. **Recovery of specific neurologic deficits**
   1. **Ambulation**
      a. Ability to ambulate at stroke onset has large influence on ability to ambulate independently at discharge from rehabilitation.
      b. Copenhagen Stroke Study found that nearly 30–40% of patients initially diagnosed with a stroke would be able to ambulate independently (Table 12).
      c. Remaining patients who were able to walk with assistance had a nearly 100% probability of independent ambulation after rehabilitation.
      d. Patients who could take a few steps with assistance or were not able to ambulate at all had a probability of 60% and 15%, respectively.
      e. Recovery of walking function and lower extremity strength occurred in most patients by 11 weeks after stroke.
      f. Olson found similar results with the majority of patients in his study, who reached their best walking function at 14 weeks.

TABLE 10. Neurologic and Functional Recovery Based on Initial Stroke Severity

Stroke Severity	Best Neurologic Recovery (wk)		Best Functional Recovery (wk)	
	80%	*95%*	*80%*	*95%*
Very severe	10	13	11.5	20
Severe	9	15	11.5	17
Moderate	5.5	10.5	7	13
Mild	2.5	6.5	3	8.5

Severity based on neurologic assessment using the Scandinavian Stroke Scale and functionally by the Barthel Index.
Data compiled from Jorgensen HS et al.[20]

TABLE 11.   Discharge Outcomes Based on Initial Stroke Severity

Stroke Severity	Mortality (%)	Severity on Admission (%)	Severity at Discharge (%)
Very severe	62	18.5	4
Severe	33	14.3	7
Moderate	12	26.4	11
Mild	3	40.8	78

Severity based on neurologic assessment using the Scandinavian Stroke Scale and functionally by the Barthel Index.
Data compiled from Jorgensen HS et al.[20]

   g. Ambulation is a complex task influenced by more than just lower extremity strength.
      i. Often deficits in cognition, balance, perception, and coordination can be equally important barriers to independent ambulation.
      ii. Stroke survivors who are unable to sit independently will not be able to walk independently, even if there are no deficits in cognition and lower extremity strength.
 2. **Upper extremity (UE) function**
   a. As with the lower extremity, functional recovery of the UE is influenced by the initial neurologic deficit.
      i. 57% of patients with severe paresis were able to improve to the next level (i.e. moderate paresis).
      ii. More pronounced results were found in patients with mild or no paresis; 78% and 70% improved to an upper level, respectively.
   b. Table 13 summarizes the Copenhagen Stroke Study data about recovery of UE function at weeks 1 and 4 of hospitalization, and recovery of UE based on initial stroke severity.
   c. Olsen found similar results in regard to UE function.
      i. For patients with gravity-eliminated active movement or less (< 2) at admission to rehabilitation, 8% had achieved independence in eating and upper extremity dressing, whereas 23% had regained independence in at least one of these ADLs at discharge.
      ii. 42% of patients with active movement against gravity or greater (> 3) were able to perform both functions, and 81% regained independence in at least one function.

TABLE 12.   Lower Extremity (LE) Neurological and Functional Recovery Based on Initial Stroke Severity

LE Severity	Initial Severity (%)	Mortality (%)	Independent Ambulation (%)	Best Level of Walking Function (wk)		Best Level of LE Strength (wk)	
				80%	*95%*	*80%*	*95%*
Paralysis	19	56	6	1	11	5	11
Severe paresis	10	33	21	5	11	5	11.2
Moderate paresis	11	29	28	3	9	3	6
Mild paresis	25	7	66	3	9	1	4
No paresis	35	7	78	1	4	NA	NA

NA = not applicable. Data compiled from Jorgensen HS et al.[19]

TABLE 13. Upper Extremity (UE) Neurologic and Functional Recovery Based on Initial Stroke Severity

UE Function (%)	Severe Paresis (n = 137)		Mild Paresis (n = 154)		No Paresis (n = 130)	
	Week 1 (%)	Week 4 (%)	Week 1 (%)	Week 4 (%)	Week 1 (%)	Week 2 (%)
Death	27	45	6	8	2	5
None	46	20	7	5	5	1
Partial	22	24	31	10	19	14
Full	5	11	56	77	74	80

Best UE Functional Recovery Based on Initial Stroke Severity

	80% (wk)	95% (wk)	80% (wk)	95% (wk)	80% (wk)	95% (wk)
Functional recovery	6	11	3	6	2	6

    d. Several studies have suggested that the majority of functional recovery takes place within the first 3 months.

      i. Copenhagen Stroke Study found that overall, 80% of patients reached best possible UE function 3 weeks after stroke. The best possible UE function was reached in 9 weeks.

      ii. Olsen also found that the best UE function was reached on average at 9 weeks, with 95% reaching their best UE function at 13 weeks.

      iii. Wade et al. followed a cohort of patients for 2 years and found no significant improvement in function after 3 months.

  3. **Aphasia**

    a. Approximately 25% of all patients with acute stroke are aphasic.

    b. Of patients who are still aphasic at 1 month, 33–55% will remain aphasic at 6 months and 25% at 1 year after stroke.

    c. Aphasia classification and initial severity are important determinants of recovery pattern.

    d. Kertesz and McCabe reported the following findings at 1-year follow-up:

      i. Global aphasics had a poorer prognosis, followed by patients with Broca's and Wernicke's aphasias.

      ii. Complete recovery was frequently seen in patients with anomic, conduction, and transcortical aphasia.

      iii. Patient's with global aphasia tended to improve rapidly and developed into severe nonfluent or anomic aphasia.

    e. Recovery pattern for aphasia tends to be slower and longer compared with motor recovery.

      i. Greatest recovery occurs in most patients within first 3–6 months after stroke.

      ii. In some groups, however, such as global aphasics, the greatest recovery took place in the latter half of the first year.

    f. As with neurologic motor deficits, no one treatment program has been shown to be more beneficial than another. Even more importantly, the value of therapeutic treatment is still unclear.

V. Stroke Rehabilitation

  A. **Goals of rehabilitation program**

    1. Each program is **patient-specific** and based on severity of neurologic deficits.

    2. **Baseline assessment** documents functional and neurologic deficits.

    3. **Elements of rehabilitation program**

a. Coordination of multidisciplinary treatment plan to upgrade patient's current functional level
b. Patient and family education
c. Assessment for appropriate adaptive equipment for mobility and ADLs
d. Secondary stroke prevention
e. Improvement in generalized deconditioning
f. Prevention and treatment of stroke comorbidities
g. Psychosocial counseling
h. Community and vocational reintegration
i. Evaluation of safe discharge options that will return patient to the maximal level of independence in the safest environment

B. **Rehabilitation settings**
   1. **Acute inpatient rehabilitation**
      a. Highest level of inpatient therapeutic intensity; provides comprehensive interdisciplinary team approach.
      b. Patients have significant neurologic deficits that prevent them from going home safely.
      c. Patients must be able to tolerate at least 3 hours of therapy per day.
      d. Patients should not need continuous or invasive monitoring (e.g., ICP monitoring or cardiac telemetry), although daily physician visits and 24-hour physician availability and nursing care are still required.
      e. Patients receive coordinated therapeutic program provided by an interdisciplinary team, which may include physical, occupational, speech, recreational and vocational therapists as well as support from social work and discharge planning/practice management teams.
      f. Rehabilitation psychology and neuropsychology may be available to evaluate and treat deficits in cognition and mood.
      g. Patients should be medically and cognitively able to sit supported for at least 1 hour and to follow one-step commands with progressive consistency.
      h. Primary focus is to achieve significant cognitive and/or physical improvements so that the patient can be transferred to the next appropriate level of rehabilitation.
      i. Discharge home or with family/friends is the optimal goal, but intensive rehabilitation can be of benefit to maximize function before discharge to a subacute or extended care facility.

   2. **Subacute rehabilitation**
      a. Provides lower level of inpatient therapeutic intensity but still involves comprehensive interdisciplinary team approach.
      b. Patients have significant neurologic deficit that prevents them from going home safely.
      c. Patient must be able to tolerate at least 1 hour of therapy per day.
      d. Medical nursing services and physician management are required, although physicians often do not evaluate patients on a daily basis (2–3 visits per week).
      e. Program consists of coordinated therapeutic intervention provided by an interdisciplinary team that may consist of physical, occupational, speech, and recreational therapies as well as psychological and social work.
      f. Patients may receive 1–3 hours of therapy per day.
      g. Placement depends on several factors, including insurance providers, bed availability, level of nursing care needed, capabilities of the facility

(e.g. management of ventilator-dependent patients), and proximity to family and friends.

   h. Primary focus is to achieve significant cognitive and/or physical improvements so that the patient can be transferred to the next appropriate level of rehabilitation.

3. **Extended care facility**
   a. Inpatient setting for patients with significant neurologic deficits that prevent a safe return to home. There are multiple nursing and ADL needs that family and friends cannot provide on a daily basis.
   b. Nursing care is provided as well as physician monitoring on an infrequent basis (1–2 times/month).
   c. Rehabilitation services and therapies are minimal and can be provided from 1 hour/day to 2–3 times/week.
   d. Duration of stay is generally indefinite or until social or functional status changes.
   e. Same placement issues as with subacute rehabilitation.

4. **Day treatment rehabilitation**
   a. Patients have significant functional loss but are able to go home safely with or without additional care.
   b. Patients are capable of community travel.
   c. Highest level of outpatient therapeutic intensity.
   d. Patients can to tolerate one-half to full day of therapies 4–5 times/week.
   e. Patients may receive weekly physician and rehabilitation nursing intervention.
   f. Patients receive coordinated interdisciplinary team approach that is similar to acute inpatient setting.
   g. May provide caregivers respite or chance to continue employment.

5. **Outpatient rehabilitation**
   a. Noninterdisciplinary program without team approach; various levels of therapeutic intensity are available.
   b. Patients have significant neurological deficit but can go home safely.
   c. Patients benefit from 1 hour of a particular therapy, 1–3 times/week, to improve current functional deficits.
   d. Intermittent physician involvement, with little-to-no rehabilitation nursing involvement.
   e. Appropriate for patients with the ability to transport to another facility and the need for continued physical, occupational, and/or speech therapies as well as rehabilitation psychology or neuropsychological intervention.

6. **Home rehabilitation**
   a. Patients have significant functional loss but can go home safely, with or without supervision.
   b. Intended for patients with enough functional independence to ensure safety or appropriate caregiver support.
   c. Patients are not capable of community travel to an outpatient facility.
   d. Intermittent physician supervision and rehabilitation nursing.
   e. Patients benefit from 1–3 hours of therapeutic intervention, 1–3 times/week, to upgrade current functional status, transfer to the next appropriate level of rehabilitation, or discontinue rehabilitation services.
   f. Limited by available equipment or resources.

C. **Therapy for motor recovery**

1. Kottke describes **four neurophysiologic phases**:
   a. Activation of nonresponsive muscles
   b. Reinforcement of feedback
   c. Inhibition of muscles not in a coordinated pattern
   d. Improved performance of the coordinated pattern
2. **Flaccid or low-tone muscle**
   a. Passive ROM once or twice daily to prevent contractures formation
   b. Appropriate positioning to maximize joint protection.
   c. Use synergy patterns to facilitate movement through flaccid stages and progress toward voluntary movement as more voluntary control returns.
3. **High-tone or spastic muscles** (see Chapter 19, Spasticity)
   a. Use neurodevelopmental techniques (e.g., Bobath Neurodevelopmental Training or Proprioceptive Neuromuscular Facilitation) to normalize tone and decrease spasticity by using special tone reducing postures.
   b. Long and slow stretching can help decrease class Ia afferent discharge rates, leading to decreased spasticity.
4. **Constraint-induced therapy**
   a. Voluntary restraint and nonuse of unaffected limb leading to central reorganization and ultimately improvement of control over the affected limb.
   b. Research is still evolving about its purpose in acute, subacute, and chronic stages. Some believe use too early may impede normal recovery.
   c. Useful in "fine-tuning" movements, even in chronic stages, as long as patient has some voluntary movement.
5. **Orthotic management**
   a. **Upper extremity**
      i. Devices for joint protection, spasticity reduction, prevention of shoulder subluxation, and contractures should be used early in recovery.
      ii. Goal of shoulder positioning should be to elevate and externally rotate scapula while maintaining proper alignment of the glenohumeral joint with the wrist and fingers in neutral position.
   b. **Lower extremity**
      i. Assistive devices, such as walkers and straight and four-pronged canes should be used for patients with impaired balance, weakness, or impaired proprioception.
      ii. Ankle-foot orthoses (AFOs) may be required when impaired ankle dorsiflexion or significant plantarflexion tone results in decreased toe clearance. A ground reaction AFO, slightly plantarflexed, may aid in knee extension weakness by facilitating knee hyperextension and increasing knee stability.
      iii. A tone-reducing AFO also may be used to control spasticity limiting the gait cycle.
6. **Mobility retraining and adaptation**
   a. Patients must have intact vision, proprioception, and inner ear function.
   b. Less affected side is used to assist with bed mobility.
   c. Patients progress to transfer training, which may include level transfers using stand-pivot (most commonly), squat-pivot, or sliding board techniques.
   d. Weight-shifting exercises are performed with appropriate fall precautions, support equipment, and supervision.
   e. For ambulation, the patient needs to meet the following requirements:

      i. Ability to follow three-step commands

      ii. Ability to maintain standing balance

      iii. No limitation by flexion contractures in his hips, knees, or ankles

      iv. Capability of antigravity voluntary hip extension to stabilize both hip and knee in extension

      v. Grossly intact proprioception in the affected extremity (not an absolute requirement)

  f. Reciprocal patterns of gait are taught with the aid of parallel bars for support as well as any necessary orthotic equipment.

  g. Ambulation with a four-point cane follows, with progression to a single-point cane.

  h. Patient progresses to higher-level ambulation skills, such as, navigation of stairs, ramps, curbs, and floor transfers.

VI. Stroke Prevention

  A. **Primary prevention** (see Table 2)

  B. **Secondary prevention:** ischemic stroke and transient ischemic attacks (Table 14)

TABLE 14. **Secondary Prevention for Patients with Prior ischemic Stroke or Transient ischemic Attacks**

Risk Factor	Goal	Recommendations
Hypertension	SBP < 140 mmHg and DBP < 90 mmHg If end-organ damage is present, SBP < 135 mmHg and DBP < 85 mmHg	Lifestyle modification and antihypertensive medications.
Smoking	Cessation	Strongly encourage patient and family to stop smoking. Provide counseling and formal cessation programs, nicotine replacement, and medications (e.g., bupropion).
Diabetes mellitus	Glucose < 125 mg/dl	Diet, oral hypoglycemics, insulin.
Lipids	LDL < 100 mg/dl	Start AHA step II diet: ≤ 30% fat, < 7% saturated fat, < 200 mg/day cholesterol; emphasize weight management and physical activity. If target goal is not achieved with these measures, add drug therapy (e.g., statin agent) if LDL > 130 mg/dl; consider drug therapy if LDL = 100–130 mg/dl. Statins are thought to produce protective effect independent of lipid-lowering effect.
Alcohol	Moderate consumption (≤ 2 drinks/day)	Strongly encourage patient and family to stop excessive drinking or provide formal alcohol cessation program.
Weight	≤ 120% of ideal body weight	Diet and exercise.
Atherosclerotic carotid disease ≥ 70% stenosis		Consider endarterectomy (definite benefit if done with acceptable morbidity and mortality). Antiplatelet agents. Angioplasty with stent is currently under evaluation.
60–69% stenosis		Carotid endarterectomy of potential benefit, depending on risk factors. Antiplatelet agents.
< 50% stenosis		Carotid endarterectomy is of no benefit. Antiplatelet agents.

Table continued on following page

TABLE 14.   Secondary Prevention for Patients with Prior ischemic Stroke or Transient ischemic Attacks *(Continued)*

Risk Factor	Goal	Recommendations
Cardiac embolism		
Definite source		Oral anticoagulants (unless contraindicated)
Nonvalvular AF		INR 2–3 (target 2.5) lifelong therapy
LV thrombus,		INR 2–3 (target 2.5) 6-month therapy
recent MI		
Prosthetic VHD		INR 3–4 (target 3.5) lifelong therapy
Possible source		Antiplatelet agents (oral anticoagulation undergoing evaluation)
Transient ischemic attack (TIA)		
Atherothrombotic		Recommended: aspirin, 50–325 mg/day
		Options: extended-release dipyridamole, 200 mg, + aspirin, 25 mg, twice daily
Atherothrombotic and aspirin-intolerant or if TIA occurs during aspirin therapy		Recommended: extended-release dipyridamole, 200 mg, + aspirin, 25 mg, twice daily
		Options: Ticlopidine, 250 mg twice daily; warfarin (INR 2–3), aspirin (50–1300 mg/day)

SBP = systolic blood pressure, DBP = disatolic blood pressure, LDL = low-density liporotein, HDL = high-density lipoprotein; TC = total cholesterol, TG = triglycerides, AF = atrial fibrillation, MI = myocardial infarction, LV = left ventricular, VHD = valvular heart disease.
Adapted from Wolf PE, et al: Preventing ischemic stroke in patients with prior stroke and transient ischemic attack: A statement for healthcare professionals from the Stroke Council of the American Heart Association. Stroke 30:1991–1994, 1999; and Albers GW,et al: Supplement to the guidelines for the management of transient ischemic attacks: A statement from the ad hoc committee on guidelines for the management of transient ischemic attacks, Stroke Council, American Heart Association. Stroke 30:2502–2511, 2000.

Bibliography

1. Adams HP Jr, Brott TG, Furlan AJ, et al: Guidelines for thrombolytic therapy for acute stroke: A supplement to the guidelines for the management of patients with acute ischemic stroke: A statement for healthcare professionals from a Special Writing Group of the Stroke Council, American Heart Association. Circulation 94:1167–1174, 1996.
2. Adams HP, et al: Baseline NIH Stroke Scale score strongly predicts outcome after stroke: A report of the Trial of Org 10721 in Acute Stroke Treatment (TOAST). Neurology 53:126–131, 1999.
3. Albers GW, et al: Supplement to the guidelines for the management of transient ischemic attacks: A statement from the ad hoc committee on guidelines for the management of transient ischemic attacks, Stroke Council, American Heart Association. Stroke 30:2502–2511, 1999.
4. Alexander M: Medical, neurologic, and functional outcome of stroke survivors. In Mills VM, Cassidy JW, Katz DI (eds): Neurologic Rehabilitation: A Guide to Diagnosis, Prognosis, and Treatment Planning. Malden, MA, Blackwell Science, 1997.
5. American Heart Association: 2000 Heart and Stroke Statistical Update. Dallas, TX, American Heart Association, 1999.
6. Blower PW: Relationship between wheelchair propulsion and independent walking in hemiplegic stroke. Stroke 26(4):606–608, 1995.
7. Brandstater ME: Stroke rehabilitation. In DeLisa JA, Gans BM (eds): Rehabilitation Medicine, 3rd ed. Philadelphia, Lippincott-Raven, 1998.
8. Broderick JP, Adams HP, Barsan W, et al: Guidelines for the management of spontaneous intracerebral hemorrhage: A statement for healthcare professionals from a special writing group of the Stroke Council, American Heart Association. Stroke 30:905–915, 1999.
9. Brott, JJ, Bogousslavsky J: Treatment of acute ischemic stroke. N Engl J Med 343:710–720, 2000.
10. Daniels S, et al: Aspiration in patients with acute stroke. Arch Phys Med Rehabil 1998, 79:14–19, 1998.
11. Dromerick A, Reding M: Medical and neurological complications during inpatient stroke rehabilitation. Stroke25:358–361, 1994.

12. Finestone HM, Greene-Finestone LS: Nutrition and diet poststroke. In Teasell RW (ed): Physical Medicine and Rehabilitation: State of the Art Reviews, vol. 12, no. 3. Philadelphia, Hanley & Belfus, 1998.
13. Frankel MR, et al: Predicting prognosis after stroke: A placebo group analysis from the National Institute of Neurological Disorders and Stroke rt-PA Stroke Trial. Neurology 55:952–959, 2000.
14. Geerts WH, Heit JA, et al: Prevention of venous thromboembolism. Chest 119:132S–175S, 2001.
15. Granger CV, et al: Quality and outcome measures for medical rehabilitation. In Braddom RL (ed): Physical Medicine and Rehabilitation. Philadelphia, W.B. Saunders, 1996, pp 239–253.
16. Heitzner, JD, Teasell RW: Clinical consequences of stroke. In Teasell RW (ed): Physical Medicine and Rehabilitation: State of the Art Reviews, vol. 12, no. 3, Philadelphia, Hanley & Belfus, 1998.
17. Hirofumi N, et al: Recovery of upper extremity function in stroke patients: The Copenhagen Stroke Study. Arch Phys Med Rehabil 75:394–398, 1994.
18. Jorgensen HS, et al: Stroke: Neurologic and functional recovery. The Copenhagen Stroke Study. Phys Med Rehabil Clin North Am 10:887–906, 1999.
19. Jorgensen HS, et al: Recovery of walking function in stroke patients: The Copenhagen Stroke Study. Arch Phys Med Rehabil 76:27–32, 1995.
20. Jorgensen HS, et al: Outcome and time course of recovery in stroke. Part I: Outcome. The Copenhagen Stroke Study. Arch Phys Med Rehabil 76:399–405, 1995.
21. Jorgensen HS, et al: Outcome and time course of recovery in stroke. Part II: Time course of recovery. The Copenhagen Stroke Study. Arch Phys Med Rehabil 1995, 76:406–412, 1995.
22. Kelly-Hayes M, Robertson JT, et al: The American Heart Association Stroke Outcome Classification. Stroke 29:1274–1280, 1998.
23. Kottke FJ: Neurophysiologic therapy for stroke. In Licht S (ed): Stroke and Its Rehabilitation. New Haven, CT, Elizabeth Licht, 1975.
24. Lowenstein DH, Alldredge BK: Status epilepticus. N Engl J Med 338:970–976, 1998.
25. McGuire JR, Harvey RL: The prevention and management of complications after stroke. Phys Med Rehabil Clin North Am 10:857–874, 1999.
26. Muir KW, Wier CJ, Murray GD, et al: Comparison of neurological scales and scoring systems for acute stroke prognosis. Stroke 27:1817–1820, 1996.
27. Nakayama H, Jorgensen HS, Raaschou HO, Olsen TS: Recovery of upper extremity function in stroke patients: The Copenhagen Stroke Study. Arch Phys Med Rehabil 75:394–398, 1994.
28. Olsen TS: Arm and leg paresis as outcome predictors in stroke rehabilitation. Stroke 21:247–251, 1990.
29. Reith J, et al: Body temperature in acute stroke: Relation to stroke severity, mortality, outcome and infarct size. The Copenhagen Stroke Study. Lancet 347:422–425, 1996..
30. Roth EJ, Harvey RL: Rehabilitation of stroke syndromes. In Braddom RL (ed): Physical Medicine and Rehabilitation, 2nd ed. Philadelphia, W.B. Saunders, 2000, pp 1117–1160.
31. Smith J: Rehabilitation Institute of Chicago Alternate Levels of Rehabilitation Care Guidelines. Chicago, Rehabilitation Institute of Chicago, 1997.
32. Teasell RW, McRae M, Finestone HM: Aspiration and pneumonia following stroke. In Teasell RW (ed): Physical Medicine and Rehabilitation: State of the Art Reviews, vol. 12, no. 3. Philadelphia, Hanley & Belfus, 1998.
33. Twitchell T: The restoration of motor function after stroke. Brain 74:443–480, 1951.
34. Wahlgren NG: Stroke scales. In Ginsberg MD, Bogousslavsky J (eds): Cerebrovascular Disease: Pathophysiology, Diagosis, and Management. Malden, MA, Blackwell Science, 1998.
35. Wiebe S, Butler JT: Poststroke seizures and epilepsy. In Teasell RW (ed): Physical Medicine and Rehabilitation: State of the Art Reviews, vol. 12, no. 3, Philadelphia, Hanley & Belfus, 1998.
36. Wiebers, DO, Feigin VL, Brown RD Jr: Handbook of Stroke. Philadelphia, Lippinicot-Raven, 1997.
37. Wolf PE, et al: Preventing ischemic stroke in patients with prior stroke and transient ischemic attack: A statement for healthcare professionals from the Stroke Council of the American Heart Association. Stroke 30:1991–1994, 1999.

Chapter 10

TRAUMATIC BRAIN INJURY

Anne G. Hartigan, M.D., and Sharon K. McDowell, M.D.

I. General Principles

A. Traumatic brain injury (TBI) is a **common comorbid condition** for many patients on the inpatient rehabilitation unit.
   1. Consequences of TBI can affect all body systems.
   2. Often subtle brain injury first becomes apparent after transfer to the rehabilitation floor.

B. **Epidemiology**
   1. Difficult to estimate because of the following factors:
      a. Many people with TBIs, especially mild TBIs, are never evaluated in hospital or doctor's office.
      b. Levels and definitions of TBI vary from study to study and center to center.
      c. TBIs in fatal accidents are not recorded.
   2. Fatal incidence
      a. 51,000 of all injury-related deaths annually involve TBI.
      b. Mortality rate for TBI: 14–30 per 100,000 population per year.
      c. Elderly population has highest mortality rate.
   3. Nonfatal incidence
      a. Estimated 1.5–2 million people in U.S. (150 per 100,000 population) suffer TBI annually.
      b. 73,152 estimated new cases of disability from brain injury in 1995 in the U.S. (28 per 100,000 population).

C. **Cost**
   1. Average lifetime cost per person: $85,000; for severe TBI, $300,000.
   2. Severely injured persons require 40 times as much financial support as mildly injured persons.
   3. In U.S. estimated $6.5 billion for care of patients with new brain injury each year; $13.5 billion for annual continuing care for existing TBIs.

D. **Risk factors**
   1. Age: 15–24 and 65–75 years.
   2. Gender: males > females.
   3. Race: African Americans, Hispanics.
   4. Low socioeconomic status.
   5. Alcohol: Kraus et al. found that 56% of adults with a diagnosis of brain injury who were tested had a positive blood alcohol concentration.
   6. Prior hospitalization for head injury.

E. **Etiology**
   1. Transportation-related (including motor vehicle, bicycle, and pedestrian accidents)

2. Falls
3. Assaults (e.g., firearms)
4. Sports and recreation (horseback riding, skateboarding, skiing, sledding, use of playground equipment)

II. Classification and Mechanisms

A. Definitions

1. **TBI:** all injuries to the brain resulting from trauma.
2. **Diffuse axonal injury (DAI):** widespread stretching of axons caused by rotation of brain around its axis; associated with diffuse brain swelling.
   a. Mechanism unclear: damage to white fiber tracts caused by acceleration-deceleration injury.
   b. Based on centripetal model → greatest force at surface of brain → cortex affected first.
   c. More severe TBI: affects deep brain, corpus callosum, and long fiber tracts.
   d. Cause of initial loss of consciousness.
   e. Head computed tomography (CT) scan may show small hemorrhagic lesions at gray-white junction of cerebral cortex and corpus callosum, deep nuclei and brainstem.
3. **Coup and contrecoup contusions:** coup contusions occur at site of impact; contrecoup contusions occur in brain tissue diametrically opposite point of contact.
   a. Usually due to acceleration-deceleration.
   b. Affect inferior frontal and anterior temporal lobes.
   c. Lesions usually bilateral.
   d. Functional defects: focal cognitive and sensory motor.

B. Classification

1. **Anatomic lesions** (Figs. 1 and 2)
   a. Closed head injury: dura intact.
   b. Open head injury: dura opened.
   c. Penetrating head injury: foreign object penetrates dura and enters brain.

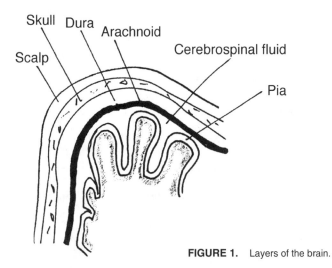

FIGURE 1.   Layers of the brain.

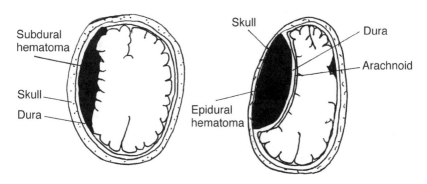

FIGURE 2. Subdural vs. epidural hematoma.

2. **Primary vs. secondary**
   a. Primary: immediate impact-related injury.
      i. Most due to acceleration-deceleration
      ii. Injuries may include scalp injury, skull fracture, surface contusions/laceration, intracranial hematoma, and DAI.
   b. Secondary: delayed injury
      i. Example: increased intracranial pressure (ICP) that leads to decreased cerebral perfusion, which in turn leads to ischemic damage.
      ii. Injuries may include hemorrhage (epidural, subdural, and intracerebral), raised ICP, edema (vascogenic or cytogenic), hypoxia, excitotoxicity (caused by increased excitatory neurotransmitters), production of free radicals, and meningitis.
3. **Focal vs. diffuse**
   a. Focal injury may involve scalp injury, skull fracture, epidural and subdural injury, intracerebral hematomas, contusions, and raised ICP.
   b. Diffuse injury may involve DAI, contusion, hypoxia-ischemia, diffuse brain swelling, and diffuse neurochemical changes.
4. **Contact vs. acceleration-deceleration**
   a. Contact injury may involve scalp lesions, skull fracture with or without extradural hematoma, surface contusions, intracerebral hemorrhage.
   b. Acceleration-deceleration injury may involve tearing of bridging veins with formation of subdural hematoma (SDH), DAI, acute vascular injury, and neurochemical changes.
III. **Acute Evaluation and Treatment**
   A. **Goals**
      1. Stabilize airway, breathing, and circulation (ABCs): provide airway, adequate ventilation and perfusion, and control blood pressure.
      2. Prevent secondary injury.
      3. Address neurologic impairments.
      4. Establish neurologic diagnosis and prognosis for recovery.
   B. **Evaluation**
      1. **Clinical signs and symptoms**
         a. Check and stabilize ABCs.
         b. Consider mannitol to decrease ICP.
         c. Neurologic evaluation

    i. Glasgow Coma Scale (See Appendix F)
- First stimulus: verbal.
- If no response, pain stimulus of heavy pressure on nailbed of little finger or great toe. Test each side to identify hemiplegia.
- If still no response, sternal rub or pressure to supraorbital area, mastoid region to identify tetraplegia.

    ii. Pupils (Table 1)

    iii. Corneal, gag, and cough reflexes to evaluate lower brainstem and pons.

    iv. Check for meningism, neck stiffness after cervical spine cleared; may develop several hours after subarachnoid hemorrhage (SAH).

    v. Motor exam: determine if weakness is lateralized.

    vi. In comatose patient, test response to deep supraorbital painful stimulation.

    vii. In awake patient, ask about details of event, memories before event, how patient arrived at hospital, and similar questions.

    viii. Complete neurologic exam when patient is stable.

2. **Diagnostic imaging/testing** (Table 2)
   a. **Immediate head CT**
      i. Identifies blood, edema, facial or skull fractures (vault fracture raises risk of intracranial complications tenfold)
      ii. Intracranial air: associated with dural tearing and communication between outside and subarachnoid space; increased risk of infection
      iii. Some patients with normal CT scan may still have diffuse injury.
   b. **Cervical spine x-rays**
   c. **Magnetic resonance imaging (MRI) of brain**
      i. More sensitive than CT to nonhemorrhagic shear injuries, but longer time required for test.
      ii. Hemorrhage within 72 hours can be difficult to detect.
      iii. A few days after injury MRI is more sensitive than CT because blood becomes hyperintense on T1-weighted images and hypointense on T2-weighted images.
      iv. Usually performed during rehabilitation phase to explain deficits.
      v. Superior test for brainstem lesion and deep lesions, such as petechial hemorrhages, seen in DAI.
      vi. Extent of DAI can be classified according to corpus callosum atrophy, regional brain volume measurements and ventricular enlargement.
   d. **Functional MRI (fMRI):** mapping of regional cerebral blood flow in response to activation due to difference in magnetic properties of deoxygenated vs. oxygenated hemoglobin.
   e. **Single-photon emission computed tomography (SPECT)**
      i. More sensitive to focal injury but insensitive to brain swelling.
      ii. Although SPECT picks up more lesions than CT, some abnormalities (e.g., contusions, SAH, SDH) are only seen on CT.
      iii. Hypoperfusion associated with poorer neuropsychological outcome.
      iv. SPECT may correlate better than structural imaging with neuropsychological outcome and deficits.
      v. May be useful for prognostication.
   f. **Electrophysiologic studies**
      i. May be useful when patient unable to interact with examiner (i.e., in coma).

TABLE 1. Eye Exam

Aspect of Exam	Finding	Rule Out	Diagnostic Test
Pupil size and light response		Asymmetry	Ipsilateral and consensual light reflex
	Unreactive, dilated pupils	Cerebral hypoxia or ischemia Drug intoxication (atropine, alcohol)	Head CT
	Bilateral pinpoint, reactive pupils	Pons lesions Thalamic lesion Narcotic overdose Metabolic encephalopathy	Head CT
	Unilateral dilation	Transtentorial/uncal herniation (ipsilateral intracranial mass)	Neurosurgical emergency Hyperventilation Mannitol Head CT
	Anisocoria (slight difference in size of pupils; present in 15–30% of population)	Mydriatics used (scopolamine, atropine)	If physiologic anisocoria, light reflex present
Eye movement	Full conjugate gaze in all 6 directions without nystagmus		Check extraocular movement
	Disconjugate gaze	Brainstem lesion	Head CT/MRI
	Head rotated left, eyes should move to right to regain central position and then follow head to right	Normal: inhibited doll's eye maneuver (brainstem intact)	Oculocephalic or "doll's eye" maneuver (if no cervical spine precautions); hold head at 30° from supine and rotate to side
	Turn head left, eyes go right	Diencephalic level of function	CT/MRI
	Turn head left, eyes can only abduct	Midbrain or pontine lesion; CN VI intact	CT/MRI
	Turn head left, eyes go left (no eye movement)	Medullary level: damaged brainstem	CT/MRI
	Cold water: eyes tonically deviate to irrigated side but have quick, saccadic eye movement in opposite direction (tonic reflex is slow, cortical saccade is fast)	Normal	Oculovestibular (caloric) tests: head at 30° from supine, at least 20 ml cold water injected into external auditory meatus by syringe
	Tonic deviation toward cold stimulus, no nystagmus	Diencephalic level injury	CT/MRI
	Tonic eye abduction only	Midbrain-pontine level (damage to MLF)	CT/MRI
Vertical gaze	No vertical gaze	Midbrain lesion Central herniation Acute hydrocephalus	Simultaneous caloric stimulation of both ears
Resting eye	Conjugate deviation	Toward hemiparesis: rule out brainstem lesion on opposite side Away from hemiparesis: rule out frontal lobe lesion contralateral to hemiparetic side	CT/MRI
Fundus		Rule out papilledema	Fundoscopic exam

CT = computed tomography, MRI = magnetic resonance imaging, CN = cranial nerve, MLF = medial longitudinal fasciculus.

Table 2. Diagnostic Imaging

Imaging Technique	Best Used to Evaluate	Advantages	Limitations
Plain x-rays	No indication		No indication
CT	Acute SAH, fractures (FLAIR better for sub-acute SAH)	Quick (monitor difficult patients) Inexpensive	Radiation Not sensitive for DAI
MRI–T1	Hematomas (EDH, SDH, intraparenchymal) > 1 mo old Sensitive to methemoglobin	Highest signal-to-noise ratio Best for anatomy	Insensitive for non–contour-deforming intraparenchymal injuries
MRI-3D-T1 (gradient)	For seizure patients:subtle cortical abnormalities	Best anatomic resolution	Very long sequence
MRI-T2	Acute intraparenchymal injury Subacute extra-axial fluid collections (EDH, SDH, hygromas)	Shows nonhemorrhagic injuries	Cannot do with contrast enhancement
MRI–T2 (gradient)	Subtle subacute hemor-rhages Hemosiderin in microfoci of DAI Rule out cavernous heman-giomas	Most sensitive to subacute hemorrhage (days) Fast sequence	Artifacts at skull base Lower resolution Lower signal-to-noise ratio Magnetically susceptible
FLAIR	Gray/white matter and periventricular abnor-malities SAH	Similar to T2 but no water signal (CSF is black	Artifacts at skull base
MTR-MRI	White matter abnormalities	Demonstrates myelin integrity	Not commonly available for clinical use
DT-MRI	DAI Assessment of mild TBI	Defines location, direction, and integrity of white matter tracts by deter-mining direction of water diffusion	Limited research with TBI
PET	Identifying injured but structurally intact regions Regional function by glu-cose uptake ([18F]-fluoro-deoxyglucose), even if structure intact (cobalt 55, C-11-diacylglycerol)	Identifies pathophysiology: (hyperglycolysis and calcium toxicity) Correlates with cognitive/behavioral disorders Images functional re-covery	Limited diagnostic/clinical utility Expensive Not widely available Radiation exposure Poor specificity
SPECT	Global/regional function by perfusion tracers (HMPAO, 123I-iodoamphetamine, technetium-99m ECD, xenon) Better assessment of lesion size	More sensitive for mild TBI Better correlation with cognitive disorders Sensitive for depression, anxiety, and learning disability	Radiation exposure No specific TBI pattern
fMRI	Indirectly measures changes in metabolic activity by blood flow (using magnetic properties of oxy-, deoxy-Hgb) Altered pattern of cognitive activation after mild TBI	No radiation exposure Better spatial/temporal resolution Noninvasive	Unknown clinical utility Few studies with TBI Several contradictions in analysis

Table continued on following page

Table 2.   Diagnostic Imaging *(Continued)*

Imaging Technique	Best Used to Evaluate	Advantages	Limitations
Proton MRS	Decreased N-acetyl aspartate in areas of DAI	Ischemic brain and penumbra Separates reversibly and irreversibly damaged brain	Long sequence Decreased spatial resolution Difficult and lengthy to reconstruct
Phosphorus MRS	Metabolic changes in brain Loss of Mg ions, which correlates with TBI severity	Measures shift in high-energy phosphates Measures change in intracellular Mg ions	
Magnetic source imaging	Integrates anatomic data using MRI Assesses magnetic fields generated by neurons	High resolution of physiology Correlates with cognitive deficits and recovery High sensitivity, acceptable specificity	Limited research

CT = computed tomography; MRI-T1 = magnetic resonance imaging, T1-weighted; MRI-3D-T1 = three-dimensional MR-T1; MRI-T2 = MRI, T2-weighted; FLAIR = fluid-attenuated inversion recovery; MTR-MRI = magnetization transfer ratio MRI: PET = positron emission tomography; SPECT = single-photon emission computed tomography; fMRI = functional MRI; MRS = magnetic resonance spectroscopy; SAH = subarachnoid hemorrhage; EDH = epidural hematoma; SDH = subdural hematoma; DAI = diffuse axonal injury; Hgb = hemoglobin; Mg = magnesium; CSF = cerebrospinal fluid, DT-MRI = diffusion tensor MRI.

  ii. Help in diagnosis of posttraumatic seizures.
  iii. Less sensitive than functional neuroimaging to localize lesion or dysfunction.
  iv. Examples
   • Electroencephalography (EEG)
   • Brainstem auditory evoked potentials (BAEP)
   • Visual evoked potentials (VEP)
   • Somatosensory evoked potentials (SSEP)
   • Multimodal evoked potentials (MEP)
   • Event-related evoked potentials
 g. Blood gas analysis
 h. Hematocrit, toxicology screen, electrolytes, alcohol level
 i. Lumbar puncture (cerebrospinal fluid [CSF])
3. **Reasons to admit patient for observation**
 a. Altered state of consciousness
 b. Prolonged loss of consciousness
 c. Nausea and vomiting
 d. Seizure
 e. Focal neurologic signs
 f. Skull fracture < 24 hours old
   • Severe headache
   • Penetrating brain injury
   • CSF rhinorrhea or otorrhea
   • Cerebral contusion or swelling intracranial hematoma
C. **Acute treatment**
1. **Goal:** to optimize cerebral homeostasis and prevent secondary injury.
2. **Monitor** ventilation, fluid balance, cerebral and systemic blood pressure, temperature.
3. **Treat elevated ICP**.
 a. **Mannitol** is first-choice therapy; there is no indication for corticosteroids in head injury.

      i. Data are insufficient to recommend one form of mannitol infusion over another

      ii. Mannitol for elevated ICP may improve mortality rates compared with pentobarbital treatment.

      iii. ICP-directed treatment shows small benefit compared with treatment directed by neurologic signs and physiologic indicators.

      iv. Data about effectiveness of prehospital administration of mannitol are insufficient to support harmful or beneficial effect.

      v. Direct comparison indicates that **bifrontal regional oxygen saturation** is better with hypothermia or osmotic agents than with barbiturates.

b. Role of **hypothermia** remains to be defined.

c. **Barbiturates**

      i. Believed to reduce intracranial pressure by suppressing cerebral metabolism, thus reducing cerebral metabolic demands and cerebral blood volume.

      ii. Also reduce blood pressure in 1 in 4 patients; hypotensive effect offsets any ICP-lowering effect on cerebral perfusion pressure (CPP).

      iii. No evidence indicates that barbiturate therapy in patients with acute severe head injury improves outcome.

g. **Hypertonic saline solution**

      i. Increase in serum sodium concentration significantly decreases ICP and increases CPP.

      ii. Hypertonic saline is effective agent to increase serum sodium concentrations.

      iii. Sustained hypernatremia and hyperosmolarity are safely tolerated in pediatric patients with TBI.

h. **Indomethacin (IND)**

      i. Case series involving severe TBI suggest that IV boluses of 30–50 mg reduce ICP by 37–52% and reduce cerebral blood flow by 22–26%, with a modest 14% increase in CPP.

      ii. Despite these encouraging results, IV IND should be considered only as experimental treatment for control of refractory ICP in TBI.

i. **Hyperventilation**

      i. Aggressive hyperventilation ($pCO_2 < 30$ mmHg), especially during first few days after severe TBI, should be avoided.

      ii. Although controversial, **optimized hyperventilation, induced systemic hypertension, and vasoconstrictive therapy** are optimally used under multimodal monitoring.

      iii. Forced hyperventilation over lengthy period seems to have unfavorable effect.

j. **Sedative or hypnotic therapy:** medications to reduce cerebral blood flow and cerebral metabolic rate to decrease ICP and brain oxygen requirements (e.g., propofol, thiopental).

4. **Treat other systemic issues.**

IV. **Severity of Injury**

A. Scales and factors useful in acute setting as **indicators of impairment and predictors of gross outcome**

1. Glasgow Coma Scale (GCS) (See Appendix F)

  a. Standardized system for assessing response to stimuli in neurologically impaired patients.
  b. Reactions are given numerical value (1–5) in three categories (eye opening, verbal responsiveness, and motor responsiveness). Three scores are then added together. Lowest values are worst clinical scores.
  c. Note best and worst GCS scores within 24 hours of injury.
  d. Severity often based on GCS at lowest point after resuscitation (Table 3).
 2. Length of coma
 3. Duration of posttraumatic amnesia (PTA): period of loss of memory after injury
  a. Galveston Orientation and Amnesia Test (GOAT) determines when patient is out of PTA (Appendix F).
  b. Follow patient with serial exams.
  c. General rule: GOAT score > 75 for 2 consecutive days indicates end of PTA.
  d. Not useful prognostic indicator in rehabilitation, but rate of cognitive recovery may have strong relationship to PTA.
 B. **Mild brain injury** (definition controversial)
 1. Includes injuries resulting from acceleration/deceleration of head, skull distortion with resultant pressure gradients, and cervical spine stretching.
 2. Definition is controversial. Mild Traumatic Brain Injury Special Interest Group of the American Congress of Rehabilitation Medicine offers following definition:
  a. Traumatically induced physiologic disruption of brain function as manifested by at least one of the following:
   i. Any period of loss of consciousness
   ii. Any loss of memory for events immediately before or after accident
   iii. Any alteration in mental state at time of accident (e.g., feeling dazed, disoriented or confused)
   iv. Focal neurologic deficits, which may or may not be transient
  b. Severity of injury does not exceed the following:
   i. Loss of consciousness of approximately 30 minutes or less
   ii. After 30 minutes, an initial Glasgow Coma Scale of 13–15
   iii. Posttraumatic amnesia for no longer than 24 hours
  c. Definition includes blows to head, head striking an object, and brain undergoing acceleration/deceleration movement (i.e., whiplash) without direct external trauma to head.
 C. **Prognostic indicators:** early prognostication of severe disability has < 60% reliability even with sophisticated testing (Table 4).

Table 3.   Severity of Closed Head Injury*

Severity	GCS Score	Description
Mild	13–15	Loss of consciousness < 20 min No TBI abnormalities on neurologic exam Normal head CT scan
Moderate	9–12	Combative or lethargic Normal neurologic exam and CT abnormality indicate moderate TBI or mild TBI with complications
Severe	3–8	Coma

* Based on Glasgow Coma Scale (GCS) at lowest point after resuscitation.

TABLE 4. Prognostic Indicators

System	PE or test	Test Information	Bad Prognostic Signs
Brainstem	CN exam		Fixed or dilated pupils
Cortical/brainstem	GCS score		Low motor score
Cerebrospinal fluid (CSF)	Intracranial pressure		> 30 mmHg for several hours
	LP with CSF analysis	Concentrations of creatinine kinase (CK) BB, lactate, catecholamines, and cytokines	Low concentrations, especially of CK-BB
Structural scanning	CT/MRI	MRI shows small, temporary lesions during first month	Early CT abnormalities MRI abnormalities after 1 month
Electrical brain activity	Continuous EEG	Compressed spectral array most predictive	Absence of activity even on high gain
	Evoked potentials	Useful only if done serially	
	Magnetic source image	Correlates with cognitive outcome	
Cerebral perfusion	Cerebral blood flow	Not reliable if flow present	Absence of cerebral blood flow
Cerebral metabolism	AVdO$_2$ studies	Not reliable	
	SPECT/PET	Correlates with cognitive recovery, good for mild TBI	
Patient's age			> 60 years

CN = cranial nerve, GCS = Glasgow Coma Scale, LP = lumbar puncture, CT= computed tomography, MRI = magnetic resonance imaging, EEG = electroencephalography, SPECT = single-photon emission computed tomography, PET = positron emission tomography.

V. Structure-Function Relationships
A. **Strain at surface of cortex:** amnesia, short-term memory deficits, high-level neuropsychological deficits.
B. **Lower brainstem injury:** respiratory irregularities, apnea, vomiting, hypertension, bradycardia.
C. **Upper pontine/mesencephalic injuries** (caused by stronger forces): loss of consciousness, corneal areflexia, pupillary areflexia, decerebration, cortical blindness from vascular hyperreactivity.
D. **Frontal lobe**
  1. Dorsolateral: executive dysfunction, disorganized thinking, cognitive rigidity, perseveration.
  2. Orbitofrontal: disinhibition.
  3. Superior medial: akinetic mutism, apathy.
  4. Inferior medial: amnesia, confabulations, disinhibition, lack of motivation, inattention, utilization behavior.
E. **Left hemisphere**
  1. Anterior: apraxia, nonfluent aphasia.
  2. Posterior: fluent aphasia.
F. **Right hemisphere**
  1. Anterior: motor inpersistence, aprosody.
  2. Posterior: neglect, visuospatial disturbance.
G. **Temporal lobe**
  1. Medial: anterograde amnesia.
  2. Anterior: retrograde amnesia.

3. Lateral: semantic amnesia.
4. Posterior (bilateral): visual agnosia.
5. Posterior (right): prosopagnosia.
   H. **Parietal lobe**
1. Left: alexia, agraphia, Gerstmann's syndrome (finger agnosia, right-left confusion, dyscalculia, and dysgraphia), ideomotor apraxia.
2. Right: unilateral neglect, geographic disorientation.

VI. Impact of TBI on Body Systems

Although TBI implies brain injury alone, practically all body systems can be affected. Common problems in patients with TBI are listed alphabetically by body system with symptoms, causes, and treatment options.
   A. **Affective disorders**
1. **Agitation:** emotional state associated with severe anxiety, fear, or uncertainty and motor restlessness.
   a. **Systemic causes:** pain, infection/fever, hypoxia, metabolic abnormalities, GI obstruction, constipation, urinary obstruction/retention, alcohol/drug withdrawal, medication toxicity or interaction.
   b. **Neurologic causes**: increased ICP, expanding mass lesion, posttraumatic hydrocephalus, posttraumatic seizures, altered sensory input, visual deficits, hearing loss, somatosensory loss (peripheral nerve injury), injury to frontal-temporal pathways, neurochemical changes.
   c. **Treatment/modifications**
      i. Rule out systemic or neurologic causes.
      ii. Provide structured environment.
         • Maintain low stimulus level (reduce light and noise, limit visitors).
         • Maintain consistent staffing.
         • Regulate daily schedule.
         • Follow day/night pattern with appropriate lighting/noise.
      iii. Reorientation
         • Provide frequent reorientation to place, time, and situation.
         • All staff should reintroduce themselves with each interaction.
         • Explain all procedures and daily routine.
         • Keep family photos in room.
      iv. Behavioral, emotional, and cognitive approaches
         • Adjust physical and cognitive demands to patient's level.
         • Actively engage patient in treatment.
         • Reassure patient.
         • Have family member present for minor procedures.
         • Have patient keep memory logbook.
         • Keep meaningful tokens or objects in room.
      v. Active interventions
         • Use de-escalation techniques.
         • Redirect patient.
         • Allow time-outs.
         • Use cubicle or vail beds.
         • Use soft restraints, posey vest.
         • Provide sitter for supervision/help in redirecting patient.
         • Use appropriate medications (see VII. Psychopharmacology).
         • Follow agitation with Agitated Behavior Scale. Ask team members to complete form after patient sessions.

    2. **Anxiety:** irritability, restlessness, decreased concentration, poor endurance.
      a. More common in left hemispheric lesions.
      b. Treat with psychotherapeutic or behavioral approach.
      c. For appropriate medications, see VII. Psychopharmacology.
    3. **Depression**
      a. Occurs in 10–60% of patients with TBI.
      b. At 1 year after injury, major depression is present in 26% of patients.
      c. May be caused by decreased serotonin pathways secondary to DAI (unproven theory).
      d. For appropriate medications, see VII. Psychopharmacology.
    4. **Posttraumatic stress disorder (PTSD)**
      a. Debatable whether PTSD and TBI can coexist.
        i. Probably more likely in mild TBI with shorter amnestic period.
        ii. Estimated to affect 20–30% of patients with TBI.
      b. Signs and symptoms include nightmares, flashbacks to causative traumatic event(s).
      c. Treatment: psychotherapeutic or behavioral approach, appropriate medications (see VII. Psychopharmacology).
  B. **Autonomic system**
    1. **Hypertension**
      a. Major symptom: headache.
      b. Causes: high ICP, catecholamine release, focal brain lesion near hypothalamus.
      c. Treatment
        i. Rule out other causes.
        ii. Use cardioselective beta blockers in acute phase (atenolol, metoprolol).
        iii. Usually self-limited; if primary hypertension is present, use least sedating medications (diuretics or clonidine [alpha agonist] patches).
    2. **Hypotension**
      a. Major symptoms: dizziness, fatigue.
      b. Causes: prolonged bed rest, orthostatic hypotension, hypopituitarism.
      c. Treatment
        i. Compression garments (TEDS, JUZOs).
        ii. Medication: ephedrine (?).
    3. **Tachycardia**
      a. Cause: catecholamine release.
      b. Treatment: beta blocker.
    4. **Temperature regulation, central fever**
      a. Major symptom: hyperthermia.
      b. Causes: infection, lesions in anterior hypothalamus with generalized decerebration, drugs, neuroleptic malignant syndrome (phenothiazines), deep venous thrombosis (DVT), diencephalic storm.
      c. Treatment
        i. Rule out infection.
        ii. Use environmental controls (cooling blankets, tepid baths, fan).
        iii. Prescribe appropriate medications.
    5. **Hypothermia**
      a. Causes: lesions in posterior hypothalamus, myxedema, hypothyroidism, barbiturates.
      b. Treatment

       i. Identify cause and correct.

       ii. Use external environmental controls.

       iii. Possible treatment with intranasal vasopressin (DDAVP).

C. **Behavioral and psychosocial impairments**

  1. **Aggression**

    a. Symptoms: disinhibited, disruptive, or combative behavior.

    b. Test for assessment and follow-up: Overt Aggression Scale (OAS).

    c. Treatment (see agitation section)

      i. Behavioral modification

      ii. Behavioral modification planning

      iii. Psychotherapy

      iv. Psychoactive medications (anticonvulsants, beta blockers, antidepressants)

  2. **Impaired awareness**

    a. Major symptom: anosognosia (failure to acknowledge neurologic deficits, denial, decreased self-awareness).

    b. No validated treatments

  3. **Sexual dysfunction**

    a. Major symptoms: hypersexuality, hyposexuality, impotence, loss of feeling of attractiveness, incapacity to engage in intimate relationships.

    b. Treatment

      i. For hypersexuality: selective serotonin reuptake inhibitors (SSRIs), anticonvulsants, beta blockers.

      ii. For hyposexuality
* Check medication side effects.
* Medication: cyproheptadine.
* Consider counseling.

  4. **Impaired social behavior**

    a. Symptoms: child-like behavior, difficulty in establishing or maintaining relationships, talkativeness, tangential expression.

    b. Treatment

      i. Group psychotherapy

      ii. Language groups with audio or videotape feedback

      iii. Recreation therapist to find new activities and modify premorbid hobbies

  5. **Substance abuse**

    a. Preinjury substance abuse prevalent in > 50% people with TBI.

    b. Treatment: specialized head injury programs for dual diagnosis of TBI and substance abuse.

D. **Cardiovascular system**

  1. **Ischemia/necrosis**

    a. Symptoms: chest pain, irregular heart beat.

    b. Causes: catecholamine release, direct trauma, increased ICP, increased cardiac work and oxygen consumption.

    c. Treatment

      i. Consult with cardiologist.

      ii. Rule out myocardial infraction.

  2. **Arrhythmias**

    a. Present in 21% of patients in study by McLeod et al.

    b. Symptoms: torsades de pointes, pulsus alternans, U-wave alternans.

    c. Cause: Myocardial damage.

    d. Treatment: check baseline EKG on admission.

3. **DVT**

    a. Symptoms: red, warm, swollen, tender extremity; Homan's sign (calf pain with dorsiflexion).

    b. 54% incidence in patients with major brain trauma, 69% incidence in patients with lower extremity orthopedic injury.

    c. Risk factors: immobility, trauma, surgery, lower extremity fractures, age > 40 yr.

    d. Prevention: graded compression stockings in conjunction with:

        i. Low-molecular-weight heparin (LMWH) 40 mg/day subcutaneously once daily, or 30 mg LMWH subcutaneously every 12 hr, or unfractionated heparin, 5000 U every 12 hr subcutaneously.

        ii. Intermittent pneumatic compression helpful, but difficult to use 24 hr/day.

        iii. Consider vena cava filter if anticoagulation is contraindicated.

    e. Treatment

        i. IV heparin or LMWH until warfarin becomes therapeutic.

        ii. Warfarin therapy, 3–6 months, for target international normalized ratio (INR) of 2–3.

E. **Cognitive deficits**

1. **Arousal:** state of preparedness to receive incoming sensory input and/or generate response.

    a. Tonic arousal: slow fluctuations due to diurnal rhythm, temperature, activity level.

    b. Phasic arousal: abrupt shifts in response to task demands and warning signals.

    c. Controlled by reticular activating system (RAS) with reciprocal cortical and subcortical feedback loops.

    d. Regulated by multiple neurotransmitter systems (norepinephrine, dopamine, acetylcholine, serotonin).

    e. Indicators: eye opening, body language, EEG spectrum, sleep pattern, changes in performance over time, slow responsiveness, infrequent response, slow processing, difficulty in coping with cognitively demanding situations.

    f. Assess and follow with Coma Emergence Scales.

    g. Treatment

        i. Experimental: collect data to validate treatment.

        ii. Behavioral: naps vs. upright position (tonic arousal), frequent task changes (phasic arousal).

        iv. Compensatory strategy: engage in tasks when most alert.

        v. Pharmacologic: stimulants, dopaminergics.

2. **Attention:** conscious, effortful processing with selective channeling of arousal and selection of specific sensory stimuli and motor responses required for facilitation.

    a. Cortical and subcortical regions involved (right parietal and prefrontal).

    b. Indicators: errors related to location/space (parietal) or time (prefrontal); unusual eye movement patterns (eyes looking away from task)

    c. Assessment and follow-up measures

        i. Observe patient to determine if he or she is easily distractable.

      ii. Check mental control: ask patient to count backward from 20, name months forward and backward.

      iii. Check sustained attention: read a random list of letters and have patient indicate when you say "A"; letter cancellation; repeat digit span.

   d. Treatment

      i. Experimental: collect data to validate treatment.

      ii. Team should agree on consistent behavioral and compensatory treatment approaches.

      iii. Carry over strategies into functional activities.

3. **Executive function:** ability to solve problems, adapt to change, anticipate outcomes, cope with new situations.

   a. Cognitive flexibility involves prefrontal cortex.

   b. Indicators: difficulty with planning, reasoning, problem solving; impulsivity; perseveration; inappropriate gestures; bizarre speech.

   c. Tests: verbal fluency, response inhibition, problem solving, perseveration, set shifting, abstractions, judgment, similarities.

   d. Treatment: no proven treatments; focus on functional tasks in all aspects of rehabilitation.

4. **Initiation**

   a. Major indicator: delay in starting requested tasks; increased or decreased amount of spontaneous behavior.

   b. Assessment: record time to beginning task after receiving instructions (may be recorded daily by therapist).

   c. Treatment

      i. Experimental: measure treatment responses.

      ii. Use structured initiation cues.

      iii. Give positive reinforcement for initiation of tasks.

      iv. Medications: psychostimulants and dopaminergic agonists.

5. **Language and communication**

   a. Dysnomia: disturbance in word-finding or object-naming; most common language disorder in TBI (dominant parietal area).

   b. Aphasia tends to resolve within 6 months.

   c. Basic functional language skills recover by 6 months, but higher-level difficulties may be first detected in challenging environment (work/school).

   d. Verbal fluency: left frontal or bifrontal lesions.

   e. Indicators: dysnomia, dysgraphia, dyslexia, dyscalculia, anomic aphasia (semantic errors, circumlocution, concretism).

   f. Assessment and follow-up

      i. Describe spontaneous speech (articulation, volume, latency, prosody).

      ii. Test and describe language characteristics: fluency, naming and recognition; repetition; comprehension; reading/writing; praxis (buccofacial, limb, axial).

   g. Treatment

      i. Use same strategies across disciplines.

      ii. Educate families.

6. **Memory**

   a. Processes: encoding, storage, and retrieval.

   b. Retrograde amnesia: inability to recall events preceding injury.

   c. Anterograde amnesia: difficulty with acquiring new information.

      i. Most common cognitive complaint of patients and families.

      ii. Areas involved: medial temporal lobes, hippocampus, thalamus.

    d. Causes: difficult to isolate cause of memory impairment; numerous possibilities include attentional deficits, impaired processing, frontal executive dysfunction.

    e. Indicators: inability to recall instructions, forgetting to perform requested tasks.

    f. Assessment and follow-up

      i. Neuropsychological testing to determine:
- If patient has disorder of functional memory (global vs. material-specific).
- Whether disorder can be attributed to attention deficits, core memory deficits, frontal organizational deficits, or prospective memory deficits.

      ii. See posttraumatic amnesia tests in Appendix F.

    g. Treatment

      i. Avoid medications that impair memory.

      ii. Consider use of cholinergic agents.

  7. **Visuospatial perception**

    a. Less common disorder after TBI (posterior brain damaged less frequently than frontotemporal regions)

    b. Indicators: neglect, difficulty in recognizing objects.

    c. Assessment and follow-up

      i. Neglect: line cancellation, line bisection, object drawing.

      ii. Construction: copy geometric design, freehand drawing, clock, Draw-A-Person.

      iii. Spatial: judgment of line orientation, map orientation.

      iv. Agnosia: visual recognition of objects, face recognition (prosopagnosia), color recognition.

    d. Treatment (few validated studies)

      i. Dopaminergic agonists

      ii. Caloric/vestibular stimulation in conjunction with therapy

      iii. Efferent motor stimulation in left hemispace

      iv. Afferent stimulation on far left with salient stimuli.

      v. Visual scanning exercises

      vi. Eye prisms

      vii. Left eye patching

      ix. Binasal occlusion

      x. Use of mirror for dressing

      xi. Use of verbal or written cues

E. **Endocrine system**

  1. **Acne or rash**

    a. Cause: endogenous or exogenous corticosteroids, allergy.

    b. Treatment: after elimination of allergic reaction, use benozyl peroxide, topical antibiotic ointments, oral antibiotics.

  2. **Appetite control**

    a. Symptoms: weight gain or loss, decreased or increased appetite.

    b. Cause: behavioral disorder or injury to hypothalamus satiety centers.

      i. Ventromedial hypothalamus (increased appetite)

      ii. Lateral hypothalamus (decreased appetite)

    c. Treatment

      i. Use behavioral modifications.

     ii. Change insulin secretion.

    iii. Change dopamine/serotonin system.

    iv. Consider amphetamines to depress appetite.

     v. Consider naltrexone, naloxone for hyperphagia.

3. **Decreased cellular immune response** (normal humeral immune response)

4. **Hyponatremia**

   a. Symptoms: mental status changes, coma, psychosis, seizures, cramps, nausea.

   b. Multiple causes (extrarenal, renal, adrenal) include cerebral salt wasting (CSW), osmotic diuresis, salt-losing nephropathy, renal tubular acidosis (RTA), hyperaldosteronism, vomiting, diarrhea, sweating, and syndrome of inappropriate secretion of antidiuretic hormone (SIADH).

   c. Usually hypotonic euvolemic (SIADH) or hypovolemic (CSW) volume status in TBI.

   d. Diagnosis

      i. Measure serum osmolality.

     ii. Determine extracellular fluid (ECF) status.

    iii. Measure urine osmolality and sodium concentration.

   e. Treatment

      i. Total increase in serum sodium concentration should not exceed 12 mEq/L in 24 hours. *Do not correct too rapidly!*

     ii. In patients with SIADH

       • Restrict fluids.

       • Promote water excretion (loop diuretic + salt tablets or hypertonic saline)

    iii. In patients with CSW, correct underlying disorder and give isotonic saline.

5. **Hypernatremia**

   a. Symptoms: polydipsia, polyuria (dilute urine), fatigue, change in mental status.

   b. Causes: central diabetes insipidus (DI), medications, impaired thirst, sodium overload, volume contraction with inadequate water replacement, osmotic diuresis. Central DI is most common cause (result of ADH deficiency due to hypothalamic or pituitary damage).

   c. Diagnosis

      i. Determine ECF volume status.

   d. To distinguish central vs. nephrogenic DI

      i. Restrict water intake for 12–18 hours.

     ii. Measure urine osmolality.

    iii. Administer 10 μg DDAVP intranasally.

    iv. Urine osmolality should increase by 50% in patients with central DI; no change in patients with nephrogenic NDI.

   e. Treatment of central DI

      i. Replace ongoing water loss.

     ii. Correct free water deficit slowly over 48–72 hours.

    iii. Replace ADH via aqueous vasopressin, lysine vasopressin nasal spray, or DDAVP nasal drops.

    iv. Other option to reduce polyuria: carbamazepine

6. **Anterior pituitary disease**
   a. Symptomatic endocrine dysfunction is rare after TBI (about 4%, according to Kalisky et al.).
   b. Symptoms: amenorrhea, decreased libido, impotence, loss of secondary sex characteristics, thyroid disease.
   c. Causes: hyperprolactinemia, growth hormone deficiency leading to increased catabolism, adrenocorticotropic hormone (ACTH) deficiency (*possibly fatal*), thyroid-stimulating hormone (TSH) deficiency, decreased levels of thyrotropic-releasing hormone (TRH).
   d. Screen for anterior pituitary dysfunction in patients with:
      i. Posterior pituitary dysfunction
      ii. Basilar skull or facial fractures
      iii. Poor neurologic improvement or regression
      iv. Persistent amenorrhea (> 6 months)
      v. Signs of endocrine dysfunction (stimulation test for TRH, luteinizing hormone-releasing hormone)
      vi. Abnormal gonadal hormones and gonadotropins
      vii. History of severe hypotension or shock
7. **Amenorrhea**
   a. Causes: stress, hormonal irregularity.
   b. Menses usually return within 6 months of injury.
   c. Amenorrhea does not always mean infertility.
   d. Educate family.
8. **Sleep irregularities**
   a. Symptoms: prolonged sleep onset, daytime sleepiness.
   b. Causes: medications, disrupted sleep/wake cycle, alteration in brain chemicals.
   c. Treatment
      i. Monitor sleep/wake cycle.
      ii. Simulate normal day with stimulating activity and infuser light during day and reduced stimulation and lighting at night.
      iii. Medications to aid sleep, including melatonin (see VII. Psychopharmacology)

F. **Gastrointestinal (GI) system**
   1. **Constipation**
      a. Symptoms: distention, hard stool
      b. Causes: inadequate fluid intake, pain medications, inactivity.
      c. Treatment: develop bowel program (see Chapter 16, Neurogenic Bowel Management).
   2. **Diarrhea**
      a. Causes: enteral feedings, infection.
      b. Treatment
         i. Rule out infection.
         ii. Use high-fiber/isoosmotic formulas.
         iii. Add fiber supplements to feedings.
         iv. Avoid antidiarrheal medications.
   3. **Bowel accidents** (loose stool, no control)
      a. Causes: neurogenic bowel, poor comprehension, *Clostridium difficile* infection.
      b. Treatment

       i. Behavioral modifications

      ii. Timed bowel program

     iii. Treatment of *C. difficile* infection with metronidazole (Flagyl), oral vancomycin.

4. **Dysphagia, neurogenic** (see Chapter 20, Speech, Language, and Swallowing Concerns)

    a. Incidence in TBI as high as 27.

    b. Symptom: difficulty swallowing.

    c. Causes: decreases in cognition, motor control and/or brainstem reflexes; change in receptors.

    d. Evaluate with videofluoroscopic swallow study when patient is alert before beginning therapeutic feeds.

    e. Treatment

       i. Trials of small spoonfuls of thickened foods, cold or acidic foods to stimulate swallow.

      ii. Dysphagia precautions and compensatory techniques such as supraglottic swallow, chin tuck, turning head, Mendelsohn's maneuver.

    f. In patients in whom oral intake is unsafe

       i. Use nasogastric (NG) or Dobhoff tube.

      ii. Use percutaneous endoscopic gastrostomy (PEG) if use of NG tube is expected to exceed 3–4 weeks.

     iii. Jejunostomy tube does not allow bolus feeding.

     iv. Try to bolus feed or cycle at night.

      v. Continuous feeds are associated with less aspiration/vomiting.

     vi. Elevate head of bed to decrease reflux.

5. **Gastroesophageal reflux disease (GERD)**

    a. Symptoms: burping, heartburn, poor tolerance of tube feeds, increased agitation after meals.

    b. Cause: decreased lower esophageal sphincter (LES) tone.

    c. Treatment

       i. Elevate head of bed with feeds.

      ii. Give H_2 receptor antagonist or proton pump inhibitor and antacids.

     iii. If LES tone is decreased, jejunal feeds may be required instead of gastric feeds.

6. **Gastritis or ulcer**

    a. GI bleed occurs in up to 80% of survivors of TBI and trauma.

    b. Symptoms: see GERD; blood in stool, drop in hemoglobin and hematocrit.

    c. Causes: increased acid due to stress response or elevated ICP.

    d. Prophylaxis: sucralfate, H_2 receptor antagonist, or proton pump inhibitor.

       i. Be cautious of cognitive side effects of cimetidine and ranitidine.

      ii. Discontinue use as soon as possible.

7. **Hepatic dysfunction**

    a. Symptoms: icteric sclera, elevated liver function tests (LFTs).

    b. Causes: anticonvulsant agents (gamma-glutamyl transferase and alanine aminotransferase most commonly affected, may be twice normal values), antispasticity agents, hepatitis, biliary obstruction, hepatic necrosis after cardiovascular shock, abdominal trauma.

    c. Treatment

       i. Monitor for symptoms.

      ii. Follow LFTs.

       iii. Consider medication modifications and/or imaging.
- 8. **Hiccups** may be be treated with acupuncture, esophagogastroduodenoscopy, rectal massage, carbamazepine, amitriptyline.
- 9. **Hypermetabolism**
  - a. Symptoms: weight loss, low serum albumin, prealbumin < 25.
  - b. Cause: increased energy expenditure and nutrition requirement.
  - c. Begin enteral feeding as soon as possible with protein-rich formula.
    - i. Use NG tube if oral ingestion is not possible.
    - ii. Use PEG if need for NG tube is expected to exceed 3–4 weeks.
    - iii. Patients with severe TBI may have decreased LES tone and increased risk of aspiration with gastric feeding. Consider jejunal feeds.
    - iv. Jejunostomy tube does not allow bolus feeding.
    - v. Try to bolus feed or cycle at night.
    - vi. Elevate head of bed to decrease reflux.
- 10. **Decreased motility**
  - a. Major symptom: constipation
  - b. Causes: cranial nerve X injury (usually corrects by third week).
  - c. Treatment: metoclopramide, erythromycin.
- 11. Increased motility
  - a. Major symptom: osmotic diarrhea.
  - b. Treatment
    - i. Rule out *C. difficile* infection.
    - ii. Change tube feed strength to one-half or one-quarter strength.
    - iii. Change to bolus feeds.
- 12. **Vomiting/nausea**
  - a. Causes: vestibular problems, injury to hypothalamus, injury to vomiting center, pancreatitis, increased ICP, intracranial hemorrhage, SAH, superior mesenteric artery (SMA) syndrome (compressed duodenum).
  - b. Treatment
    - i. Check complete blood count (CBC), amylase, lipase.
    - ii. Consider decompression and placement of NG tube.
    - iii. Position patients with SMA syndrome in left lateral decubitus position.
    - iv. If tube feeds are used, try continuous rather than bolus feedings.
- G. **Genitourinary system**
  - 1. **Loss of cortical urinary control**
    - a. Symptoms: incontinence, frequency.
    - b. Cause: frontal injury.
    - c. Treatment: timed voids, trial of anticholinergic agent. Avoid Foley or condom catheter.
  - 2. **Bladder dyssynergia**
    - a. Major symptom: small, frequent voids.
    - b. Cause: subcortical damage.
    - c. Treatment
      - i. Test by checking postvoid residuals.
      - ii. Try cholinergic agent (urecholine).
      - iii. Clean intermittent catheterization (CIC) may be required.
  - 3. **Urinary tract infection**
    - a. Incidence in patients with TBI: 38%.
    - b. Symptoms: urgency, frequency, dysuria.
    - c. Treatment: antibiotics.

4. **Neurogenic bladder** (see Chapter 15, Neurogenic Bladder Management)
   a. Major symptoms: incontinence, frequency.
   b. Causes
      i. Uninhibited detrusor hyperreflexia (frequent voiding of small amounts).
      ii. Urinary retention during acute care may lead to myotonic bladder with inadequate emptying, overflow incontinence.
      iii. Detrusor hyporeflexia secondary to bladder overdistention (due to obstruction).
      iv. Behavioral disorder.
   c. Treatment
      i. Initiate timed voids.
      ii. Use external collection device (diaper, condom catheter) only if patient is unable to participate in timed void.
      iii. Patients with detrusor hyporeflexia or coexisting spinal cord injury, may need CIC or Foley catheter.
      iv. Behavioral disorder: use token economies.
H. **Neurologic system**
   1. **Auditory disorder**
      a. Major symptom: hearing loss.
      b. Causes: temporal bone trauma leading to:
         i. Conductive hearing loss (tympanic perforation, hemotympanum, ossicular disruption)
         ii. Sensorineural hearing loss (acute cochlear concussion, perilymphatic fistula)
      c. Management: auditory testing and evaluation.
   2. **Olfactory disorder**
      a. Major symptoms: no taste, no smell, altered feeding behavior, associated with CSF rhinorrhea.
      b. Most common CN injury in TBI: CN I (olfactory nerve) injury due to cribriform plate disruption.
      c. Diagnosis
         i. Scratch-and-sniff odor panel
         ii. Trial of smelling coffee grounds
         iii. Alcohol pad sniffing stimulates other receptors; hence *not* diagnostic.
   3. **Diplopia**
      a. Cause: CN III, IV, or VI damage.
      b. Treatment: consider unilateral or alternating eye patching.
   4. **Eye movement abnormalities**
      a. Symptoms: poor eye movement, ptosis.
      b. Causes: CN III, IV, or VI damage, damage to nuclei, cerebral hemispheric stroke, damage to basal ganglia.
   5. **Motor disturbances**
      a. Ataxia, poor coordination (cerebellar or basal ganglia lesion)
      b. Tremor, bradykinesia, parkinsonism (basal ganglia or substantia nigra lesion)
      c. Slowed motor processing (slowed central processing)
      d. Diagnosis
         i. Rule out peripheral neuropathy.
         ii. Diagnose tremor in relation to action, rest, and sleep.

  e. Treatment
    i. Consider trial of levodopa for movement disorders or propranolol for tremors.
    ii. Consider trials of wrist weights to decrease tremor amplitude.
    iii. Train in limb length shortening during use to decrease amplitude of ataxia/tremor motor "overshoot."

6. **Neglect**
  a. Major symptoms: neglect of body parts, poor spatial awareness.
  b. Causes: disruption of attentional, intentional and representational mechanisms.
  c. Treatment: no unequivocally effective protocols. Suggested strategies include scanning, cuing, vestibular stimulation, eye patching, prisms, or medication (dopaminergic agents or stimulants).

7. **Peripheral nerve injury**
  a. Incidence in TBI: 34%; in study by Garland and Bailey, 11% of rehabilitation patients presented with undiagnosed peripheral nerve injury.
  b. Symptoms: numbness, tingling, paresthesias, pain, weakness.
  c. Causes
    i. Spasticity and contractures (e.g., elbow injury may lead to ulnar mononeuropathy, severe wrist flexion to carpal tunnel syndrome)
    ii. Positioning (e.g., risk for peroneal neuropathy, especially in prolonged ICU stay)
    iii. Postoperative complications
    iv. Trauma (e.g, midshaft humerus fracture that leads to radial nerve injury)
    v. Heterotopic ossification
    vi. Iatrogenic (e.g., improper cast fit)
  d. Diagnosis
    i. Perform neurologic exam.
    ii. Identify motor/sensory deficits, asymmetric hyperreflexia, atrophy, fasciculations.
    iii. Order electromyography (EMG) and nerve conduction studies.
    iv. Imaging (e.g., MRI to rule out mechanical lesion for brachial plexopathy)
  e. Treatment
    i. Use orthotic devices for contracture prevention, support.
    ii. Position patient to avoid pressure on nerve.
    iii. Direct therapies to avoid further stretch on nerve in patients with traction injury.
    iv. Neurosurgical evaluation if appropriate (e.g., brachial plexopathy).

8. **Posttraumatic hydrocephalus**
  a. Hydrocephalus is enlargement of ventricles due to impairment of flow and absorption of CSF.
  b. Incidence: 1–8%.
  c. Patients with SAH at greatest risk.
  d. Symptoms: incontinence, dementia, ataxia, deep coma (remember 3 Ws: wobbly, wacky, and wet).
  e. Treatment
    i. Arrange neurosurgical consultation.
    ii. Order serial monthly CT scans to confirm diagnosis.

    iii. Consider lumbar puncture to check opening pressure and determine whether shunt or drain may be helpful.

9. **Posttraumatic seizures**
   a. Symptoms: clonic movements, unresponsiveness, staring spells.
   b. Causes: brain damage, any irritant to brain tissue, electrolyte disorders, hypoglycemia, CNS infection.
   c. Patients with depressed skull fracture, intracranial hemorrhage, or early seizure at greatest risk for developing disorder.
   d. Seizure prophylaxis usually determined on an individual basis.
      i. In patients with no structural brain abnormality, usually for 1 week, then discontinued.
      ii. Phenytoin often used in acute setting, but switch to carbamazepine or lamotrigine as soon as possible (fewer cognitive and sedating side effects).

10. **Sensory deficits**
    a. Plan treatment around sensory deficit.
    b. Strengthen remaining sensory capabilities.

11. **Sleep disorder**
    a. Symptoms: sleep cycle reversal, poor sleep maintenance, poor dreaming, high sleep latency, apnea, restless leg syndrome, excessive daytime sleepiness.
    b. Causes: hypophysis bruised in TBI, disruption of neurotransmitter tracts from DAI, alterations in 5-HT and norepinephrine/dopamine systems.
    c. Treatment
       i. Sleep initiation problems: improvements in sleep hygiene, melatonin, zolpidem (short-term usage).
       ii. Sleep maintenance problems: trazodone, nortriptyline.
       iii. Poor-quality sleep: light therapy in morning, trial of nasal oxygen or continuous positive airway pressure (if sleep study reveals apnea), dopamine agonists for restless leg syndrome.

H. Neuromuscular system

1. **Contractures**
   a. Major symptom: hard endpoint with range of motion (ROM); not velocity-dependent.
   b. Causes: increased tone, heterotopic ossification.
   c. Prevention: ROM exercises, splinting, treatment of tone.
   d. Treatment: serial casting, traction, ultrasound, surgical intervention (only after other methods fail).

2. **Rigidity**
   a. Symptoms: increased resistance to movements of all velocities, slower movements, loss of postural stability.
   b. Causes
      i. Decorticate posturing: lesion of cortex, internal capsule, basal ganglia, or thalamus.
      ii. Decerebrate posturing: injury to midportion of brainstem or higher.
   c. Treatment
      i. Positioning techniques in bed (foam wedges to promote knee flexion)
      ii. Appropriate seating
      iii. Head straps
      iv. Passive ROM

      v. Serial casting
     vi. Neurolytic procedures with phenol
    vii. Chemodenervation with botulinum toxins

3. **Parkinsonism**
   a. Symptoms: bradykinesia, rest tremor, loss of postural reflexes, rigidity; perioral movements develop gradually in drug-induced disease.
   b. Causes
      i. Posttraumatic parkinsonism: degeneration of pars compacta of substantia nigra.
      ii. Pugilistic parkinsonism: cumulative brain trauma with neurofibrillary degeneration of substantia nigra and medial temporal cortex, accelerated beta-amyloid deposits.
      iii. Drugs: dopamine depletors, metoclopramide, clebopride.
   c. Treatment
      i. Medications
         - First-line choice: levodopa or levodopa/carbidopa.
         - Dopamine agonists (bromocriptine, pergolide) cause fewer dyskinesias.
         - Anticholinergic agents: help tremor but with more side effects and less efficacy in patients with TBI.
         - Selegiline and vitamins C and E delay disability in early stages.
         - Propranolol for drug-induced disease: slow response.
      ii. Therapy
         - Rigidity: ROM, strengthening, and coordination training.
         - Consider relaxation techniques.
         - Bradykinesia: proprioceptive neuromuscular facilitation (PNF), biofeedback, neurodevelopmental treatment (NDT).
         - Adaptive equipment for mobility (avoid rolling walkers, which may cause festination).
         - Occupational therapy (OT): fine motor coordination and adaptive equipment for writing, activities of daily living (ADLs).
         - Speech and langauge therapy for breath support and amplification of speech.

4. **Tremor**
   a. Types: resting, intention, action (postural, kinetic, position-specific, isometric).
   b. Causes
      i. Lesions of cerebellar outflow pathways (dentate nucleus and superior cerebellar peduncle): ipsilateral tremor.
      ii. Lesions above decussations of cerebral peduncles in midbrain: contralateral tremor.
      iii. Slow tremors: brainstem injuries.
      iv. Isolated episodic tremors: TBI.
      v. Delayed onset from axonal sprouting, altered receptor receptivity, or neuronal degeneration.
   c. Treatment
      i. Medications
         - Clonidine (desynchronizes tremor by increasing amplitude; fewer side effects than beta blockers)

- Propranolol (may have central mechanism; best for physiologic and action tremors).
- Arotinolol (essential tremor)
- Clonazepam, primidone, and lorazepam
- Valproic acid
- Levodopa (rubral tremor)
- Mysoline
  ii. Procedures: botulinum toxin injections, surgery.
  iii. Therapies: weighting of limbs, thalamic stimulation.
5. **Akathisia**
   a. Symptoms: motor restlessness (also dysphoria) associated with neurogenic pain.
   b. Causes: dopamine blockade in prefrontal cortex, antipsychotic medications.
   c. Treatment
      i. Bromocriptine (may increase psychiatric symptoms)
      ii. Anticholinergics (unproven efficacy and side effects in TBI)
      iii. Amantadine (patients develop tolerance)
      iv. Benzodiazepines (limited use)
      v. Beta blockers (may help)
6. **Ataxia**
   a. Symptoms: irregular, discoordinated movements.
   b. Causes: cerebellar, sensory, labyrinthine, psychogenic; abnormal midbrain signal on MRI,
   c. Therapeutics: coordination activities, weighting utensils.
   d. Medications: beta blockers, acetazolamide, TRH, choline/ lecithin.
7. **Athetosis**
   a. Symptoms: continuous slow, writhing movements (slow chorea); more common in children.
   b. Cause: injury to basal ganglia; phenytoin disrupts basal ganglia receptors.
   c. Treatment
      i. Surgery (ventrolateral thalamotomy, lesioning of dentate nucleus)
      ii. Electrical stimulation (anterior cerebellum)
8. **Ballismus**
   a. Symptoms: large-amplitude flinging/flailing in proximal muscles; usually unilateral; onset weeks after TBI.
   b. Causes: lesion in contralateral subthalamic nucleus or striatum; cerebrovascular accident (CVA) in bilateral basal ganglia; excessive levodopa administration; rare after TBI.
   d. Treatment: surgery (stereotactic thalamotomy), valproate and other anticonvulsants.
9. **Chorea**
   a. Symptoms: rapid, involuntary, irregular, purposeless movements that flow from one body part to another; can be suppressed temporarily; presents in persistent or paroxysmal form; rare after TBI.
   b. Causes: lesions in contralateral subthalamic nucleus, striatum, or thalamic nuclei; bilateral lesions lead to general chorea; phenytoin may cause disruption of basal ganglia receptors.
   c. Treatment: valproic acid, phenobarbital, stereotactic destruction of dentate nucleus of cerebellum.

10. **Dystonia**
    a. Types: athetotic, myoclonic, single body part, segmental, cranial, laryngeal.
    b. Symptoms: sustained, repetitive twisting movements of variable speed, anywhere in body; delayed onset; muscle tone worsens, sleep relieves.
    c. Causes
        i. Side effect of phenytoin, neuroleptics, buspirone
        ii. Disrupted pathways between striatum and thalamus (with corticospinal tracts intact)
        iii. Peripheral trauma and nerve damage
        iv. Hemiparesis and striatal damage
    d. Treatment
        i. Spasmodic or laryngeal dystonia: botulinum toxin injection into vocalis complex.
        ii. "Sensory tricks" (proprioceptive feedback alters dystonia)
            • Hold side of head for nuchal dystonia.
            • Thumb abduction for hand dystonia.
11. **Cranial dystonia**
    a. Symptoms: blepharospasm; Meig's syndrome (eye and mouth dystonia).
    b. Treatment
        i. Open mouth or manually open eyes.
        ii. Surgery (involves complications and possible recurrence): myectomy of orbicularis, facial nerve sectioning, brow lift.
        iii. Botulinum toxin injection: first-line treatment.
        iv. Tetrabenazine with lithium to improve results.
12. **Oromandibular dystonia**
    a. Symptoms: trismus, retraction of corners of mouth, tongue protrusion, jaw opening.
    b. Treatment
        i. Medications (limited effectiveness, significant cognitive side effects): clonazepam / lorazepam, baclofen, trihexiphenidyl.
        ii. Submental botulinum toxin injections
13. **Cervical dystonia/spasmodic torticollis**
    a. Symptoms: twisting head movements, pain from continuous contractions (75% of patients).
    b. Treatment
        i. Physical therapy (PT)/ROM exercises to prevent contractures.
        ii. Drugs give little relief (diazepam, lorazepam, clonazepam, cyclobenzaprine, carbamazepine).
        iii. Peripheral nerve denervation (may recur)
14. **Hemidystonia**
    a. Symptoms: delayed-onset nocturnal paroxysmal dystonia.
    b. Causes: aberrant neuronal sprouting, neuroleptics (2.5% of cases).
    c. Treatment
        i. Botulinum toxin injections: first-line treatment but temporary.
        ii. Most medications (e.g., trihexiphenidyl, tetrabenazine, ethopropazine) are not helpful.
        iii. Most effective drugs are muscle relaxants and anticholinergics, which help other patients with dystonia but are not tolerated by patients with TBI (tardive dyskinesias).

    iv. Systemic treatment with levodopa may be helpful.
    v. Intrathecal baclofen may be used for generalized dystonia.
    vi. Thalamotomy provides mild, transient relief.
    vii. Experimental: electrical stimulation of ventroposterolateral thalamus, dopamine-depleting agents (tetrabenazine).
    viii. Surgery may be indicated for severe cases in which botulinum toxin is not effective.
      • Unilateral thalamotomy (some relief of distal symptoms)
      • Bilateral dystonia (may cause dysarthria)

15. **Progressive supranuclear palsy**
  a. Symptoms: bradykinesia, rigidity, postural instability, hypophonia, vertical gaze limitations, hypometric saccades, facial muscle contractions, symmetric symptoms; no resting tremor.
  b. Causes: atrophy of midbrain, pontine tegmentum, substantia nigra, and/or subthalamic nuclei; normal striatum.
  c. Treatment
    i. High-dose levodopa, amitriptyline, desipramine; fluoxetine may improve postural stability.
    ii. Not responsive to dopaminergic medications.

16. **Stereotypy (tardive dyskinesia)**
  a. Symptoms: repetitive, voluntary, purposeless movements (simple or complex).
  b. Causes: amphetamine administration, increased dopamine.
  c. Treatment: dopamine antagonist (haloperidol).

17. **Tics**
  a. Rare (simple or complex) in TBI.
  b. Major problem is patient discomfort.
  c. Causes: aberrant peripheral nerve sprouting, dopamine antagonists, methylphenidate.
  d. Treatment
    i. Medications: clonazepam (gamma-aminobutyric acid [GABA] agonist), clonidine (noradrenergic).
    ii. Psychological intervention only for coping skills.

18. **Psychogenic movement disorders**
  a. Rule out organic disorders.
  b. Psychotherapy is treatment of choice; medication is inappropriate.

19. **Drug-induced movement disorders**
  a. Causes: generally pre- or postsynaptic dopamine antagonists. Examples include anticonvulsants, tricyclic antidepressants, neuroleptics (haloperidol, fluphenazine, or pimoxide), metoclopramide (increased dystonia), levodopa and CNS stimulants.
  b. Treatment: dopamine agonists (bromocriptine, amantadine).

20. **Myoclonus**
  a. Symptoms: sudden irregular, rhythmic muscle jerks; hypoxic myoclonus also associated with ataxia, dementia, postural deficits, and seizures.
  b. Causes
    i. Pathologic: hypoxia, abnormal metabolism, toxins.
    ii. Anatomic: cortex, brainstem, and spinal cord involved; palatal: lesion of cerebellorubro-olivary tract, medulla.

        iii. Chemical: acetylcholine system in palatal/essential myoclonus; GABA system in cortical myoclonus, hypoxic myoclonus.

    c. Treatment

        i. Cortical: clonazepam or valproate facilitates GABA system.

        ii. Palatal: clonazepam or carbamazepine.

        iii. Brainstem myoclonus: clonazepam.

        iv. Hypoxic myoclonus: 5-hydroxy-tryptophan (serotonin precursor, difficult to obtain clinically), clonazepam, carbamazepine, valproic acid, or primidone; propranolol if tremor also present.

        v. Reflex myoclonus: clonazepam, piracetam, valproate, primidone.

21. **Spasticity**

    a. Major symptom: velocity-dependent increase in muscle tone.

    b. Complications include joint subluxation, heterotopic ossification, acquired peripheral neuropathy.

    c. Treatment (see also Chapter 19, Spasticity)

        i. ROM exercises

        ii. Splinting, serial casting

        iii. Heat, ultrasound, biofeedback

        iv. Injections (focal)

        v. Medication (systemic spasticity)

I. **Orthopedic system**

  1. **Fractures**

    a. Major symptoms: pain, deformity.

    b. 11% incidence of undiagnosed fractures at admission to rehabilitation, according to study by Garland and Bailey.

    c. Acute screening x-rays include cervical and thoracic spine, pelvis, hips, knees; consider bone scan to detect fractures.

    d. Avoid casting in flexed position.

  2. **Heterotopic ossification** (see Chapter 14, Heterotopic Ossification)

    a. Definition: formation of mature lamellar bone in soft tissue.

    b. Major symptoms: decreased ROM, painful ROM.

    c. 10–20% incidence; etiology uncertain.

    d. Affects periarticular region of large joints: hip > elbows > shoulders > knees.

J. **Complex regional pain syndrome** (see Chapter 11, Acute and Chronic Pain)

    a. Symptoms: diffuse distal limb pain of burning quality out of proportion to initial event, loss of function, and objective evidence of autonomic dysfunction. Other symptoms include swelling, joint contracture, trophic skin changes, vasomotor instability.

    b. Causes: autonomic, especially sympathetic instability.

    c. Common predisposing events include neurologic insult, such as TBI.

    d. Diagnosis: triple-phase bone scan, sympathetic blockade associated with pain decrement; x-rays of little use for early diagnosis.

    d. Treatment

        i. Avoid sedating medications.

        ii. Control pain.

        iii. Decrease sympathetic activity.

        iv. Restore function.

        v. Medications such as steroids in acute phase, tricyclic antidepressants.

        vi. Stellate ganglion block.

K. **Postconcussive syndromes**
   1. **Cervical acceleration /deceleration injuries**
      a. **Acute**
         i. Signs and symptoms: straightened lordotic curve on x-ray, neck pain, headache, decreased neck ROM. Less common symptoms include dizziness, weakness, paresthesias.
         ii. Causes: strain/tears of ligaments supporting cervical spine (longus colli muscle tear, anterior longitudinal ligament tear, retropharyngeal hematoma), additional cervical rotational torque (zygapophyseal joint capsules, alar ligament complex, intervertebral discs).
         iii. Treatment: trigger-point injections, cervical stretching, gentle traction, manual mobilizations.
      b. **Chronic**
         i. Causes: anterior/posterior cervical myofascial dysfunction, upper shoulder myofascial dysfunction.
         ii. Reversal of lordotic curve/cervical spondylolysis may be indicators for poor recovery; unrelated to gender or litigation.
      c. **Cranial nerve injuries**
         i. Symptoms: face, neck, and shoulder dysesthesias; with damage to CN V, facial sensory changes (vibration, temperature); with C2–C3 zygapophyseal joint injury, chronic cervical pain.
         ii. Damage to upper cranial nerve injuries (greater auricular, superficial cervical, supraclavicular nerves)
         iii. Damage to descending CN V fibers in cervical cord or pons/medulla.
      d. **Greater occipital neuralgia**
         i. Symptoms: altered sensation over face, scalp, and neck; retro-orbital/periorbital eye pain.
         ii. Causes: traction injury to C2 dorsal rami (shoulder harness in motor vehicle accident); relationship between C2 and CN V in medulla; myodystonia of semispinalis capitis or trapezius.
      e. **Third occipital injury**
         i. Major symptom: headache.
         ii. Cause: C3 dorsal ramus injury.
      f. **Anterior cervical myofascial pain**
         i. Symptoms
            • Sternal trigger points refer pain to vertex, occiput, cheek, eye, throat, and sternum as well as produce autonomic changes (ipsilateral eye, nose, and ear)
            • Clavicular trigger points produce postural dizziness, vertigo, syncope, disequilibrium.
         ii. Cause: sternocleidomastoid muscle strain
         iii. Treatment
            • Acute: immobilization (soft collar), ice, NSAIDs, muscle relaxants
            • Subacute: heat, gradual mobilization, cervical traction, correction of biomechanics.
            • Long-term: active mobilization, isometric strengthening, interruption of pain cycle (spray and stretch, trigger point injections, electrical stimulation, ultrasound, ischemic pressure, pulsed electromagnetic therapy, acupuncture), phasic exercises (rapid eye, head, neck, and arm movements).

g. **Posterior cervical myofascial pain**
   i. Symptoms
      • Upper trapezius trigger points refer pain to posterolateral neck, posterior ear and temple.
      • Lower trapezius trigger points refer pain to high cervical, suprascapular, and interscapular regions.
      • Splenius refers pain to vertex, eye, neck angle.
      • Semispinalis refers pain to posterior occiput, ipsilateral frontotemporal area behind orbit.
      • Multifidus refers pain to suboccipital and upper shoulder girdle.
      • Scalene refers pain to anterior chest and ipsilateral arm.
      • Temporalis refers pain to frontal, upper dentition and behind orbit.
   ii. Causes: injury to trapezius, splenius capitis and cervicus, semispinalis capitis and cervicus, scalene muscle; most common = multifidi/rotators.
h. **Neurovascular entrapment of brachial plexus and subclavian vein/artery**
   i. Symptoms: ulnar hand pain and edema.
   ii. Diagnosis by imaging, vascular studies.
2. **Cervicogenic dizziness**
   a. **Vertebrobasilar insufficiency**
      i. Symptoms: diplopia, dizziness, drop attacks, dysmetria, headache.
      ii. Cause: constriction of vertebral artery at C2 level.
      iii. Treatment of dizziness is an art, not a science; no proven treatment; possible surgery.
   b. **Collet-Sicard syndrome:** caused by stretch of CNs IX–XII .
   c. **Nonvertiginous dizziness**
      i. Symptoms: cervical trigger points, postural sway toward hypertonic neck muscles; no peripheral/central vestibular dysfunction.
      ii. Causes: abnormal afferents from positional proprioceptors in cervical/lumbar areas, cervical sympathetic hyperexcitation, vertebral artery compromise, cervicolumbar hypertonicity.
   d. **Anterior cervical sympathetic dysfunction** (Bernard-Horner syndrome) is associated with myosis, ptosis, and anhydrosis.
   e. **Posterior cervical sympathetic dysfunction** (Barré-Lieou syndrome) (controversial)
      i. Symptoms: vertigo, tinnitus, occipital headaches, blurry vision, dysphonia.
      ii. Causes: irritation of posterior cervical sympathetics (vertebral nerve and cervical sympathetic plexus); transient ischemia to pons and occipital lobe, degeneration of cervical spine.
      ii. Treatment
         • Decrease cervical myodystonia.
         • Decrease soft tissue inflammation.
         • Increase cervical spine mobility (myo-oligomentous and osseus).
   f. **Vestibular dysfunction**
      i. 30–65% patients with TBI suffer symptoms of vestibular pathology, according to study by Shumway-Cook.
      ii. Symptoms: positive Hallpike-Dix maneuver, episodic vertigo, nausea.

        iii. Caused by calcium carbonate crystals lodged in macula of utricle.

        iv. Treatment: Epley repositioning maneuver (vestibular therapy).

3. **Head pain/headache**

  a. **Postconcussive vascular headache**

     i. Symptoms: pain, photophobia, dizziness, ataxia.

     ii. Cause: posttraumatic vertebrobasilar insufficiency.

     iii. Treatment

       • Usually resolves within 1 year.

       • Medications: midrol or antidepressants for cluster headache; Midrin; beta blockers and other migraine medications for migraine symptoms; NSAID's or muscle relaxants. Avoid narcotics.

       • PT: active mobilization followed by isometric strengthening; cervical traction; spray and stretch, trigger point injections, ischemic pressure, manual mobilizations (controversial), electrical stimulation, ultrasound, pulsed electromagnetic therapy.

  b. **Vertebrobasilar insufficiency**

     i. Symptoms: diplopia, dizziness, drop attacks, dysmetria, headache.

     ii. Caused by constriction of vertebral artery at C2 level.

  c. **Collet-Sicard syndrome:** CN IX–XII stretched.

  d. **Basilar artery migraine**

     i. Symptoms: intense vascular headache, posterior circulation prodrome (visual impairment, ataxia, dysarthria, paresthesias, vertigo, drop attacks, and weakness).

     ii. Cause: altered basilar vascular flow.

     iii. Treatment: migraine headache medications, anticonvulsants.

  e. **Greater occipital neuralgia**

     i. Symptoms: altered sensation over face, scalp, and neck; retro-orbital/periorbital eye pain.

     ii. Cause: Traction injury to C2 dorsal rami (shoulder harness in motor vehicle accident), relationship between C2 and CN V in medulla; chronically, myodystonia of semispinalis capitis or trapezius. Temporalis refers pain to frontal, behind orbit, and upper dentition.

  f. **Third occipital neuralgia:** caused by injury to C3 dorsal ramus.

  g. **Temporomandibular joint derangement**

     i. Symptoms: pain in muscles of mastication, ROM restrictions, muscle tenderness with or without joint crepitation and subluxation; due to intra-articular derangement that leads to pathology of disk glenoid fossa, condylar head, or synovial linings of joint.

     ii. Rule out dental or facial fractures, myofascial disorder of muscles of mastication.

     iii. Dental treatment/oral prosthesis.

  h. **Facial sensory changes** (vibration, temperature) with damage to CN V in cervical cord or pons/medulla.

  i. **Optic nerve injury**

     i. Symptoms: blurry vision, blindness, inattention.

     ii. Cause: injury to optic nerve or tracts, occipital region, cortex.

     iii. Distinguish optic nerve lesion from cortical blindness, hemi-inattention, visual agnosia.

      iv. Treatment: neuro-ophthalmology consultation, more detailed acuity testing when patient can cooperate.

L. **Pulmonary system**

  1. **Airway management** (decannulation)

    a. Perform laryngoscopy on all symptomatic or unresponsive patients (RL III or below) before decannulation.

    b. No standard process for decannulation.

    c. Downsize tracheostomy tube when uncuffed tube is tolerated (e.g., downsize from Shiley size 6 to 4). This allows air to move around tube.

    d. Gradually plug tracheostomy and follow oxygen saturation values.

    e. If patient has strong cough, can manage secretions, and is asymptomatic, remove tube and place occlusive dressing.

  2. **Airway obstruction**

    a. Symptoms: decreased oxygen saturation, fatigue. Patients with severe TBI may not show stridor, dyspnea on exertion, or diminished exercise tolerance.

    b. Causes: food, tracheal stenosis, tracheal malacia, pneumonia, decannulation, asthma, others.

    c. Treatment: standard ABCs approach.

  3. **Tracheal granulomas**

    a. Occur in up to 56% of patients with TBI and tracheostomies for > 1 month, according to study by Law et al.

    b. Irritation of skin by tracheostomy tube results in overgrowth of epithelial tissue, usually on anterior portion of trachea.

    c. Treatment: direct excision or laser ablation; ear, nose, and throat consultation.

  4. **Hypoxemia/respiratory failure**

    1. Symptoms: hypoxia, tachypnea.

    2. Causes: aspiration, depression of central respiratory drive, pulmonary/chest wall injury, neurogenic pulmonary edema, infection, fat embolus or pulmonary embolism.

    3. Treatment: monitor arterial blood gases; consider tracheostomy.

M. **Skin**

  1. **Skin breakdown and pressure sores:** see Chapter 18, Skin Care.

  2. **Perioral redness**

    a. Cause: Poor control of secretions, drooling.

    b. Treatment: control secretions, avoid allowing skin surface to remain wet; consider anticholinergic medication.

VII. **Psychopharmacology**

A. **Short-term medications for acute management of posttraumatic agitation**

  1. Directed agitation: agitation directed at a particular object, source, cause. (e.g., splint application, tube feeds).

    a. Lorazepam, 0.5–2 mg, or haloperidol, 0.5–2 mg, as needed every hour up to 4 doses.

    b. If > 4 doses are needed within 24 hours, start scheduled dose regimen.

  2. Nondirected agitation: general agitation that occurs regardless of changes in environment or interaction with patient; no direct cause or trigger identified.

    a. Lorazepam, 0.5–2 mg, or haloperidol, 0.5–2 mg.

    b. Schedule dosing on alternating basis: lorazepam at 6 AM, 2 PM, and 10 PM; haloperidol at 2 AM, 10 AM, and 6 PM.

    c. Continue for 48 hours, then taper and reassess.

B. **Long-term symptom-guided medication for persistent posttraumatic agitation**
   1. **Aggression**
      a. Trazodone, 25 mg at bedtime (increased dosing/day: 25 mg; range: 25–400 mg/day)
      b. Fluoxetine, 5 mg/day (increased dosing/day: 5 mg; range: 10–40 mg/day)
      c. Propranolol, 10–20 mg test dose, then 60 mg/day (increased dosing/day: 60 mg; range: 60–1000 mg/day)
   2. **Anxiety**
      a. Carbamazepine, 100 mg 2 times/day (increased dosing/day: 100 mg; range: 200–600 mg/day)
      b. Buspirone, 7.5 mg 2 times/day (increased dosing/day: 5 mg; range: 30–60 mg)
   3. **Nondirected (nonspecific) confusion**
      a. Trazodone, 25 mg at bedtime (increased dosing/day: 25 mg; range: 25–400 mg)
      b. Amitriptyline, 25 mg at bedtime (increased dosing/day: 25 mg; range: 75–100 mg/day)
      c. Fluoxetine, 10 mg /day (increased dosing/day: 10 mg; range: 10–40 mg/day)
   4. **Depression** (Table 5)
   5. **Disinhibition/emotional lability**
      a. Carbamazepine, 100 mg 2 times/day (increased dosing/day: 100 mg; range: 200–600 mg)

TABLE 5. Treatment for Depression

Category	Mechanism	Drug	Starting dose	Side effects
SSRI	Inhibit reuptake of serotonin (5-HT)	Fluoxetine Paroxetine Sertraline Citalopram	10 mg/day 10 mg/day 25 or 50 mg/day 10 mg/day	GI, sexual dysfunction, mild parkinsonism, sweating, sedation or insomnia, teeth grinding
Atypical	Inhibits NE and DA reuptake	Bupropion	100–150 mg 2 times/day	Seizures, anorexia, no sexual side effects
	Inhibits 5-HT, NE, and DA reuptake	Venlafaxine	22.5 mg/day	Many side effects; titrate slowly; if paresthesias, stop immediately.
	5-HT and NE antagonist	Nefazodone	50 mg/day	Fewer sexual side effects, sedation.
	5-HT$_2$ antagonist	Mirtazapine	15 mg at bedtime	Fewer sexual side effects, weight gain.
TCAs		Nortriptyline Desipramine Amitriptyline Doxepin		Avoid amitriptyline and doxepin because of memory problems and anticholinergic effects.
Stimulants		Methylphenidate	5 mg at 8 AM and noon	
		Dextroamphetamine Amantadine	10 mg (patient-specific)	High abuse potential, weight loss, anorexia
ECT				

SSRI = selective serotonin reuptake inhibitor, TCA = tricyclic antidepressant, NE = norepinephrine, DA = dopamine, ECT = electroconvulsive therapy.

      b. Fluoxetine, 10 mg/day (increased dosing/day: 10 mg; range: 10–40 mg)

      c. Propranolol, 10–20 mg test dose, then 60 mg/day (increased dosing/day: 60 mg; range: 60–1000 mg)

  6. **Motor restlessness**

      a. Amantadine, 100 mg at 8 AM and 2 PM (increased dosing/day: 100 mg; range: 200–400 mg/day)

      b. Bromocriptine, 2.5 mg at 8 AM and 2 PM (increased dosing/day: 2.5 mg; range: 10–30 mg/day)

      c. Propranolol, 10–20 mg test dose, then 60 mg/day (increased dosing/day: 60 mg; range: 60–1000 mg/day)

  7. **Low attention or arousal**

      a. Amantadine, 100 mg at 8 AM and 2 PM (increased dosing/day:100 mg; range: 200–400 mg/day)

      b. Methylphenidate, 5 mg at 8 AM and noon (increased dosing/day: 10 mg; range: 10–60 mg/day

      c. D-amphetamine, 1.25 mg at 8 AM and noon (increased dosing/day: 2.5 mg; range: 2.5–40 mg/day)

C. **Medications to avoid in brain-injured patients**

  1. **Anticonvulsants**

      a. Phenytoin (sedating)

      b. Phenobarbital (decreases information processing)

  2. **Antihypertensives**

      a. Propranolol (decreases cognition)

      b. Metoprolol (sedating)

      c. Methyldopa

  3. **Antispasmodics**

      a. Baclofen (decreases cognition, sedating)

      b. Diazepam (long-acting)

  4. **Psychoactive agents**

      a. Neuroleptics (haloperidol, thorazine; delayed outcome in brain recovery)

      b. Amitriptyline (may decrease arousal due to anticholinergic effects)

      c. Doxepin and imipramine (as for amitriptyline)

  5. **GI drugs**

      a. Cimetidine (sedating)

      b. Metoclopramide (impairs memory)

VIII. Neurologic Recovery

A. **Stages of recovery from diffuse injury**

  1. Coma: state in which patient does not open eyes; no evidence of cognition, such as following commands or speaking

  2. Vegetative state

  3. Minimally conscious state

  4. Confusional state

  5. Postconfusional-evolving independence

  6. Intellectual and social competence

B. **Neurologic assessment measures** (Table 6)

C. **Functional assessment measures**

  1. **Rancho Los Amigos Scale** (RLAS; level of cognitive functioning scale) (see Appendix F)

      a. Original nomenclature for stages of cognitive recovery.

      b. Scale to describe behavioral impairments and follow stages of recovery.

TABLE 6. Neurologic Assessment Measures

Population	Cognition Scale	Used for:	Correlates with:	Test Time	Administration	Reliability
Coma emergence scales						
Coma emerging	Glasgow Coma Scale	Depth/duration of coma through responsiveness Most widely used Easy, minimal training	Survival Functional outcome	5–10 min	Hourly/ daily	High
RLAS II-V	Western Neuro-Sensory Stimulation Profile	Determining emergence from coma and start of interactions with environment Used during early stages of PTA	RLAS Predicts improvement	30 min	Weekly	Variable
RLAS II-IV	Coma/Near-Coma Scale	Measuring small clinical changes in low-level patients	DRS Evoked potentials	< 30 min		High
RLAS II-IV	Coma Recovery Scale	Assessing subtle changes in responsiveness	GCS DRS Predicts improvement	30 min		Lower
RLAS II-III	Rader Scale (sensory stimulation assessment measure)	Measuring responses to structured sensory stimulation program used for coma stimulation programs	GCS DRS RLAS	30–45 min	During sensory stimulation program	High
Posttraumatic amnesia scales (PTA)						
RLAS IV-VI	Galveston Orientation and Amnesia Test	Assess progress through PTA Temporal orientation Duration of retrograde/ anterograde amnesia Detects TBI in patients with spinal cord injury	Orientation Group Monitoring System Severity on GCS CT scan pathology Predicts 6-mo outcome	5 min	Daily	High
RLAS IV-VII	Orientation Group Monitoring System	Evaluation of clearing PTA during orientation group	GOAT MMSE Simple RT Choice RT Medical complications Decreased agitation	30 min	Daily	High
RLAS IV-VII	Westmead Post-Traumatic Amnesia Scale	Measures clearance from PTA Not used much	Cognitive outcome	5 min	Daily	Undocumented
Behavior Scales						
RLAS-IV	Neurobehavioral Rating Scale	Screening tool for psychiatric/affective disturbance after TBI Monitor improvement	TBI severity Frontal lobe injury	30 min structured interview	Daily	Adequate with training

Table continued on following page

TABLE 6. Neurologic Assessment Measures *(Continued)*

Population	Cognition Scale	Used for:	Correlates with:	Test Time	Admini-stration	Reli-ability
Behavior scales *(continued)*						
RLAS-IV	Agitated Behavior Scale	Serial measurement of agitation Monitor improvement		30 min		High

RLAS = Rancho Los Amigos Scale, GCS = Glasgow Coma Scale, GOAT = Galveston Orientation and Amnesia Test, MMSE = Mini-Mental Status Exam, DRS = Disability Rating Scale, RT = reaction time.

2. **Functional Independence Measure** (FIM)
   a. Most commonly used measure of personal independence.
   b. Based on motor and cognitive abilities.
   c. 7-point scale (complete dependence to complete independence).
   d. Excellent reliability and validity.
   e. Useful during inpatient rehabilitation but insensitive to gains made in postacute period.
3. **Functional Assessment Measure** (FAM)
   a. 12 items added to FIM.
   b. Attempts to improve assessment of cognition, psychosocial adjustment, and communication.
4. **Craig Handicap Assessment and Reporting Technique** (CHART)
   a. Originally developed for patients with spinal cord injury.
   b. Assesses functional status in physical independence, mobility, occupation, social integration, and economic self-sufficiency.
   c. Good reliability; correlates with scores from CIQ (see below).
   d. Sensitive to treatment effects of postacute brain rehabilitation.
5. **Community Integration Questionnaire** (CIQ)
   a. Assesses home integration, social integration, productive activities.
   b. Good reliability; correlates with CHART.
   c. Sensitive to treatment effects of postacute brain rehabilitation.
6. **Disability Rating Scale** (DRS)
   a. Assesses general, not specific functional status.
   b. Attempts to reflect functionally significant changes over time.
   c. Can track person from coma to community reintegration.
   d. Advantages: 8 items, easy to use, brief (<5 minutes).
   e. Poor sensitivity to extremes of functional deficits (mild TBI or severe impairment).
   f. Sensitive to improvement in inpatient TBI rehabilitation.

IX. **Additional TBI Rehabilitation Issues**
  A. **Goals**
   1. Control secondary medical problems.
   2. Prevent complications.
   3. Maximize functional and cognitive recovery.
  B. **Rehabilitation settings and community reintegration**
   1. Important team questions to help identify optimal rehabilitation setting to maximize function and community reentry:
      a. Does patient need 24-hour supervision?
      b. How severe are medical problems?
      c. Is 24-hour skilled nursing care necessary?

2. Family support:
    a. Can family and friends commit to and manage 24-hour supervision?
    b. Have family members been actively involved in learning patient's care and participating in therapies?
    c. What financial resources are available?
    d. Is home accessibility adequate?
    e. How is transportation to and from rehabilitation center managed?
    f. Are local day treatment programs available?
  C. **Discharge dispositions** (see Chapter 9, Stroke Rehabilitation)

Bibliography

1. Binder LM: A review of mild head trauma. Part II: Clinical implications. J Clin Exp Neuropsychol 19:432–457, 1997.
2. Cunitz G: Early management of head-brain trauma patients. Anaesthesist 44(5):369–391, 1995.
3. De Lisa JA (ed): Rehabilitation Medicine: Principles and Practice, 2nd ed. Philadelphia, J.B. Lippincott, 1993.
4. Erhard J, et al. Preclinical diagnosis and management in severe craniocerebral trauma. Unfallchirurg 99(8):534–540, 1996.
5. Garland D, Bailey S: Undetected injuries in head injured adults. Clin Orthop 155:162, 1981.
6. Geerts W, et al: A prospective study of venous thromboembolism after major trauma. N Engl J Med 331:1601, 1994.
7. Grabois M, et al (eds): Physical Medicine and Rehabilitation: The Complete Approach. Oxford, Blackwell Science, 2000.
8. Graham DI: Pathophysiological aspects of injury and mechanisms of recovery. In Rosenthal M, et al (eds): Rehabilitation of the Adult and Child with Traumatic Brain Injury. Philadelphia, F.A. Davis, 1999, p. 20.
9. Hagen C, Malkmus D, Durham P: Levels of cognitive function. In Downey CA (ed): Rehabilitation of the Head-Injured Adult: Comprehensive Physical Management. Professional Staff Association, Rancho Los Amigos Hospital, 1979.
10. Horn P, Munch E, Vajkoczy P et al: Hypertonic saline for control of elevated intracranial pressure in patients with exhausted response to mannitol and barbiturates. Neurol Res 21(8) p 758–764, 1999.
11. Kalisky A, et al: Medical problems encountered during rehabilitation of patients with head injury. Arch Phys Med Rehabil 66:25, 1985.
12. Khanna S, et al: Use of hypertonic saline in the treatment of severe refractory posttraumatic intracranial hypertension in pediatric traumatic brain injury. Crit Care Med 28(4):1144–1151, 2000.
13. Kraus JF, McArthur DL: Incidence and prevalence of, and costs associated with, traumatic brain injury. In Rosenthal M, et al (eds): Rehabilitation of the Adult and Child with Traumatic Brain Injury. Philadelphia, F.A. Davis, 1999, pp 5–8.
14. Kraus J, et al: Alcohol and brain injuries: Persons blood-tested, prevalence of alcohol involvement, and early outcome following injury. J Public Health 79:294, 1989.
15. Law JH, et al: Increased frequency of obstructive airway abnormalities with long-term tracheostomy. Chest 104:136, 1993.
16. Levin HS, O'Donnell VM, Grossman RG: The Galveston Orientation and Amnesia Test: A practical scale to assess cognition after head injury. J Nerv Mental Dis 167(11):675–684, 1979.
17. McLeod A, et al: Cardiac sequelae of acute head injury. Br Heart J 47:221, 1982.
18. Miller JD: Evaluation and treatment of head injury in adults. Neurosurg Q 2:28, 1992.
19. Nara I, et al. Comparative effects of hypothermia, barbiturate, and osmotherapy for cerebral oxygen metabolism, intracranial pressure, and cerebral perfusion pressure in patients with severe head injury. Acta Neurochirurgica (Suppl) 71:22–26, 1998.
20. National Institutes of Health: Rehabilitation of Persons with Traumatic Brain Injury. NIH Consensus Statement 16(1):1–41, 1998.
21. O'Dell M, et al. Standardized assessment instruments for minimally-responsive, brain-injured patients. NeuroRehabil 6:45, 1996.
22. Roberts I: Barbiturates for acute traumatic brain injury. Cochrane Database of Systematic Reviews (computer file). (2):CD000033, 2000.
23. Roper SN, et al: An analysis of cerebral blood flow in acute closed-head injury using technetium-99m-TC-HM-PAO-SPECT and computed tomography. J Nucl Med 32:1684, 1991.

24. Rosenthal M, et al: Rehabilitation of the Adult and Child with Traumatic Brain Injury, 3rd ed. Philadelphia, F.A. Davis, 1999.
25. Schierhout G, Roberts I: Mannitol for acute traumatic brain injury. Cochrane Database of Systemic Reviews (computer file). (2):CD001049, 2000.
26. Slavik RS, Rhoney DH: Indomethacin: A review of its cerebral blood flow effects and potential use for controlling intracranial pressure in traumatic brain injury. Neurol Res 21:491–499, 1999.
27. Shumway-Cook A: Rehabilitation of vestibular dysfunction in traumatic brain injury. Phys Med Rehab Clin North Am 3:2, 1992.
28. Teasdale G, Jennett B: Assessments of coma and impaired consciousness: A practical scale. Lancet 2:81, 1974.
20. Woo BH, Nesathurai S (eds): The Rehabilitation of People with Traumatic Brain Injury. Boston Medical Center, Blackwell Science, 2000.
30. Zasler ND: Mild traumatic brain injury: Medical assessment and intervention. J Head Trauma Rehabil 8(3):13–29, 1997.

Website

www.tbims.org

Chapter 11

ACUTE AND CHRONIC PAIN

Andrew J. Haig, M.D.

I. General Principles

A. Few heart surgeons have undergone sternotomy, and few radiation oncologists have experienced the side effects of their treatment. Their lack of experience is a double-edged sword. Perhaps they feel less empathy, but they are not biased by their own personal baggage.

B. All of us have experienced pain. On one hand, knowledge of pain can help clinicians understand what patients are experiencing. On the other hand, they may be tempted to make erroneous assumptions, judging pain on their own terms.

   1. At some level clinicians relate a patient's fractured femur to their own sprained ankle.

   2. At some level the doctor brought up in a stoic family misunderstands the emotional patient's verbalization of pain.

   3. Physicians may be blindsided by the emotionality of pain in a person brought up in an abusive household, the extent to which a narcotic-seeking patient will go to deceive, or the amount of pain a patient with cancer is willing to tolerate to stay fully alert.

C. Clinicians need to recognize that **pain is what the patient says it is**.

   1. Pain is just one of many discomforts that patients may experience.

   2. Other discomforts—whether insomnia or bankruptcy—interact and modify the pain experience, making it less tolerable.

   3. Pain is not equivalent to nociception. It does not readily correlate with disability.

D. **Definitions**

   1. **Pain:** defined by the International Association for the Study of Pain (IASP) as "an unpleasant sensory and emotional experience associated with actual or potential tissue damages or described in terms of such damage."

   2. **Nociception:** the sensation that a stimulus is painful.

   3. **Allodynia:** pain related to a stimulus that usually does not cause pain (e.g., a light touch causes substantial pain to a burn patient).

   4. **Hyperalgesia:** exaggerated response to a stimulus that is usually painful.

   5. **Hyperpathia:** exaggerated pain (especially in duration) in response to a stimulus.

   6. **Dysesthesia:** an abnormal sensation, whether spontaneous or evoked, that is unpleasant.

   7. **Paresthesia:** an abnormal sensation, whether spontaneous or evoked, that is not unpleasant.

   8. **Radiating pain:** pain in a nerve distribution, caused by stimulation of that nerve.

9. **Referred pain:** pain in an area where the stimulation is not occurring, but not radiating pain (not in the distribution of a nerve that is irritated).
10. **Sympathetically mediated pain:** pain associated with sympathetic phenomena, such as redness or sweating.
11. **Nonsympathetically mediated pain:** pain not associated with sympathetic phenomena.
12. **Complex regional pain syndrome I** (CRPS I): pain, allodynia, or hyperalgesia greater than expected for the tissue injury.
13. **Complex regional pain syndrome II** (CRPS II): pain, allodynia, or hyperalgesia greater than expected and not limited to the distribution of a traumatized nerve.
14. **Causalgia:** same as CRPS II.
15. **Reflex sympathetic dystrophy**: pain, vasomotor insufficiency, and dystrophy. Numerous other synonyms exist. The entity is poorly defined, and other terms (e.g., CRPS) are preferred.

II. Pain Pathophysiology

A. The science of pain is evolving quickly. The chemical soup and myriad axonal connections defy easy understanding, but a simple model of pain may serve as a framework.

B. **Peripheral nervous system**
   1. Tissue damage or nerve stimulation without tissue damage.
   2. Depolarization traverses the myelinated A-delta fibers (which cause a sharp, focussed pain sensation) and unmyelinated C fibers (which cause a burning pain) to the dorsal horn of the spinal cord.

C. **Spinal cord**
   1. Countless axons interact with nerve transmission in the spinal cord, including, among others, substance P, beta endorphins, enkephalins, amino acids, and neuropeptides.
   2. "Wind-up" involves facilitation of transmission and increased sensitivity.
   3. The gate theory of Melzack and Wall, although not proven, suggests that other sensory input along faster traveling nerve fibers can inhibit pain at the spinal level, essentially "distracting" the system from the pain.

D. **Brain**
   1. Relevant neuropathways include spinal thalamic tract to lateral thalamic nuclei, rubrospinal tract to medial thalamic nuclei, and thalamus to sensory cortex, the site where pain is consciously "felt."
   2. Numerous other central nervous system factors (e.g., emotions, alertness) can be effective inhibitors.

E. **Adaptations to chronic pain**
   1. Once pain is chronic, research indicates that it becomes a learned behavior. Chemical changes in everything from the dorsal horn to the frontal cortex cause a more complex response.
   2. Pain is amplified when it persists beyond removal of the painful stimulus, when a small pain stimulus causes severe pain reactions, or when pain distribution extents beyond the area of the stimulus.

III. General Approach to Treatment

A. Physicians and health care teams should proactively develop **strategies to prevent pain**.

B. When pain is noted, its **cause** should be determined.
   1. If the cause for pain cannot be eliminated, treatment is chosen.

3. Nonpharmacologic measures are first line of treatment for all patients.
4. Medications are typically the second line of therapy.
5. Interventional treatments may also be indicated.
C. If complete relief is not achieved through a physical medicine approach, a **rehabilitation approach** is taken.
   1. Evaluate for secondary causes of impairment, disability, and handicap.
   2. Establish the patient's goals, and treat with the objective of increasing quality of life.
D. **Discontinuation of treatment**
   1. As an important last step, the physician acknowledges and informs the patient that reasonable and appropriate medical treatment has failed to completely relieve pain and restore quality of life.
   2. This concrete endpoint allows the patient to focus energies away from treatment of pain toward other life activities.

IV. **Timing and Circumstances of Pain**
A. **Acute vs. chronic pain**
   1. In the first days or weeks after onset of pain, there appears to be a strong relationship between the amount of tissue damage and the pain levels.
   2. As pain lasts longer and longer, neural mechanisms amplify the pain and streamline the path that it takes to the brain.
   3. Pain becomes bigger than life, and the brain becomes preoccupied with looking for, fearing, and avoiding the pain.
   4. Behavioral consequences—rewards or punishments at the most basic level—change the interpretation of pain.
B. **Predicting and preventing pain**
   1. Pain may present suddenly, but its presence is rarely a surprise.
   2. Physiatrists, because of their role as team leaders, are in a position to develop proactive strategies for pain.
   3. Physiatrists with administrative roles often develop hospital or clinic strategies to detect and minimize pain.
   4. New Joint Commission on Accreditation of Health Care Organizations (JCAHCO) standards require that health care systems develop proactive strategies for the detection, treatment and management of pain.
   5. Physician administrators can affect pain management and prevention in following ways:
      a. **Posttraumatic pain:** educate emergency department personnel about appropriate pain medication prescription and administration practices.
      b. **Intraprocedural pain:** assign pain monitoring and treatment duties to someone other than the proceduralist.
      c. **Postoperative pain:** educate patients preoperatively; establish a plan for postoperative treatment preoperatively.
      d. **Activity-related musculoskeletal pain:** train nurses and aides about proper techniques, warm-up exercises. Educate nurses about appropriate use of medications prior to activities, including mobility and activities of daily living (ADLs).
      e. **Pain related to inactivity:** frequent position changes, stretching, ergonomically appropriate beds and chairs.
      f. **Recurrent procedural pain** (e.g., dressing changes): teach biofeedback, use hypnosis and other psychological supports.
C. **Pain that will predictably resolve**

1. When the pain is minor, patients and physicians should choose less aggressive treatments, viewing the risks as not worth the benefit.
2. When the pain is severe, patients and physicians may do the opposite—treat aggressively, because they know that the treatment side effects will not be a longstanding issue.

D. **Pain in terminal illness**
   1. Long-term side effects or risks of pain treatment are of little consequence (e.g., narcotic analgesics, permanent nerve ablation).
   2. Patient's goals may be different from those of other pain patients.
      a. Pain relief may take precedent over function.
      b. Alertness may take precedent over pain relief.
   3. **Physician strategies**
      a. Certain side effects (e.g., constipation, nausea) of other treatments may be worsened by pain medications. Medical safety, addiction, or lack of proof is less of an issue.
      b. Adequate pain relief can be obtained in most patients with terminal illness.
      c. Reassurance and emotional support are powerful pain management strategies.

V. **Diagnosing Pain**
A. **Overall strategy**
   1. First obligation is to determine cause of pain, if possible.
   2. Pain, especially in inpatient setting, may be warning sign of something ominous.
   3. Pain behavior may appear irrational in a number of systemic disorders that affect the brain
      a. Primary acute hospital service—busy with saving patient's life—may miss hidden injury or disease process.
      b. Numerous treatable diagnoses are not obvious to casual observer.

B. **"Pain all over" syndromes**
   1. Central pain syndrome
   2. Spinal cord pain
   3. Polyneuropathy
   4. Myopathy
   5. Polyarthritis
   6. Cryoglobulinemia
   7. Syndromes that also may be associated with delirium
      a. Metastatic cancer
      b. Hypercalcemia in immobilized teens
      c. Drug withdrawal
      d. Thyroid disease
      e. Sickle cell crisis
      f. Showering emboli
      g. Vasculitis
      h. Drug reaction
      i. Psychiatric diseases

C. **Common or important regional pain syndromes**
   1. **Head**
      a. Migraines
      b. Spinal headache
      c. Stress-related myofascial pain
      d. Tooth pain
      e. Temporomandibular junction pain
      f. Glaucoma/eye disease
      g. Tumor
      h. Infection
      i. Aneurysm
      j. Secondary to hypoxia, hypoglycemia, hypotension, or anemia

2. **Neck**
   a. Mechanical neck pain
   b. Undetected spinal trauma
   c. Meningitis
   d. Retropharyngeal abscess
   e. Postintubation throat pain
   f. Fungal esophagitis
3. **Chest**
   a. Aortic aneurysm
   b. Myocardial infarction
   c. Pulmonary embolus
   d. Pneumonia/abscess
   e. Tietze's syndrome or costo-chondritis
   f. Mechanical rib dysfunction
   g. Undetected spinal trauma
4. **Low back**
   a. Mechanical related to bed rest
   b. Undetected spinal trauma
   c. Exacerbation of premorbid pain syndrome
   d. Retroperitoneal hematoma
   e. Aneurysm
   f. Psoas abscess
   g. Urinary tract infection
   h. Gynecologic disorder
5. **Abdomen/pelvis**
   a. Acalculus cholecystitis
   b. Aneurysm
   c. Appendicitis
   d. Stress ulcer
   e. Bowel infarction
   f. Bowel obstruction
   g. Bowel venous insufficiency
   h. Constipation
   i. Superior mesenteric artery syndrome (in spinal cord injury)
   j. Postsurgical infection or bleed
   k. Urinary retention/infection
   l. Renal disease
   m. Pancreatitis
   n. Gynecologic disorders
   o. Heterotopic ossification
6. **Upper limb**
   a. Cardiac/pulmonary referred pain
   b. Mechanical joint pain
   c. Strain/sprain
   d. Shoulder-hand syndrome
   e. Missed/new trauma
   f. IV filtration/compartment syndrome
   g. Nerve palsy related to needle trauma
   h. Cervical radiculopathy
   i. Positioning-related radial or ulnar nerve palsy
7. **Lower limb**
   a. Lumbar radiculopathy
   b. Injection or surgical sciatic trauma
   c. Peroneal nerve pressure
   d. Compartment syndrome
   e. Ischemia
   f. Pressure sore
   g. Gout
   h. Mechanical joint pain
   i. Strain/sprain
   j. Deep venous thrombosis

V. **Measurement of Pain**
  A. **Proving the existence of pain**
   1. While the cause of pain can often be diagnosed, pain itself cannot be diagnosed.
   2. Many of the components of the pain cascade can be disrupted or corrupted. Examples include the following:
      a. Although fractured toes are typically quite painful, many diabetics walk around oblivious to x-ray findings. In this case the tissue damage released appropriate chemicals, but the nerves were not present to transmit the signal.
      b. Pain radiating below the knee is typical of disc herniation syndrome. But radiating pain also can occur with noxious stimulation of muscles, joints, and ligaments.

  i. Referred pain is not highly selective or specific.

  ii. Surgical study showed that light stimulation of a nerve root does not cause radiating pain in general, but persons whose sciatica has resolved feel radiating pain when the previously affected root is stimulated.

  ii. Thus it appears that the nervous system reorganizes based on previous pain experiences.

3. There is a great disparity between pain behavior and pain itself.

  a. Patients may report pain when they want to abuse narcotics, want to win a lawsuit, or want attention from nursing staff. They may deny pain when they want to be discharged from the hospital.

  b. Physical and verbal pain behaviors vary both personally and culturally.

  c. Physician's personal experiences and culture result in varied interpretation of pain behaviors.

  d. Objective measures such as tachycardia or diaphoresis, seen in severe acute pain, also occur in numerous other medical disorders.

B. **Methods for measurement of pain**

 1. **Assumptions**

  a. Patient's report of pain is genuine.

  b. Other motivating factors are constant.

 2. **Three common measures of pain**

  a. **Visual Analog Pain Scale** is useful in quantifying extent of pain.

   i. 10-cm line with anchors of 0 and 10 at either end. At 0 is the phrase "no pain whatsoever" and at 10 is the phrase "worst pain imaginable." The patient is asked to place an X on the line at the point that represents his or her pain.

   ii. Variations ask for the average, best, and worst pain in the past week.

   iii. Main problem with a visual analog scale is that it has a ceiling. The patient who marked 10 last week and now feels that the pain is worse has nowhere to go. A follow-up visual analog scale can place "same as last week" at the 5 position, with "complete improvement" at 0 and "completely worse" at 10.

  b. **McGill Pain Scale** considers various qualities of pain.

   i. Patients circle words describing various aspects of their pain—sensory, affective, evaluative, and miscellaneous categories.

   ii. Significant problem with McGill Scale is the relatively high literacy level needed to circle descriptors such as "lancinating."

   iii. Useful research tool but has clinical limitations.

  c. **Westhaven Yale Multidimensional Pain Inventory** (WHYMPI or MPI) is useful in determining effect of pain on patient's life.

   i. MPI looks at pain from multiple perspectives.

    • Person's experience with pain (pain interference in life activities, how supported patient feels, pain severity, life control, and affective distress).

    • Responses given by others to patient's pain (negative, solicitous, or distracting) and activity levels (household chores, outdoor work, activities away from home, social activities, and general activity).

    • Combination scores can categorize patient's responses in terms of ability to adapt to pain—adaptive "copers" will likely do well, whereas dysfunctional or interpersonally distressed persons may need more support.

   ii. MPI can predict responses to rehabilitation and detect barriers to success.
3. **Miscellaneous other scales**
   a. Alternative measures of pain
      i. Facial expression
      ii. Body language
      iii. Pictures and scales for children or persons with reading or language problems
   b. Other facets of pain commonly measured
      i. Fear and avoidance of pain (avoidance predicts performance better than pain alone).
      ii. Locus of control (external locus of control, in which patient blames others, is bad prognostic sign).
      iii. Pain related quality of life (overall goals of pain program typically relate to this facet).
      iv. Attributes and beliefs about interventions (belief in certain treatments or lack of agreement with or among physicians results in poor prognosis).
      v. Self-rating of prognosis (highly predictive of outcome).
4. **Clinical use of pain scales**
   a. Scales do not drive treatment; they are used to monitor treatment.
   b. Example: Pain at 8/10 does not suggest a certain medication or even a certain level of aggressiveness. But a change from 8 to 5 is a good thing.

VI. Chronic Pain Syndromes
A. **General issues**
   1. Acute pain is generally proportional to tissue damage. It "makes sense" to the clinician. Chronic pain is often out of proportion to tissue damage. It can be confusing but appears less so when one takes into account behavioral adaptations that must occur for many patients to cope with pain.
   2. Patients learn to avoid pain by avoiding movements. As a result, they become deconditioned, which affects strength, endurance, flexibility, and coordination. Deconditioning itself becomes disabling and causes pain under circumstances that would not cause pain to others.
   3. Patients become vigilant; that is, they search for ways to avoid pain.
   4. When pain is truly unavoidable, vigilance is frustrated, often resulting in anxiety. Anxiety, coupled with life stresses and sleep deprivation, results in depression.
B. **Psychopathology and chronic pain**
   1. Premorbid psychopathology is common in persons with chronic pain.
   2. Chronic pain has its rewards for persons with psychosocial dysfunction.
   3. Social rewards, such as financial secondary gain, are often involved.
   4. Especially in hospitalized patients with chronic pain, hysteria, malingering, or factitious disorders are always possible.
   5. **Specific psychosocial correlates of chronic pain**
      a. **Premorbid**
         i. Personality disorders
         ii. Dysthymia or depression
         iii. Anxiety disorder
         iv. Thought disorders
         v. Alcohol and drug abuse

     vi. Hysteria

     vii. Malingering

     viii. Fictitious disorders

     ix. Tendency to avoid pain

     x. Mistrust or excessive faith in health care providers

     xi. Physical, sexual, or emotional abuse

     xiii. Impending major social change (e.g., layoff, divorce)

  b. **Resultant**

     i. Fear

     ii. Posttraumatic stress disorder

     iii. Anxiety

     iv. Depression

     v. Financial or legal secondary gain

     vi. Secondary social gain (e.g., spouse support, staff attention, avoidance of military service)

     vii. Sleep disorders

     viii. Medication-related delirium

     ix. Unrealistic medical goals

     x. Abandonment

     xi. Financial crisis

     xii. Social handicap

  6. Successful treatment looks beyond severe or obvious psychiatric diagnoses to personality traits and coping styles. These factors may be assets or barriers in different circumstances.

C. **Complex regional pain syndrome (CRPS)**

  1. **Clinical perspective**

    a. Chronic pain out of proportion to injury, often associated with disuse and autonomic changes.

    b. Has existed for hundreds of years under a hundred different names.

    c. Use of term "reflex sympathetic dystrophy" is discouraged, because reflex and sympathetic components have not been established and not all patients have dystrophy. However, it is ingrained in medical literature.

    d. Commonly seen as "shoulder-hand syndrome" in cardiac patients in 1950s, but became rare when increased activity was encouraged.

    e. Now shoulder-hand syndrome is seen occasionally in inpatients with stroke or other neurologic syndromes, perhaps related to trauma, traction, or disuse.

    f. Children develop CRPS. Unlike in adults, it affects leg more commonly than arm and seldom causes disability.

  2. **Stages of CRPS**

    a. **Acute phase** (first 3–6 months): pain, tenderness, swelling, and vasomotor changes.

    b. **Dystrophic phase** (3–6 months): continued pain and trophic changes to skin and bone; classically a shiny hand, nail bed changes, and patchy osteopenia.

    c. **Atrophic phase:** skin is cool, tight and shiny, with atrophy and contractures of muscles. The limb is painless but often useless.

    d. Stages of shoulder-hand syndrome are well ingrained in most physiatrists, but probably do not actually occur in sequence or in all patients.

3. **Diagnosis of CRPS**
    a. No diagnostic tests are specific to CRPS; painless disuse often has similar findings. Patients who are symptomatically cured continue to exhibit the findings.
    b. Triple-phase bone scan is abnormal in early-to-middle phases.
    c. X-rays show patchy osteopenia in middle-to-late phases.
    d. Thermography or skin temperature measurements may show difference > 2°C—either cooler or warmer—on affected limb.
4. **Treatment of CRPS**
    a. Physical therapy
        i. Range-of-motion exercises
        ii. Desensitization
        iii. Physical modalities (classically, paraffin baths)
    b. Oral and injected medications
        i. Pain medications
        ii. Oral steroids appear effective in short term, but their effect on prognosis is unknown.
        iii. Sympathetic ganglion blocks are commonly used but have not been shown effective in a randomized trial.
        iv. Bier blocks with reserpine and other medications are commonly used.

VII. **Treatment of Pain**
  A. Treatment of pain can be described in various terms (e.g., more or less aggressive, more or less invasive), but there is no established hierarchy of treatment. Depending on the cause, severity, duration, and functional consequences of the pain, treatment may or may not progress from noninvasive to invasive.
  B. **Psychological treatment**
    1. Relaxation, biofeedback and hypnosis
        a. Especially helpful when pain will recur, as with dressing changes.
        b. Less helpful when patient must concentrate on other tasks such as therapy or work.
    2. Patient education is a powerful psychological factor.
        a. Patients who incorrectly associate pain with tissue damage, future harm, or more dangerous disease experience more pain.
        b. Physicians are powerful and credible players in counseling, but professional counselors are often necessary.
        c. Psychological treatment of associated disorders is obvious and important. Physicians can assist with medications as needed.
  C. **Physical modalities**
    1. Examples: heat, cold, electricity, and vibration.
    2. Modalities can decrease pain in short term.
    3. Therapist-applied modalities have little use in outpatient setting. Most studies show no long-term effect and no substantial difference among modalities for pain management. The cost of therapist-applied modalities is high.
    4. Therapist-applied modalities may be useful in inpatient setting.
        a. Patients are often unable to self-apply modalities.
        b. More generous use of modalities may help avoid medications that can complicate medical disease.
        c. When possible, patient control over use and timing of modalities increases effectiveness.

      d. Nursing staff is often unfamiliar with nuances of physical modalities. They should be encouraged to use modalities before as-needed medications if there is a chance that they will be effective.

C. **Active physical therapy**
1. Hands-on physical therapy and exercise are often effective.
2. Common forms of manual therapy
    a. Mobilization without impulse
    b. Muscle energy technique
    c. High-velocity, low-amplitude thrust
    d. Functional (indirect) techniques
    e. Myofascial release
    f. Craniosacral techniques
3. Other therapist interventions
    a. Massage is often performed by nurses or persons with less training than desirable, but it can still be effective.
    b. Active or passive stretching relieves painful contractures and spasm.
    c. Strengthening exercises can relieve pain and spasm.
    d. More specific techniques for back pain, such as McKenzie approach, are well established in outpatient setting.

D. **Medication**
1. **Scheduled medications are more effective than as-needed medications.**
    a. Patients who have to assess the level of their pain in order to obtain medication feel the pain more.
    b. Availability of medication is not immediate.
    c. Pain prevention is more effective than treating pain after it has caught the patient's attention.
    d. Additional doses for breakthrough pain are appropriate.
    e. Choice of medication depends on severity and duration of pain and risk of side effects.
2. **Potential problems with standing as-needed pain medication orders.**
    a. Important medical diagnoses may be missed.
    b. Medications may be used instead of nursing assessment and treatment of cause of discomfort.
    c. Medications may be used instead of more benign physical modalities.
    d. Medications may be used after pain occurs rather than prophylactically.
    e. Physicians may not be aware of variable or large doses of pain medications causing side effects.
3. **Specific medications** (for dosages, side effects, and other issues, see chapter Chapter 23, Pharmacology).
    a. **Acetaminophen.** Because of its low side-effect profile, acetaminophen is usually the first-line medication for pain, although often it is underutilized by staff members who look for something "more powerful." But 24-hour coverage with acetaminophen is surprisingly effective. Hepatic dysfunction, including substantial alcohol use, precludes extensive use. Overdosing can occur when acetaminophen is continued simultaneously with "next-step" opiate analgesics that also contain acetaminophen.
    b. **Nonsteroidal anti-inflammatory drugs (NSAIDs)** theoretically are advantageous because of their anti-inflammatory properties. In terms of pain alone, they have not been shown to be more effective than acetaminophen. Their side-effect profiles, including homeostatic, hepatic,

renal, and gastrointestinal (GI) problems, are serious, especially for elderly patients. Caution must be taken to switch from long-acting NSAIDs preoperatively, because the risk of bleeding increases. Still, there is no question that they are effective—and for some patients may be more effective than acetaminophen. In elderly patients or patients with GI risks, the newer cyclooxygenase (COX) II inhibitors may be safer.

c. **Muscle relaxants.** Medications commonly known as muscle relaxants include carisoprodol, cyclobenzaprine, and others. They may have an effect on pain, but no evidence suggests that they are more effective for "muscle spasm" (a poorly defined entity) than for other pain problems. Physical modalities, trigger-point injections, and stretching may be more specific treatments for sore muscles. Central nervous system (CNS) side effects can be significant.

d. **Opiate analgesics** are a mainstay of hospital treatment of severe pain. They are highly effective for acute pain syndromes and quite useful in malignancy-related pain. Choice of medication depends on severity of pain. Oral medications typically are used for less severe pain, intravenous or intramuscular medications for more severe pain. Alternative routes such as suppository or patches (for long-term maintenance) may be appropriate in some cases. Continuous or on-demand opiate analgesia, either IV or epidural, is quite useful for severe pain, especially in the postoperative period. Important side effects include depression, delirium, respiratory depression, constipation, and urinary retention.

e. **Opiates for chronic, nonmalignant pain**

   i. Use of opiates for chronic benign pain is controversial.

   ii. In the rehabilitation setting it is often not clear when patients make the transition from "acute" to "chronic."

   iii. When patients with chronic pain present for hospitalization, choice as to whether to detoxify the patient or to continue medications depends on the reason for hospitalization and long-term management strategies.

   iv. Prehospital physicians often do not begin narcotic analgesia in a logical manner. Hospital physicians should be cautioned to avoid validating or continuing erroneous decisions during hospitalization or at discharge.

   v. The hospital is a good place for objective assessment and restructuring of opiate use.

   vi. **Policy for chronic opiate use**

      • Screen for history of alcohol or drug abuse and contraindications or possible adverse effects.

      • Make a contract with the patient. The agreement should include the understanding that only one physician and one pharmacy will be involved, that increasing dosage will not be allowed without communication with the physician, that refills will be given only on schedule, and that objective measures of medication effectiveness (such as continued employment or outside activity) must be demonstrated.

      • Reassess use, function, and side effects at 1 month and then at least every 6 months.

      • Longer-acting opiates may be more appropriate.

      • Strongly consider an annual month-long drug holiday to assess continued need, compliance, and effect of medication on function.

f. Other chronic pain medications
i. General principles
- Pain medications do not cure pain. They dampen it. Choices must be realistic.
- Many agents require consistent use for weeks.
- Most agents have poorly defined therapeutic dosages; it is a common practice to titrate the medication until side effects occur.
- If second or third medication is chosen, choose from drugs with different mechanisms of action (Table 1) and consider not discontinuing the first used medication to promote an overlapping effect.

TABLE 1.   Mechanisms of Action of Medications Used for Chronic Pain

Mechanism	Symptoms	Target	Drug
Sodium channel accumulation, redistribution, altered expression	Spontaneous pain paresthesias, neuroma sign	Sodium channels sensitive to tetrodotoxin, sodium channel resistant to tetrodotoxin	Sodium channel blockers Antiepileptic drugs (carbamazepine, lamotrigine) Antiarrhythmic agents (mexiletine, TCAs) Blockers with greater analgesic than anticonvulsant index* Ion channel-selective blockers*
Central sensitization	Tactile (dynamic) hyperalgesia, cold hyperalgesia, pin prick hyperalgesia	NVDA-R Neurokinin 1-R Neuronal nitric oxide synthase Protein kinase gamma	NMDA antagonists Ketamine Dextromethorphan Amantadine Glycine site antagonists* Subunit specific antagonists[†] Neurokinin 1-R antagonists[†] Neuronal nitric oxide synthase Protein kinase C inhibitors
Peripheral sensitization	Pressure (static) hyperalgesia Thermal hyperalgesia Spontaneous pain Neurogenic inflammation	Varilloid receptor-1 desensitization Sodium channels resistant to tetrodotoxin Nerve growth factor	Capsaicin Neurokinin 1-R antagonists[†] Blockers of sodium channels resistant to tetrodotoxin[†] Nerve growth factors
Alpha-receptor expression, sympathetic sprouting	Spontaneous pain	Alpha-receptor antagonists	Phentolamine Guanethidine Nerve growth factor antagonists[†]
Increased transmission, reduced inhibition	Spontaneous pain Hyperalgesia	N-type calcium channels Receptors (MDR alpha$_2$, GABA, Neurokinin 1, adenosine, P2X$_2$, kainate, MgluR, cholecystokinin, rAChR	Conatoxin Opiates Gabapentin TCAs SNRIs

* In clinical development.
[†] In preclinical development.
From Woolf CJ, Manton RJ: Neuropathic pain: Etiology, symptoms, mechanisms, and management. Lancet 353:1959–1964, 1999, with permission.

ii. **Common choices**
- **Tricyclic antidepressants (TCAs).** The more anticholinergic the drug, the better the response. Use very low doses for elderly patients; most patients respond by levels of 50 mg/day. TCAs may be better for aching pain than neuropathic pain.
- **Seizure medications.** Gabapentin has the best side-effect profile. Carbamazepine is well studied; phenytoin and most others have been tried. New agents are coming out. Seizure medications may be better for neuropathic pain than aching pain.
- **Benzodiazepines.** Whether due to anxiolytic, amnestic, central pain effects, or unproven effect on muscle spasm, they have been used for chronic pain, although the addiction potential is high.
- **Capsaicin.** Topical cream is most effective at 0.075%, but it may hurt more and actually damage neurons.
- **Sympathetic blockers**
- **Beta blockers** (propranolol), **alpha blockers** (phenoxybenzamine), **alpha and beta blockers** (guanethidine), Alpha agonist (clonidine).
- **Calcium channel blockers**
- **Calcitonin.** Intranasal administration may have a direct antipain effect, but is used for bony pain, including compression fractures and spinal stenosis.

4. **Medications to treat associated conditions**
   a. **Depression.** Selective serotonin reuptake inhibitors (SSRIs) probably do not affect pain directly but do affect depression.
   b. **Sleep disturbances.** Typically TCAs are useful; anxiety or phobia components of posttraumatic stress disorder.
   c. **Obsessive aspects** of pain may respond to SSRIs.

E. **Injections**
   1. Relatively benign **trigger-point injections** can be useful for tight muscles. They are best reserved for patients who cannot relieve trigger points with stretching (e.g., patients in a halo brace on inpatient rehabilitation unit).
   2. **Botulinum toxin** injections for muscle spasm (not spasticity) are not yet proven. Long-term consequences of injection need to be weighed against potential benefits. For painful spasticity, either botulinum or phenol blocks may be appropriate, however.
   3. **Spinal injections** (see Chapter 24, Physiatric Procedures).
   4. **Sympathetic blockade.** CRPS is often treated with sympathetic ganglion blocks. Bier blocks are performed with exsanguination of the limb, followed by IV injection of medications such as reserpine.
   5. **Destructive nerve blocks.** Malignant pain in patients with poor prognosis suggests more invasive and destructive means of pain relief. For instance, phenol block of intercostal nerves or other pain generating nerves can substantially improve quality of life.

F. **Surgery.** Surgery for pain itself is not common but takes many forms.
   1. **Implanted morphine pumps** are used for chronic pain after failure of other methods and demonstrated success of a trial injection.
   2. **Electrical stimulators** are also implanted in the spinal canal for pain. Like implanted morphine pumps, they have been available for decades. Neither has taken hold as mainstream treatment; both are costly.

3. **Surgical ablation** of a pain-generating nerve may be appropriate for malignant pain. For benign pain this approach is usually futile. An exception is relief from phantom pain secondary to neuroma after limb amputation.
4. Amputation of a limb for pain alone, spinal cord section, and thalamotomy are now obscure treatments.
5. Surgical relief of painful lesions such as disc herniation

G. **Alternative treatments**
1. **When to use alternative treatments for pain.** Almost by definition, alternative means unproven. Even when specific effectiveness is questioned, the placebo effect of such treatments can be quite large for pain. Choice of alternative therapy may be based on face validity to the patient, but risk of harm—physical, emotional, or financial—must be considered.
2. **Common categories**
   a. Movement-related: yoga, tai-chi, Alexander technique, Pilates, Feldenkrais.
   b. Medication-like: herbs, naturopathy, homeopathy, aroma therapy.
   c. Passive treatments: acupuncture, massage, chiropractic, sclerotherapy, moxibustion.
   d. Mind-body therapies: meditation, crystals, astrologic counseling, religious interventions.

IX. Rehabilitation of Chronic Pain

A. **Basic concepts**
1. Rehabilitation of chronic pain (minimizing disability and handicap) is separate from treatment of chronic pain.
2. There is little relationship between pain and disability. However, factors such as pain avoidance and perception of harm are related to disability.
3. Secondary factors, including psychiatric disease and deconditioning, are common reversible causes of disability.
4. The patient must have a need to succeed functionally—whether personal, financial, or social.

B. **Rehabilitation programs** (typically outpatient programs)
1. Multidisciplinary programs aimed at improving function, regardless of pain, appear to be highly effective.
2. Multidisciplinary program includes:
   a. Assessment of social history, patient goals, physical and psychosocial functioning.
   b. Assessment of barriers to success (e.g., legal, personal, financial, other medical problems, language).
   c. Education, exercise, counseling, and planning for the future.
   d. Concrete, time-limited program with specific weekly goals for therapy.
   e. Long-term program for independent management.
   f. Scheduled long-term (typically 1-, 3-, 6-, and 12-month) follow-up (not on as-needed basis)

X. When Nontreatment of Pain Is Acceptable

A. Joint Commission on Accreditation of Healthcare Organizations (JCAHO) recently mandated assessment and management of pain as a "vital sign" in all patients.
B. This policy raises pain relief above other potentially important issues, such as functional ability, psychiatric status, and quality of life, which are not mandated "vital signs."

C. Especially in regard to medication prescription, physicians must feel comfortable *not* treating pain when other goals are in conflict.
   1. When further attempts at treatment are unlikely to make a significant difference in quality of life.
   2. When pain relief measures may interfere with assessment or treatment of medical problems.
   3. When acute pain relief measures interfere with an overall plan to manage functional abilities and independence of patients with chronic pain.
   4. When pain relief measures interfere with management of psychiatric disorders such as drug abuse or depression.
   5. When side effects of pain relief measures interfere with goals more valued by the patient. Examples may include alertness (e.g., in a terminal patient), learning of new skills (e.g., in physical therapy), brain plasticity (during recovery from head injury or stroke), balance, appetite, and continence.

Bibliography

1. Foley KM: Advances in cancer pain. Arch Neurol 56:413–417, 1999.
2. IASP Subcommittee on Taxonomy: Classification of chronic pain: Descriptions of chronic pain syndromes and definitions of pain terms. Pain 3(Suppl):S1–S225, 1986.
3. Kingery WS: Complex regional pain syndrome. In Grabois M, Garrison SJ, Hart KA, Lemkuhl LD (eds): Physical Medicine and Rehabilitation: The Complete Approach. Malden, MA, Blackwell Science, 2000, pp 1101–1123.
4. Loeser JD (ed): Bonica's Management of Pain, 3rd ed. Philadelphia, Lippincott Williams & Wilkins, 2001.
5. Turk DC, Melzack R: Handbook of Pain Assessment. New York, Guilford Press, 1992.
6. Woolf CJ, Mannion RJ: Neuropathic pain: Etiology, symptoms, mechanisms, and management. Lancet 353:1959–21964, 1999. (Lancet volume 353 [full text on Medline] has a strong series of articles reviewing many aspects of pain and pain management.)

Chapter 12

DECONDITIONING AND BED REST

Henry C. Tong, M.D., and Christopher M. Brammer, M.D.

I. **Definition:** Deconditioning is defined by DeLisa as reduced functional capacity of the musculoskeletal and other body systems.

II. **Effects by System**

A. **Cardiovascular system**

1. Bed rest → fluid shift from legs to trunk (central fluid shift) → increased venous return to the heart → stretched carotid and aortic baroreceptors and cardiopulmonary mechanoreceptors → decreased aldosterone and antidiuretic hormone → diuresis → decreased plasma volume (about 5% in 25 hours, 10% in 6 days, 20% in 14 days).

2. **Cardiac changes**

   a. **Stroke volume** (SV): decreased by up to 30% with both submaximal and maximal exercise.

   b. **Heart rate** (HR)

      i. At rest: increased by about $\frac{1}{2}$ beat/minute each day for 3–4 weeks, then plateaus.

      ii. With exercise: abnormally large increase in heart rate with submaximal exercises.

   c. **Cardiac output** (CO)

      i. Because of increased heart rate and decreased stroke volume, resting cardiac output (SV × HR) is unchanged or slightly decreased.

      ii. Maximal CO is decreased at maximal exercise by up to 26%.

   d. **Maximum oxygen consumption** ($\dot{V}O_2$max): decreased with exercise by up to 28%.

   e. **Orthostatic hypotension**

      i. Cause: may be due to decreased cardiac vagal tone, decreased plasma volume, or impaired cardiac baroceptor reflex response.

      ii. Signs and symptoms: dizziness, tachycardia, light-headedness, fainting.

      iii. Diagnosis: during transfer from lying to sitting or standing position, systolic blood pressure (BP) falls by 30 mmHg *or* diastolic BP falls by 10 mmHg *and* patient has symptoms.

      iv. Prevention: early mobilization, sitting at bedside.

      v. Treatment: active exercise with physical/occupational therapy and therapeutic recreation when medically safe.

      vi. Recovery time frame: at least twice as long as duration of bed rest.

3. **Vascular effects**

   a. **Decreased blood flow in muscles** due to decreased muscular pumping action.

    b. **Increased blood viscosity** (plasma loss faster than red blood cell mass decrease, resulting in increased hematocrit and blood viscosity).

    c. **Increased platelet adhesiveness**

    d. **Increased fibrinogen level**

    e. **Increased risk for deep vein thrombosis (DVT) and pulmonary embolism (PE)** (see Chapter 13, Deep Venous Thrombosis)

B. **Respiratory system**

    1. Supine position → abdominal contents push diaphragm → diaphragm elevation → decreased space for lung expansion → decreased residual lung volume → decreased breathing → **increased atelectasis.**

    2. In paraplegic patients with **paralysis of thoracic respiratory muscles**, diaphragm elevation in supine position may improve ventilation (see Chapter 8, Spinal Cord Injury Rehabilitation).

    3. **Increased VQ mismatch** in supine position leads to decreased oxygenation.

    4. **Increased respiratory rate**

    5. **Increased forced vital capacity**

    6. **Diaphragm elevation**

    7. **Increased risk of nosocomial pneumonia**

        a. In critically ill or ventilator-dependent patients.

        b. Postulated causes: increased mucus plugging, decreased ciliary action, and decreased cough (due to weak abdominal musculature), compromised immunity.

        c. Signs and symptoms: fever, cough, yellow-green sputum.

        d. Diagnosis: chest x-ray, complete blood count (CBC) with differential, sputum culture/throat swab; bronchoalveolar lavage may be required.

        e. Prevention: early mobilization, frequent position changes, incentive spirometry, deep breathing, adequate hydration, good dental care, chest percussion with postural drainage (CPPD).

        f. Treatment: antibiotics.

C. **Central nervous system**

    1. **Changes in affect** (depression, anxiety, and fear), **cognition** (decreases in concentration, judgment, problem-solving), and **perception** (delirium and decreased pain threshold) may result from bed rest and sensory deprivation in unfamiliar hospital room.

    2. **Delirium**

        a. Diagnostic criteria (according to Diagnostic and Statistical Manual of Mental Disorders, Fourth Edition [DSM-IV])

            i. Altered consciousness that decreases attention.

            ii. Altered cognition (e.g., disorientation, hallucinations) not explained by dementia.

            iii. Fluctuation of deficits during day.

        b. Evaluation should look for causes.

            i. General medical condition (myocardial infarction, stroke, DVT)

            ii. Medication (e.g., narcotics, antiepileptics, anticholinergics)

            iii. Substance withdrawal

        c. Treatment

            i. Treat medical causes of delirium.

            ii. Stop medications that may cause changes in mental status.

            iii. Frequently orient patient to time and place.

            iv. Put patient in semiprivate room.

  v. Encourage visits from family and friends, who also may bring favorite pictures, music, books.
  vi. Encourage clergy visits (if appropriate).
  vii. Encourage group activities, and take patient outside.
  viii. Keep patient's hearing aids and glasses easily available (if applicable).
D. **Peripheral nervous system:** compression neuropathies may occur (see Appendix B for common entrapment sites).
E. **Musculoskeletal system**
  1. **Muscles**
    a. **Decreased muscle strength**
      i. Strength decreases by 0.5–1.7% day. Mueller noted loss of 1.0–1.5% of isometric strength per day of bed rest over 2 weeks. Cast immobilization of the arm resulted in loss of 1.3-5.5% per day over 2 weeks.
      ii. Strength loss relatively more rapid during early part of bed rest, plateaus at about 20–50%.
      iii. Strength loss generally greater in legs than arms (according to study by Dietrick, in which healthy volunteers were placed in bivalved body casts for 6 weeks).
      iv. Antigravity muscles (e.g., gastrocsoleus and back muscles) lose more strength.
      v. Signs and symptoms: impaired transfers, ambulation, and activities of daily living (ADLs).
      vi. Evaluation should focus on physical mobility and strength. Medical Research Council grades:
        • 5 = normal strength
        • 4 = full active range of motion (AROM) against gravity and moderate resistance
        • 3 = full AROM against gravity
        • 2 = full AROM in "gravity-eliminated" position
        • 1 = trace visual/palpable contraction
        • 0 = no contraction
      vii. Prevention and treatment
        • Relatively intense exercises (isotonic or iskoinetic) in bed help maintain muscle strength..
        • Daily ROM exercise of muscles delays atrophy.
        • Early mobilization and weight-bearing activity (when safe). After mobilization is started, it may take twice as along as duration of immobilization to recover muscle strength.
        • Minimal type and amount of exercise needed are not known. In Mueller's study, daily muscle contractions of 30–50% of maximal tension for several seconds maintained muscle strength.
    b. **Decreased muscle fiber mass/atrophy**
    c. **Decreased tendon strength**
    d. **Histologic changes**
      i. Decreased adenosine triphosphate (ATP) and glycogen stores → increased muscle fatigability.
      ii. In animal studies by Appell, predominantly type I slow-twitch fibers were affected, but 30-day bed-rest study by Dudley found little difference between type I fiber atrophy and type II fiber atrophy.
      iii. Increased relative collagen content and cross-linkage.

iv. Prolonged immobilization causes replacement of loose connective tissue with dense connective tissue with type I collagen fibers.

v. Decreased strength at myotendinous junction.

2. **Joints**
   a. **Decreased joint ROM → contractures.**
      i. **Anatomic classification of joint contractures**
         - Arthrogenic contracture (due to pathology in joint itself): cartilage damage (degenerative joint disease, trauma, Charcot joints); synovial proliferation (effusion or synovitis/connective tissue disease), and faulty positioning of capsule or ligaments (fiber shortening, infection).
         - Soft-tissue or extra-articular contracture: due to soft tissue changes around joint from inflammation (e.g., scleroderma or burns), trauma and scar formation, infection, Dupuytren's contracture, or immobilization.
         - Myogenic contracture: due to muscle fiber shortening from inflammation (myositis), trauma (intramuscular hemorrhage), immobilization (paralysis or bed rest), or muscle imbalances (spasticity or weakness). Initial cause of muscle shortening: perimysium tightness; later cause: decreased number of sarcomeres in series. Two-joint muscles typically more affected (e.g. gastrocnemius).
         - Mixed arthrogenic, soft tissue, and myogenic changes also noted.
      ii. Signs and symptoms: decreased ADLs due to decreased AROM.
      iii. Diagnosis: clinical exam.
      iv. Clinical sequelae (Table 1)
      v. Prevention and treatment include early mobilization, proper positioning, static splinting (foot board or positioning ankle-foot orthosis [AFO] to prevent ankle plantarflexion contracture), and active and passive ROM to full ROM.
         - No consensus about minimum frequency of ROM exercises, needed, but daily to twice daily seems to be effective.
         - ROM exercises stretch tight muscles/connective tissues and strengthen antagonist muscle to help maintain gains.
         - Low-force, long-duration stretches favor permanent viscous deformation.
         - Heating connective tissue (40–43°C) increases viscous properties and maximizes effect of stretching.

TABLE 1.   Clinical Sequelae of Muscle Contractures

Contracture	Clinical Sequelae
Hip flexion	Lumbar lordosis, knee flexion, short steps
Knee flexion	Toe-walking, crouch gait
Ankle plantarflexion	Genu recurvatum, absence of heel strike
Shoulder internal rotation	Protracted shoulders, shoulder impingement
Elbow flexion	Only major joint where contracture of moderate severity minimally affects basic ADLs
Wrist flexion	Weakened power grip
Finger flexion	Difficulty in grasping large objects

- Contraindications to stretching: bony block, cartilage damage, loose body, joint incongruity, fracture, dislocation, cancer in bone.
  b. **Cartilage degeneration**
     i. Prolonged-contact surfaces develop pressure necrosis and erosions occur.
     ii. Noncontact surfaces develop fissures and lose smoothness.
  c. **Fibrofatty connective tissue infiltration**
  d. **Synovial atrophy**
  e. **Subchondral bone deterioration**
  f. **Fusion/ankylosis** in severe cases of extra-articular connective tissue contracture
  g. **Osteoarthritis** (controversial)
3. **Bones**
  a. **Cortical thinning at ligament insertion sites**
  b. **Osteoporosis**
     i. More significant in weight-bearing bones such as vertebral bodies, long bones of the legs, calcaneous, metacarpals.
     ii. Bone mineral density (BMD) in vertebral bones decreases by about 1% per week of bed rest.
     iii. If due to short-term (3–6 months) immobilization, osteoporosis may be reversible; if due to long-term sedentary lifestyle, it may not be reversible.
     iv. Causes: decreased weight-bearing (in animal models, bone loss plateaus at about 50% of original mass); postmenopausal hormonal changes.
     v. Signs and symptoms: asymptomatic until fracture occurs.
     vi. Diagnosed with dual-energy x-ray absorptiometry (DEXA).
     vii. World Health Organization criteria for diagnosis
        - Osteoporosis: BMD ≥ 2.5 standard deviations (SD) below average for 25-year-old woman.
        - Osteopenia: BMD = 1–2.5 SD below average for 25-year-old woman.
     viii. Prevention and treatment
        - Early weight-bearing to stimulate bone formation. Minimum amount of weight-bearing/force needed is unknown.
        - Isometric and isotonic bed exercises minimally affect bone loss.
        - Intranasal calcitonin (Miacalcin): 1 spray (200 IU)/day; alternate nostrils to decrease irritation.
        - Bisphosphonates: alendronate (Fosamax), 10 mg every morning orally; risedronate (Actonel), 5 mg every morning orally. Both drugs should be taken first thing in morning on empty stomach with full glass of water. Patients should sit upright for 30 minutes before taking food, beverage, or other medication to decrease risk of esophageal erosions.
        - Calcium carbonate: 1000 mg/day orally for premenopausal women; 1500 mg/day orally for postmenopausal women because of decreased GI absorption.
        - Adequate vitamin D intake or supplement, 400–800 IU/day.
        - In postmenopausal women, estrogen replacement or raloxifine (when safe) (Table 2).

TABLE 2. **Prevention and Treatment of Osteoporosis in Postmenopausal Women**

1. Conjugated estrogens: 0.625 mg once a day orally.
2. If uterus is intact: Prempro (estrogen, 0.625 mg once a day orally, and medroxyprogesterone, 2.5 mg once a day orally) or Premphase (estrogen, 0.625 mg once a day orally and medroxyprogesterone, 5 mg once a day orally) on days 14–28 in 28-day cycle.
3. Raloxifene (Evista): 60 mg once a day orally.

    4. **Tendons and ligaments**
        a. **Decreased tensile strength:** according to study by Noyes, primates may lose up to one-third of strength with 8 weeks of immobilization.
        b. **Increased collagen turnover**
        c. **Decreased collagen mass**
        d. **Histologic changes**
            i. Longitudinal stress to connective tissues fosters parallel alignment of collagen fibers.
            ii. With bed rest, newly formed collagen is laid down in haphazard arrangement.
F. **Metabolic and endocrine systems**
    1. **Body composition** (results of study by Krebs with 5 weeks of bed rest)
        a. Total body weight is not changed.
        b. Lean body mass decreases, and percentage of body fat increases.
        c. Appetite and water intake decrease.
        d. Energy absorption from food is unchanged.
    2. **Metabolic changes**
        a. Basal metabolic rate (BMR): some studies show unchanged BMR, some show decreased BMR.
        b. Body temperature is unchanged by bed rest alone.
        c. Nitrogen
            i. Urinary excretion increases starting 5 days after immobilization and parallels loss of muscle.
            ii. With exercise, excretion decreases below normal values, then normalizes by sixth week.
        d. Calcium
            i. Immobilization hypercalcemia: rarely seen with bed rest alone, but when it occurs, it is usually seen in adolescent males with trauma or spinal cord injury (see Chapter 8, Spinal Cord Injury Rehabilitation).
            ii. Urinary/fecal excretion increases and parallels loss of bone mass.
            iii. With exercise, calcium excretion also decreases below normal, with a trough at sixth week, then gradually normalizes.
    3. **Endocrine changes:** glucose tolerance decreases within 3 days of bed rest.
        a. Hospitalized diabetics may require more insulin than they normally use at home because of decreased activity; others may not change because of better diet control.
        b. Glucose intolerance may be ameliorated with both isotonic and isometric exercise. In a study by Fluckey, outpatients with insulin-dependent diabetes showed improved insulin response 18 hours after one exercise session. Therefore, on admission to rehabilitation unit, do not try to achieve tight sugar control, because the first few days of exercise may cause the patient to become hypoglycemic.

G. **Integumentary system** (see Chapter 18, Skin Care)
1. **Capillary blood pressure** = about 30 mmHg; higher pressures compromise blood flow to local tissue.
2. **Pressures while sitting and lying**
   a. Sitting: 150–500 mmHg over ischial tuberosities.
   b. Supine lying: 10–50 mmHg over sacrum; pressure is also increased over occiput and heels.
   c. Side lying: pressure increased over greater trochanters.
3. **Intrinsic factors predisposing to development of pressure sores**
   a. Abnormal skin sensation
   b. Abnormal mental status or decreased consciousness
   c. Advanced age
   d. Increased local tissue metabolic rate
   e. Previous pressure sore
   f. Muscle and skin atrophy
   g. Scars
   h. Edema
   i. Malnutrition
   j. Anemia
   k. Sedative medication
   l. Obesity
   m. Skin grafts
   n. Infection
4. **Extrinsic factors for developing pressure sores**
   a. Duration of pressure
   b. Direction of pressure
   c. Vertical pressure
   d. Shear force
   e. Moisture and skin maceration

H. **Gastrointestinal (GI) system**
1. **Constipation**
   a. Prevalence is 12% among elderly people in the community and 41% among hospitalized elderly.
   b. Risk increased by decreased GI motility due to decreased mobility and fluid intake.
   c. Certain medications can lead to constipation, including narcotics, aluminum hydroxide antacids, anticholinergics, and iron supplements.
   d. Hypercalcemia and hypothyroidism also increase risk.
   e. Signs and symptoms: abdominal pain, bloating, hard or infrequent stools (compared with patient's normal frequency).
   f. Diagnosis is based on clinical history and physical exam.
      i. Abdominal x-ray used to evaluate fecal impaction.
      ii. Endoscopy may be required for suspected tumor.
   g. Prevention and treatment
      i. Use toilet or bedside commode when possible instead of bed pan.
      ii. Encourage early mobilization.
      iii. Use high-fiber diet or fiber supplementation.
      iv. Ensure adequate fluid intake.
      v. Decrease constipating medications, such as narcotics.
      vi. Consider stool softeners: docusate sodium/Colace: 50 mg, 1 or 2 tablets daily or twice daily orally.
      vii. Consider senna/Senokot, 2 tablets once a day orally.
      ix. Enemas (if needed): tap-water enema, Fleet enema, or glycerin enema daily as needed.
      x. Laxatives (if needed): bicacodyl/Dulcolax, 10 mg rectal suppository as needed; lactulose, 15–30 ml once a day orally as needed; magnesium citrate, 150–300 ml once a day orally as needed; milk of magnesia, 30 ml twice a day orally as needed.

2. **Gastroesophageal reflux disease (GERD)**
   a. Causes: lying supine; may be aggravated by fatty foods, sweets, alcohol, peppermint, coffee, tea, anticholinergics, calcium channel blockers, and theophylline.
   b. Signs and symptoms: retrosternal burning sensation that radiates upward and worsens after large meals and with supine position.
   c. Diagnosis is based on clinical history. If myocardial ischemia is suspected, rule out myocardial infraction first.
   d. Prevention and treatment
      i. Elevate head of bed.
      ii. Use antacids: calcium carbonate, 500 mg orally every 22 hours as needed.
      iii. Consider H_2 blockers: famotidine (Pepcid), 20 mg twice a day orally; ranitidine (Zantac), 150 mg twice a day orally; nizatidine (Axid), 150 mg twice daily orally; or cimetidine (Tagamet), 400 mg twice daily orally.
      iv. Consider proton pump inhibitors: lansoprazole (Prevacid), 15–30 mg once-twice a day orally, or omeprazole (Prilosec), 20–40 mg once a day orally; esomeprazole (Nexium), 20–40 mg once-twice a day orally; rabeprazole (Aciphex), 20 mg once-twice a day orally.

I. **Genitourinary system**
   1. **Increased urination initially**, as noted in cardiovascular section.
   2. **Later, decreased urination/urinary stasis**, hypercalciuria, and hyperphosphaturia may increase the risk for calcium-containing renal stones.
   3. **Decreased spermatogenesis** in primates, but no proven effects on reproduction in humans.
   4. **Urinary incontinence**
      a. Prevalence among elderly is 5–15% in community and 40–50% in hospital.
      b. Causes: not direct physiologic effect of bed rest, but risk factors include:
         i. Immobility
         ii. Intravenous lines
         iii. Inability of staff to respond quickly enough
         iv. Medication effects
         v. Altered mental status
      c. Prevention and treatment
         i. Institute timed void program.
         ii. Use toilet/bedside commode instead of bed pan when possible.
         iii. Ensure proper fluid intake and avoid unnecessary medications that affect kidney and bladder functioning.
         iv. Maximize mental status.
         v. Institute intermittent catheterization program, if needed.
         vi. If neurogenic bladder is present, see Chapter 15, Neurogenic Bladder Management.

Bibliography
1. Amiel D, Akeson WH, Harwood FL, Mechanic GL: The effect of immobilization on the types of collagen synthesized in periarticular connective tissue. Connect Tissue Res 8:27–32, 1980.
2. Appell H: Muscular atrophy following immobilization. Sports Med 10:42–58, 1990.

3. Buschbacher RM, Porter CD. Deconditioning, conditioning, and the benefits of bed rest. In Braddom RL (ed): Physical Medicine and Rehabilitation, 2nd ed. Philadelphia, W.B. Saunders, 2000, pp 702–726.
4. Dietrick JE, Whedon GD, Shorr E: Effects of immobilization upon various metabolic and physiologic functions of normal men. Am J Med 4:3–36, 1948.
5. Fluckey JD, Hickey MS, Brambrink JK, et al: Effects of resistance exercise on glucose tolerance in normal and glucose-intolerant subjects. J Appl Physiol 77:1087–1092, 1994
6. Halar E: Complications of bedrest, inactivity and prolonged immobilization. In Stolov W (ed): Chronic Disease and Disability: Evaluation and Treatment.Seattle, ASUW Publishing, 1983, pp 41–49.
7. Halar EM, Bell KR. Immobility: Physiological and functional changes and effects of inactivity on body functions. In DeLisa JA, Gans BM (eds): Rehabilitation Medicine: Principles and Practice, 3rd ed. Philadelphia, Lippincott-Raven, 1998, pp 1015–1034.
8. Hilton J: On the Influence of Mechanical and Physiological Rest in the Treatment of Accidents and Surgical Diseases, and the Diagnostic Value of Pain. London, Bell & Daldy, 1863.
9. Houston ME, Bentzen H, Larsen H: Interrelationships between skeletal muscle adaptations and performance as studied by detraining and retraining. Acta Physiol Scand 105:163–170, 1979.
10. Krebs JM, Schneider VA, Evans H, et al: Energy absorption, lean body mass, and total body fat changes during 5 weeks of continuous bed rest. Aviat Space Environ Med 61:314–318, 1990.
11. Means KM: Rehabilitation of joint contractures. In Grabois M, Garrison SJ, Hart KA, Lehmkuhl LD (eds): Physical Medicine and Rehabilitation: The Complete Approach. New York, Blackwell Science, 2000, pp 859–870.
12. Mueller EA: Influence of training and of inactivity on muscle strength. Arch Phys Med Rehabil 51:449–462, 1970.
13. Noyes FR: Functional properties of knee ligaments and alterations induced by immobilization. Clin Orthop 123:210–242, 1977.
14. Saltin B, Blomquist g, Mitchell JH, et al: Response to exercise after bed rest and after training. A longitudinal study of adaptive changes in oxygen transport and body composition. Circulation 38(Suppl 7):VII1-VII78, 1968.
15. Shankar K, Jain S: Deconditioning and bed rest. In Grabois M, Garrison SJ, Hart KA, Lehmkuhl LD (eds): Physical Medicine and Rehabilitation: The Complete Approach. New York, Blackwell Science, 2000, pp 831–847.
16. Welch WH: Thrombosis. In Clifford AT (ed): A System of Medicine, Vol. 6. London, MacMillan & Co., 1899, pp 155–228.
17. Young JL: Scientific principles of sports medicine. Phys Med Rehabil Clin North Am 11(2): 251–305, 2000.

Chapter 13

DEEP VENOUS THROMBOSIS

Lisa A. DiPonio, M.D.

I. Risk Assessment

A. **Virchow's triad** for risk of deep venous thrombosis (DVT) includes venous stasis, hypercoagulability, and vessel wall damage.

1. Many rehabilitation inpatients have hemiplegia, paraplegia, or other causes of immobility and venous stasis.
2. Many patients had traumatic events causing widespread vessel wall damage.
3. Malignancies, dehydration, altered blood elements, increased platelet aggregation, and other conditions contribute to hypercoagulability.
4. Given these facts, you will be hard pressed to find a rehabilitation inpatient who is *not* at risk. Therefore, appropriate prophylaxis and clinical suspicion must be the rule rather than the exception.
5. Virchow did not describe immobility as the single risk factor for venous thrombosis. Therefore, mobility alone is not enough to justify withholding prophylaxis. You must assess the risk of each and every patient, mobile or not, and treat appropriately.

B. **Common risk factors**

1. **General:** malignancy, increased age, obesity, immobility (including bed rest, stroke, and paralysis), history of DVT, varicose veins, major surgery (especially abdominal or pelvic), central venous catheters, cardiac dysfunction, pregnancy or childbirth, estrogen treatment, and nephritic syndrome.
2. **Neurologic:** stroke, hemiparesis, spinal cord injury (SCI), and traumatic brain injury (TBI).
3. **Trauma:** notably lower extremity or pelvic fractures, but also including face, chest, and upper extremities.
4. **Orthopedic:** joint replacement surgery, fractures, and other procedures in the lower extremities.
5. **Hypercoagulable states:** pregnancy, estrogen replacement, paraneoplastic syndrome, inflammatory bowel disease, hyperhomocystinemia, antiphospholipid antibodies or lupus anticoagulant, and nonhemorrhagic myeloproliferative disorders (e.g., polycythemia vera).
6. **Inherited thrombophilia:** deficiency of antithrombin, protein C, protein S, plasminogen, or plasminogen activator; dysfibrinogenemia.
7. **Activated protein C resistance** (factor V Leiden mutation) carries greater risk for DVT and less risk for pulmonary embolism (PE).

C. **Risk stratification**

1. **Low risk:** age < 40 years, with history of minor trauma or surgery and no other clinical risk factors (ambulatory status, normal coagulability, no significant vessel wall damage). No specific prophylaxis recommended.

2. **Moderate risk:** > 40 years old, especially with history of moderate surgery, and no other clinical risk factors (ambulatory status, normal coagulability).
3. **High risk:** > 40 years old with history of major surgery and additional clinical risk factors (bed rest > 3 days).
4. **Very high risk:** > 40 years old with history of malignancy or major surgery, and high associative risk factors, such as stroke, hip or knee fractures, hip or knee replacement, spinal cord injury, history DVT, or age > 60.

II. Prophylaxis

A. Mechanical

1. **Graded elastic compression stockings** (GECS)
   a. Not sufficient for prophylaxis.
   b. Can reduce incidence of postphlebitic syndrome if applied correctly.
   c. Significant hand dexterity and strength are needed for correct application.
   d. Incorrect application can cause tourniquet effect.
2. **Sequential compression device** (SCD) or **intermittent pneumatic compression** (IPC)
   a. Studies have shown effectiveness in low-to-moderate risk patients for preventing DVT when applied correctly and left in place.
   b. Reducing venous stasis and enhancing fibrinolysis are the proposed mechanisms of action.
   c. Some argue that they are useful only when left in place > 23 hours/day, limiting their effectiveness in patients who take them off to attend therapy sessions.
   d. Theoretically, there is a risk of converting DVT into PE.
   e. Should be strongly considered when chemical prophylaxis is contraindicated.
3. **Inferior vena cava (IVC) filter** (e.g., Greenfield filter)
   a. Prophylaxis for PE, not DVT.
   b. Indications for filter include proximal DVT or PE in the setting of contraindication to anticoagulation and/or failure of anticoagulation.

B. Chemical

1. **Heparins**
   a. Low-dose unfractionated heparin (LDUH)
      i. Typical dosage is 5000 units subcutaneous (SQ) 2–3 times/day.
      ii. Binds to antithrombin III (AT III), effectively converting it from slow thrombin inhibitor into rapid inhibitor of both thrombin and factor Xa. Thrombin is approximately ten-fold more sensitive to inhibition by the heparin-thrombin complex than factor Xa.
   b. Adjusted-dose unfractionated heparin (ADUH)
      i. Initial dose: approximately 3500 units SQ every 8 hours.
      ii. Adjust upward or downward by increments of 500 units per dose to keep partial thromboplastin time (PTT) at high normal values.
   c. Low-molecular-weight heparins (LMWH)
      i. Differ from unfractionated heparin in that they are not bound to plasma proteins, endothelial cells, or macrophages. This difference contributes to longer half-life and consistent, predictable clearance.
      ii. No monitoring is required.
      iii. Adjust dose when creatinine is > 2.0.
      iv. PTT does not measure anticoagulant effect.

     v. Cost is 8–10 times that of unfractionated heparin.

     vi. Have more significant effect on factor Xa than thrombin (factor IIa) compared with unfractionated heparin.

     vii. Different LMWH formulations are classified by ratio of anti-Xa to anti-IIa activity (e.g., enoxaparin ratio is 4:1, whereas dalteparin ratio is 2:1).

   d. Danaparoid: low-molecular-weight heparinoid with anti-Xa to anti-IIa ration of 28:1.

  2. **Warfarin**

   a. Clinically viewed as highly effective despite lack of good evidence.

   b. Limited usefulness due to late onset of effectiveness and need for invasive monitoring.

   c. International normalized ratio (INR) of 2–3 is recommended, although ongoing research may reveal INR < 2.0 to be effective for DVT prophylaxis.

  3. **Aspirin:** not recommended for DVT prophylaxis because of more effective alternatives.

  4. **Persantine:** no role in DVT prophylaxis.

C. **Contraindications to chemical prophylaxis**

  1. Spinal puncture or epidural anesthesia. Use caution in following situations:

   a. Epidural catheter placement, removal, or lumbar puncture should be done at least 12 hours after dosing LDUH or LMWH, not with oral anticoagulants or antiplatelet agents, and heparinoid agents should be withheld for at least 2 hours afterward.

   b. LDUH or LMWH should be avoided with traumatic ("bloody") tap.

  2. Intracranial hemorrhage (ICH) or severe head trauma within preceding 4 weeks or increased risk of ICH for any other reason.

  3. Thrombocytopenia

  4. Coagulopathy

  5. Active hemorrhage from wounds or surgical drains

  6. Heparin contraindicated in heparin-induced thrombocytopenia

  7. Warfarin contraindicated in pregnancy

  8. Recent craniotomy (preceding 4 weeks)

  9. Retroperitoneal bleeding

  10. History of severe gastrointestinal bleeding

  11. Contraindicated by clinical judgement

D. **Duration of prophylaxis**

  1. Not many data support any particular length of treatment or end-point after which withholding prophylaxis is considered safe.

  2. Patients may still be at high risk even if they are walking 100 feet/day.

  3. Some studies suggest that DVT risk after major surgery persists for 4–5 weeks; others recommend at least 7–10 days of prophylaxis. Debate probably will increase in coming years.

  4. It is reasonable to consider prophylaxis for duration of inpatient rehabilitation in moderate-risk patients; in high-risk patients, consider extending prophylaxis beyond discharge.

III. **Recommendations for Prevention in Specific Conditions**

A. **General surgery**

  1. **Low risk**

   a. Definition: minor procedure, < 40 years of age, no additional risk factors.

   b. Recommendation: no specific treatment other than early ambulation.

2. **Moderate risk**
   a. Definitions
      i. Minor procedures with additional risk factors.
      ii. Age 40–60 with no additional risk factors.
      iii. Age < 40, no other risk factors, major procedures.
   b. Recommendation
      i. LDUH, 5000 U SQ every 8–12 hr, *or*
      ii. LWMH
         • Dalteparin, 2500 U SQ 1–2 hr before surgery and once daily post-operatively, *or*
         • Enoxaparin, 20 mg SQ 1–2 hr before surgery and once daily post-operatively, *or*
         • Nadroparin, 2850 U SQ 2–4 hr before surgery and once daily postoperatively, *or*
         • Tinzaparin, 3500 U SQ 2 hr before surgery and once daily postoperatively, *and*
      vii. IPC
3. **High risk**
   a. Definitions
      i. Age 40–60, major procedures.
      ii. Age > 60 without additional risk factors, nonmajor surgery.
   b. Recommendation
      i. LDUH, 5000 U SQ every 8–12 hr, *or*
      ii. LMWH
         • Dalteparin, 5000 U SQ 8–12 hr before surgery and daily, starting 12–24 hours postoperatively, *or*
         • Danaparoid, 750 U SQ 1–4 hr before surgery and every 12 hr postoperatively, *or*
         • Enoxaparin, 40 mg SQ 1–2 hr before surgery and daily postoperatively, *or*
         • Enoxaparin, 30 mg SQ every 12 hr, starting 8–12 hr postoperatively, *and*
      vii. IPC
      viii. In high-risk patients with greater than usual risk of bleeding, use IPC and GECS.
4. **Very high risk**
   a. Definition: multiple risk factors.
   b. Recommendation: pharmacologic agents (as in high-risk patients) combined with mechanical agents (IPC and GECS).
B. **Orthopedic surgery**
   1. **General recommendations**
      a. Optimal duration of prophylaxis is uncertain, but at least 7–10 days is recommended and longer in high-risk patients.
      b. Routine duplex screening before discharge in asymptomatic patients is not recommended.
   2. **General suggested dosing of LMWH** (see below for optimal timing in specific conditions)
      a. Dalteparin, 5000 U SQ every 8–12 hr preoperatively and daily, starting 12–24 hr postoperatively.
      b. Dalteparin, 2500 U SQ 6–8 hr postoperatively; then 5000 U/day SQ.

    c. Danaparoid, 750 U SQ 1–4 hr preoperatively and every 12 hr postoperatively.

    d. Enoxaparin, 30 mg SQ every 12 hr, starting 12–24 hr postoperatively.

    e. Enoxaparin, 40 mg/day SQ, starting 12–24 hr postoperatively.

    f. Nadroparin, 38 U/kg SQ 12 hr preoperatively, 12 hr postoperatively, and daily on postoperative days 1, 2, and 3; then increase to 57 U/kg/day SQ.

    g. Tinzaparin, 75 U/kg/day SQ, starting 12–24 hr postoperatively.

    h. Tinzaparin, 4500 U SQ 12 hr preoperatively and daily postoperatively.

3. **Elective total hip arthroplasty**

    a. LMWH started 12 hr before surgery and 12–24 hours after surgery (half dose at 4–6 hr after surgery, then continue at regular dose in very-high-risk patients).

    b. ADUH is an acceptable alternative.

    c. GECS or IPC may provide additional benefit.

    d. LDUH is *not* recommended.

4. **Elective total knee arthroplasty**

    a. LMWH or adjusted-dose warfarin (INR range: 2–3).

    b. IPC may provide additional benefit.

    c. LDUH is *not* recommended.

5. **Surgical repair of hip fracture**

    a. LMWH or adjusted-dose warfarin.

    b. LDUH is an alternative.

    c. Aspirin alone is not recommended.

C. **Neurologic/neurosurgical conditions**

1. **Neurosurgical patients**

    a. IPC with or without GECS is highly recommended for patients undergoing intracranial surgery.

    b. Postoperatively, LDUH or LMWH is acceptable alternative when weighed against the risk of intracranial hemorrhage.

    c. Concomitant mechanical and pharmacologic interventions are recommended in high-risk patients.

2. **Ischemic cerebrovascular accident**

    a. Routine use of LDUH, LMWH, or danaparoid is recommended.

    b. Mechanical prophylaxis recommended if anticoagulation is contraindicated.

D. **Trauma**

1. Patients with multiple trauma and identifiable risk factor: LMWH as soon as safety allows, within 36 hours of the injury.

2. Recommendation: enoxaparin, 30 mg SC twice daily, starting 12–36 hr after injury in hemodynamically stable patient.

3. When early LMWH prophylaxis is contraindicated, start mechanical prophylaxis as soon as possible.

4. When LMWH has been withheld during the 36 hours after injury, consider duplex ultrasound screening.

5. Consider IVC filter when proximal DVT is demonstrated and anticoagulation is contraindicated, not as primary prophylaxis.

6. **Contraindications to anticoagulation** include intracranial hemorrhage, perispinal hematoma with incomplete spinal cord injury, ongoing and/or uncontrolled bleeding, and uncorrected coagulopathy.

E. **Acute spinal cord injury**
1. Recommendation: LMWH
   a. Enoxaparin, 30 mg SQ twice daily
   b. Duration: 8 weeks for uncomplicated motor complete injuries and 12 weeks for motor complete and other risk factors.
   c. LDUH, GECS, and IPC are relatively ineffective when used alone.
   d. GECS and IPC may have added benefit in combination with heparin or if early anticoagulation is contraindicated.
   e. Continue anticoagulation with LMWH or oral anticoagulation during rehabilitation phase.

F. **General medical procedures**
1. Use criteria similar to general surgery.
2. Recommendation: LDUH, 5000 U SQ every 8–12 hr, or LMWH when risk factors are present.
3. Recommended LMWH dosing
   a. Dalteparin, 2500 U/day SQ
   b. Danaparoid, 750 U SQ every 12 hr
   c. Enoxaparin, 40 mg/day SQ
   d. Nadroparin, 2850 U/day SQ

IV. Diagnosis of Acute DVT

A. Diagnosis is challenging because most cases of DVT are asymptomatic. A **high index of suspicion** is essential.

B. **Physical examination**
1. Neither sensitive nor specific.
2. **Most cases of DVTs**, especially proximal ones, are **clinically silent**. Normal physical exam alone does not justify withholding prophylaxis.
3. **Possible findings**
   a. Unilateral lower extremity edema or erythema.
   b. Fever of unknown source.
   c. Asymmetry of calf circumference measured 10 cm below inferior patellar pole.
   d. Homan's sign: pain with passive ankle dorsiflexion (not highly accurate).
   e. Palpable cord in calf or popliteal fossa.
   f. Tachypnea, tachycardia, and shortness of breath may be presenting signs if PE has occurred.

C. **Venous ultrasound**
1. Although not considered a gold standard, it is the standard of care at many institutions.
2. Noninvasive and relatively inexpensive.
3. Sensitivity is reduced in cases of asymptomatic DVT.
4. Results are technician-dependent.

D. **Venography**
1. Once considered the gold standard of diagnosis.
2. Associated with significant rate of nondiagnostic studies. and many of the thrombi detected are of questionable clinical significance.
3. Invasive and expensive; also involves dye load, which is a potential risk.

E. **Magnetic resonance imaging** (MRI)
1. Sensitivity: about 90%; specificity: approximately 97%.
2. Seldom used routinely because of cost.

F. **Radioiodine [^{125}I]-labeled fibrinogen uptake test**
   1. No longer used in U.S.
   2. Lacks sensitivity and specificity (10–30% false-positive rate).
G. **Plethysmography**
   1. Detects differences in limb volume due to venous obstruction.
   2. Has low specificity in the setting of other causes of lower extremity edema, such as congestive heart failure, postoperative edema, or pregnancy.

V. **Treatment of Acute DVT**
   A. **Activity**
      1. After diagnosis, 48 hours of relative inactivity with therapeutic anticoagulation is generally accepted.
      2. Recent studies, however, found no difference in rate of PE when patients were randomized to early ambulation or immobilization.
   B. **Drugs**
      1. **UFH**
         a. Start with unfractionated heparin bolus of 5000 U, continue drip at 1000 U/hr.
         b. Alternatively, start with bolus of 80 U/kg and continue drip at 18 U/kg/hr.
         c. PTT must be checked at least every 6 hours while patient is taking heparin and adjusted according to normogram:
            i. PTT < 35: rebolus with 80 U/kg, increase drip by 4 U/kg/hr.
            ii. PTT 35–45: rebolus with 40 U/kg, increase drip by 2 U/kg/hr.
            iii. PTT 46–70: no action needed.
            iv. PTT 71–90: reduce drip by 2 U/kg/hr.
            v. PTT > 90: hold drip for 1 hr, decrease drip by 3 U/kg/hr.
      2. **LMWH**
         a. Enoxaparin, 1mg/kg SQ twice daily or 1.5 mg/kg/day SQ.
         b. Dalteparin, 200 U/kg/day SQ.
         c. Nadroparin calcium, 86 anti-Xa U/kg twice daily for 10 days or 171 anti-Xa U/kg/day SQ.
         d. Tinzaparin sodium, 175 anti-Xa U/kg/day SQ.
      3. **Warfarin:** once heparin is at therapeutic level, titrate dose to keep INR between 2 and 3 with target of 2.5 for duration of 3–6 months. Many clinicians believe that 6-month treatment is superior.
      4. **Others**
         a. Hirudins
            i. Inhibit thrombin independently of antithrombin (AT).
            ii. Theoretically inhibit fibrin deposition in interstices of developing thrombus better than larger heparin-AT complex.
            iii. Agents include lepirudin and argatroban. Initial studies appear promising.
         b. Danaparoid: LMWH with high anti-Xa/IIa ratio (28:1).

VI. **Complications of Anticoagulation Therapy**
   A. **Hemorrhage: risk factors**
      1. Higher intensity of anticoagulation effect is most important risk factor.
         a. Therapeutic dosing carries higher risk than low-dose prophylactic use.
         b. Risk of intracranial hemorrhage increases dramatically with INR > 4.0, regardless of indication for therapy.
      2. Past GI bleeding, especially during warfarin therapy.

3. Peptic ulcer disease alone, without history of bleeding, has not been associated with higher risk of bleeding during anticoagulation therapy.
4. Comorbid diseases associated with bleeding during warfarin therapy are malignancy, renal insufficiency, treated hypertension, and cerebrovascular disease.
5. Age > 75 years.
6. Concomitant use of aspirin.
7. Prolonged period of anticoagulation therapy.

B. **Heparin-induced thrombocytopenia** (HIT)
1. Caused by antibody formation to heparin.
2. Should be suspected in patients with otherwise unexplained drop in platelet count > 50% or skin rash at injection site.
3. Usually a complication of UFH; theoretically *not* a risk with very-low-molecular-weight heparin (reviparin) and less of a risk with other LMWHs.
4. Diagnosed clinically and serologically by activation assays and antigen assays to detect HIT antibodies.
5. Treatment: prophylactic platelet transfusions not recommended.
6. Heparin and LMWH contraindicated in patients with existing HIT.
7. If HIT is associated with thrombosis or DVT, treatment with danaparoid, lepirudin, or argatroban is recommended until adequate anticoagulation is achieved with platelet count >100,000, followed by warfarin.

C. **UFH overdose or need for reversal**
1. Give IV protamine in ratio of 1 mg per 100 units UFH (e.g., 10 mg reverses 1000 mg bolus of heparin).
2. Since half-life of heparin is about 1 hour, only amount infused intravenously over proceeding 2–3 hours needs to be reversed.
3. Infuse protamine over 1–3 minutes to avoid hypotension and bradycardia.
4. Allergic reactions to protamine are rare but possible in patients with exposure to Hagedorn insulin, vasectomy, or hypersensitivity to fish.

D. **LMWH overdose or need for reversal**
1. Protamine preferentially reverses anti-IIa (thrombin) activity of LWMH, with incomplete reversal of factor Xa inhibition.
2. Dose depends on specific LMWH; check product labeling. For enoxaparin, give 1 mg protamine for each 1 mg of enoxaparin given in the previous 8 hours.
3. Be aware of risk of allergy to protamine (see 4 above).

E. **Warfarin overdose or need for reversal:** give vitamin K (phytonadione), 10 mg SQ injection, or fresh frozen plasma.

Bibliography
1. Aschwanden M, Labs KH, Engel H, et al: Acute deep vein thrombosis: Early mobilization does not increase the frequency of pulmonary embolism. Thromb Haemost 85:42–46, 2001.
2. Bounameaux H: Factor V Leiden paradox: Risk of deep-vein thrombosis but not of pulmonary embolism [commentary]. Lancet 356:182–183, 2000.
3. Brandjes DP, Buller HR, Heijboer H, et al: Randomised trial of effect of compression stockings in patients with symptomatic proximal-vein thrombosis [see comments]. Lancet 349:759–762, 1997.
4. Consortium for Spinal Cord Medicine: Clinical Practice Guidelines: Prevention of thromboembolism in spinal cord injury. Washington, DC: Paralyzed Veterans of America, 1999.
5. Comerota AJ, Chouhan V, Harada RN, et al: The fibrinolytic effects of intermittent pneumatic compression: Mechanism of enhanced fibrinolysis. Ann Surg 226:306–313; discussion, 313-314, 1997.

6. Gans BM: Rehabilitation care settings and deep vein thrombosis. Am J Phys Med Rehabil 79(Suppl):S1–S2, 2000.
7. Geerts WH, Heit JA, et al: Prevention of venous thromboembolism. Chest 119:132S–175S, 2001.
8. Greenfield LJ, Proctor MC: Recurrent thromboembolism in patients with vena cava filters. J Vasc Surg 33:510–514, 2001.
9. Hirsh J, Dalen JE, et al: Oral anticoagulants: Mechanism of action, clinical effectiveness, and optimal therapeutic range. Chest 119:8S–21 S, 2001.
10. Hirsh J, Dalen J, Guyatt G: The sixth (2000) ACCP guidelines for antithrombotic therapy for prevention and treatment of thrombosis. Am Coll Chest Physicians Chest 119:1S–2S, 2001.
11; Hirsh J, Warkentim TE, et al: Heparin and low-molecular-weight heparin: Mechanisms of action, pharmcokinetics, dosing, monitoring, efficacy, and safety. Chest 119:64S–94S, 2001.
12. Levine MN, Raskob G, et al: Hemorrhagic complications of anticoagulant treatment. Chest 119:108S–S121, 2001.
13. Merli GJ: Low-molecular-weight heparins versus unfractionated heparin in the treatment of deep vein thrombosis and pulmonary embolism [review]. Am J Phys Med Rehabil 79(Suppl 5):S9–S16, 2000.
14. Landefeld CS, Goldman L: Major bleeding in outpatients treated with warfarin: Incidence and prediction by factors known at the start of outpatient therapy. Am J Med 87:153–155, 1989.
15. Nelson PH, Moser KM, Stoner C, Moser KS: Risk of complications during intravenous heparin therapy. West J Med 136(3):189–197, 1982.
16. Trowbridge A, Boese CK, Woodruff B, et al: Incidence of posthospitalization proximal deep venous thrombosis after total hip arthroplasty: A pilot study. Clin Orthop 299:203–208 1994.
17. Wells PS, Lensing AW, Davidson BL, et al: Accuracy of ultrasound for the diagnosis of deep venous thrombosis in asymptomatic patients after orthopedic surgery. A meta-analysis. Ann Intern Med 122:47–53, 1995.
18. Weitz JI, Hudoba M, Massel D, et al: Clot-bound thrombin is protected from inhibition by heparin-antithrombin III but is susceptible to inactivation by antithrombin III-independent inhibitors. J Clin Invest 86:385–391, 1990.

Chapter 14

HETEROTOPIC OSSIFICATION

Andrew R. Briggeman, D.O., and Anita S. Craig, D.O

I. **General Principles**
   A. Heterotopic ossification (HO) is frequently overlooked and misdiagnosed in inpatient rehabilitation units
   B. HO is defined as the formation of new osseous material in tissues where bone formation does not usually occur.
      1. Bone is trabecular, may be unilateral or bilateral, and forms in periarticular tissue usually within the planes of surrounding soft tissue layers.
      2. Bone can cause significant loss of range of joint motion. Marked loss of function may occur if HO is not diagnosed early and treated properly or prophylactically.

II. **Epidemiology**
   A. Ossification of soft tissues near and around joint regions occurs most commonly after spinal cord injury, traumatic brain injuries, burns, general trauma, total joint surgeries, and occasionally in pediatric amputation patients.
   B. Although each condition has different rates of occurrence, associated risk factors, and comorbidities, all are similar in that homeostasis within certain periarticular tissues is unexplainedly disrupted and acute/chronic bone formation begins to occur.
   C. **Specific conditions**
      1. **Spinal cord injury** (SCI)
         a. Incidence of 15–40%, with severe functional impairment in 8–12%.
         b. Most common at hip, followed by knees.
         c. Increased incidence if SCI is complete, secondary to trauma, and associated with tetraplegia.
         d. Usually worse on side with more significantly abnormal tone (whether it be flaccidity or spasticity) and generally occurs below level of lesion.
         e. Peak incidence occurs at approximately 8–12 weeks after injury; HO can develop as early as 18 days and as late as 1 year after injury.
      2. **Traumatic brain injury** (TBI)
         a. Incidence of 10–20%.
         b. Most common at hips, followed by elbows and shoulder.
         c. Incidence correlates with extent and severity of neurologic injury and residual deficits, specifically with presence of increased tone in involved extremity, fractures, joint injury, immobilization, and prolonged coma (usually > 2 weeks).
         d. Peak occurrence around 4–12 weeks.
      3. **Burns**
         a. Incidence ranges from 0.1% to 35%.

  b. Most common at elbows, followed by shoulder (adults) and hip (children).
  c. Development associated more commonly with full-thickness burns, burns affecting > 20% total body surface area, immobility, repeated minor trauma/pressure to involved areas, and wounds that are left open for prolonged periods.
  d. Site of ossification does not necessarily coincide with location of burn.
  e. Average occurrence is 8–12 weeks after burn.
 4. **Trauma/surgery**
  a. Incidence differs with types of injury: general fractures, 15–20%; acetabular fracture, 30–50% after open reduction-internal fixation (ORIF); elbow dislocation, 3%.
  b. Also common after total hip arthroplasty, direct muscle trauma, posterior spinal fusion, forcible stretching, organ transplantation in patients with encephalopathy (after prolonged use of wrist restraints), and pediatric amputation (distal end of amputated bone).
 5. **Amputation**
  a. Found at ends of the long amputated long bones with tenderness, warmth, and erythema.
  b. Most commonly affects humerus, fibula, tibia, and femur.
 6. **Other:** encephalitis, meningitis, myelitis, tetanus, tumors, HELLP syndrome (**h**emolysis, **e**levated **l**iver enzymes, **l**ow **p**latelet count), stroke, polio, tabes dorsalis, multiple sclerosis, and epidural abscesses.
III. Etiology
 A. Unclear; thought to result from disruption of homeostasis due to neurologic injury, trauma, burns, surgery, infection, and presence of inducing agents (bone morphogenic protein, osteogenin, and prostaglandins).
 B. Disruption of homeostasis leads to proliferation of noncirculatory pluripotent mesenchymal cells to form chondroblasts and osteoblasts and subsequent formation of bony material in areas permissive to osteogenesis (muscle and fascia, healthy periarticular soft tissue, damaged periosteum and soft tissue).
 C. Some researchers believe that forcible manipulation of joints causes formation of localized hematomas, which are potential areas for beginning of ossification.
 D. Other documented predisposing factors include male gender, comorbidities (spasticity, pressure ulcers, fractures, decreased preoperative hip motion), history of HO or preexisting HO, large osteophyte formation in affected joints, increased age, genetics (alleles HLA B18, B27, DW7), and history of surgical soft tissue releases.
IV. Clinical Presentation
 A. **Signs and symptoms**
  1. Hallmark feature of early HO: loss of range of motion (ROM) or stiffness in affected area.
  2. Pain with ROM and palpation.
  3. Swelling, heat, and warmth at affected area.
  4. Inflammatory signs subside and localized edema becomes more indurated after acute phase (7–10 days); then palpable mass forms and further limits ROM.
  5. During later stages (weeks to months later), edema may be noted distal to lesion secondary to venous compression.
  6. Preexisting spasticity may increase in affected limbs.

B. **Associated complications**
1. Severe limitation of joint motion or joint ankylosis
2. Pressure ulcers near affected areas
3. Neurovascular compression/peripheral nerve entrapment
4. Deep venous thrombosis (DVT) from narrowing of veins in affected area
5. Spasticity

V. **Diagnosis**

A. **Differential diagnosis**

1. Thrombophlebitis
2. Cellulitis
3. Osteomyelitis
4. Septic arthritis
5. Complex regional pain syndrome
6. Impending pressure ulcer
7. Local trauma with hemarthrosis or fracture

B. **Rule out emergent causes**
1. In most cases, ultrasound can accurately rule out DVT.
2. Joint aspiration must be performed to rule out septic arthritis.
3. Clinical exam, complete blood count, erythrocyte sedimentation rate, blood/tissue cultures, and nuclear and radiographic studies help eliminate or confirm majority of more acutely threatening diagnoses.

C. **Radiographs**
1. Show hazy, shell-like appearance at lesion site similar to what an immature callus looks like on plain films of healing fractures.
2. May detect HO as early as 3 weeks after injury, although usually they are not confirmatory until 2 months after injury; also may show lesion 7–10 days after clinical symptoms arise.
3. Good for locating and grading lesion, checking response to treatment, and serially evaluating for maturation of HO; used in combination with serum alkaline phosphatase levels and physical examination.

D. **Triple-phase bone scan** (^{99m}technetium-methylene diphosphonate)
1. Phases I and II (indicative of hyperemia and blood pooling) are most sensitive for detection of early HO.
2. 90% sensitive 2–4 weeks after injury; may precede x-ray findings by 3 weeks.
3. Can be used serially to assess maturity of HO; uptake eventually decreases or plateaus with HO maturity.

E. **Computed tomography (CT)/magnetic resonance imaging (MRI)**
1. Primarily used by surgical specialists for preoperative localization of HO and its relationship to muscles, nerves, and vessels before resection.
2. MRI is better than CT for soft tissue discrimination.

F. **Laboratory evaluation**
1. **Serum alkaline phosphatase**
   a. Usually begins to elevate with increasing HO activity but does not correlate with severity of lesion.
   b. Usually elevates after 3 weeks and stays above normal for average of 5 months.
   c. Always precedes radiographic findings and is used for diagnosis and assessment of HO activity, progression toward maturity, and response to treatments in conjunction with other studies.
   d. Also may be elevated in presence of fractures and hepatic disease, among other conditions.
2. **Serum calcium:** usually decreases below normal during first week and returns to normal at 3 weeks after injury.

VI. Treatment
A. Nonsteroidal anti-inflammatory drugs (NSAIDs)
1. Suppress prostaglandin-mediated inflammation along with mesenchymal cell differentiation into osteogenic cells.
2. Examples include indomethacin, aspirin, ibuprofen, and naproxen.
   a. Indomethacin, 25 mg orally 3 times/day, is commonly used for at least 4–6 weeks (along with disodium etidronate) for indications above. Indomethacin has most support in literature.
   b. Ibuprofen, 300–400 mg orally 3 time/day.
   c. Aspirin, 650 mg orally 3 times/day.
B. Diphosphonates
1. Inhibit growth of calcified hydroxyapatite crystals.
2. Disodium etidronate, 20 mg/kg/day for 2 weeks, followed by 10 mg/kg/day for 10 weeks or 20 mg/kg/day for 6 months, provides treatment/prophylaxis in TBI, SCI, burn, trauma, and occasionally surgical patients (total hip arthroplasty, acetabular repair).
C. Radiotherapy
1. Prevents cell proliferation by altering DNA in rapidly producing cells.
2. Usually performed as prophylaxis in high-risk patients within 48–72 hours after total hip arthroplasty, acetabular ORIF, and other complicated joint surgeries.
3. Used prophylactically in conjunction with NSAIDs in above patients.
4. Occasionally used for prevention in patients with SCI as well.
D. Physical therapy
1. Therapies should consist of either immobilization in functional position or gentle active-assisted ROM exercises, especially during acute inflammatory phase; they generally help to prevent ankylosis and promote better overall function.
2. Gentle active-assisted ROM within pain-free range is essential in preventing ankylosis and significant loss of function in all patients with HO, whether they be trauma, burn, SCI, TBI, postsurgical, or even postossification resection (72 hours after procedure).
3. Manipulation under general anesthesia typically has been reserved for patients with TBI and is done a maximum of 3 times, at least 1–2 months apart.
E. Surgical resection
1. Usually wedge resection is delayed until osseous lesion has matured.
2. Maturity is determined by serial x-rays/bone scans (lack of progression/activity), serum alkaline phosphatase levels (return to normal range); typically occurs 6 months after trauma, 1 year after SCI, and 12–18 months after TBI.
VII. Prognosis
A. Significant loss of function occurs in approximately 8–12% of patients diagnosed with HO.
B. Patients do not benefit from surgical resection if it is delayed for too long (usually > 2 years after onset).
C. If HO is diagnosed early and proper therapies and procedures are managed in a timely fashion, patients tend to have fewer long-term residual deficits and less reoccurrence.
D. Poor prognosis is associated with poor neurologic recovery, persistent spasticity, premorbid decreased joint ROM, and prolonged elevation of serum alkaline phosphatase levels (1–2 years after injury).

Bilbiography

1. DeLisa J: Rehabilitation Medicine: Principles and Practice. Philadelphia, J.B. Lippincott, 2000.
2. Ellerin BE, Helfet D, Parikh S, et al: Current therapy in the management of heterotopic ossification of the elbow: A review of case studies. Am J Phys Med Rehabil 78:259–271, 1999.
3. Freebourn TM, Barber DB, Able AC: The treatment of immature heterotopic ossification in spinal cord injury with combination surgery, radiation therapy, and NSAID. Spinal Cord 3:50–53, 1999.
4. Garland D: A clinical perspective on common forms of acquired heterotopic ossification. Clin Orthop 263:13–25, 1991.
5. Lal S, Hamilton B, Heinemann A, Betts H: Risk factors for heterotopic ossification in spinal cord injury. Arch Phys Med Rehabil 70:387–389, 1989.
6. Peterson S, Mani M, Crawford C, et al: Postburn heterotopic ossification: Insights for management decision making. J Trauma 29:365–369, 1989.
7. Subbarao J, Garrison S: Heterotopic ossification: Diagnosis and management, current concepts and controversies. J Spinal Cord Med 22:272–283, 1999.
8. Wittenberg RH, Peschke U, Botel U: Heterotopic ossification after spinal cord injury: Epidemiology and risk factors. J Bone Joint Surg 74B:215–218, 1992.

Chapter 15

NEUROGENIC BLADDER MANAGEMENT

Ann T. Laidlaw, M.D., and Anthony Chiodo, M.D.

I. General Principles

A. Voiding dysfunction is a common problem in rehabilitation patients.

B. Dysfunction may result from medications, cognitive changes, physical impairments, and neurologic etiologies.

C. Recognizing the problems, understanding the etiology, and prescribing appropriate treatment should be the focus of the rehabilitation specialist.

D. **Anatomy**

1. **Fundus**

a. Detrusor muscle: smooth muscle composing the walls of the bladder; expands freely up to 300–500 ml.

b. Transitional epithelium: mucosal lining; allows considerable stretching with bladder filling.

2. **Trigone**

a. Triangular area at base of bladder.

b. Defined by entrance of ureters superiorly and urethra inferiorly.

c. Acts as funnel during micturition.

d. Relatively unexpandable.

3. **Uretovescicular junction:** oblique penetration of ureters through detrusor muscle within trigone prevents reflux of urine.

4. **Urethra**

a. **Male**

i. Preprostatic (smooth muscle, prevents retrograde ejaculation; "internal sphincter")

ii. Prostatic

iii. Membranous (external sphincter composed of striated muscle, pelvic floor)

iv. Penile (spongy, cavernous)

b. **Female**

i. Approximately 4 cm in length

ii. Incomplete external sphincter

iii. Continence maintained primarily by pelvic floor, which acts as sling and helps with "stress."

E. **Innervation**

1. **Supraspinal**

a. Frontal cortex provides volitional control (inhibitory influence on sacral micturition center).

b. Pontine micturation center acts as coordination center.

    c. Additional connections via impulses through pontine micturition center or directly to sacral segments.

i. Medial frontal lobe	iv. Hypothalamus
ii. Corpus callosum	v. Basal ganglia
iii. Limbic system	vi. Cerebellum

  2. **Sacral micturition center** (responsible for detrusor contraction)

  3. **Peripheral pathways** (Figs. 1 and 2)

    a. **Sympathetic:** T10–L2 via hypogastric nerve

      i. Alpha-adrenergic
- Supplies bladder neck (internal sphincter).
- Stimulation causes contraction of bladder neck (promotes urinary continence and prevents retrograde ejaculation).

      ii. Beta-adrenergic
- Supplies detrusor (fundus) of bladder.
- Stimulation inhibits detrusor contraction and thereby assists in urine storage.

    b. **Parasympathetic:** S2–S4 via pelvic (inferior splanchnic) nerve

      i. Supplies detrusor (fundus) of bladder.

      ii. Stimulation facilitates detrusor contraction and voiding.

    c. **Somatic:** S2–S4 via pudendal nerve; innervates external urethral sphincter (striated muscle).

II. Normal Micturition

  A. **Functions of the bladder**

    1. Storage of urine

    2. Emptying of urine

  B. **Voiding requirements**

    1. Peripheral nervous system

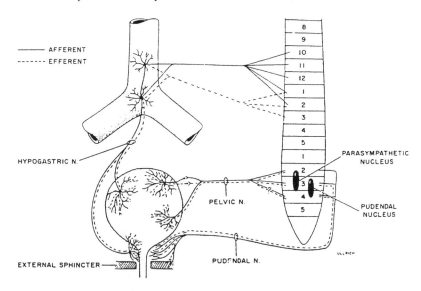

FIGURE 1. The parasympathetic, sympathetic, and somatic nerve supply to the bladder, urethra, and pelvic floor. (From Blaivas JG: Management of bladder dysfunction in multiple sclerosis. Neurology 30(2):12–18, 1980, with permission.)

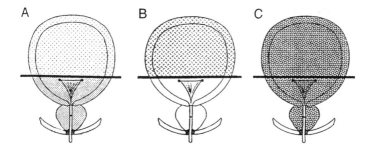

FIGURE 2.   *A,* Distribution of the alpha-adrenergic receptors, with few in the dome of the bladder and more in the base of the bladder and prostate. *B,* Distribution of the beta receptors, which are largely in the dome. *C,* Distribution of the cholinergic receptors, which are widely distributed throughout the dome and the base of the bladder and the urethra. (From Cardenas DD, Mayo ME: Management of bladder dysfunction. In Grabois M, et al (eds): Physical Medicine and Rehabilitation: The Complete Approach. Malden, MA, Blackwell Science, 2000, with permission.)

    2. Sacral micturition center
    3. Pontine micturition center
    4. Cerebral cortex
  C. **Filling phase (storage)**
    1. **High compliance** allows bladder to accommodate to increasing volume without increasing intravesical pressure.
      a. Compliance is due to viscoelastic properties of bladder wall and intact beta-adrenergic sympathetic innervation.
      b. Compliance is reduced by fibrotic change secondary to chronic infection and/or neurologic lesion.
      c. Reduced compliance leads to increased pressures during filling.
    2. **Cerebral cortex** allows bladder storage by suppressing parasympathetic sacral micturation center.
    3. **Holding reflex:** reflexive contraction of external urethral sphincter to prevent urine leakage during vigorous sudden activity (e.g., jumping, coughing).
    4. **Guarding reflex:** external sphincter contraction reflexively relaxes detrusor.
    5. **Sensation of filling** at 100 ml.
    6. **Sensation of fullness** sensed by brain (frontoparietal cortex) at 300–400 ml.
      a. Sensation can be depressed, resulting in inhibiton of micturition, *or*
      b. Voiding can be initiated voluntarily.
  D. **Voiding phase**
    1. **Detrusor-sphincter synergia**
      a. Voluntary relaxation of external urethral sphincter and pelvic floor.
      b. Followed by detrusor muscle contraction → urine expelled.
      c. Pontine micturation center coordinates relaxation and contraction.
    2. **Detrusor contraction**
      a. Results from increased sacral parasympathetic outflow to bladder via pelvic nerve.
      b. Decreased sympathetic outflow to detrusor allows relaxation and "funneling" of bladder neck and proximal urethra.

III. Abnormal Voiding
  A. **Anatomic classification**
    1. **Supraspinal lesion**
       a. Located above pons (i.e., head injury, stroke, brain tumor, multiple sclerosis).
       b. Characteristics
          i. Detrusor hyperreflexia: low capacity bladder with involuntary contractions due to lack of inhibition by cerebral cortex on sacral (parasympathetic) micturition center.
          ii. Sensation often absent.
          iii. High intravesicular pressure with hypertrophy.
          iv. No sphincter dyssynergia because pontine micturition center is intact.
       c. Symptoms include frequency, urgency, and incontinence.
    2. **Suprasacral lesion**
       a. Located between pons and conus medullaris (i.e., traumatic cord injury, transverse myelitis, syringomyelia).
       b. Characteristics
          i. Detrusor external sphincter dyssynergia: pathologic, hyperactive holding reflex during attempted voiding.
          ii. Detrusor hyperreflexia.
          iii. Sensation often absent.
          iv. High intravesicular pressure.
          v. Detrusor and sphincter are *not* coordinated; therefore, risk for vesicoureteral reflux is high.
    2. **Infrasacral lesion**
       a. Located below conus medullaris and involving sacral micturition center or peripheral nerves (i.e., cauda equina injury, diabetes mellitus, Guillain-Barré syndrome).
       b. Characteristics
          i. Detrusor areflexia: decreased to absent detrusor contractions.
          ii. Sensation often absent.
          iii. Large-volume bladder.
          iv. May progress to low-volume, high-pressure bladder over time.
          v. Do not confuse with spinal shock.
  B. **Specific voiding dysfunction**
    1. **Cerebrovascular accidents** (CVAs)
       a. High incidence of voiding dysfunction initially.
       b. Spontaneous resolution in most patients over 6–12 months.
       c. Variety of voiding dysfunctions; urinary incontinence is most common.
    2. **Multiple sclerosis**
       a. Voiding dysfunction often changes with remission or exacerbation.
       b. Combination of supraspinal and suprasacral lesions influences the type of bladder dysfunction.
       c. Frequent reevaluation is needed.
    3. **Parkinson's disease:** detrusor hyperreflexia.
    4. **Advanced age**
       a. Women
          i. Laxity of pelvic muscles → incontinence
          ii. Atrophic urethritis
       b. Men: outlet obstruction.
       c. Other factors include cognition, mobility, and medications.

IV. Evaluation of the Neurogenic Bladder

A. **History** of voiding problem (i.e., trauma, surgery)

B. **Description** of voiding problem (i.e., frequency, urgency)

C. **Comorbidities** (i.e., CVA; impaired mobility; cognitive deficits; prostatic hypertophy; infection, especially recurrent urinary tract infections; atrophic urethritis; stool impaction/incontinence)

D. **Medications** (i.e., diuretics, antidepressants)

E. **Neurologic exam**
   1. Mental status exam
   2. Sensory level, including sacral segments
   3. Digital exam for tone and voluntary contraction
   4. Reflexes
      a. Bulbocavernosus: anal contraction with squeeze of glans or clitoris
         i. Present in all normal persons and patients with SCI if lesion is above conus.
         ii. Absent in spinal shock and lesions below conus.
      b. Cremasteric

F. **Functional history**
   1. Activities of daily living (ADL's): hand function, transfers, dressing.
   2. Mobility – transfers, ambulation, wheelchair.

G. **Diagnostic studies**
   1. **Urinalysis**
   2. **Urine culture and sensitivity testing**
   3. **Postvoid residual** (PVR)
      a. Determines ability of bladder to empty.
      b. "Balanced bladder" has < 100 ml PVR with > 2 hours between reflex voids.
   4. **Renal ultrasound**
      a. Noninvasive anatomic study of kidneys, ureters, and bladder.
      b. Demonstrates space-occupying lesions, hydronephrosis, and postvoid residuals.
   5. **Intravenous pyelogram** (IVP)
      a. Radiologic study using contrast agent to visualize upper and lower urinary tract.
      b. Demonstrates:
         i. Renal function: creatinine > 7 mg/dl or blood urea nitrogen (BUN) > 70 mg/dl results in poor study (kidneys cannot concentrate dye for proper visualization).
         ii. Space-occupying lesions (cyst, tumor, stones)
         iii. Hydronephrosis
         iv. Vesicoureteral reflux
         v. Bladder stones
   6. **Voiding cystourethrogram** (VCU)
      a. Last stage of IVP or dye introduced directly into bladder via catheter.
      b. Demonstrates:
         i. Bladder size, diverticula, trabeculations
         ii. Vesicoureteral reflux
         iii. Sphincter competence, ability to start/stop micturition, and adequate sphincter opening
         iv. PVR
   7. **Cystometrogram** (Fig. 3)

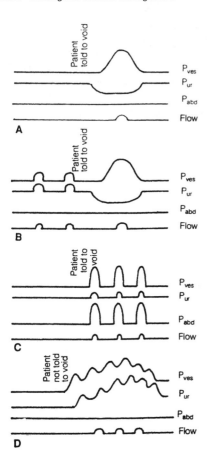

FIGURE 3. Schematic representation of various voiding patterns. *A*, Normal. *B*, Uninhibited contractions occur with filling. The sphincter is attempting to inhibit contractions. Patient has a normal voiding phase. *C*, No bladder contractions. Rises in bladder pressure are due to rises in abdominal perssure (i.e., Valsalva voiding). *D*, Uninhibited contractions occur with simultaneous sphincter contractions (i.e., detrusor sphincter dyssynergia). P_{abd} = intra-abdominal pressure, P_{ur} = uretheral sphincter pressure, P_{ves} = intravesical pressure). (From Lisenmeyer TA, Stone JM: Neurogenic bladder and bowel dysfunction. In DeLisa JA (ed): Rehabilitation Medicine: Principles and Practice. Philadelphia, Lippincott Williams & Wilkins, 1998, with permission.)

  a. Assesses bladder sensation, capacity, compliance (pressure), and activity.
  b. Bladder filled with gas or liquid.
  c. Pressures are measured in bladder and abdomen (via rectum).
     i. Intravesicular pressure = bladder pressure – abdominal pressure.
     ii. Normal pressure increases 10–15 cmH_2O with bladder filling; pressure increases > 20 cmH_2O are abnormal (suggest hyperreflexive bladder).
  d. Coupled with electromyography (EMG) of external sphincter.
  e. May cause autonomic dysreflexia in patients with higher-level SCI; precautions should be taken (see Chapter 8, Spinal Cord Injury Rehabiliation).
  8. **Cystoscopy**
  a. Direct visualization of bladder wall and urethra.
  b. Used to obtain tissue biopsy and to remove stones from distal ureter or bladder.
V. **Management Strategies**
  A. **Behavioral strategies**
    1. **Timed voids**
      a. Voiding at set intervals rather than waiting for sense of fullness
      b. Useful for patients with:

      i. Hyperreflexia producing urgency or incontinence.

      ii. Sphincter weakness, because incontinence is worse when bladder is full.

      iii. Normal bladder function, but incontinence due to poor cognition, aphasia, or impaired mobility.

2. **Bladder stimulation**
   a. Crede's maneuver
      i. Forceful surface palpation over bladder mechanically pushes urine out.
      ii. Usually performed by attendant for patients with tetraplegia.
   b. Valsalva's maneuver
      i. Bladder emptying via increased intra-abdominal pressure.
      ii. Used by patients with areflexia and some denervation of pelvic floor.
      iii. Over time, may worsen stress incontinence.
   c. Both Crede and Valsalva maneuvers may exacerbate hemorrhoids, rectal prolapse, or hernia; avoid using in patients with detrusor sphincter dyssynergia and vesicoureteral reflux.
   d. Suprapubic tapping or jabbing
      i. Mechanical stretch of bladder wall triggers bladder contraction.
      ii. Used by paraplegic patients who have good upper extremity function in conjunction with condom catheters.

3. **Pelvic floor exercises (Kegel)**
   a. May be effective in neurologically intact women with mild incontinence due to sphincter.
   b. Number of recommended exercise contractions varies by author from 8–160 per day.
   c. Effects may not be seen for 4–8 weeks.

B. **Urine collection devices**
   1. **Undergarments (diapers)**
      a. Absorbs urine, facilitates care, allows social integration.
      b. Potential for skin breakdown; change every 2–4 hours
      c. Expensive, difficult to get off/on.
      d. Often used in incontinent demented patients with adequate bladder emptying.
   2. **Condom catheters**
      a. Advantages over diapers: changed only once per day, less bulky.
      b. Potential disadvantages include wearing a leg bag, penile skin breakdown, slight increase in bladder infection rate.
   3. **Indwelling catheters**
      a. May be urethral or suprapubic.
      b. Used when other programs have failed or patient is unable to perform clean intermittent catheterization or for patient convenience.
      c. Important management principles
         i. Copious fluid intake (at least 2 L/day).
         ii. Catheter changes every 2–4 weeks.
         iii. Avoid traction on catheter.
         iv. Sterilize collecting bag with bleach.
         v. Prevent reflux of urine into bladder.
         vi. Prevent tearing or tissue irritation from external catheter pulling on urethra or glans.

    d. Long-term use associated with increased incidence of squamous cell carcinoma of bladder; therefore, yearly cystoscopy is recommended after 10 years (5 years in patients with increased risk factors, such as smoking).

C. **Clean intermittent catheterization** (CIC)

  1. Sterile technique introduced by Guttmann in 1950s for management of patients with SCI.

  2. Clean technique proposed by Lapides in 1972 proved successful; easier to perform and more practical than sterile technique.

  3. Requires low-pressure bladder of > 300 ml capacity; may be combined with anticholinergics if bladder is hyperreflexic.

  4. Catheterize frequently enough to prevent bladder overdistention (< 400–500 ml).

  5. Timing based on fluid intake/output records; usually start trial at frequency of every 4–6 hours.

  6. Minimum of 3 catheterizations per 24 hours is recommended; longer intervals may increase risk of symptomatic bacteriuria.

  7. Functionally can be managed by men with lesions at C6 and below and by women with lesions at C7 and below.

  8. Common problems

    a. Symptomatic bacteriuria

    b. Urethral trauma

      i. Often due to sphincter spasm; try extra lubrication, local anesthetic gel, curved (coude) catheter.

      ii. Repeated urethral bleeding may suggest false passage.

    c. Incontinence

D. **Medication by functional problem** (Table 1)

  1. **Incontinence due to hyperreflexic bladder**

    a. Anticholinergic medications relax detrusor by blocking acetylcholine receptors competitively (propantheline bromide, oxybutynin [Ditropan], tolterodine [Detrol]).

    b. Tricyclic antidepressants (TCAs) cause urinary retention because of anticholinergic effects (imipramine, amitriptyline).

  2. **Incontinence due to outlet or sphincter incompetence**

    a. Alpha agonists (ephedrine, phenylpropranolamine, pseudoephedrine)

    b. TCAs

  3. **Retention caused by bladder areflexia:** cholinergic agonists (bethanechol)

  4. **Retention caused by sphincter contraction**

    a. Alpha-adrenergic blocker

      i.. Doxazosin (selective alpha$_1$ adrenoceptor blocker)

      ii. Terazosin (selective alpha$_1$ adrenoceptor blocker)

      iii. Prazosin (postsynaptic alpha adrenoceptor blocker)

    b. Lioresal

    c. Dantrolene sodium

E. **Surgical treatments**

  1. **Suprapubic catheter**

    a. Alternative to indwelling Foley catheter.

    b. Indication: patients with urethral stricture, fistual, abscess, or perineal skin breakdown; female patients with difficulty performing CIC because of adductor spasticity or obesity.

TABLE 1. Drugs Used in the Treatment of Neurogenic Bladder

Drug	Action	Indication	Side Effects	Contraindications	Dosage
Propantheline (Pro-Banthine)	Anticholinergic (muscarinic receptor antagonist) Decreases frequency and amplitude of bladder contractions; increases total bladder capacity	Incontinence due to hyperreflexic bladder-	Dry mouth, mydriasis, blurred vision, tachycardia, drowsiness, nervousness, decreased GI motility, impotence	Glaucoma, urinary or GI obstruction, acute paralytic ileus, severe colitis, myasthenia gravis	7.5–15 mg orally 30 min before meals 3 times/day and 30 min before bedtime
Tolterodine (Detrol)	Anticholinergic (competitive muscarinic receptor antagonist)	Incontinence due to hyperreflexic bladder with urinary frequency, urgency, or urge incontinence	Same as propantheline	Same as propantheline	2 mg orally 2 times/day; 1 mg 2 times/day if patient has impaired hepatic function
Oxybutynin (Ditropan)	Decreases frequency of uninhibited bladder contractions, increases bladder capacity; decreases urgency, frequency, and urge continence; also decreases dysuria	Incontinence due to hyperreflexic bladder	Same as propantheline	Same as propantheline	5 mg orally 2, 3, or 4 times/day
Tricyclic antidepressants	Anticholinergic; sphincter contraction by potentiating adrenergic responses Urinary retention via inhibitory effect on bladder smooth muscle and increased outlet obstruction	Incontinence due to hyperreflexic bladder or sphincter incompetence Imipramine may be used for children with nocturnal enuresis of nonorganic etiology	Same as propantheline as well as rash, increased liver function tests, agranulocytosis, fine tremor, postural hypotension, delirium	Use of monoamine oxidase inhibitors	Imipramine, 50–150 mg orally at bedtime Amitriptyline, 10–25 mg orally 3 times/day or 20–75 mg orally at bedtime
Ephedrine	Predominantly alpha agonist, some mild beta-agonist activity Increases urethral resistance	Stress incontinence, postprostatectomy incontinence, enuresis	Hypertension, anxiety, palpitations, arrhythmias, respiratory difficulty, insomnia	Hypertension, angina, hyperthyroidism, obstructive prostatism	25–50 mg 4 times/day

Table continued on following page

TABLE 1. Drugs Used in the Treatment of Neurogenic Bladder *(Continued)*

Drug	Action	Indication	Side Effects	Contraindications	Dosage
Estrogen cream		Stress incontinence in postmenopausal women due to atrophic urethritis		Breast cancer, pregnancy, genital bleeding, thromboembolic disease	2–4 gm (0.625 mg/gm) applied intravaginally daily for 4–6 weeks
Bethanechol (Urecholine)	Muscarinic cholinergic agonist Increases detrusor tone but probably does not stimulate physiologic bladder contraction	Urinary retention, detrusor atony	Flushing, headache, salivation, nausea, vomiting, bronchospasm, difficulty with visual accommodation, hypotension with reflex tachycardia	Sphincter detrusor dyssynergia, bowel or bladder outlet obstruction, asthma, peptic ulcer disease, hyperthyroidism, coronary artery disease, parkinsonism, cardiac arrhythmia	10–50 mg 2–4 times/day; maximum: 150 mg/day
Alpha antagonists	Alpha blocker Decreases urethral resistance	Sphincter detrusor dyssynergia or prostate outlet obstruction; also decreases frequency of autonomic dysreflexia associated with bladder distention	Orthostatic hypotension, reflex tachycardia, impotence	Situations in which hypotension is undesirable	Terazosin, 1 mg orally at bedtime; increase stepwise to maximum of 20 mg at bedtime Prazosin, 1 mg orally 2 or 3 times/day up to 40 mg/day Doxazosin, 1–16 mg/day orally
Lioresal (Baclofen)	Binds to GABA receptors in spinal cord to decrease striated muscle spasticity	Spastic external sphincter	Drowsiness, dizziness, ataxia, nausea, hypotension, personality disturbance, hallucinations, hepatic dysfunction Sudden withdrawal may lead to seizures, hallucinations	Epilepsy	30–100 mg/day divided in 3 or 4 divided doses
Dantrolene sodium (Dantrium)	Inhibits release of calcium from sarcoplasmic reticulum	Spastic external sphincter	Long-term hepatotoxicity, weakness, drowsiness, dizziness, malaise	Amyotrophic lateral sclerosic, liver disease	25 mg 2 times/day; increase slowly to maximum of 400 mg/day

    c. Technique: suprapubic catheterization with bladder neck closure.

    d. Drawbacks: complications similar to those of Foley catheter.

2. **Bladder augmentation**

    a. Goal: increase bladder capacity and lower intravesical pressures.

    b. Indication: patients with severe detrusor hyperreflexia, decreased compliance or ongoing upper tract damage who failed conservative management.

    c. Technique: portion of bladder is removed and replaced with segment of bowel.

    d. Drawbacks: may require long-term CIC because of inefficient bladder emptying; increased mucus in urine due to bowel segment can be annoying.

3. **Bladder augmentation with continent stoma**

    a. Goal: increase bladder capacity and form continent, catheterizable channel that opens onto abdominal wall.

    b. Indication: women who have difficulty with intermittent self-catheterization (IC) because of leg adductor spasticity, body habitus, severe urethral incontinence, or need to transfer from wheelchair; men who are unable to do IC because of strictures, false passages, or fistulas.

    c. Technique: bowel is used to increase bladder capacity and form continent, catheterizable stoma; terminal ileum and ileocecal valve work well.

    d. Drawbacks: patient must be compliant with CIC because bowel segment can rupture internally before overflow incontinence occurs through urethra or stoma.

4. **Denervation procedures**

    a. Indication: bladder hyperreflexia; not widely used.

    b. Technique: interrupt innervation to bladder at root (sacral rhizotomy) or peripheral nerve (unilateral pudendal nerve block) or by removing perivesical ganglia.

    c. Drawbacks: impotence, worsening of bowel evacuation problems; detrusor hyperreflexia may return.

5. **Implantable electrical stimulation**

    a. Goal: stimulate detrusor contraction *or* relax hyperreflexic bladder.

    b. Technique: electrodes implanted on bladder wall, pelvic nerve, pudendal nerve, sacral roots (most common), or conus.

    c. Investigational and controversial.

6. **Injection therapy**

    a. Indication: stress incontinence.

        i. Technique: autologous fat and bovine collagen injected in urethra.

        ii. Low potential side effects.

        iii. Suitable for elderly and poor surgical-risk patients.

    b. Indication: detrusor dyssynergia.

        i. Technique: botulinum toxin (Botox) injected into striated sphincter.

        ii. Drawbacks: effects last only a few months; experimental.

7. **Fascial sling procedure**

    a. Goal: improve urethral support and position.

    b. Indication: women with incontinence due to pelvic floor laxity.

    c. Technique: strip of fascia is taken from rectus abdominis or tensor fascia lata, wrapped around bladder neck, and fixed anteriorly to abdominal fascia or pubic tubercle.

    d. Drawbacks: postoperative retention, possibly requiring intermittent catheterization; inability to void using Valsalva maneuver.

8. **Artificial urethral sphincter**
   a. Indication: selective injury affecting only sphincter (i.e., pelvic fracture, children with myelodysplasia, SCI with detrusor areflexia).
   b. Technique: cuff is implanted around bladder neck with pressure-regulating balloon; control pump in labia or scrotum allows patient to open cuff to void.
   c. Drawbacks: mechanical failure, cuff erosions, and infection.
9. **Sphincterotomy**
   a. Indication: men with SCI and detrusor sphincter dyssynergia.
   b. Technique: ablation of striated sphincter, usually by incision.
   c. Drawbacks: impotence; incontinence requiring collecting device (i.e., condom catheter with leg bag); recurrent obstruction due to stricture; recurrent dyssynergia; irreversible procedure.

VI. **Functional Classification of Voiding Dysfunction and Management Options**
   A. **Incontinence (failure to store)**
      1. **Due to bladder hyperreflexia**
         a. Behavioral: timed voids
         b. Collection devices: diapers, indwelling catheter, condom catheter, CIC
         c. Medications: anticholinergics, TCAs
         d. Surgery: augmentation, denervation, continent diversion
      2. **Due to outlet or sphincter**
         a. Behavioral: timed voids, pelvic floor exercises
         b. Collection devices: diapers, indwelling catheter, condom catheter
         c. Medications: alpha-adrenergic agonists, imipramine, estrogen cream
         d. Surgery: fascial sling, artificial sphincter, collagen injection
   B. **Retention (failure to empty)**
      1. **Due to bladder areflexia**
         a. Behavioral: timed voids, suprapubic tapping, Valsalva maneuver, Crede's maneuver
         b. Collection devices: indwelling catheter, CIC
         c. Medications: cholinergic agonists
      2. **Due to outlet or sphincter dyssynergia**
         a. Behavioral: suprapubic tapping, anal stretch void
         b. Collection devices: indwelling catheter, CIC
         c. Medications: alpha-adrenergic blockers, striated muscle relaxants (lioresal, dantrolene, diazepam)
         d. Surgery: sphincterotomy, pudendal neurectomy, bladder outlet surgery (prostate resection, bladder neck incision)

VII. **Complications of Voiding Dysfunction**
   A. **Urinary tract infections**
      1. Common source of morbidity
      2. Signs and symptoms
         a. Dysuria, frequency, urinary incontinence, hematuria
         b. In patients with SCI, look for fever, increased spasticity, new onset of urinary incontinence, autonomic dysreflexia, cloudy and odorous urine, malaise, lethargy, or sense of unease.
         c. In elderly, presentation may be subtle (i.e., confusion and lethargy).
      3. Asymptomatic bacteriuria
         a. Prophylactic antibiotics for patients on intermittent catheterization program or with indwelling Foley is controversial.

    b. Treatment warranted in patients with high-grade reflux, hydronephrosis, or urea-splitting organisms (associated with stone formation).

4. Symptomatic bacteriuria
    a. Obtain urine culture and treat empirically with antibiotics.
    b. Mild illness: nitrofurantoin or trimethroprim/sulfamethoxazole commonly used; *Pseudomonas aeruginosa* not covered.
    c. Mild-to-moderate illness: oral fluoroquinolones (ciprofloxacin, levofloxacin, or ofloxacin) provide coverage against most expected pathogens, including *P. aeruginosa.*
    d. More seriously ill patients (high fever, dehydration, or autonomic dysreflexia)
      i. Broad-spectrum coverage (e.g., ampicillin plus gentamicin or imipenem)
      ii. Oral or IV hydration
      iii. Foley catheter to keep bladder decompressed

B. **Vesicoureteral reflux**
1. Causes
    a. High intravesicle pressures associated with detrusor-sphincter dyssynergia.
    b. Anatomic changes in oblique course of ureters through bladder wall perpendicular course due to bladder thickening and trabeculation.
    c. Recurrent cystitis
2. Associated with renal deterioration
3. Treatment goals: lower intravesical pressures, eradicate infections

C. **Hydronephrosis:** caused by ureteral dilation secondary to high detrusor pressures, high PVRs, bladder outlet obstruction, mechanical obstruction (e.g., stone or stricture).

D. **Renal stones**
1. Significant risk factor for renal deterioration.
2. 8% of patients with SCI develop renal stones.
3. 98% composed of:
    a. Calcium (due to hypercalcuria of immobilization) *or*
    b. Struvite (magnesium ammonium phosphate due to alkaline urine from urease-producing organisms)
4. May require surgical removal to prevent obstruction.
    a. Extracorporeal shock wave lithotripsy for stones < 3 cm in diameter.
    b. Percutaneous approach for stones > 3 cm in diameter.

E. **Pyelonephritis**
1. Associated with vesicoureteral reflux, kidney stones and obstruction.
2. Can lead to renal deterioration.
3. Perform diagnostics to rule out correctable cause (IVP; renal ultrasound; x-rays of kidney, ureters, and bladder; renal scan; 24-hour urine creatinine clearance).

F. **Bladder stones**
1. Associated with an indwelling Foley catheter or prolonged urinary retention.
2. Occasionally caused by foreign body (e.g., pubic hair).
3. May result in hematuria, persistent UTI, autonomic dysreflexia, or obstruction.
4. Not associated with renal deterioration.

G. **Penoscrotal complications**
1. Usually due to catheters.
2. Abscess, fistula, diverticula, strictures, epididymitis.

H. **Bladder cancer**
   1. Usually squamous cell carcinoma.
   2. More prevalent in patients with SCI and indwelling Foley for >10 years.
   3. Monitor with cystoscopy, cell cytology, bladder biopsy of suspicious areas.
 I. **Autonomic dysreflexia**
   1. Commonly precipitated by full bladder or blocked urinary catheter.
   2. Other urologic sources include urinary tract infection and bladder stones.
VIII. **Long-term Care of the Neurogenic Bladder**
   A. **Routine evaluation**
      1. Annually for first 5 years, then every other year if condition is stable.
      2. Testing should include:
         a. Renal ultrasound and x-rays of kidney, ureters, and bladder
         b. Creatinine clearance, 24-hour urine collection
         c. PVR unless indwelling catheter in place
         d. Others as indicated
            i. IVP or CT if indicated by ultrasound or clinically
            ii. Urodynamics
   B. **Cystoscopy**
      1. After 10 years of chronic catheterizations
      2. Earlier (at 5 years) in patients at high risk
         a. Heavy smoker
         b. Age > 40 years
         c. History of complicated urinary tract infections

Bibliography
1. Cardenas DD, Mayo ME: Management of bladder dysfunction. In Grabois M (ed): Physical Medicine and Rehabilitation: The Complete Approach. Malden, MA, Blackwell Science, 2000, pp 561–577.
2. Linsenmeyer TA, Stone JM: Neurogenic bladder and bowel dysfunction. In DeLisa JA (ed): Rehabilitation Medicine: Principles and Practice. Philadelphia, Lippincott Williams & Wilkins, 1993, pp 733–758.
3. Nesathurai S: Bladder management. In Nesathurai S (ed): The Rehabilitation of People with Spinal Cord Injury: A House Officer's Guide. Boston, Arbuckle Academic Publishers, 1999, pp 39–46.
4. Perkash I: Urologic disorders in rehabilitation. In O'Young B, Young M, Stiens S (eds): Physical Medicine and Rehabilitation Secrets. Philadelphia, Hanley & Belfus, 1997, pp 464–470.
5. Tan JC: Practical Manual of Physical Medicine and Rehabilitation. St. Louis, Mosby, 1998, pp 538–552.

Chapter 16

NEUROGENIC BOWEL MANAGEMENT

Ann T. Laidlaw, M.D., and Anthony Chiodo, M.D.

I. General Principles

A. Neurogenic bowel can be a primary disabling feature for patients with conditions such as spinal cord injury (SCI), stroke, amyotrophic lateral sclerosis, multiple sclerosis, diabetes mellitus, myelomeningocele, and muscular dystrophy.

B. Because of widespread presentation in rehabilitation patients, rehabilitation specialists must familiarize themselves with the presentation and treatment of bowel dysfunction.

C. **Anatomy of gastrointestinal (GI) tract**

1. **Colon:** closed tube that is bound proximally by the ileocecal valve and distally by the anal sphincter.
2. **Smooth muscle:** inner circular layer and outer longitudinal layer.
3. **Internal anal sphincter** (IAS): formed by thickening of smooth muscle layers.
4. **External anal sphincter** (EAS): consists of circular band of striated muscle that is part of pelvic floor; its contraction is under both reflex and voluntary control.
5. **Innervation** (Fig. 1)
   a. Intrinsic system coordinates peristalsis.
      i. Auerbach's (myenteric) plexus, located between the muscle layers, serves primarily a motor function. Stimulation increases gut activity, including force and velocity of contractions.
      ii. Meissner's plexus, located in submucosa, serves primarily a sensory function and coordinates gut wall movements and secretion of digestive juices.
   b. Parasympathetic system
      i. Via cranial (vagus nerve) and sacral (pelvic nerve) divisions.
      ii. Increased parasympathetic tone stimulates gut wall.
   c. Sympathetic system
      i. Through hypogastric nerve via superior mesenteric, inferior mesenteric, and celiac ganglia.
      ii. Stimulation relaxes ileocecal valve, gut wall, and contracts IAS.
   d. Somatic system
      i. Via pudendal nerve (S2–S4).
      ii. Supplies EAS and pelvic floor muscles.

D. **Continence**

1. **Maintenance:** by tonic activity of IAS and acute angle of anorectal canal produced by puborectalis sling.
2. **Tone:** increased via sympathetic discharges.

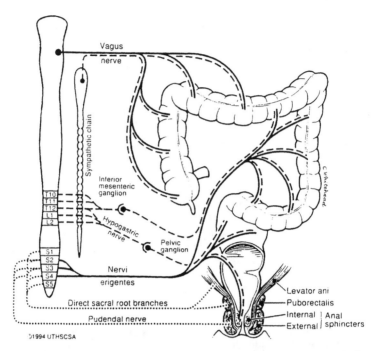

FIGURE 1. Neurologic levels and pathways for the sympathetic, parasympathetic, and somatic nervous system innervation of the colon and anorectum. Not shown is the enteric nervous system, which travels along the bowel wall from esophagus to internal anal sphincter and forms the final common pathway to control the bowel wall smooth muscle. (From King JC, Stiens SA: Neurogenic bowel: Dysfunction and management. In Grabois M, et al (eds): Physical Medicine and Rehabilitation: The Complete Approach. Malden, MA, Blackwell Science, 2000, p 586, with permission.)

    3. **IAS tone:** inhibited via rectal dilation by stool or digital stimulation.
    4. **Reflex contraction of EAS and puborectalis** prevents incontinence with cough or Valsalva maneuver.
  D. **Propulsion and defecation** (Fig. 2)
    1. **Transit time** from cecum to anus is 12–48 hours with normal bowel function.
    2. **Reflex activity**
      a. Giant migratory contractions advance stool through colon to rectum.
      b. Gastrocolic reflex refers to increased colonic activity that occurs 30–60 minutes postprandially.
      c. Rectorectal reflex occurs when bowel proximal to distending bolus contracts and distal bowel wall relaxes, propelling the bolus further caudal.
      d. Rectoanal inhibitory reflex occurs as stool distends rectum and IAS relaxes, triggering conscious urge to defecate.
      e. Holding reflex occurs as EAS and puborectalis muscle contract to retain stool.
    3. **Peristalsis** pushes stool into rectum.
    4. **"Urge":** sensation of rectal fullness that triggers rectoanal inhibitory reflex.
    5. **Defecation:** initiated with voluntary relaxation of EAS and puborectalis muscles and contraction of levator ani, abdominals, and diaphragm.

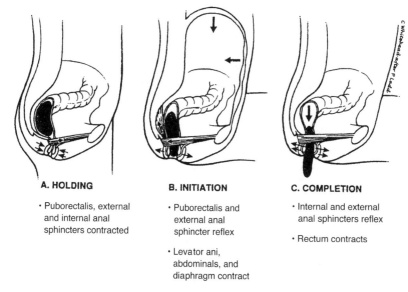

A. HOLDING	B. INITIATION	C. COMPLETION
• Puborectalis, external and internal anal sphincters contracted	• Puborectalis and external anal sphincter reflex	• Internal and external anal sphincters reflex
	• Levator ani, abdominals, and diaphragm contract	• Rectum contracts

FIGURE 2. *A,* Defecation is prevented by a statically increased tone of the internal anal sphincter and puborectalis as well as by the mechanical effects of the acute anorectal angle. Dynamic response of the external anal sphincter and puborectalis to rectal distention reflexes or increased intra-abdominal pressures further impede defecation. *B,* To initiate defecation, the puborectalis muscle and external anal sphincter relax while intra-abdominal pressure is increased by the Valsalva maneuver, which is facilitated by squatting. The levator ani helps reduce the acute anorectal angle to open the distal anal canal to receive the stool bolus. *C,* Intrarectal reflexes result in continued internal anal sphincter relaxation and rectal propulsive contractions, which help expel the bolus through the open canal. (From King JC, Stiens SA: Neurogenic bowel: Dysfunction and management. In Grabois M, et al (eds): Physical Medicine and Rehabilitation: The Complete Approach. Malden, MA, Blackwell Science, 2000, p 582, with permission.)

6. **Evacuation:** process of pushing stool out of rectum by continued peristalsis and increased abdominal pressure via squatting and Valsalva maneuver.
II. **Pathophysiology of Dysfunction**
   A. **Supraspinal lesions** (lesion above pons)
      1. Characterized by cortical dysfunction with normal lower tract function, but without voluntary control.
      2. Treatment: establish bowel regimen similar to that for patients with SCI.
   B. **Upper motor neuron bowel** (UMNB)
      1. Central nervous system (CNS) lesion between pons and conus medullaris.
      2. Characterized as "spastic" because of excessive colonic wall activity.
      3. Underactive propulsive peristalsis.
      4. Hyperactive holding reflex due to spasticity of pelvic floor with inability to voluntarily relax EAS (modulates descending inhibition).
      5. Stool retention.
      6. Key issue: requires mechanical or chemical stimulus to trigger reflex defecation.
      7. Goal of treatment: soft-formed stool that can be readily evacuated with rectal stimulation.

C. **Lower motor neuron bowel** (LMNB)
  1. Results from lesions at or distal to conus medullaris.
  2. Characterized as "relaxed."
  3. No spinal cord-mediated reflex peristalsis occurs.
  4. Slow stool propulsion coordinated by myenteric plexus alone.
  5. Increased transit time results in increased moisture absorption, producing dry, rounder stool.
  6. EAS has low or absent tone.
  7. Key issues: fecal incontinence, constipation, and difficulty with evacuation.
  8. Goal: firmly formed stool that can be retained between bowel care routines, yet easily evacuated manually.

III. **Evaluation**
  A. **History**
    1. Fluid and fiber intake, diet, activity, medications.
    2. Bowel care: frequency, duration, technique of defecation, and stool consistency.
    3. Associated predefecatory activities: time of day, effect of position, trigger foods, effect of bowel medications or facilitative techniques.
    4. Premorbid bowel function.
    5. Ability to prevent stool loss during Valsalva activities (laughing, sneezing, coughing).
    6. Problems with stool consistency, incontinence, bleeding.
    7. Effect of problems on work, travel, interaction with others, and activities of daily living.
    8. Medical history: pregnancies, traumatic deliveries, anorectal or GI surgery, trauma to perineum or spinal cord, neurologic disease, diabetes, radiation therapy, neurogenic bladder, impotence.
  B. **Physical examination**
    1. **Abdominal exam**
      a. Inspection for hernias, distention.
      b. Palpation for masses and tenderness as well as detection of hard stool in right colon (should not be present).
    2. **Anal inspection**
      a. Anal buttock contour is flattened or scalloped in patients with LMNB due to loss of EAS muscle bulk; normal with UMN lesions.
      b. Anal opening: patulous, gaping orifice suggests history of overdistention and trauma by bowel regimen.
      c. Perineal descent with Valsalva maneuver.
    3. **Digital exam of anus and rectum**
      a. Tone and voluntary squeeze strength of the EAS
      b. Tone of IAS
      c. Palpable ridge of puborectalis sling (absence suggests LMN lesion)
      d. Anocutaneous reflex
      e. Bulbocavernosus reflex
      f. Anal closing reflex: normally brisk when finger withdrawn
    4. **Functional mobility**
      a. Assess patient's gait.
      b. Assess time required for position change and ambulation.
      c. Assess ability to manipulate clothing in preparation for toileting.

C. **Diagnostic tests**
1. Laboratory studies to consider if disorder of GI tract is suspected: complete blood count, electrolytes, stool culture, stool analysis for ova and parasites, stool assay for *Clostridium difficile* toxin.
2. Anatomic studies if lesions or GI obstruction is suspected.
   a. Endoscopy
   b. Radiologic studies: barium enema, computed tomography (CT), magnetic resonance imaging (MRI)
   c. Biopsy
3. Functional studies
   a. Electromyography (EMG)
   b. Manometry
   c. Rectodynamics
   d. Defecography
   e. Serial radiographs of radiopaque beads to evaluate colonic transit time
4. Anal continence studies: rectally infused saline continence test, solid sphere retention test

IV. **Management: Establishing Bowel Program for Patients with New SCI**
A. **Preliminary considerations**
1. Ascertain premorbid bowel function: time of day, frequency, use of bowel medications (e.g., laxative dependency).
2. Minimize medications that decrease gut motility, such as narcotics, anticholinergics, and tricyclics.
3. Begin with empty gut.
4. If obstipation is present, manual disimpaction or osmotic laxatives/enemas may be used but should not be used chronically. Examples include magnesium citrate, milk of magnesia, Fleet Phosphosoda, Fleet Phosphosoda enema, GoLytely, lactulose.

B. **Control stool consistency.**
1. **Ideal consistency** is soft, well-formed stool.
   a. Hard stool may result in hemorrhoids, abscess, or impaction.
   b. Unformed stool may cause bowel accidents.
2. **Diet** is integral determinant of stool consistency.
   a. Fiber provides bulk and eases transit.
      i. Goal intake: 15 gm/day.
      ii. Goal should be achieved gradually based on premorbid fiber intake and symptoms of intolerance, such as flatulence or abdominal distention.
      iii. Sources include:
         • Fruit with tough skins or seeds (e.g., apples, berries, dates, figs grapes, plums, prunes, raisins).
         • Nuts
         • Whole grain breads, bran cereal, granola
         • Raw vegetables, potato skins, corn, and cooked beans
   b. Fatty foods and dairy products may impair gut mobility.
   c. Caffeinated beverages, prune juice, and apricot nectar may aid in bowel evacuation.
3. **Fluid intake** is also essential to bowel program.
   a. 500 ml/day more than standard guidelines for general public is recommended.

b. 1 ml fluid/kcal of energy needs + 500 ml/day *or*

c. 40 ml/kg body weight + 500 ml/day

4. **Medications**

a. Used on individual basis if consistency cannot be controlled by diet alone.

b. Stool softeners prevent formation of hard stool and are first-line medication.

c. See below for other adjunctive medication.

C. **Timing**

1. Schedule bowel care at same time at least once every 2 days.

a. Irregular patterns may result in bowel accidents.

b. Some patients may require daily program; some may go every third day.

c. Longer than every third day may result in fecal impaction and, over long term, chronic colorectal overdistention.

2. Establish program at time that is convenient for the patient and caregiver (if one is needed), taking into consideration premorbid timing.

3. Take advantage of gastrocolic reflex by scheduling bowel program approximately 30 minutes after ingestion of food or hot caffeinated beverages.

D. **Techniques and positioning**

1. Upright sitting with forward-leaning position is optimal for elimination.

a. Hips and knees flexed.

b. Footstool can be used to put knees slightly higher than hips.

c. Gives maximal gravity assist and mechanical advantage of abdominal muscles.

2. Left lateral position is second best, if upright position is not possible.

3. Valsalva maneuver

4. Digital bowel stimulation

a. May be done with or in place of suppository.

b. Facilitates reflex defecation by increasing peristalsis and relaxing EAS.

c. Insert gloved, lubricated finger into rectum and move it in gentle circular motion while maintaining mucosal contact until bowel wall relaxes (30 seconds to 2 minutes).

d. Start 20 minutes after using suppository, if applicable.

5. Manual disimpaction

a. Used if digital stimulation has failed or to remove stool before insertion of suppository against rectal mucosa for reflexive bowel care.

b. Use caution to prevent overstretching of sphincter or anorectal injury.

c. Lidocaine gel may help decrease nocioceptive sensory input for patients predisposed to autonomic dysreflexia (AD).

E. **Modifications**

1. Change only one program element at a time (e.g., diet or frequency or time of bowel care).

2. Allow 3–5 cycles to assess pattern before making further changes.

V. **Medications to Augment Bowel Program** (also see Chapter 23, Pharmacology)

A. **Laxatives**

1. Used to achieve optimal stool consistency and/or increase intestinal peristalsis and stool frequency.

2. **Surfactant laxatives** (e.g., docusate sodium [Colace])

a. Softens stool without adding bulk or increasing peristalsis.

b. Not habit-forming.

c. Used when straining should be avoided (e.g., after surgery, angina, hemorrhoids, prone to AD).

3. **Lubricant laxatives** (e.g., mineral oil)
   a. Coats stool and allows easier passage.
   b. Used for short-term management of constipation.

4. **Stimulant laxatives**
   a. Stimulate peristalsis.
   b. Senna (Senokot): effects seen in 6–10 hr.
   c. Pericolace: Casanthrol combined with docusate.
   d. Bisacodyl (Dulcolax): effects seen 6–12 hr after oral dose; 15–60 minutes after rectal administration.

5. **Bulk-forming agents**
   a. Maintain stool moisture and consistency.
   b. Taken with water or juice.
   c. Effects seen within 12–24 hr.
   d. Examples: psyllium powder (Metamucil), methylcellulose (Citrucel), polycarbophil (Fibercon).

6. **Osmotic laxatives**
   a. Indicated for immediate evacuation.
      i. Start of bowel-training program.
      ii. Bowel preparation for surgery, endoscopy, or radiologic studies.
   b. Should *not* be used chronically.
   c. Saline-based agents
      i. Magnesium salts (e.g., magnesium citrate, milk of magnesia)
         • Effects seen in 3–4 hr.
         • Caution: hypermagnesemia in patients with renal failure.
      ii. Sodium phosphates (e.g., Fleet Phosphosoda)
      iii. Polyethylene glycol (e.g., GoLytely)
   d. Hyperosmotics
      i. Glycerin
         • Bowel evacuation within 30 minutes.
         • Applied rectally to soften stool and lubricate rectum.
      ii. Lactulose

B. **Mini-enemas**
   1. Produce bowel movement within 15 minutes.
   2. Low volume (~ 4 ml).
   3. Theravac = docusate + glycerin/polyethylene glycol ± benzocaine anesthetic.
      a. Triggers peristalsis, provides lubrication, and softens stool.
      b. Commonly used in SCI to minimize nocioceptive stimuli that may induce AD.

C. **Enemas**
   1. Bowel cleansing in preparation for surgery or diagnostic procedure.
   2. Use sparingly to prevent bowel complications.
   3. Use when more conservative care has failed.

D. **Prokinetic agents:** metoclopramide (Reglan), erythromycin

VI. **Surgery**
A. **Colostomy**
   1. **Procedure of last resort** for treatment of fecal incontinence or difficulty with evacuation.

2. **Indications**
   a. Conservative bowel care has failed.
   b. Intrinsic bowel deficits such as Hirschsprung's disease, Chagas' disease, or "cathartic colon."
   c. Pressure ulcers or other skin lesions that cannot heal due to frequent soiling.
   d. Recurrent urinary tract seeding by repetitive bowel impactions.
3. **Sigmoid colostomy vs. ileostomy:** choice is based on transit-time studies.
   a. If entire colon is atonic, ileostomy is chosen.
   b. If markers accumulate in rectosigmoid colon, sigmoid colostomy is chosen.

B. **Catheterizable appendicocecostomy stoma**
1. **Indications**
   a. Prolonged bowel care time.
   b. Recurrent fecal impactions.
   c. Poor or intermittent response to rectal medications to initiate bowel care.
2. **Antegrade continence enema**
   a. Stoma is catheterized and infused with 200–600 ml tap water.
   b. Triggers propulsive colonic peristalsis and defecation in 10–20 minutes.

C. **Anal sphincter repair:** indicated for patients with deficient EAS without neurologic damage (e.g., aging).

D. **Muscle transplant surgery**
1. Indicated for patients with deficient EAS and sacral nerve deficits.
2. Involves transposition of innervated muscle or free muscle graft (gracilis, adductor longus, gluteus maximus, palmaris longus) to replace puborectalis, levator ani, or EAS functions.

E. **Myotomy**
1. Indicated for patients with constipation due to incomplete EAS relaxation during defecation.
2. Involves IAS and partial EAS incision.
3. Not popular.
4. Relieves constipation in 62%, but results in fecal incontinence in 16%.

VII. Complications of Neurogenic Bowel
A. **Fecal impaction**
1. Affects 80% of patients with SCI by 5 years after injury.
2. May be manifest by overflow diarrhea.
3. May trigger AD.
4. May lead to perforated viscus.
5. Treatment
   a. Prevention with stool softeners, diet, fluids.
   b. Manual disimpaction in conjunction with laxatives or enemas.
   c. If repeatedly associated with AD, ileostomy or colostomy may be indicated.

B. **Traumatic superficial mucosal erosion**
1. Most common cause of bright red rectal bleeding after SCI.
2. Characterized by streaks of blood on glove or stool.
3. Treat conservatively.

C. **Hemorrhoids**
1. Caused by increased rectal pressures associated with prolonged efforts to remove hard stool.
2. Exacerbated by suppositories, enemas, or digital stimulation.

3. Treatment
   a. Prevention with stool softeners or gel or air cushion to support pelvic floor and evenly distribute pressure over entire perineum.
   b. Frequent digital stimulation to minimize time to complete bowel care.
   c. Symptomatic treatment with topical steroid ointments and medicated suppositories.
   d. Surgical consultation
      i. Indications
         • No response to conservative treatment.
         • Bleeding characterized by dripping into commode or passing clots.
         • Mucus soilage
         • Difficulty with hygiene
      ii. Procedures
         • Rubber band ligation
         • Operative hemorrhoidectomy

D. **Rectal prolapse**
   1. Associated with overstretched, patulous sphincter due to passage of very large hard stool secondary to LMNB.
   2. Treatment
      a. Avoid straining and stretching of atonic bowel.
      b. Stool softening with diet or medications.
      c. Avoid Valsalva maneuver.
      d. *Gentle* manual disimpaction if needed to protect denervated structures.
      e. Temporary colostomy allows overdistended bowel to regain tone.

E. **Rectal bleeding**
   1. Common causes include traumatic superficial injury and hemorrhoids.
   2. Consider and rule out other sources, if indicated (e.g., colorectal cancer).

F. **Bloating, abdominal distention, and flatulence**
   1. May be severe in patients with anorectal dyssynergia (increased EAS tone in response to rectal distention).
   2. Treatment
      a. Increase frequency of bowel program.
      b. Avoid gas producing foods (e.g., beans).
      c. Digital release of flatus.
      d. Antiflatulent medications (containing simethicone).

G. **Premature diverticulosis**

H. **Megacolon**
   1. Needs eventual decompression; surgical consultation is warranted for possible surgical intervention.
   2. Nothing by mouth is indicated with upper GI decompression; nasogastric tube for continuous suction should be considered.

I. **Autonomic dysreflexia** (see Chapter 8, Spinal Cord Injury Rehabilitation)

VIII. **Long-term Care**

A. **Screening:** indicated in patients > 45 years old for colorectal cancer.
   1. Flexible sigmoidoscopy: if polyps or tumor is seen, perform full colonoscopy.
   2. Fecal occult blood test: good for initial screening but may be of little value because of frequency of rectal bleeding.

B. **Strive for regular and predictable bowel emptying**

1. Improves quality of life
2. Reduces risk of chronic GI problems

Bibliography
1. Bergman SB: Bowel management. In Nesathurai S (ed): The Rehabilitation of People with Spinal Cord Injury: A House Officer's Guide. Boston, Arbuckle Academic Publishers, 1999, pp 47–52.
2. Consortium for Spinal Cord Medicine: Neurogenic Bowel Managemente in Adults with Spinal Cord Injury. Washington, DC, Paralyzed Veterans of America, 1998.
3. King JC, Stiens SA: Neurogenic bowel: Dysfunction and management. In Grabois M (ed): Physical Medicine and Rehabilitation: The Complete Approach. Malden, MA, Blackwell Science, 2000, pp 579–590.
4. Linsenmeyer TA, Stone JM: Neurogenic bladder and bowel dysfunction. In DeLisa JA (ed): Rehabilitation Medicine: Principles and Practice. Philadelphia, Lippincott Williams & Wilkins, 1993, pp 733–758.
5. Stiens S, Goetz L: Neurogenic bowel dysfunction. In O'Young B, Young M, Stiens S (eds): Physical Medicine and Rehabilitation Secrets. Philadelphia, Hanley & Belfus, 1997, pp 460–464.
6. Tan JC: Practical Manual of Physical Medicine and Rehabilitation. St. Louis, Mosby, 1998, pp 553–579.

Chapter 17

REHABILITATION PSYCHOLOGY AND NEUROPSYCHOLOGY CONSULTATION

Seth Warschausky, Ph.D., Jeffrey E. Evans, Ph.D., and Anne Bradley, Ph.D.

I. General Principles

A. **Rehabilitation psychology** addresses the health and well-being of persons with disabilities. On the inpatient service, rehabilitation psychology and neuropsychology (RPN) provide:

1. Assessment of psychological and neuropsychological status, including monitoring cognitive recovery
2. Psychological intervention
3. Family education and treatment
4. Team-level support, education, and information critical to interventions (e.g., awareness of deficits, competence and safety)
5. Discharge planning recommendations

B. **Pediatric and adult services:** numerous key distinctions differentiate the role of RPN in adult vs. pediatric inpatient services.

1. Psychological needs on adult service include addressing:
   a. Stress associated with change in ability to meet adult responsibilities (e.g., occupational and caregiving roles)
   b. Reactions to change in independence
   c. Reactions to increased morbidity and mortality risks
   d. Effects on marital and other family relationships.
2. Psychological needs of pediatric inpatients include addressing:
   a. Age-specific understandings of medical implications, including death or permanent disability
   b. Separation from family during hospitalization
   c. Family reactions and education regarding psychological and social implications and changes in family roles necessary to compensate for new deficits
   d. School-related needs
   e. Peer reactions

II. Neuropsychological Status: Recovery and Progress

A. **Overview**

1. RPN provides serial assessments of neuropsychological status that differ from those of other disciplines, such as speech/language pathology or occupational therapy, by providing broad overview of relative strengths and weaknesses in context of a patient's personality and emotional functioning.

2. In addition, RPN provides information critical to team decisions about safety and competence and education for family and team about patient status, recovery, and prognosis across basic neuropsychological domains, which include:

   a. **Arousal:** level of alertness.

   b. **Processing speed:** rates of information processing and responding.

   c. **Attention:** ability to select information for processing, span of apprehension, vigilance and complex mental tracking.

   d. **Executive functions:** control of information processing, as in task switching, working memory, goal formulation and planning.

   e. **Memory:** retention, learning, and retrieval.

   f. **Verbal functions:** expressive and receptive language and reasoning.

   g. **Perceptual functions:** visual and tactile skills and reasoning.

   h. **Manual sensorimotor functioning:** fine motor speed and dexterity.

3. RPN consults with physicians about need for psychopharmacologic intervention and assists in assessing effects of medication over time.

B. **Neurocognitive assessment: nonstandardized procedures**

   1. Clinical interview of patient and family to assess awareness, attention, safety, strengths and weaknesses.

   2. Naturalistic and structured observation to assess competency; perceptual, sensory, verbal, and visual/spatial processing; executive functioning.

C. **Common measures specific to neurocognitive domain(s) by age**

   1. **Adults and older adolescents**

      a. Aphasia screening, including multilingual aphasia examination (MAE)

      b. Boston Naming Test: expressive naming/vocabulary

      c. Category Test: executive functions

      d. Cognistat: screening of range of functions

      e. California Verbal Learning Test (CVLT): verbal memory, learning

      f. Controlled Oral Word Association (COWA): word fluency

      g. Digit Symbol Test: processing speed

      h. Dementia Rating Scale (DRS): domains affected by dementia

      i. Galveston Orientation and Amnesia Test (GOAT)

      j. Rey-Osterrieth Test: visual construction and memory

      k. Symbol Digit Modalities Test (SDMT): processing speed

      l. Spatial Span Test: immediate and working memory

      m. Stroop Test: inhibition, executive function

      n. Test of Everyday Attention (TEA): range of attention functions

      o. Trail-Making Test: complex attention

      p. Developmental Test of Visuo-Motor Integration (VMI): visual construction, graphomotor function

      q. Wechsler Adult Intelligence Scale–Third Edition (WAIS)/Wechsler Abbreviated Scales of Intelligence (WASI): IQ estimate and range of functions

      r. Recognition Memory Test (RMT): memory

      s. Wechsler Memory Scale (WMS): attention and memory functions

      t. Wisconsin Card-Sorting Test (WCST): executive functions

   2. **Younger adolescents and children**

      a. Children's Orientation and Amnesia Test (COAT): orientation and immediate memory

      b. CVLT for Children (CVLT-C): verbal memory, learning

    c. Children's Memory Scale (CMS): attention and memory functions

    d. Coding: processing speed

    e. NEPSY: range of neurocognitive functions

    f. Peabody Picture Vocabulary Test–Third Edition (PPVT): receptive vocabulary, naming

    g. Rey-Osterreith Test: visual construction and memory

    h. SDMT: processing speed

    i. Spatial Span Test: immediate and working memory

    j. TEA for Children (TEA-Ch): range of attention functions

    k. Trail-Making Test: complex attention

    l. VMI: visual-motor integration

    m. Wide Range Assessment of Memory and Learning (WRAML): attention and memory functions

    n. Wechsler Intelligence Scale for Children (WISC)/WASI: IQ estimate and range of function

  3. **Preschoolers and infants**

    a. Bayley Scales of Infant Development: range of cognitive and sensorimotor functions

    b. Child Development Inventory (CDI): developmental questionnaire

    c. McCarthy Scalest: range of cognitive functions

    d. NEPSY: range of neurocognitive functions

    e. Wechsler Preschool and Primary Scale of Intelligence (WPPSI): range of cognitive functions

D. **Prognostic indicators** for neurobehavioral recovery

  1. Depth of coma (Glasgow Coma Scale)

  2. Duration of posttraumatic amnesia

  3. Cerebral perfusion pressure

  4. Pupillary reactivity

  5. Presence of hemispatial neglect

  6. Age

  7. Awareness of deficit

  8. Psychosocial history

E. **Neuropsychological screening**

  1. Inpatient neuropsychological testing typically takes the form of screening via interview, observation, and brief qualitative and quantitative measures.

    a. Depending on referral question, screening can have breadth of coverage or focus on one or more functions (e.g., executive functioning, attention, memory, perception, construction, praxis, language).

    b. Neuropsychological screening contributes to team's assessment of awareness, attention, safety, strengths and weaknesses, and competence.

    c. Patients with suspected mild traumatic brain injury (TBI) should be referred to RPN if they report any alteration in consciousness at scene of injury or complain of cognitive or emotional sequelae.

  2. Full-battery assessment involves 1 day of testing, often after hospital discharge. Goals include the following:

    a. Update treatment plan.

    b. Provide baseline for comparison with future assessments.

    c. Form recommendations about supports or interventions needed to return to higher levels of functioning, such as independent living, work, or school.

    d. Breadth and depth of coverage allow more thorough evaluations, including estimates of premorbid ability and postacute motivation for rehabilitation.

F. **Screening for awareness and attention**

  1. **Diminished awareness** is common problem in brain injury, particularly when injury involves right hemisphere or frontal lobes.

    a. Anosagnosia (diminished awareness of deficit) affects patients' ability to participate fully in rehabilitation therapy because of their incomplete awareness that anything is wrong.

    b. Quality and extent of anosagnosia is typically assessed by interview and observation.

    c. Patients also may exhibit diminished awareness of their general life circumstances, not limited to deficits. This has important implications for their ability to make decisions that require the normal broad understanding of what is going on in their own lives.

  2. **Impaired attention** compromises learning and memory with implications for participation in therapy and safety at home.

    a. Hemispatial neglect (hemi-inattention) is a disorder of attention and perception affecting the side of space contralateral to cerebral lesion. Patients are typically inattentive to affected side and are often unaware of it as well.

    b. Neglect is common in focal lesions, particularly of right hemisphere, such as seen in stroke and TBI, and is usually evaluated on basis of perceptual-motor tasks.

    c. Safety is major concern in neglect; severe, persistent neglect suggests poor prognosis for return to independent functioning.

G. **Screening for safety**

  1. In addition to attention and awareness, memory, visual-spatial ability, global judgment, and neurobehavioral symptoms are central to screening for safety, especially when patients will be home alone.

  2. **Memory disorders** are common in all forms of brain injury or illness and can be limited to a single modality (e.g., verbal, visual), include multiple modalities, or be global.

    a. Short-term memory (minutes) is particularly vulnerable to injury, but long-term or even remote memory (years) also can be affected.

    b. Screening tests for memory emphasize short-term verbal and visual modalities.

    c. Posttraumatic amnesia (PTA), the global inability to form accurate new memories (including of place, time and circumstance), is common in acute phase of recovery from TBI.

    d. Persisting PTA suggests need for 24-hour assistance for safety.

  2. **Visual-spatial ability** governs functions such as tool use, hand-eye coordination, and judgment of relative position of objects in space.

    a. Impairment is common in right hemisphere injury but may accompany brain injury to other loci.

    b. Typical screening tests include drawing and block construction.

    c. Patients with impairment are often discharged with restrictions on activities that may pose danger.

  3. **Global judgment** refers to ability to behave or respond appropriately in given context.

    a. Impairment is common in frontal lobe injury and typically is assessed via interview and observation.

b. It is central to maintenance of social relationships and other complex involvements of daily life.

c. For some patients, assistance with judgment involves constant supervision; for others, it involves assistance at certain times or with certain functions.

4. Prominent **neurobehavioral symptoms** include impulsivity (acting too quickly or acting before thinking) and akinesia (acting too slowly or not at all). Impulsivity is of particular concern, especially when it coexists with poor judgment, impaired awareness or perceptual difficulties.

H. **Screening for strengths and weaknesses**

1. In rehabilitation therapy, which helps patients compensate for areas of deficiency, it is important to gauge cognitive strengths as well as weaknesses. To accomplish this goal, breadth of coverage of modalities and cognitive domains is required in a screening battery.

2. If patient performs poorly on verbal but not visual memory tasks, it is possible that transforming verbal material to be remembered into a visual format will improve memory functioning.

3. If patient is impulsive but responds well to verbal cues to slow down and has a good memory, it is possible that self-cueing can be developed.

4. If patient has left hemispatial neglect but some awareness of the fact, it is possible to train orientation of gaze to left so that left side of space may be brought into intact visual field.

5. Screening for strengths and weaknesses can assist with treatment planning for both inpatients and outpatients. It can also assist with patient and family education, especially in improving understanding of the disorder and ultimately increasing motivation and cooperation with treatment.

I. **Screening for competence**

1. Questions of competence arise frequently in inpatient rehabilitation and generally refer to ability to handle important life activities or make important decisions.

2. In question may be concrete tasks, such as keeping checkbook, or more global activities, such as financial management, dispensing own medication, general medical decision-making, deciding where to live, or deciding if to live.

3. Issues of awareness, neglect, judgment, and diminished intellectual capacity are primary in questions of competence; which competencies are in question determines appropriate modes and methods of assessment.

III. **Referrals for Psychological Assessment and Treatment**

A. **Emotional and behavioral characteristics that put family and patient at risk** for poor participation in rehabilitation and ability to cope include premorbid and present traits.

1. **Premorbid risk factors**

a. **Patients**

i. Impaired insight

ii. Drug or alcohol abuse

iii. Impulsive behavior

iv. Failure to follow through on medical treatment

v. Poor judgment that endangers self or others

vi. Recent history of important emotional losses

vii. Paucity of coping resources, including social isolation and rigid coping style

viii. Prior diagnosis of psychopathology or mood disorder

  b. **Families**
     i. History of neglect, child or elder abuse, domestic violence
     ii. Discord between patient and spouse/partner
     iii. Spouse/partner of patient with significant cognitive deficits
     iv. Parents of child patient with significant cognitive deficits
  2. **Present risk factors**
     a. **Patients**
        i. Behavioral and emotional symptoms of adjustment disorders which, while not clinically significant, have impact on ability to function
        ii. Psychological symptoms that are severe enough to reach clinical diagnosis (e.g., depressive episode, posttraumatic stress disorder)
        iii. Inability to consider long-term consequences
        iv. Denial of severity of impact of deficits
        v. Poor insight into deficits
     b. **Families**
        i. Exacerbated conflict among family members, particularly those in care-taking role
        ii. Inappropriate levels of conflict with medical staff
        iii. Inability to take in new information
        iv. Inability to consider long-term consequences
        v. Denial of severity of impact of deficits
  B. **Treatment**
     1. Assess at what point common adjustment symptoms become **indicators of need for intervention** (Table 1).
     2. **Patient and family education and treatment**
        a. Education covers such issues as:
           i. Ongoing feedback about neurocognitive and psychological recovery from injury
           ii. Patient's current status in relation to typical recovery patterns
           iii. Emotional, family, and community resources necessary to optimize functioning while in rehabilitation and after discharge
           iv. Emotions underlying behavioral difficulties and emotional symptoms common to adjustment
        b. Psychotherapy
           i. Given limited lengths of stay, goal of therapeutic intervention is to address acute issues impeding patient's and family's ability to participate in rehabilitation and make transition to life outside hospital.
           ii. RPN services often do not have resources, and patients and families are often not hospitalized long enough, to address effectively long-standing premorbid psychological issues during the inpatient stay.
           iii. RPN can address how long-standing issues affect current adjustment to trauma and how trauma affects even well-functioning individuals and families. Recommendations should be made for appropriate follow-up on discharge.
           v. Focus during inpatient stay is often two-fold: to increase coping and to reduce stress (Table 2).
IV. **Team Resources and Treatment**
  A. Rehabilitation patients and their families often are in acute crisis, with intense emotional distress and disorganized behavior that is confusing and anxiety-provoking.

TABLE 1.   Indicators of Need for Intervention

Domain	Distressed but Adaptive	Questionable	Coping Overwhelmed
Sleeping	Restless but sufficient sleep within 24-hr period	Insufficient sleep in 24-hr period; catch-up within few days	Arousal, energy, and emotional regulation impaired
Eating	Eating less or more than usual, but takes in mini-mally sufficient nutrition	Nutritional intake is insufficient but vari-able or occasionally seeks out food as soothing	Nutritional intake is chronically insufficient or compulsively ex-cessive
Attention/ concentration/ memory	Preoccupied and needs reminders but able to learn and participate in care	Needs frequent remin-ders but can partici-pate in care	Difficulty with learning new skills, taking in new information, participat-ing meaningfully in care
Depressed mood/affect	Transitory periods of sad affect, able to perceive positive aspects and has hope	More time spent ex-hibiting sad than positive affect, but recognizes hopeful aspects	Flat affect, little enjoy-ment of day-to-day positive aspects of life, little hope
Frustration tolerance	Occasionally irritable in pro-portion with irritating situa-tion/event	Fairly easily irritated, variable persistence in face of challenges	Chronically irritable, un-able to tolerate small day-to-day frustrations, gives up easily/with-draws
Anxiety	Tense but able to soothe self enough to have periods of calm	Needs soothing from others to have periods of calm	Disorganized behavior, does not respond to soothing from others easily, causes anxiety in others
Behavioral control	Flees tense situations or engages in infrequent mild/moderate conflicts	Engages in periodic mild/moderate con-flicts	Engages in frequent mild/moderate con-flicts or any severe conflict
Initiation	Procrastinates but makes decisions or acts when needed	Needs reminders/dead-lines to make deci-cision or act	Does not meet deadlines for decisions or actions

TABLE 2.   Common Means of Assisting Ability to Cope with Acute Trauma

Increase Coping Repertoire	Decrease Sources of Stress
• Develop new resources; highlight alerting function of emotional distress or dis-rupted behavior and assist in activation of premorbid coping mechanisms	• Provide education about hospital environment to reduce unknown
• Provide emotional support as new coping resource	• Normalize emotional distress and limitations on ability to meet socially sanctioned role expectations
• Remove internal or external impediments to premorbid coping resources	• Process and integrate new information, assisting with integration into preexisting conceptual frameworks
• Redirect ineffective use of coping resour-ces to more effective expression	• Act as mediator between family and medical staff
• Refer for psychotherapeutic or psychiatric interventions for long-standing premorbid pathology	

B. Intense emotions tend to reverberate from one person to another, creating emotionally stressful work environment. RPN professionals bring skills to the rehabilitation team that can help with managing both chronic and acute work stressors. As well as being versed in the functioning of individuals, psychologists are trained in the functioning of human systems, whether families or work units.

C. **Team intervention**
   1. **Common indicators of need**
      a. Team or team member makes mistake that is distressing to team or team member.
      b. Team or team member lashes back at family in distress.
      c. Patient dies.
      d. Team members' manner of interacting with each other starts to parallel self-defeating patterns of interaction among members of family being served.
      e. Team is caught in repetitive, never-resolving cycles of conflict over particular issue.
   2. **Methods of intervention**
      a. Typically informal.
      b. RPN professionals are usually most effective in making sure that team's preferred methods of coping are available to members rather than providing direct services.
      c. RPN professionals act as coworkers who have particular expertise in dealing with emotions and interpersonal relationships.
   3. **Specific issues and situations that preclude intervention by RPN team member and necessitate outside intervention**
      a. Problem involves RPN professional on team.
      b. Team members are having difficulty performing and are not comfortable with using RPN or each other as coping resource.
      c. RPN professional is not able/willing to act as informal resource because of his or her own coping needs.
      d. Team member exhibits signs of psychopathology, clinical levels of emotional dysfunction, or substance abuse that impairs work performance.

V. **Discharge Planning Recommendations**
   A. **Need for outpatient psychological services** as well as specific information about the following:
      1. Psychological status at time of discharge
      2. "Frontal" symptomatology
         a. Distinction between lack of initiation/motivation stemming from psychological or environmental factors vs. organic executive dysfunction.
         b. Organic contributions to other types of affective or behavioral difficulties, including anxiety and aggression.
      3. Psychological and neuropsychological factors in social functioning.
   B. **Family desires and capabilities**
      1. Motivation to meet patient's needs.
      2. Ability to cope with stress specific to patient's home care needs.
      3. Ability to provide supervision and appropriate levels of structure and routine.
      4. Ability to advocate for services and resources.
   C. **Implications of patient's status for community reintegration**
      1. Psychological and neuropsychological factors in performance of activities of daily living

2. Employment and vocational training
3. Education, including specific special educational needs
4. Social integration needs, including focused interventions

Bibliography

1. Broman SH, Michel ME (eds): Traumatic Head Injury in Children. New York, Oxford University Press, 1995.
2. Frank RG, Elliott TR (eds): Handbook of Rehabilitation Psychology. Washington, D.C., American Psychological Association, 2000.
3. Lezak M: Neuropsychological Assessment, 3rd ed. New York, Oxford University Press, 1995.
4. Prigatano GP, Schacter DL: Awareness of Deficit After Brain Injury: Clinical and Theoretical Issues. New York, Oxford University Press, 1991.
5. Rosenthal M, Griffith ER, Bond MR, Miller JD (eds): Rehabilitation of the Adult and Child with Traumatic Brain Injury, 2nd ed. Philadelphia, F.A. Davis Company, 1990.
6. Spreen O, Strauss E: Compendium of Neuropsychological Tests, 2nd ed. New York, Oxford University Press, 1998.

Chapter 18

PRESSURE ULCERS: PREVENTION AND CARE

David Klipp, M.D., M. Catherine Spires, M.D., and Paula M. Anton, R.N., M.S.A.

I. General Principles

A. Pressure ulcers (decubitus ulcers) are a persistent problem of hospitalized rehabilitation patients, prolonging length of stay, delaying return to home, and altering patient's function and lifestyle.

B. Problem is increasing, especially in present health-care system, which is focused on cost containment.

C. Good news is that increasing treatment modalities and preventative measures can be implemented .

D. Term "decubitus" is derived from Latin adjective meaning "lying down." Pressure ulceration can result from any prolonged, unchanged position.

E. Pressure ulcers are clinical manifestation of local tissue death and catabolism.

F. Ulcers are found most frequently over bony prominences exposed to compressing surfaces.

G. Geriatric patients are at high risk because of epidermal thinning, decreased elasticity, loss of dermal blood vessels, and flattening of dermal-epidermal ridges associated with aging.

H. All strategies for prevention need to be continued during pressure ulcer treatment. Same risk factors that cause pressure ulcers may prevent them from healing.

I. Pressure ulcers should be staged according to severity. Classification systems are based on depth. Table 1 offers system consistent with recommendations of National Pressure Ulcer Advisory Panel (NPUAP).

II. Epidemiology

A. **Incidence** varies widely by hospitalized population.

1. 7.7% of hospitalized patients develop pressure ulcers within 21 days of admission.

2. Within orthopedic and geriatric subpopulations, incidence rates are as high as 24%.

3. Incidence among patients with spinal cord injury (SCI) ranges from 24% to 59% and correlates with severity of paralysis.

4. Incidence is controllable: one rehabilitation hospital reported zero incidence in controlled studies.

B. **Prevalence**

1. Rehabilitation population overall has prevalence of 25% at admission from acute care settings.

TABLE 1.   Pressure Ulcer Classification System

Stage I	Pressure-related area of intact skin with nonblanchable erythema compared with adjacent or opposite area on body; may include changes in one or more of following: skin temperature; tissue consistency; and/or sensation. Ulcer appears as defined area of redness in light skin or red, blue or purple hues in darker skin (also known as "the heralding lesion of skin ulceration"). This lesion should not be confused with reactive hyperemia (see main text, below), which resolves with removal of occlusion to blood flow to affected area.
Stage II	Partial-thickness skin ulcer, superficial lesion resembling abrasion, blister, or shallow crater, involving less than total loss of epidermis and/ or dermis
Stage III	Full-thickness skin loss with damage or necrosis of underlying tissue. Stage III extends down to, but not through, underlying fascia. Resembles deep crater with or without undermining of adjacent tissue.
Stage IV	Full-thickness skin loss with extensive destruction, tissue necrosis, or damage to muscle, tendon, bone, or supporting structures. Undermining and tunneling should be expected and rigorously assessed.

Note: Pressure ulcers with slough or eschar cannot be staged because full extent or depth of ulcer cannot be determined without debridement of slough or eschar.

General caveat: Staging classification system cannot be used to monitor progress over time. Pressure ulcer healing does not progress in reverse staging order (i.e., "the ulcer was stage III but now looks like stage I" is an incorrect assessment). A healing stage III or IV ulcer may resemble the depth of a stage II ulcer; it must, however, be documented as a healing stage III or IV ulcer. By so doing, both ongoing and postdischarge care can be provided and reimbursed appropriately.

    2. Patients with SCI have reported prevalence of 25–40%.

    3. Geriatric population has overall prevalence of 17.4%; among elderly patients admitted from acute care, prevalence is 83.4%.

  C. **Role in health care economy**

    1. Considered major preventable problem by Agency for Health Care Policy and Research (AHCPR).

    2. 836 million health care dollars spent with pressure ulcers as primary diagnosis in 1992.

    3. 500 million health care dollars spent with pressure ulcers as secondary diagnosis.

    4. More prevention and aggressive treatment are needed to reduce human and economic costs.

III. Prevention

  A. **Understanding of etiologic factors**

    1. **Pressure**

      a. Consider both duration and intensity.

        i. Inverse pressure-time relationship: low pressure over long periods is more damaging than high pressure for short periods.

        ii. If thresholds of duration and intensity are exceeded, damage will continue despite relief.

      b. Average capillary inflow pressure is 32 mmHg.

      c. Skin pressure support at < 32 mmHg prevents ischemia.

      d. Relief of pressure is characterized by bright red flush to area (called **reactive hyperemia**).

    2. **Shear**

      a. Occurs with movement of underlying tissues with skin adherent or stationary (e.g., sacral skin adherent to bed linens)

    b. Skin ischemia results in "shear ulcer" characterized by wide undermining around base of visible ulcer

    c. Common causes

        i. Poor sitting position

        ii. Poor bed positioning

        iii. Spasticity

        iv. Sliding instead of lifting patient for transfers

  3. **Friction** (e.g., skin tears, abrasions)

  4. **Secondary factors**

    a. Mobility   f. Smoking

    b. Nutrition   g. Elevated body temperature

    c. Age   h. Impaired mental status

    d. Moisture/incontinence

    e. Diabetes

  5. Some of these criteria have been used to develop a scale to help identify patients at risk (Table 2).

B. **Primary prevention** focuses on relief from prolonged, positional pressure.

  1. Figure 1 indicates areas of high risk in sitting, supine, and side-lying positions. Pressure over these sites should be avoided or reduced to a minimum.

  2. For patients who need assistance with transfers or bed mobility, manually lift patient; avoid sliding patient's body across surfaces

TABLE 2. Dutch Consensus Meeting for the Prevention of Pressure Sores Risk Score*

Variable	Score			
	0	1	2	3
Mental status	Normal	Listless, depressed, frightened	Severely depressed, psychotic, apathetic	(Semi)comatose
Neurologic status	Normal	Minor disorders, minor loss of strength	Loss of sensation, partial hemiparesis (points × 2)	Hemiparesis (points × 2) Paraparesis below T5 (× 3) Paraparesis above T6 (× 4)
Mobility	Normal	Limited, walks with help	Nonambulatory	Always in bed
Nutritional status	Good	Moderate, no food for several days	Poor, no food for 1 week	Emaciated
Nutritional intake	Normal, good appetite	Parenteral	No appetite, insufficient feeding	None
Incontinence	None	Occasionally urinary	No control but catheter in place	Fecal and urinary
Age (yr)	< 50	50–59	60–69	> 70
Temperature (°C)	> 35.5 < 37.5	> 37.4 < 38.5	> 38.4 < 39.0	< 35.6 > 38.9
Medication	None	Corticosteroids, sedatives, anticoagulants	Tranquilizers, chemotherapy, oral antibiotics	Parenteral antibiotics
Diabetes	None	Diet-controlled	Diet and oral medication control regimen	Diet and insulin regimen

* Score > 8 indicates that patient is at risk.
From Hofman A, Geelkerken RHK, Wille J, et al: Pressure sores and pressure-decreasing mattresses: Controlled clinical trial. Lancet 343:458–571, with permission.

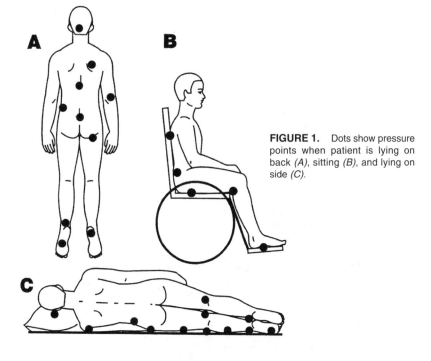

FIGURE 1. Dots show pressure points when patient is lying on back *(A)*, sitting *(B)*, and lying on side *(C)*.

    3. Patient should be repositioned every 2 hours.
    4. Inspect and assess skin with each turning.
    5. **Requirements for wheelchair-using patients**
      a. Maximal support over available seated area.
      b. Position foot plates to avoid excessive pressure over ischium, transferring weight to thighs.
      c. Position changes every 15–20 minutes
      d. Weight shifting or relief
        i. Anterior, lateral, and press-up weight-shifting techniques
        ii. Patients with SCI may benefit from power tilt or reclining mechanism, which allows relative independence in weight shifting.
  C. **Support surfaces** (Table 3)
    1. Patients who are at risk for ulcers at time of discharge from hospital should be prescribed bed and mattress with pressure relief system, such as gel inserts.
    2. It is cost-effective for hospitals and other inpatient facilities to select mattresses with built-in pressure relief systems. Initial investment is high, but benefit of reduced incidence of pressure sores and financial burden will prove cost effective in long run.
IV. Wound Assessment and Classification
  A. **Area**
    1. Initial size of wound is important factor in determining rate of healing.
    2. Measure and document size in centimeters by length, width, and depth.
    3. Large shallow wounds, like skin-graft donor sites, are covered with new epithelium at about same rate as small shallow wounds, especially if kept moist.
    4. In contrast, large deep wounds take longer to heal than small deep wounds.

TABLE 3. Support Surfaces

Type	Advantages	Disadvantages
Static surfaces		
Foam	Inexpensive, lightweight, versatile	Poor durability, absorbs odors and liquids, one patient use
Air-filled cushion or mattress	Easily cleaned, lightweight, good pressure relief	More expensive, less stable, susceptible to puncture/rupture, requires monitoring for proper inflation
Flotation (gel or water)	Adjusts to patient's movement, provides good pressure relief	Expensive, retains body heat, heavy
Combination cushions (e.g., gel mattress on foam base)	Provides good pressure relief, supports good posturing of patient	Expensive, retains body heat, heavy
Mattresses/beds		
Dynamic overlays	Portable, good moisture control, cleaned easily	Expensive, require powering, considered "noisy"
Low-air-loss bed/ overlays	Good pressure relief, reduces friction/shear; overlays may be portable; good moisture control	Expensive
Air-fluidized beds	Good fluid/moisture absorption, good pressure relief, bacteriostatic glass beads reduce nosocomial infections	Expensive, may dehydrate patient, reported sensory deprivation in patient, transfers more difficult

B. **Depth**
  1. Wound depth profoundly affects rate of healing.
  2. Wounds healing by secondary intention or formation of granulation tissue are classified by depth.
  3. To measure depth of deep wounds, gently insert gloved finger into deepest part of the wound bed; mark and measure against centimeter ruler; measure wound dimensions regularly; compare with previous measurement

C. **Wound bed**
  1. Condition of wound bed provides information about progress of healing and effectiveness of treatment.
  2. Significant amount of fibrin slough or necrotic tissue in wound bed suggests inadequate wound debridement, an impediment to wound healing.
  3. Appearance of red-to-pink circumferential, granulation tissue indicates that healing is progressing.

D. **Exudate:** visually appraise amount and character (color, viscosity, odor) of wound drainage.

E. **Integrity of surrounding skin**
  1. Monitor and document wound margins for signs of maceration or inflammation (erythema, edema, pain).
  2. Inflammation may be caused by unrelieved pressure and/or adverse reactions to wound care treatment.
  3. Skin maceration
     a. Caused by prolonged contact of wound fluid with skin.
     b. Sign that topical wound treatment is inappropriate for patient.

F. **Induration:** hardened tissue that can be palpated on intact skin around pressure ulcer or wound.

G. **Infection**
   1. Cardinal signs of wound infection are warmth, pain, erythema, edema, induration, purulence.
   2. Assess surrounding wound tissue for cellulitis.
   3. Tissue biopsy should be obtained to confirm infection and isolate infective organisms.
   4. Osteomyelitis must be considered.
H. **Additional complications of pressure ulcers**
   1. Cellulitis
   2. Septic arthritis
   3. Sinus tract infection or abscess
   4. Fistula formation
   5. Sepsis (endocarditis; meningitis)
   6. Heterotopic ossification
   7. Maggot infestation (however, in some parts of world, maggots are accepted therapeutic option because they ingest only necrotic tissue)
   8. Pseudoaneurysm
   9. Squamous cell carcinoma (requires years to develop)
   10. Sequelae of treatment modalities (toxicities, allergic reactions)
V. **Assessing the Three Stages of Normal Healing Process**
   A. **Inflammatory phase**
      1. **Findings on physical exam:** edema, erythema, warmth and pain.
      2. Typically lasts for about 3 days.
      3. Vasoconstriction occurs in first seconds and lasts for short period; platelets and thrombin aggregate along injured vessels; initiation of coagulation cascade.
      4. Vasodilatation; prostaglandin release; leakage of proteins.
      5. Leukocyte migration
         a. Neutrophils for first 3 days.
         b. Macrophages release growth factors, facilitate chemotaxis.
         c. Phagocytosis "debrides" wound.
      6. Fibrinogen sequesters lymphatics and tissue spaces to prevent spread of infection; scab is caused by dehydration of fibrin network.
      7. Goals of treatment
         a. To initiate hemostasis and prevent spread of infection
         b. To clean area
         c. To lay groundwork for repair
   B. **Proliferative phase**
      1. **Findings on physical exam:** pink-to-red granulation tissue circumscribes wound.
      2. **Granulation tissue:** beefy red appearance; fibroblasts actively synthesize collagen, elastic fibers, and fibronectin "scaffold" over which epidermal migration occurs.
      3. **Epithelialization:** thin silvery appearance circumscribes red granulation tissue; migrates inward, covering wound.
      4. **Wound contraction:** caused by fibroblasts transforming into myofibroblasts with contractile properties pulling margins of wound together.
         a. Begins during inflammatory phase and continues through maturation.
         b. Function is to resurface and strengthen wound.
         c. Formation of granulation tissue, epithelialization, and contraction of wound borders.

C. **Maturation phase**
   1. **Findings on physical exam:** scar tissue shrinkage and paling of wound site.
   2. Begins within 3 weeks and may continue over months to years.
   3. Final phase of wound healing, in which scar forms and fades, often called "remodeling."
   4. Strengthening and reorganization of collagen into scar.
   5. Capillary regression after healing is responsible for decreased erythema.

VI. **Wound Management Priorities**
   A. **Reduce or eliminate causative factors** (refer to Section III, above).
   B. **Provide systemic support for wound healing.**
      1. Tissue perfusion and oxygenation
      2. Nutritional and fluid support
         a. Optimal nutrition is imperative for wound healing.
         b. Obtain nutritional assessment to determine if patient intake is adequate.
         c. 30–50% of inpatients in U.S. hospitals are malnourished.
         d. Baseline laboratory evaluation should include serum albumin and pre-albumin.
            i. Serum albumin level reflects nutritional status 2–3 weeks before because half-life of albumin is 15–19 days.
            ii. Prealbumin reflects status within past few days (half-life of prealbumin is 1.9 days).
         e. Other indicators of poor nutrition include total protein, cholesterol, triglyceride, creatinine, blood urea nitrogen, total lymphocyte count and beta carotene levels.
         f. Patients who are malnourished are more likely to have pressure ulcers.
         g. All patients should receive basic requirements of vitamins and trace elements.
            i. Zinc is required for protein synthesis and repair.
            ii. Vitamin C is needed for collagen synthesis.
            iii. Adequate fluid intake is required
      3. Control of systemic conditions affecting wound healing
         a. Diabetes mellitus   c. Immunosuppression
         b. Hematopoietic abnormalities   d. Renal failure
   C. **Initiate appropriate therapy.**
      1. Debridement
      2. Identify and eliminate infection.
         a. All ulcers above grade 1 become colonized with bacteria.
         b. Regular cleansing and dressing changes are effective in controlling colonization.
         c. If infection is suspected, do not use swab cultures; perform wound biopsy or obtain fluid with needle aspiration.
            i. Perform wound biopsy or obtain fluid with needle aspiration.
            ii. Wound with $> 10^5$ bacteria per gram of tissue are considered infected; wound healing will not occur until bacteria count is reduced.
            iii. If bacterial count is elevated, meticulous wound cleansing, debridement, and possible trial of topical antibiotic should be considered.
            iv. Any signs of systemic involvement demand IV antibiotics.
         d. If wound fails to progress properly after 2–21 days of optimal therapy, consider trial of topical antibiotic (Table 4) even if not obviously infected.

TABLE 4.   Topical Antibiotics

Drug	Effective Against	Comment
Combination (e.g.,. neomycin, bacitracin, and polymixin B)	Gram-negative and gram-positive organisms	Enhances epidermal healing, but also may sensitize tissue
Silver sulfadiazine	Gram-negative and gram-positive organisms	Enhances epidermal healing. Softens necrotic debris. May macerate wound and surrounding tissues. Leukocytopenia may be seen
Mafenide acetate	Gram-negative and gram-positive organisms	Penetrates eschar. Frequent reports of pain or burning sensation on application. May excoriate newly healing skin. Leukocytopenia may occur.
Mubirocin	Staphylococci and streptococci in impetigo and superficial skin infections	Effective against methicillin-resistant *Staphylococcus aureus*
Gentamicin	Highly active against gram-negative organisms	Nosocomially may promote increased resistance of flora
Bacitracin	Gram-positive organisms	Increases epidermal healing but my also sensitive tissue
Metronidazole	Effective against aerobic organisms	Also for anti-inflammatory effect as expedient to healing

3. Obliterate dead space.
4. Absorb excessive exudate.
5. Maintain moist wound surface.
6. Provide thermal insulation.
7. Protect healing wound.

D. **Education**
  1. Health care professionals, patients, and caregivers need to be educated about prevention as well as wound care.
  2. Education programs and materials should be appropriate to target audience and its level of sophistication.
  3. Patient and caregiver information should include ulcer prevention, risk factors, and methods of wound cleansing, dressing and monitoring for deterioration or serious complications

VII. **Debridement**
  A. **Definition:** removal of necrotic tissue from ulcer.
  B. **Different methods** are used concurrently or in succession (e.g., sharp debridement followed by chemical or wet-to-dry debridement).
  C. **Autolytic debridement** refers to natural process of allowing eschar to self-digest by action of enzymes in wound fluid.
    1. Patients with impaired immune function may not be able to mount adequate response.
    2. Examples of dressings that promote moisture retention and autolytic debridement include transparent film, hydrocolloid, hydrogel, and continuously moist gauze.
  D. **Mechanical debridement** is removal of debris and necrotic tissue by physical forces.

1. Wet-to-dry dressings
2. Wound irrigation
3. Whirlpool

E. **Chemical debridement** is topical application of enzymes to dissolve dead tissue (e.g., collagenase [Santyl]).
    1. Concurrent use of Polysporin powder decreases risk of infection.
    2. As necrotic tissue separates from wound, patient is at higher risk for developing sepsis.

F. **Surgical debridement or sharp debridement** is removal of devitalized tissue by instruments such as a scalpel or surgical scissors.
    1. Sharp debridement is usually most effective method to remove thick eschar and heavy coagulum.
    2. Sterile instruments must be used.
    3. Large wounds with likely require extensive debridement should not be debrided at bedside but require operative setting.
    4. Grade IV lesions also may require bone biopsy to determine if osteomyelitis is present.
    5. Heel ulcers with dry eschar without sign of infection do not need debridement. In patients with erythema, fluctuance, drainage, or any other evidence suggesting infection, debridement should be done
    6. After sharp debridement patient may experience pain. Treat pain appropriately.

VIII. **Wound Cleansing**
    A. **Goal of cleansing** is to remove devitalized tissue, metabolic waste, and discharge.
    B. **Cleansing agent and method** must provide effective cleansing with minimal mechanical or chemical trauma.
    C. **Principles of wound cleansing**
        1. Wounds must be cleaned regularly to maintain healthy wound bed and avoid infection; wound should be cleansed at each dressing change.
        2. Wound should be treated gently to avoid trauma, balanced with need to remove necrotic tissue, excessive coagulum, and drainage.
        3. Irrigation can be used to cleanse debris but must deliver 4–15 pounds per square inch (psi) to be effective.
            a. 8 psi is considered ideal.
            b. Excessive pressure traumatizes wound, may drive pathogens deeper into local tissues.
            c. Whirlpool is indicated for wounds with heavy or extensive eschar, coagulum or debris; avoid direct pressure from water jets; contraindicated in dry gangrene.
        4. Normal saline can be used to clean most wounds.
            a. Antiseptic solutions (Table 5) are usually not indicated because they are cytotoxic
            b. Toxicity index (Table 6) refers to dilution needed to preserve phagocytosis and viability of white blood cells.

IX. **Dressing Types and Characteristics**
    A. **General principles**
        1. Dressing must be biocompatible, support physiology of wound healing, and preserve integrity of healthy tissue.
        2. Therapeutic goals to keep in mind in selecting wound dressing
            a. Maintain moist wound bed; avoid desiccation of the wound.

TABLE 5. Generic Antiseptic Solutions

Agent	Action	Comments
Saline solution	Provides moisture to enhance autolytic debridement Gauze enhances mechanical debridement	Safest topical solution and effective when used to cleanse and maintain wounds
Chemical cleansers	Soften debris, antiseptic action	Caustic to healing tissue
Hypochlorite solutions (Chlorpactin, Dakin's)	Effective against most micro-organisms, including staphylococci and streptococci Dissolve necrotic tissue, controls odor	Toxic to fibroblasts in normal dilutions Contact may break down surrounding intact skin Drying action may dessicate wound
Povidone-iodine preparations	Broad-spectrum effectiveness when used on intact skin or small clean wounds Questionable effectiveness in infected wounds	Toxic to fibroblasts in normal dilutions May cause iodine toxicity when used in large wounds over prolonged periods
Hydrogen peroxide	Provides mechanical cleansing and some debridement by effervescent action	Can cause ulceration of newly formed tissue. Toxic to fibroblasts Should *not* be used to pack sinus tracts—may cause air embolism Shoult *not* be used for forceful irrigation—may cause subcutaneous emphysema, which mimics gas gangrene
Acetic acid (rarely used except as component of "thirds solutions (1/3 acetic acid, 1/3 saline, 1/3 hydrogen peroxide)	Effective against *Pseudomonas aeruginosa* in superficial wounds	Toxic to fibroblasts in standard dilutions Whitens exudate and so may provide false assurance for elimination of infection Drying action may dessicate wound

TABLE 6. Toxicity for Brand-Name Wound and Skin Cleansers

Agent	Toxicity Index
Shur Clens	1:10
Briolex	1:100
Saf Clens	1:100
Cara Klenz	1:100
Ultra Klenz	1:1000
Clinical Care	1:1000
Uri Wash	1:1000
Ivory Soap (0.5%)	1:1000
Constant Clens	1:10,000
Dermal Wound Cleanser	1:10,000
Puri-Clens	1:10,000
Hibiclens	1:10,000
Betadine Surgical Scrub	1:10,000
Techni-Care Scrub	1:100,000
Bard Skin Cleanser	1:100,000
Hollister	1:100,000

    b. Surrounding skin should stay dry without evidence of maceration.

    c. Control drainage without drying the wound bed.

    d. Eliminate dead space to avoid abscess formation; gently pack cavities and areas of tracking or undermining.

  3. Select dressing that is "caregiver friendly," not labor-intensive or unusually complicated for caregivers to perform.

  4. Most wounds can be managed with dressing changes 1–3 times/day

    a. Wounds with excessive drainage should be evaluated for infection.

    b. Keep dressings clean and avoid cross-contamination.

    c. Body fluid precautions must be observed.

    d. Most contaminated wounds should be dressed last; change gloves as necessary.

    e. Clean gloves should be used for each patient.

B. **Specific dressing types and their characteristics**

  1. **Hydrogel:** crosslinked polymers, 90% water; transparent and nonadhering. Maintain moist wound environment, ease pain and inflammation; facilitate autolysis of devitalized tissue and eschar; can be used occlusively or nonocclusively.

  2. **Hydrocolloid:** hydrophilic (absorbent) particulate, usually pectin, integrated with hydrophobic adhesive matrix covered by outer film or foam layer. Dressings adhere, forming occlusive soft gel by interacting with wound exudates; absorb excessive exudate; maintain moist wound environment; facilitate autolysis of devitalized tissue and eschar; and provide barrier to external contaminants.

  3. **Polymeric:** nonadhering, absorbent, and semipermeable, allowing evaporation of exudates; can be made occlusive by addition of outer dressings or tape. Good alternative to hydrogel, hydrocolloid, or other occlusive dressing. Use when surrounding skin is macerated or when wound is hypergranulating. **Composite polymeric dressings** combine other features (e.g., occlusive layers or adhesives with absorbent dressing).

  4. **Transparent adhesive:** fosters moist wound healing. Semipermeable membranes that prevent bacterial invasion from environment because of size of membrane pores. Permeability allows water vapor to escape; permits oxygen to diffuse into wound bed. *Note:* Presence of exudate can prevent both evaporation and oxygen diffusion; exudate under dressing can cause maceration of both wound and surrounding skin and should be removed.

  5. **Absorptive dressings:** fill wound, absorbing excessive exudate and maintaining moist wound environment.

    a. **Wound gels:** polymers, water, humectants, preservatives, and moisturizers. Used primarily to maintain moist environment within wound, thus facilitating autolytic debridement. Most gels absorb small amount of exudate.

    b. **Copolymer starch/beads:** absorb exudate, facilitate autolytic debridement, and maintain moist wound environment.

    c. **Alginates:** soft, naturally occurring polysaccharides. Useful in wounds with excessive drainage; absorb up to 20 times their weight in fluid. Place directly into wound and secure with secondary dressing. Alginate forms gel that maintains moist wound environment, promoting autolytic debridement. Easily removed from wound; saline irrigation recommended. Frequency of dressing changes reduced.

    d. **Gauze:** absorbs excessive drainage and maintains moist wound environment, thus facilitating autolytic debridement. Coarse weave facilitates mechanical debridement. Fine mesh weave facilitates healthy granulation tissue growth. Moistened with normal saline or other appropriate topical solution before placement on or in wound.
6. **Enzymatic debriding agents:** biochemically lyse necrotic tissue; may damage healthy tissue; require prescription. Used within moist environment, usually saline-moistened, coarse gauze. Require frequent assessment for debridement progress and to prevent extant tissue debridement.
C. **Selection of appropriate dressing** (Tables 7 and 8)

X. Surgery
A. **Indications**
1. Noninfected grade III or IV ulcer that has not healed even with optimal nonsurgical wound care.
2. Medically stable and well-nourished patient.
3. Patient desires surgery and understands expected outcome and risks and is willing to invest necessary time to recover from surgery and complete postoperative rehabilitation program.
4. Quality of life, life style, and risks of recurrence have been considered and judged favorable.
5. Patient who uses nicotine is willing to participate in smoking cessation program.
6. Bowel and bladder incontinence is managed appropriately; in some cases diverting colostomy may be required to prevent fecal contamination.
B. **Contraindications**
1. Patient who is unwilling to participate in surgical wound care program postoperatively.

TABLE 7. Guide to Selection of Appropriate Dressing

Dressing Type	Debrides Necrotic Tissue	Protects From Infection	Obliterates Dead Space	Absorbs Excessive Exudate	Maintains Moist Wound Surface	Provides Thermal Insulation	Protects Healing Wound
Hydrogel	**x, A**		x	x, L	x		x
Polymeric				x	x, L	x	x
Hydrocolloid	**x, A**	x		x	x	x	x
Transparent adhesive	x, A	x			x		x
Absorptive Wound gels	**x, A**		x	x, L	x		x
Copolymer starch/beads	x, A		x	x	x		x
Alginates	**x, A**		x	x	x	x	x
Gauze (coarse mesh)	**x, A, M**		x	x	**x, M**	x	x
Gauze (fine mesh			x	x	x	x	x
Enzymatic debriding agents	x						

Boldface = significant effects.
A = Autolytic, M = if kept moist, L = some do to limited extent.

TABLE 8.   Brand Names and Manufacturers

Dressing Type	Brand Name (Manufactuer)
Hydrogel	Cutinova (Beiersdorf), Elasto Gel (Southwest Technologies). Geliperm Wet (Fougera), Vigilon (Bard)
Polymeric and composite polymeric	Allevyn (Smith & Nephew), BioBrane (Winthrop), Curafoam (Kendall), Lyofoam (Ultra), Transorb (Brady Medical)
Hydrocolloid	Comfeel (Coloplast), DuoDerm (ConvaTec), RepliCare (Smith & Nephew), Sween-a-peel (Sween), Tegasorb (3M), Restore Plus (Hollister)
Transparent adhesives	Bioclusive (Johnson & Johnson), BlisterFilm (Sherwood Medical), Opsite (Smith & Nephew), Polyskin (Kendall), Tegaderm (3M)
Asborptive dressings	
Wound gels	Carrasyn (Carrington), DuoDerm (ConvaTec), Solosite (Smith & Nephew)
Copolymer starch/ beads	Bard Absorption Dressing (Bard), Comfeel (Coloplast), Debrisan (Johnson & Johnson)
Alginates	AligiDerm (ConvaTec), Kaltostat (Calgon-Vestal), Sorbsan (Dow)
Enzymatic debriding agents	Biozyme (Armour Pharmaceutical), Elase (Parke-Davis), Santyl (Knoll Pharmaceuticals), Travase (Travenol)

2. Medical and surgical risks (e.g., severe cardiac disease) outweigh benefits.
3. Poorly nourished patients (may become candidates once nutritional status is corrected).

C. **Type of surgery**
   1. Determination of type of flap or repair is surgeon's decision (based on his or her expertise and preference)
   2. Generally radical bone resection is not recommended because of risk of infected bone.
   3. Location of ulcer often dictates type of repair.

D. **Postoperative care**
   1. Specialized bed to avoid pressure over surgical site and other areas of risk often needed.
      a. Typical beds include air-loss mattress system, fluidized mattress.
      b. May require immobilization in bed 2 weeks or more as determined by condition of surgical site.
   2. Meticulous wound monitoring and wound care.
   3. Adequate nutrition (prealbumin level can indicate current nutritional status).
   4. Patient education stressing wound care and prevention of recurrence.
   5. Once surgeon agrees, carefully designed seating protocol is initiated after sacral and ischial wound repair, beginning with 10–15 minutes of sitting or pressure on operative site.
      a. Physical therapy to assist with prescribed sitting protocol.
      b. Sitting or pressure over operative site is increased in increments of 10–15 minutes/day unless there is evidence of breakdown, such as redness that does not resolve after pressure removed or does not blanch, separation of wound, or evidence of infection.
   6. If wound is due to problems with sitting, prescribe physical therapy to teach patient and caregivers pressure-relieving techniques and assist in wheelchair and cushion selection.

7. Physical therapist should review patient's transfer technique to determine if poor technique is contributing to ulcer formation; ideally this should be done preoperatively.
8. Occupational therapist should assess patient's dressing technique and other activities of daily living.

E. **Postoperative complications**
   1. **Wound dehiscence** is most common complication.
   2. **Hematoma** formation: risk is decreased with use of postoperative drains during first 3–4 days.
   3. **Ulcer recurrence**
      a. Incidence rate ranges from 19% to 33%.
      b. Risk factors
         i. Substance or alcohol abuse
         ii. Unemployment
         iii. Lower socioeconomic status

XI. **New Treatments**
   A. **Growth factors**
      1. Proteins secreted by platelets and macrophages that direct repair of tissue.
      2. Platelet-derived growth factor (PDGF) is chemotactic.
         a. Fibroblasts
         b. Mononuclear cells
         c. Smooth muscle cells
      3. Precipitate inflammatory response and matrix synthesis.
      4. Derivation
         a. Autologous from patient's platelet-rich plasma
         b. Recombinant DNA
      5. Commercially available but very expensive; some insurance companies deny payment.
      6. Require clean, noninfected wound.
      7. Once-daily application with saline-moist dressing
   B. **Electrical therapy**
      1. Electrotherapy can enhance healing rate of grade III and IV ulcers.
         a. Proper equipment and experienced personnel required.
         b. Established protocols that are shown to be safe and effective: low-intensity current and high-voltage monophasic pulsating current.
      2. Side effects are limited to local stinging or tingling sensation.
      3. Research is limited and has involved primarily grade III and IV wounds that were unresponsive to standard therapy.
      4. Benefit is hypothesized to result from:
         a. Improving transcutaneous partial pressure of oxygen
         b. Bactericidal properties
         c. Increasing protein and adenosine phosphate synthesis
         d. Increasing calcium uptake
   C. **Anabolic steroids**
      1. Controversial—further research is needed.
      2. Recommended by some authorities for nonvoluntary weight loss and non-healing wounds.
   D. **Hyperbaric oxygen therapy**
      1. Costly treatment
      2. Research not definitive; improved healing has not been validated.

E. **Ultrasound**
   a. Reportedly facilitates inflammatory phase, which should herald earlier pro-liferative response.
   b. Enhances chemotaxis and cellular secretion of release of growth factors
F. **Ultraviolet (UV) light**
   a. Used for many skin conditions
   b. Research does not unequivocally substantiate use of UV light therapy for wound healing.
   c. Contraindications
      i. Small vessel vascular disease
      ii. Systemic lupus erythematosus, scleroderma
      iii. Concomitant use of UV-sensitizing medications, such as tetracycline
      iv. Cardiac or renal failure

Bibliography

1. Bergstrom N, Bennett MA, Carlson CE, et al: Treatment of Pressure Ulcers. Clinical Practice Guideline No 15. Rockville, MD, U.S. Department of Health and Human Services. Public Health Service, Agency for Health Care Policy and Research. AHCPR Publication No. 95-0652, 1994.
2. Berkwits L, Yarkony GM, Lewis : Marjolin's ulcer complicating a pressure ulcer: Case report and literature review. Arch Phys Med Rehabil 67:831–833, 1986.
3. Demling RH, DeSanti L: Involuntary weight loss and the nonhealing wound: The role of ana-bolic agents. Adv Wound Care 12(Suppl 1):1–14, 1999.
4. Gentzkow GD, Pollack SV, Kloth LC, Stubbs HA: Improved healing of pressure ulcers using dermapulse, a new electrical stimulation devise. Wounds 3(5):158–170, 1991.
5. Griffin JW, Tooms RE, Mendius RA, et al: Efficacy of high voltage pulsed current for healing of pressure ulcers in patients with spinal cord injury. Phys Ther 71:433–442, 1991.
6. Maklebust J, Sieggreen M: Pressure Ulcers: Guidelines for Prevention and Management, 3rd ed. Springhouse, PA, Springhouse Corp., 2001.
7. Pinchcofsky-Devis GD, Kaminski MU Jr: Correlation of pressure sores and nutritional status. J Am Geriatr Soc 34:435–440, 1986.
8. Rousseau P: Pressure ulcers in an aging society. Wounds 1:135–141, 1989.
9. Sanchez S, Eamegdool S, Conway H: Surgical treatment of decubitus ulcers in paraplegics. Plast Reconstr Surg 43;25–28, 1969.
10. Sapico FL, Ginunas VJ, Thornhill-Joynes M, et al: Quantitative microbiology of pressure sores in different stages of healing. Diagn Microbiol Infect Dis 5:31–38, 1986.
11. Schryvers OI, Stranc MF, Nance PW: Surgical treatment of pressure ulcers: 20-year experience. Arch Phys Med Rehabil 81:1556–1562, 2000.
12. Young MM, Ehrenpreis ED, Young MA: Nutrition and dietary issues in rehabilitation. In O'Young BJ, Young MA, Stiens SA (eds): Physical Medicine and Rehabilitation Secrets. Philadelphia, Hanley & Belfus, 2002.

Chapter 19

SPASTICITY

Liza B. Green, M.D., Edward A. Hurvitz, M.D., and Rita N. Ayyangar, M.D.

I. General Principles

A. **Definitions**

1. **Spasticity:** motor disorder characterized by velocity-dependent increase in muscle tone with exaggerated tendon jerks resulting from hyperexcitability of stretch reflex, as one component of upper motor neuron syndrome.

2. **Tone:** sensation of resistance felt as one manipulates a joint through its range of motion with subject trying to relax.

B. **Components of spasticity**

1. Musculotendinous unit has properties such as plasticity and viscoelasticity that, when altered, can cause stiffness and contracture. These properties may be particularly important in patients with chronic spasticity.

2. Segmental reflex arc is altered in some way to increase muscle activation in response to stretch.

   a. Motor neurons are influenced by many converging presynaptic inputs, both excitatory and inhibitory. Some of these are part of monosynaptic or polysynaptic spinal reflex pathways that originate with peripheral receptors and their afferent nerves (Fig. 1), whereas others are part of descending pathways originating in brain.

   b. In spasticity, balance of the excitatory and inhibitory inputs is changed so that net input to motor neuron favors excitation.

   c. Reticulospinal and vestibulospinal tracts are intricately involved in spasticity.

   d. Gamma aminobutyric acid (GABA) is inhibitory neurotransmitter that modifies reflex arc. Agonists, particularly of GABA-B receptor, are used to treat spasticity.

   e. Adrenergic neurotransmitters are excitatory and also modify reflex arc. Alpha adrenergic blockers are often used in treatment of spasticity.

C. **Spasticity is part of an upper motor neuron syndrome.**

1. Includes positive symptoms or abnormal behaviors such as increased resistance to stretch and various reflex release phenomena.

2. Also negative symptoms or performance deficits, such as decreased dexterity, weakness, and fatigability.

3. Often other components of upper motor neuron syndrome are more disabling than increased tone associated with spasticity.

D. **Quantification of spasticity**

1. **Ashworth and Modified Ashworth Scales** (Table 1)

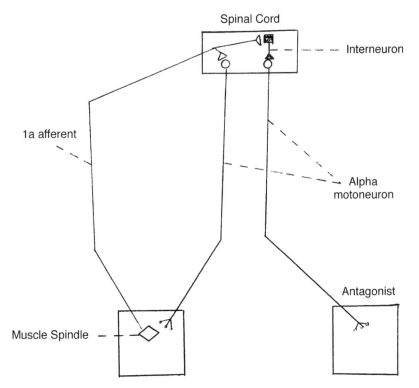

Spinal Cord

Interneuron

1a afferent

Alpha
motoneuron

Antagonist

Muscle Spindle

FIGURE 1. Stretch reflex. When the muscle is stretched, 1a afferent fibers that surround the intrafusal fibers of muscle spindles are excited. These 1a afferent neurons make monosynaptic excitatory connections with alpha motoneurons that innervate the muscle from which the 1a afferents originated. The 1a afferents also synapse with inhibitory interneurons, which then synapse with alpha motoneurons that innervate antagonistic muscles. Thus, when a muscle is stretched, it is stimulated to contract and the antagonistic muscles are stimulated to relax.

      a. Most frequently used clinical scale.
      b. Subjective scales that measure joint stiffness.
      c. Modified Ashworth scale provides greater qualitative assessment.
  2. **Boyd Modification of the Tardieu Scale** (Table 2)
      a. Used to assess dynamic muscle length and helps separate static/fixed from dynamic/elastic component.
      b. Slow passive joint range of motion (ROM) measured with standard goniometry gives indication of muscle length at rest (R2).
      c. Point of resistance to quick or rapid velocity stretch is measured as a "catch," and the angle (R1) is measured by goniometry.
      d. Large difference between R1 and R2 indicates large dynamic/elastic component, whereas small difference indicates predominantly fixed contracture in muscle.
      e. This scale also rates reaction to stretch at specified velocity with two parameters: quality of muscle reaction (X) and angle of muscle reaction (Y).
  3. **Electromyographic and biomechanical measures** also have been developed, but they are generally used only for research.

TABLE 1. Modified Ashworth Scale for Spastic Hypertonia

0	No increase in tone
1	Slight increase in muscle tone, manifested by catch and release or by minimal resistance at end of the range of motion when affected part(s) is moved in flexion or extension.
1+	Slight increase in muscle tone, manifested by catch, followed by minimal resistance throughout remainder (less than half) of range of motion.
2	More marked increase in muscle tone through most of range of motion, but affected part(s) easily moved.
3	Considerable increase in muscle tone, passive movement difficult
4	Affected part(s) rigid in flexion or extension

From Bohannon RW, Smith MB: Interrater reliability on Modified Ashworth Scale of muscle spasticity. Phys Ther 67:207, 1987, with permission.

E. Beneficial effects of spasticity
1. Deep venous thrombosis prophylaxis and prevention of muscle atrophy by constant muscle tone.
2. Sometimes patients can use spasticity to provide some increase in function (e.g., paraplegic who uses lower extremity spasticity for transfers).

F. Negative effects of spasticity
1. Musculoskeletal problems (e.g., contractures, hip dislocation, scoliosis).
2. Spasticity often prevents normal function and may make tasks such as hygiene more difficult.
3. Spasticity also may cause neurogenic bowel and bladder.

TABLE 2. Modified Tardieu Scale

Velocity of stretch: once velocity is chosen for a muscle, it remains the same for all tests
V1	As slow as possible (slower than natural drop of limb segment under gravity)
V2	Speed of limb segment falling under gravity
V3	As fast as possible (faster than rate of natural drop of limb under gravity)

Quality of muscle reaction (X)
0	No resistance throughout the course of the passive movement
1	Slight resistance throughout course of passive movement, no clear catch at precise angle
2	Clear catch at precise angle, interrupting passive movement, followed by release
3	Fatigable clonus (< 10 s when maintaining pressure) appearing at a precise angle
4	Unfatigable clonus (> 10s when maintaining the pressure) at a precise angle
5	Joint unmovable

Angle of muscle reaction (Y)
Measured relative to position of minimal stretch of muscle (corresponding to angle zero) for all joints except hip, where it is relative to resting anatomic position
Lower limb: to be tested in a supine position at the recommended joint positions and velocities
Hip	Extensors (knee extended, V3)
	Adductors (hip flexed/knee flexed, V3)
	External rotators (knee flexed 90°, V3)
	Internal rotators (knee flexed 90°, V3)
Knee	Extensors (hip flexed 90°, V2)
	Flexors (hip flexed, V3)
Ankle	Plantarflexors (knee flexed/extended 90°, V3)

Grading is always done at the same time of day, using a constant position of limb. Other joints, particularly the neck, also must remain at a constant position throughout the assessment and from one test to another.

From Boyd RN, Graham HK: Objective measurement of clinical findings in the use of botulism toxin A in the management of children with cerebral palsy. Eur J Neurology 6:523–536, 1999, with permission.

Table 3. Factors Influencing Decision Making in Spasticity Management

Chronicity	Temporary: use temporary treatments such as oral medications or local chemodenervation. Chronic: use long term treatments such as baclofen pump or surgical treatment.
Severity	Mild: risks often outweigh benefits except for physical modalities. Severe: often requires more long-term treatments, such as orthopedic surgeries.
Locus of injury	Spinal cord origin often responds better to baclofen. Patients with cerebral palsy often are considered for dorsal rhizotomy.
Comorbidities	Poor motor control: generally no gain in function with treatment. Cognitive deficits: patients have trouble with compliance and with taking advantage of spasticity reduction. Medical problems: patients who cannot tolerate intensive rehabilitation; illness may limit function. Lack of available care and support: inability to follow through on range-of-motion exercises and follow-up.

II. Spasticity Management
A. General considerations
1. Spasticity should be treated only if it is interfering with patient's function, care, or comfort and only if it is not useful for patient in some way.
2. Spasticity should be treated only after careful consideration of what contribution it makes to patient's limitations and only after careful examination of patient to locate muscles that are most troublesome.
3. First it is necessary to treat reversible factors that aggravate spasticity. Examples include urinary tract infection, urolithiasis, stool impaction,

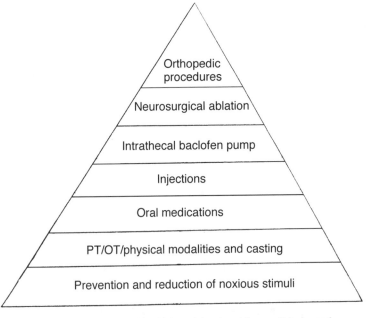

FIGURE 2. Relative frequency with which each treatment for spasticity is used.

pressure sore, fracture, dislocation, ingrown toe nail, clothing that is too tight, and heterotopic ossification.

4. Table 3 summarizes factors that influence decision making in spasticity management; Figure 2 shows relative frequency with which each treatment is used.

B. **Range of motion (ROM) exercises**
   1. Can reduce severity of spastic tone for several hours.
   2. Carry-over may result from mechanical changes in muscle itself or from plasticity of central nervous system.
   3. Habituation or adaptation of stretch reflex to repeated stretching has been shown to occur.
   3. Effect of stretching is temporary and may not affect voluntary movements.

C. **Physical modalities:** often used alone or in combination with other treatments.
   1. **Cryotherapy**
      a. Refers to use of topical cold to decrease muscle stretch reflex excitability.
      b. Reduces clonus, increases ROM, and improves power in antagonistic muscle group.
      c. Accomplished in part by decreasing sensitivity of cutaneous receptors and slowing nerve conduction.
   2. **Casting and splinting**
      a. Improves ROM of joint due to hypertonic contractures.
      b. Positioning limb in tonic stretch decreases reflex tone.
      c. Elongation of musculotendinous unit contributes to decreased tone.
      d. Orthotic devices can be made with tone-reducing features that decrease nocioceptive stimulation to reflexogenic areas.
   3. **Functional electrical stimulation of peripheral nerves**
      a. Shown to improve function in patients with spasticity.
      b. Improves standing, walking, and exercise training as well as decreases upper extremity contractures.
      c. Appears to improve motor activity in agonistic muscles and reduce tone in antagonistic muscles.
      d. Therapeutic effect may last for > 1 hour after stimulation has been stopped, probably because of neurotransmitter modulation within reflex arc.

D. **Systemic therapy with oral medications**
   1. Used to treat spasticity that involves many muscle groups throughout body.
   2. Table 4 lists oral medications most commonly used to treat spasticity with their mechanism of action, side effects, and pharmacology and dosing.
   3. Medications reduce spasticity and tone, but most have not been proved to provide functional benefit for patients in clinical trials.
   4. Because all medications have side effects, some of which are serious, they should be prescribed only when they clearly provide some benefit.
   5. It is especially important to consider cognitive and sedating side effects in treating patients with brain injury.
   6. There are special considerations for treating patients who have seizures. Baclofen lowers seizure threshold.
   7. Many seizure medications have adverse effects on liver; spasticity agents with similar adverse effects should not be used in conjunction.

E. **Local injections**
   1. **General considerations**
      a. May be helpful when spasticity is focal or when regional problem overlies generalized spasticity.

TABLE 4. Medications Used to Treat Spasticity

Drug	Potential Uses	Mechanism of Action	Side Effects and Precautions	Pharmacology and Dosing
Baclofen	Especially useful in decreasing spasticity in multiple sclerosis spinal cord injury. Patients with spasticity of cerebral origin seem to benefit less and to experience more significant side effects.	Binds to gamma-aminobutyric acid (GABA)-B receptor, causing inhibition of monosynaptic and polysynaptic spinal reflexes.	Sedation, confusion, nausea, dizziness, muscle weakness, hypotonia, ataxia, and paresthesias. Can cause difficulty with memory and attention in elderly and brain-injured patients. Can cause loss of seizure control. Withdrawal can produce seizures, confusion, rebound hypertonia, fever, and even death	Rapidly absorbed after oral administration, mean half-life of 3.5 hr. Excreted mainly through kidney, with 15% metabolized in liver. Begin with 5 mg 3 times/day and increase gradually to therapeutic level. Recommended maximum dose: 80 mg/day in 4 divided doses. Doses as high as 150 mg/day have been used. In children, starting dose is usually 2.5–5 mg/day. Dose can be increased to 30 mg (in children 2–7 years of age) or 60 mg (in children 8 and over).
Diazepam	Useful in spasticity of spinal cord origin. Also helpful in patients with cerebral palsy. In patients with hemiplegia, benefit generally outweighed by adverse effects.	Like all benzodiazepines, facilitates postsynaptic effects of GABA. Exerts indirect GABA-mimetic effect when GABA transmission is functional, resulting in increased presynaptic inhibition in brainstem reticular formation and spinal postsynaptic pathways.	Central nervous system depression, causing sedation, decreased motor coordination, and impaired attention and memory. Overdoses cause somnolence leading to coma. Withdrawal symptoms can occur if drug is stopped too abruptly (e.g. anxiety, agitation, irritability, tremor, nausea, hypersensitivity to light and sound, insomnia, seizures, psychosis, death).	Well-absorbed after oral dose, mean half-life of 20–80 hr; extensively protein-bound. Metabolized mainly in liver. Begin with nocturnal dose of 5–10 mg. Daytime therapy generally begun at 2 mg 2 times/day. Titrate upward to maximum of 60 mg/day or more. Pediatric doses range from 012 to 0.8 mg/kg/day in divided doses.
Clorazepate dipotassium	Believed to have longer potency in patients with multiple sclerosis or spinal cord injury.	Another benzodiazepine; see diazepam above.	Sedation is less common than with diazepam.	Transformed to desmethyldiazepam in gastric juice. Half-life: 106 hr. Oral dose: 5 mg twice daily.
Ketozolam	As effective as diazepam. Approved in Canada, but not yet in U.S.	Another benzodiazepine; see diazepam above.	Sedation is less common than with diazepam.	Dosage: 30–60 mg/day; does not need to be divided.

Table continued on following page.

TABLE 4. Medications Used to Treat Spasticity *(Continued)*

Drug	Potential Uses	Mechanism of Action	Side Effects and Precautions	Pharmacology and Dosing
Clonazepam	Generally used for suppression of nighttime spasms.	Another benzodiazepine; see diazepam above.	More sedating than diazepam.	Generally prescribed s 0.5–1 mg at night but can be increased to 3 mg at night.
Vigabatrin	Improves spasticity in multiple sclerosis and spinal cord injury.	Increases GABA levels by inhibiting its catabolism.	Drowsiness, fatigue, weight gain, and behavioral disturbances.	Dosage: 2–3 gm/day.
Gabapentin	Improves spasticity in multiple sclerosis and spinal cord injury.	Analog of GABA, but does not act on any known GABA receptor; exact mechanism of action unknown.	Drowsiness, dizziness, ataxia, nystagmus	Half-life: 5–7 hr; excreted by kidneys. Dosage generally at least 1200 mg/day in 3 divided doses. One study noted increased effect with dosages up to 3600 mg/day.
Dantrolene sodium	Reduces muscle tone, tendon reflexes, and clonus and increases passive range of motion. Works well in spinal cord injury and spasticity of cerebral origin. Has greater effect in children than in adults.	Works on muscle to reduce action potential-induced calcium release from sarcoplasmic reticulum, which in turn reduces force produced by muscle during contraction. Reduces activity of phasic stretch reflexes more than tonic ones. Has greatest effect on fast-twitch fibers, at lower frequencies of neural stimulation and shorter muscle lengths; little effect on smooth and cardiac muscles.	Most important side effect is hepatotoxicity, which may lead to hepatonecrosis and even death; liver enzymes should be monitored. Other side effects: mild sedation, nausea, vomiting, dizziness, diarrhea, and paresthesias. Can also cause muscle weakness.	Sodium salt is about 70% absorbed in small intestine; half-life is about 15 hr after oral dose and 12 hr after intravenous dose. Largely metabolized in liver, although 15–25% of nonmetabolized drug is excreted in urine. Begin at 25 mg/day, and titrate slowly upward to maximum of 100 mg 4 times/day. Pediatric doses begin at 0.5 mg/kg 2 times/day to maximum of 3 mg/kg 4 times/day
Tizanidine	As effective at reducing spasticity as baclofen in multiple sclerosis and spinal cord pathology. Also useful in spasticity of cerebral origin.	Imidazoline derivative with agonistic effects at central alpha₂-adrenergic sites. Prevents release of excitatory amino acids from spinal interneurons and may facilitate action of glycine, an inhibitory neurotransmitter. Reduces tonic stretch reflexes and polysynaptic reflexes.	Dry mouth, sedation, dizziness, visual hallucinations, elevated liver enzymes, insomnia, and muscle weakness. Risk of symptomatic hypotension; must be used with care in patients on antihypertensive therapy.	Well absorbed orally but has extensive first-pass metabolism in liver. Half-life of 2.5 hr. Begin with single dose of 2–4 mg at bedtime; titrate upward to maximum of 36 mg/day.

Table continued on following page

TABLE 4. Medications Used to Treat Spasticity *(Continued)*

Drug	Potential Uses	Mechanism of Action	Side Effects and Precautions	Pharmacology and Dosing
Clonidine	May be useful by itself or as adjunct to baclofen in treatment of spasticity due to spinal cord pathology, but few convincing studies have been done.	Adrenergic agonist that acts in both brain and spinal cord to enhance presynaptic inhibition of sensory afferents.	Bradycardia, hypotension, dry mouth, drowsiness, dizziness, constipation, and depression are fairly common and lead one-half of patients to discontinue drug.	Well absorbed orally. Half is metabolized in liver and half in kidney. Half-life of 5–19 hr. Begin at 0.05–0.1 mg 2 times/day, and titrate slowly to maximum of 0.1 4 times/day. Patch form delivers 0.1 or 0.2 mg/day for 7 days.
Cryptoheptadine	Decreases clonus and increases walking speed in patients with gait limited by clonus and patients with spasticity of spinal cord origin. As effective as baclofen in spinal cord injury.	Histamine and serotonin antagonist with direct inhibitory effect on motor neurons by decreasing spinal and supraspinal serotoninergic excitatory inputs.	Sedation and dry mouth.	Begin with 4 mg at bedtime, and titrate upward slowly to maximum of 36 mg/day.
Cannabinoids	Decreases electromyographic response to stretching as well as subjective grading of spasticity.	Some evidence suggests that cannabinoids exert specific antispastic effect and not just a general relaxation response.	Sleepiness, decreased short-term memory, attention, balance, depersonalization, hallucinations, delusions, paranoia, antimotivational syndrome, temporal disintegration, increased hunger, dry mouth. Tolerance and addictive potentials not adequately studied.	2–50% available after smoking; peak concentration 7–10 minutes after; effects last as long as 2–3 hr. Peak concentration after oral dose is one-half to 1 hour. Metabolized in liver into active and inactive compounds. Dosage information not available.
Phenytoin	Reduces tone in patients with various diagnoses but provides no additional benefits over other antispasticity drugs and side-effect profile is difficult to tolerate.	Inhibitory effect on repetitive firing of action potentials by slowing sodium channel recovery.	Nausea, vomiting, tremor, ataxia, dizziness, confusion, blurred vision, somnolence, headache, insomnia, gingival hyperplasia, liver toxicity, arrhythmias, hypotension.	Usual dose is 300–400 mg/day divided into 3 or 4 doses. Therapeutic blood level is 10–20 µg.ml. Absorbed slowly after oral dose; peak concentration after 3–12 hr. Extensively protein-bound and metabolized primarily by liver in dose-dependent manner.

b. Best used in combination with aggressive physical therapy and/or casting or splinting to help lengthen muscle.

c. It is important to understand that to provide benefit, injected substance generally must weaken target muscle.

2. **Commonly used local agents** (Table 5)

   a. **Local anesthetics**

      i. **Potential uses:** often for diagnostic purposes or before casting/splinting to ensure maximal possible benefits.

      ii. **Mechanism of action:** local anesthetics, which are reversible and short-acting, block nerve conduction by decreasing membrane permeability to sodium ions. This action is fully reversible and does not cause damage to nerve structure.

      iii. **Risks and side effects:** local anesthetics are generally safe. However, it is necessary to have resuscitation equipment available when injecting local anesthetics because of serious effects that may occur when they are inadvertently injected into systemic circulation.

      iv. **Technique**
      - Can be done either intramuscularly or perineurally.
      - Intramuscular injections, also called motor-point blocks, are most effective when they are done near the neuromuscular junction. They are more painful than perineural injections.
      - Most accurate way of finding optimal location for injection is to use exploratory stimulation technique in which needle used to inject drug is also used to transmit repetitive stimulation to targeted nerve or muscle. Location at which minimal stimulation is required to elicit appropriate muscle twitch or paresthesia is site for injection.
      - Onset of action is within minutes and depends on which anesthetic is used. Duration of action is hours and can be prolonged by additional use of local vasoconstrictors such as epinephrine.

   b. **Ethyl alcohol**

      i. **Potential uses:** alcohol reduces spasticity for months to years in animal and human studies when it is injected either perineurally or intramuscularly, as either motor-point block or intramuscular wash.

      ii. **Mechanism of action:** alcohol denatures proteins, thus precipitating and denaturing protoplasm. Local coagulation necrosis in muscle is followed by granulation tissue formation and fibrosis and finally by recovery.

      iii. **Risks and side effects** include pain at site of injection, phlebitis, chronic dysesthesias and pain (especially with perineural injections), permanent peripheral nerve palsy, skin irritation, muscle necrosis, and systemic effects of intoxication.

      iv. **Technique**
      - Alcohol is most often used in 35–60% dilutions. Some use 10% dilution in children.
      - Probably works best when injected with exploratory stimulation technique described above, although muscle-wash techniques have been described.

   c. **Phenol (benzyl alcohol)**

      i. **Potential uses:** phenol is used in patients with any form of spasticity, especially in large, proximal muscles. It is often used in combination

TABLE 5. Summary of Local Injections

Substance Injected	Potential Uses	Mechanism of Action	Risks and Side Effects	Onset, Duration, and Dosing
Local anesthetics	Efficacy test before long-term block Muscle relaxation before casting.	Ion channel block	Central nervous system and cardio-vascular toxicity Hypersensitivity	Onset: minutes Duration: hours Lidocaine (0.5–2%): < 4.5 mg/kg Bupivacaine (0.25–0.75%): < 3 mg/kg Etidocaine (1–1.5%): < 6 mg/kg
Ethyl alcohol	Proximal and large muscles Sensory integrity not primary concern Hygiene and comfort Combination with botulinum toxin	Tissue destruction and circulatory damage	Pain at injection Chronic dysesthesia and pain Vascular complications Permanent peripheral nerve palsy Intoxication	Onset: < 1 hr Duration: 2–36 months Dosing: 10–50% concentration
Phenol (> 3%)	Proximal and large muscles Sensory integrity not primary concern Hygiene and comfort	Tissue destruction and circulatory damage	Pain at injection Chronic dysesthesia and pain Vascular complications Permanent peripheral nerve palsy	Onset: < 1 hr Duration: 2–36 months Dosing: < 1 gm (10 ml of 5% phenol)
Botulinum toxin	Muscles accessible for intra-muscular injection Sensory integrity indispensable In combination with neurolytic agents	Presynaptic block of acetylcholine release	No major side effects; safety in children not established.	Onset: days Duration: 3–6 months Dosing: Botox: ≤ 400 units within 3 months Myobloc: 2500–5000 units per visit

with botulinum toxin injections. Phenol is injected perineurally to block large muscles that are too big to be blocked by botulinum toxin because of dosage concerns. Botulinum toxin is used to block smaller, more distal muscles.

iii. **Mechanism of action:** phenol denatures proteins and causes tissue necrosis. It results in more extensive injury than alcohol. Recovery is due to regeneration of nerve fibers, but more long-term effects may be due to vascular injury and muscle necrosis.

iv. **Risks and side effects** include pain during the injection, chronic dysesthesias, and/or chronic pain. Patient usually experiences burning paresthesia, which typically lasts several weeks but may be permanent. Repeat injections can alleviate pain. Other side effects include peripheral edema, deep venous thromboses, injury to intima of small arteries and veins, and excessive motor weakness and sensory loss. Overdoses cause tremor, convulsions, CNS depression and cardiovascular collapse. Lethal dose starts at 8.5 gm, but generally no more than 1 gm is injected in 1 day for antispasticity procedures.

v. **Technique**
   - Exploratory stimulation technique described under local anesthetics should be used. Children often require sedation or general anesthesia for this technique.
   - Intramuscular blocks work best when injected close to endplate band. EMG can localize this band by locating characteristic electrical potentials in resting muscle.
   - Usually 4–6% phenol solution is injected in amounts of 1–10 ml. Phenol diffuses approximately 2 mm from site of injection. Reported duration of effect ranges from 1 month to 2 years or more.

vi. Phenol injections compared with botulinum toxin
   - Advantages of phenol include early onset of action, possibly longer duration of effect, low cost, lack of antigenicity, and better stability.
   - Disadvantages include lack of selectivity for motor neurons, tissue-destructive effect, painful injections, and possibility of chronic painful dysesthesia.

d. **Botulinum toxin**

i. **Potential uses:** reduces spasticity in patients with wide variety of diagnoses, including multiple sclerosis, spinal cord injury, cerebral palsy, stroke, and traumatic brain injury. In some cases, reduction in spasticity also has provided some functional benefit, such as improved gait or improved function of the upper extremity.

ii. **Mechanism of action:** blocks neuromuscular transmission by inhibiting the release of acetylcholine, which causes reversible denervation atrophy.
   - Seven serotypes of botulinum toxin are labeled alphabetically from A to G. All work in same manner. Only two serotypes are commercially available, A and B.
   - Unit of measurement for botulinum toxin is the mouse unit, which is defined as amount of toxin that kills 50% of group of specific type of mouse. Trade name for American form of serotype A is Botox, which is not equal in potency to European form, called Dysport. Trade name for serotype B is Myobloc.

    iii. **Risks and side effects:** botulinum toxin treatment is remarkably safe. Fever, excessive weakness, local irritation, pain, and bruising may occur. Botulinum toxin should not be used when a patient is taking aminoglycoside antibiotics or in patients with preexisting diseases of the neuromuscular junction. Long-term safety in children has not been established, but the drug often is used in children.

    iv. **Technique**
- Because of its predilection for binding to presynaptic neurons and because of its ability to diffuse through muscle tissue, botulinum toxin can be injected into belly of target muscle, but effect is greatest when it is injected closest to motor endplate band.
- Electromyographic and electrical stimulation techniques can be used to locate target muscle more precisely when target muscle is deeper or located close to muscles where no toxin effect is desired.
- Usually Botox is diluted to 5–10 U/0.1 ml, and up to 0.5–1 ml is injected per site. The maximum recommended dose is 300–400 U/visit. Botox is reconstituted in the vial with normal saline without preservative. Gently swirl, but do not shake vial. Therapeutic effect begins within 24–72 hours with peak effect occurring at 2 weeks.
- Suggested adult and pediatric dosing can be found in Tables 6 and 7. Dosing must be adjusted based on results. It also must be based on number of muscles that clinician wishes to inject because total amount of toxin injected must be kept within maximum recommended dose.
- Occasionally patients become resistant to effects of Botox. Often such patients have antibodies to toxin in their serum. When antibodies are present, evidence suggests that one of other serotypes of toxin may work. To avoid immunoresistance, use smallest possible effective dose, extend interval between treatment as long as possible (at least 3 months), and avoid booster injections.
- When patient fails to respond to therapy, it is also possible that inadequate dose was used or that it was not injected at correct site.
- Myobloc (serotype B form of botulinum toxin) can be used as alternative to Botox. Dosage is 2500–5000 U/visit. Myobloc comes in 3.5-ml glass vials, which contain 5000U toxin/ml solution. Myobloc is particularly useful in patients who are resistant to Botox.
- Staged injections may be required to treat all affected muscle groups; generally done in proximal-to-distal order.

F. **Orthopedic surgery**
1. **Potential uses:** surgery is done in patients who have been refractory to more conservative measures and patients whose recovery after central nervous system insult has plateaued.
2. **Mechanism of action:** orthopedic surgery alters musculotendinous unit in way that decreases tension. It is often used when spasticity has progressed to contracture.
3. **Risks and side effects:** risks are the same as for any surgery. Bleeding and infection are possible. These procedures are most permanent forms of spasticity management and there is always the concern that, if used inappropriately, they may cause permanent decrease in function.

TABLE 6. Suggested Adult Dosing for Botox

Clinical Pattern	Potential Muscles Involved	Average Starting Dose/Units	Botox Dose Units/Visit	Number of Injections
Upper limbs				
Adducted/internally rotated shoulder	Pectoralis complex	100	75–150	4
	Latissimus dorsi	100	50–150	4
	Teres major	50	25–75	1
	Subscapularis	50	25–75	1
Flexed elbow	Brachioradialis	50	25–75	2
	Biceps	100	50–200	4
	Brachialis	50	25–75	2
Pronated forearm	Pronator quadratus	25	10–50	1
	Pronator teres	40	25–75	1
Flexed wrist	Flexor carpi radialis	50	25–100	2
	Flexor carpi ulnaris	40	10–50	2
Thumb in palm	Flexor pollicis longus	15	5–25	1
	Adductor pollicis	10	5–25	1
	Opponens	10	5–25	1
Clenched fist	Flexor digitorum superficialis	50	25–75	4
	Flexor digitorum profundus	15	25–100	2
Intrinsic plus hand	Lumbricales interossei	15	10–50/hand	3
Lower limbs				
Flexed hip	Iliacus	100	50–150	2
	Psoas	100	50–200	2
	Rectus femoris	100	75–200	3
Flexed knee	Medial hamstrings	100	50–150	3
	Gastrocnemius	150	50–150	4
	Lateral hamstrings	100	100–200	3
Adducted thighs	Adductor brevis/longus/magnus	200/leg	75–300	6./leg
Extended knee	Quadriceps mechanism	100	50–200	4
Equinovarus foot	Gastrocnemius medial/lateral	100	50–200	4
	Soleus	75	50–100	2
	Tibialis posterior	50	50–200	2
	Tibialis anterior	75	50–150	3
	Flexor digitorum longus/brevis	75	50–100	4
	Flexor hallucis longus	50	25–75	2
Striatal toe	Extensor hallucis longus	50	20–100	2
Neck	Sternocleidomastoid (SCM)*	40	15–75	2
	Scalenus complex	30	15–50	3
	Splenius capitis	60	50–150	3
	Semispinalis capitis	60	50–150	3
	Longissimus capitis	60	50–150	3
	Trapezius	60	50–150	3
	Levator scapulae	80	25–100	3

* Dose should be reduced by 50% if both SCM muscles are injected.
From Robinson R, Ruesch L: Spasticity: Etiology, evaluation, management, and role of botulism toxin type A. Muscle Nerve Suppl 6:5214, 1997, with permission.

   4. **Techniques**.
      a. Tenotomy involves transection of tendon.
      b. Neurectomy involves excision of part of nerve.
      c. Tendon transfer involves moving tendon from one insertion site to another.
      d. Tendon lengthening involves sectioning tendon with step-like incision and then sewing longest pieces together, again resulting in increased tendon length.
      e. Fusion involves locking joint in fixed position (generally an operation of last resort).
      f. Bony surgeries, such as rotational osteotomy, are occasionally done.

TABLE 7. Suggested Pediatric Dosing for Botox

Clinical Pattern	Potential Muscles Involved	Botox Dose Units/Visit	Number of Injections
Upper limbs			
Adducted/internally rotated shoulder	Pectoralis complex	2	2–3
	Latissimus dorsi	2	2
	Teres major	2	1–2
	Subscapularis	1–2	1–2
Flexed elbow	Brachioradialis	1	1
	Biceps	2	2–3
	Brachialis	2	1–2
Pronated forearm	Pronator quadratus	1	1
	Pronator teres	1	1
Flexed wrist	Flexor carpi radialis	1–2	1
	Flexor carpi ulnaris	1–2	1
Thumb in palm	Flexor pollicis longus	1	1
	Adductor pollicis	1	1
	Opponens	1	1
Clenched fist	Flexor digitorum superficialis	1–2	1–2
	Flexor digitorum profundus	1–2	1–2
Intrinsic plus hand	Lumbricales interossei	0.5–1	1
Lower limbs			
Flexed hip	Iliacus	1–2	1
	Psoas		
	Rectus femoris	3–4	2
Flexed knee	Medial hamstrings	3–6	3–4
	Gastrocnemius	3–6	2–4
	Lateral hamstrings	2–3	1–2
Adducted thighs	Adductor brevis/longus/magnus	3–6	1–2
Extended knee	Quadriceps mechanism	3–6	4
Equinovarus foot	Gastrocnemius medial/lateral	3–6	1–2
	Soleus	2–3	1–2
	Tibialis posterior	1–2	1
	Tibialis anterior	1–3	1
	Flexor digitorum longus/brevis	1–2	1
	Flexor hallucis longus	1–2	1
Striatal toe	Extensor hallucis longus	1–2	1

Dosage guidelines
Total maximum body dose/visit = lesser of 12 unit/kg or 400 units.
Maximum dose per large muscle per visit = 3–6 units/kg
Maximum dose per small muscle per visit = 1–2 units/kg
Maximum does per injection site = 50 units
Maximum volume per site - 0.5 ml with some exceptions
Reinjection > 3 months
From Robinson R, Ruesch L: Spasticity: Etiology, evaluation, management, and role of botulism toxin type A. Muscle Nerve Suppl 6:5189, 1997, with permission.

5. **Orthopedic intervention for spastic upper extremity**
  a. **Shoulder**
    i. Adducted/internally rotated shoulder: pectoralis major/subscapularis tendon release
    ii. Painful shoulder subluxation: biceps tendon sling
  b. **Elbow**
    i. Flexor spasticity: step-cut lengthening of brachioradialis, biceps, and brachialis
    ii. Extensor spasticity:V-Y lengthening of triceps
  c. **Wrist and hand**
    i. Flexor spasticity

- Fractional lengthening of flexor digitorum superficialis and flexor digitorum profundus
- Step-cut lengthening of flexor pollicis longus
- Overlengthening of flexor carpi radialis and flexor carpi ulnaris
- Flexor-pronator origin release
- Sublimis to profundus transfer

    ii. Thumb in palm deformity: release of thenar and adductors

6. **Orthopedic intervention for spastic lower extremity**
   a. **Functional deformities**
      i. Limb scissoring: obturator neurectomy
      ii. Crouched gait: iliopsoas recession, hamstring lengthening
      iii. Stiff knee gait: selective quadriceps release in select patients
      iv. Equinovarus foot: Achilles tendon lengthening, split anterior tibial tendon transfer
      v. Release of extrinsic/intrinsic toe flexors
      vi. Spastic valgus foot: release and transfer of peroneus longus
   b. **Static deformities**
      i. Hip adduction contracture: release of adductor longus, gracilis
      ii. Hip flexion contracture: release of sartorius, rectus femoris, tensor fascia lata, iliopsoas, pectineus
      iii. Hip extension: release of proximal hamstrings
      iv. Knee flexion contracture: release of distal hamstrings
      v. Knee extension: V-Y-plasty to lengthen quadriceps
      vi. Foot: as for functional deformities. Other options include release of plantar fascia and triple arthrodesis.

G. **Neurosurgical procedures**
1. **Rhizotomy**
   a. Surgery that involves interrupting spinal roots.
   b. Rhizotomy surgeries can be open or closed, complete or selective, and anterior or posterior. Anterior rhizotomies cause severe denervation atrophy of all innervated muscles and are no longer performed except occasionally in patients with complete spinal cord injury.
   c. In **radiofrequency rhizotomy**, radiofrequency wave is used to heat needle that burns individual dorsal roots that are localized under fluoroscopy. Often this procedure results in significant sensory loss.
   d. **Selective dorsal rhizotomy** involves ablation of select proportion of dorsal rootlets.
      i. **Potential uses:** often performed in lumbosacral roots of children with spastic cerebral palsy. Most surgical series report favorable outcome with improvements in both range of motion and gait, but many patients still have difficulties with motor control. Intensive therapy is needed to maximize long-term functional gains. Some studies suggest that these therapies rather than surgery itself provide much of the benefit seen after dorsal rhizotomy. Table 8 lists favorable selection criteria for selective dorsal rhizotomy.
      ii. **Mechanism of action:** excitatory input to motor neuron is reduced when dorsal rootlets are sectioned; thus, spasticity is reduced while sensation is preserved.
      iii. **Risks and side effects:** hypotonia, weakness, sensory changes, and bladder dysfunction have been reported.

TABLE 8. Favorable Selection Criteria for Selective Dorsal Rhizotomy

Pure spasticity (limited dystonia/athetosis)
Function limited primarily by spasticity
Adequate truncal balance/righting responses
Not significantly affected by primitive reflexes/movement patterns
Absence of profound underlying weakness
Selective motor control
Some degree of spontaneous forward locomotion
Spastic diplegia
History of prematurity
Minimal joint contracture and spine deformity
Adequate cognitive ability to participate in therapy
No significant motivational/behavioral problems
Age 3–8 years
Supportive and interactive family

      iv. **Technique:** dorsal aspect of thecal sac is exposed, dorsal roots are stimulated, and responses are recorded from ipsilateral and contralateral muscles of various myotomes. Various criteria are used to distinguish afferent rootlets that cause spastic responses in muscles from those that do not. These selected rootlets are then ablated. This technique usually allows bladder and bowel function to be spared. Usually 25–80% of the rootlets are ablated. Most frequently involved roots are at L5 and S1.

  2. **Myelotomy and cordotomy**
    a. **Potential use:** advocated as treatment modalities in most severe cases of spasticity; rarely performed except occasionally in patients with complete spinal cord injury.
    b. **Mechanism of action:** myelotomy is complete disruption of some spinal cord tracts; cordectomy is complete transection of spinal cord.
    c. **Side effects:** loss of bowel and bladder function, muscle wasting, and loss of erectile function.

 H. **Intrathecal baclofen (ITB) pump**
  1. **Potential uses:** to treat moderate and severe spasticity of both spinal and cerebral origin in patients who are either refractory to oral medications or who experience intolerable side effects to high doses of medications necessary to manage spasticity.
    a. Decreases lower extremity spasticity and, to a much lesser degree, upper extremity spasticity
    b. Also used to treat dystonia.
    c. Decrease in spasticity improves gait in ambulatory patients as well as upper extremity function.
    d. Patients are more comfortable and easier to care for.
    e. Need for lower extremity contracture surgery is decreased.
    f. Also may have beneficial effect on bladder management by loosening external sphincter, but often aggravates constipation.
  2. **Mechanism of action**
    a. Like oral baclofen, intrathecal baclofen binds to gamma-aminobutyric acid (GABA)-B receptors causing inhibition of monosynaptic and polysynaptic spinal reflexes.

b. Intrathecal dosing concentrates drug in spinal cord at lumbar-to-cervical ratio of 4:1, allowing much greater effect on spasticity with much lower systemic dose and much greater decrease in lower extremity than upper extremity spasticity.

3. **Risks and side effects**
   a. Most common side effects are drowsiness, dizziness, nausea, hypotension, and headache, but they are much less common with intrathecal dosing than with oral dosing.
   b. Like oral baclofen, intrathecal baclofen can cause excessive weakness.
   c. Other risks include pain, small chance of bleeding, and infection.
   d. Overdose may occur with incorrect filling or programming of pump and may result in respiratory depression and reversible coma.
   e. Withdrawal also may occur if intrathecal baclofen dosing is stopped inadvertently by tube dysfunction, pump failure, or incorrect programming of pump. This may cause increased spasticity, severe hyperthermia, and rhabdomyolysis, followed by multisystem failure and even death.

4. **Technique**
   a. Screening trial includes injection via a percutaneous lumbar puncture (LP). If decrease in spasticity is satisfactory (> 2-point drop in average lower limb Ashworth scores for spinal origin spasticity and > 1- point drop in spasticity of cerebral origin), surgery is scheduled.
   b. For patients with dystonia, continuous infusion trial may be necessary, requiring implantation of intrathecal catheter that is connected to either subcutaneous port or external pumping device.
   c. Surgery involves implanting pump subcutaneously in abdominal wall and tunneling catheter through to back, where catheter is placed in subarachnoid space.
   d. Pump is refilled when necessary by simple subcutaneous injection.
   e. Two types of pumps are available.
      i. Infusaid Corporation: constant-rate, gas-powered pump.
      ii. Medtronic: SynchroMed Drug Infusion Pump; used for ITB treatment; electronic and programmable to deliver drug in boluses at any time during day as well as by continuous infusion.
   f. Initial dose is usually 50–100 mg/day. Dose is titrated upward 2–3 times/week until satisfactory results are obtained. Average effective dose is 200–500 mg/day but may be high as 1500 mg/day.

5. **Practical considerations**
   a. **During screening trial**
      i. Consider withholding oral dose of baclofen on morning of trial to maximize ability to detect change in spasticity. If patient has severe spasticity even on oral baclofen and/or other medications, this step is not necessary.
      ii. Encourage good fluid intake on night before trial and after injection; lying flat for at least first 4 hours helps minimize side effects such as urinary retention and spinal headaches.
      iii. For patients who have previously had dorsal rhizotomy, try to avoid entering intrathecal space through scar tissue. Go above or below scar. Use of lumbar roll/pressure dressing over LP site reduces chance of cerebrospinal fluid leak.

    iv. Use same evaluator before and after injection for improved assessment of response.

    v. In patients with severe scoliosis or previous fusion surgery, perform LP under fluoroscopy.

    vi. Patients with severe athetosis or other movement disorder may need short-acting anesthetic to allow LP.

    vii. For very obese patients, initiate counseling and weight loss program before pump placement because refills can be quite difficult.

b. **During surgery**

    i. Dose of IV antibiotic just before incision and for 1–2 doses after surgery reduces chances of postoperative infections.

    ii. Abdominal binder, placed immediately after surgical procedure, may help reduce swelling and chances of cerebrospinal fluid leak.

    iii. Obese patients may need removal of adipose tissue to allow appropriate pump placement.

c. **Immediate postoperative period**

    i. Patient should lie flat for first 24 hours, then gradually sit up.

    ii. Monitor bowels closely; place on bowel program with stool softeners/enemas to avoid constipation.

    iii. Programming additional bolus after priming bolus appears to help with postoperative pain management while patient is tapered off oral baclofen.

d. **Discharge**

    i. Include prescription for oral baclofen for emergency use in case of pump failure.

    ii. Review signs and symptoms of acute baclofen withdrawal (give emergency card); also advise about Medic Alert bracelet.

e. **Follow-up**

    i. Application of EMLA disk or cream at least 1–1.5 hours before refill procedure helps greatly with patient acceptance of procedure.

    ii. Holding off aggressive physical therapy and using only safe, gentle range-of-motion exercises for first 3 weeks helps with wound healing.

6. **Drug-related problems**

a. **Overdose**

    i. Symptoms: drowsiness, dizziness, ascending hypotonia, somnolence, respiratory depression, seizures, progressive loss of consciousness, coma.

    ii. Therapeutic actions

      • Maintain airway, breathing, and circulation. Intubation/mechanical ventilation may be needed.

      • Stop pump with programmer. If no programmer available, empty reservoir using 22-gauge needle and needle-guiding template to stop drug flow. Record amount withdrawn. If no template is available, remember that pump has diameter of 6.4 cm. Center of reservoir can be determined by feeling edges of pump and going in 3.2 cm from outside edge. Raised edge of central port may be palpable.

      • Give IV physostigmine. In adults, 1–2 mg over 5–10 minutes. Pediatric dosage: 0.02 mg/kg slowly; no more than 0.5 mg/minute to maximum of 2 mg. Can induce seizures or bradycardia and may not be effective in reversing large overdoses.

- If not contraindicated, withdrawal of 30–40 ml of cerebrospinal fluid can further reduce baclofen concentration. May be done via LP or through catheter access port of pump using 25-gauge needle.
- Monitor closely for response, and note recurrence of symptoms. If recurrence is noted, repeat physostigmine, 1 mg or 0.01 mg/kg IV every 30–60 minutes, to maintain respiration. If response is inadequate, intubate and ventilate.
- Notify Medtronic Technical Services at 1-800-328-0810.

b. **Acute withdrawal of baclofen**

   i. Early symptoms: itching, dysphoria, irritability, dramatic increase in spasticity, tachycardia, fever, hypo or hypertension. Initiate early treatment with oral baclofen in high doses of 15–20 mg every 4–6 hours.

   ii. Progressive symptoms (irreversible cascade starts in 72 hours after onset of early symptoms): hyperthermia (temperatures up to 107°F), rhabdomyolysis, seizures, confusion, hallucinations, coma, multiple organ failure. Benzodiazepines, such as diazepam or lorazepam, can be used IV. Best treatment is rapid reinitiation of ITB via catheter port. Bolus injection may be given via LP, if catheter is thought to be nonfunctional.

7. **Troubleshooting** (Table 9)

TABLE 9.   Trouble-Shooting for Intrathecal Baclofen Pumps

Symptoms	Possible Cause
Sudden increase in spasticity	Noxious stimulus/concomitant illness (e.g,. bowel impaction, urinary tract infection, pressure ulcer, ear infection, pneumonia, appendicitis, sinusitis, pump pocket infection, meningitis)
	Improper programming of pump: particularly after recent refill or reprogramming
	Catheter problems: dislodgement, migration, kink, disconnection
	Pump malfunction: underinfusion, motor stops, battery dies
	Reservoir volume drops to below 2 ml: slowing infusion rate; alarm should sound (soft, continuous, chirping sound)
	Drug tolerance
	Advancement of disease (e.g., progressive conditions such as multiple sclerosis, worsening of spinal tumor, arteriovenous malformation)
Rostrally progressive hypotonia or other signs of overdose	Error in programming
	Pump malfunction
	Overdose during dye study
Pocket problems	
Swelling over pump	Seroma, hematoma, cerebrospinal fluid leak, infection of pocket cavity, drug extravasation
Erosion/dehiscence	Pump pocket too small, concomitant disease or treatment causes instability of skin
Suspected leakage of cerebrospinal fluid (headache, dizziness, nausea, swelling along catheter path/over pump, redness, pain at catheter incision site)-	Multiple punctures during placement of catheter
	Incomplete seal around catheter,
	Dislodgment, migration, disconnection, or puncture of catheter
	If fibrin glue is used to help seal catheter at back and pump incision sites, it will soften in about 2–3 weeks. Fluctuant puffiness may be noted at incisions, but it will not continue to increase
Difficulty in accessing reservoir port	Very obese patient (may need longer needle than that provided)
	Seroma, pocket infection
	Flipped pump

    a. Patient-related problems: infections, bowel impaction, skin infection-pump pocket/incision infections, worsening disease.

    b. System-related problems: history of recent fall should raise suspicion for catheter break/dislodgment.

    c. Programmer-related problems: least likely but known to occur; examples include battery and alarm problems.

Bibliography

1. Bohannon RW, Smith MB: Interrater reliability on modified Ashworth scale of muscle spasticity. Phys Ther 67:207, 1987.
2. Boyd RN, Graham HK: Objective measurement of clinical findings in the use of botulism toxin A in the management of children with cerebral palsy. Eur J Neurol 6:523–556, 1999.
3. Glenn MB, Whyte J: The Practical Management of Spasticity in Children and Adults. Philadelphia, Lea & Febiger, 1990.
4. Katz RT: Spasticity. In O'Young BJ, Young MA, Stiens SA (eds): PM&R Secrets, 2nd ed. Philadelphia, Hanley & Belfus, 2002, pp 442–446.
5. Katz RT, Dewald JPA, Schmit BD: Spasticity. In Braddom RL (ed): Physical Medicine and Rehabilitation. Philadelphia, W.B. Saunders, 2000, pp 592–615.
6. Robinson R, Ruesch L: Spasticity: Etiology, evaluation, management, and the role of botulinum toxin type A. Muscle Nerve 20(Suppl 6):5114–5231, 1997.

Chapter 20

SPEECH, LANGUAGE, AND SWALLOWING CONCERNS

Lynn E. Driver, M.S., CCC, and Karen B. Kurcz, M.A., CCC

I. General Principles

A. Speech-language pathologists provide diagnostic, treatment, and educational services to children and adults with impairments of speech, language, voice, fluency, communicative-cognitive, memory and swallowing skills.

B. Speech-language disorders can be divided into three categories: congenital, developmental, and acquired (Table 1).

II. Motor Speech Disorders

A. Collection of communication disorders involving retrieval and activation of motor plans for speech or execution of movements for speech production.

B. Occur in both children and adults.

C. **Congenital:** identifiable etiology presents at birth, causing processing impairment that affects speech acquisition.

TABLE 1.   Overview of Speech-Language Pathology

	Congenital	Developmental	Acquired
Motor speech disorders	Dysarthria	Phonologic disorder Verbal apraxia Articulation disorder	Dysarthria Verbal apraxia Articulation disorder
Language disorders	Aphasia	Aphasia Language delay Language disorder	Aphasia
Voice disorders	Aphonia Dysphonia	Aphonia Dysphonia	Aphonia Dysphonia
Fluency disorders		Dysfluency/stuttering Nonfluency	Dysfluency/stuttering
Communicative-cognitive disorders		Learning disabilities Autism	Traumatic brain injury Right hemisphere dysfunction Language of confusion Language of generalized intellectual impairment
Memory disorders			Short-term memory deficit Long-term memory deficit Verbal learning deficit
Swallowing disorders	Oral dysphagia Pharyngeal dysphagia Oropharyngeal dysphagia		Oral dysphagia Pharyngeal dysphagia Oropharyngeal dysphagia

D. **Developmental:** no specific, identifiable etiology to explain delays in speech acquisition and development.

E. **Acquired:** adverse event (usually neurologic) impedes continuation of previously normal speech acquisition.

F. **Subcategories** include dysarthria, oral apraxia, and apraxia of speech.

    1. **Dysarthria** (congenital, developmental or acquired)

        a. Group of related motor speech disorders resulting from disturbed muscular control of speech mechanism and manifested as disrupted or distorted oral communication due to paralysis, weakness, abnormal tone or incoordination of muscles used in speech.

        b. Oral and speech movements may be impaired in force, timing, endurance, direction, and range of motion.

        c. **Sites of lesion** include bilateral cortex, basal ganglia, cerebellum, and cranial nerves.

        d. **Parameters of speech** affected with dysarthria include:

            i. Respiration: respiratory support for speech, breathing-speaking synchrony, sustained phonation.

            ii. Phonation/voice: loudness, quality.

            iii. Articulation: precision of consonants and vowels.

            iv. Resonance: degree of airflow through nasal cavity.

            v. Prosody: melody of speech, use of stress and inflection.

        e. **Causes**

            i. Cerebrovascular accident (CVA)   vi. Myasthenia gravis

            ii. Tumor   vii. Encephalopathy

            iii. Aneurysm   viii. Seizure disorder

            iv. Progressive neurologic disease   ix. Cerebral palsy (CP)

            v. Traumatic brain injury (TBI)   x. Spinal cord injury (SCI)

        f. **Types**

            i. Different types of dysarthria depend on etiology and site of lesion.

            ii. Various classification systems have been devised for differential diagnosis of dysarthria.

            iii. Table 2 lists common dysarthrias and associated characteristics.

        g. **Evaluation**

            i. Hearing

            ii. Head/neck strength, speed and range of motion for depression, elevation, rotation

            iii. Oral motor: assessment of strength, speed, range, and coordination of movement

              • Facial

              • Labial

              • Mandibular

              • Lingual

              • Palatal

              • Oral agility: rapid repetitions of /pa/, /ta/, /ka/ and /pataka/ in 5-second trials

              • Perceptual speech analysis: respiration, phonation/voice, articulation, resonance, prosody

    2. **Oral apraxia**

        a. Impairment of voluntary ability to produce movements of facial, labial, mandibular, lingual, palatal, pharyngeal, or laryngeal musculature.

TABLE 2. Types of Dysarthria

	Spastic	Hypokinetic	Hyperkinetic	Ataxic	Flaccid	Mixed
Site of lesion	Bilateral upper motor neuron	Extrapyramidal system	Extrapyramidal system	Cerebellum	Unilateral or bilateral lower motor neuron	Multiple sites
Associated features	Spasticity of orofacial muscles	Ridigity of orofacial muscles	Involuntary movements of orofacial muscles		Flaccidity of orofacial muscles	Depends on site of lesion
	Imprecise articulatory contacts	Imprecise articulatory contacts	Imprecise articulatory contacts	Irregular articulatory breakdown	Imprecise articulatory contacts	
	Strained/strangled voice quality	Hypophonia	Harsh voice quality	Harsh vocal quality	Breathy voice quality	
	Monopitch	Monopitch	Incoordination of respiratory stream	Incoordination of respiratory strearm	Low vocal volume	
	Reduced stress	Reduced stress and inflection		Excessive and equal stress pattern	Reduced stress and inflection	
	Reduced rate	Transient increased rate/rapid rate	Transient increased rate	Reduced rate	Hypernasality	
Example	Pseudo-bulbar palsy	Parkinson's disease	Dystonia	Friedreich's ataxia	Bulbar palsy	ALS

ALS = amyotrophic lateral sclerosis.

   b. Site of lesion is left Rolandic fissure, anterior insula, and adjacent superior temporal region.
 3. **Verbal apraxia** (also called apraxia of speech [AOS])
   a. Impairment of motor speech is characterized by diminished ability to program positioning and sequencing of movements of speech musculature for volitional production of speech sounds.
   b. Apraxia does not result from muscle paralysis or weakness but may lead to perceptual disturbances of breathing/speaking synchrony, articulation, and prosody.
   c. Site of lesion is generally left precentral motor or insular areas.
 4. **Developmental verbal apraxia** (also called developmental apraxia of speech [DAOS])
   a. Motor speech disorder resulting from delay or deviance in processes involved in planning and programming movement sequences for speech in absence of muscle weakness or paralysis.
   b. Associated characteristics of verbal apraxias
     i. Receptive better than expressive language.
     ii. Presence of oral apraxia (may or may not exist with DAOS).
     iii. Phonemic errors (often sound omissions).
     iv. Difficulty in achieving initial articulatory configuration.
     v. Difficulty with transitions in place and manner of articulation.
     vi. Increase in errors with increase in word length or phonetic complexity.

      vi. Connected speech poorer than single word production.

     vii. Inconsistent error patterns.

    viii. Groping and/or trial-and-error behavior.

     ix. Vowel errors.

  c. Children with motor speech disorders may demonstrate impaired phonologic systems because their ability to acquire sound system of their language is undermined by difficulties in managing intense motor demands of connected speech.

5. **Phonologic disorder**

  a. Subset of sound production disorders in which linguistic and cognitive factors rather than motor planning or execution are thought to be central to observed difficulties (commonly associated etiologic variables include otitis media with effusion, genetics, psychosocial factors).

  b. Developmental phonologic processes are patterns seen in normal development that resolve at predictable ages. Examples include velar fronting: "tee"/ "key," "mate"/"make."

  c. Nondevelopmental phonologic processes are hallmark of disordered vs. delayed phonologic development, and rarely seen in normal development. Examples include initial consonant deletion: "ee"/"key," "ake"/"make."

III. Language Disorders

A. **Aphasia**

1. Impairment of language secondary to damage of dominant hemisphere (left in most patients).

2. Small percentage of left-handed people have reversed or mixed dominance.

3. Disturbance of ability to formulate and comprehend language symbols is not caused by disruption of sensory, motor or thought processes.

4. **Differential diagnosis** is aided by assessment of comprehension, repetition, and naming skills as described by Goodglass and Kaplan (Boston system).

5. **Causes**

  a. CVA   d. TBI

  b. Tumor   e. Arteriovenous malformation (AVM)

  c. Aneurysm

6. **Aphasia types** (Table 3)

  a. Differential diagnosis of the aphasias relates to skills of naming, repetition, and comprehension.

  b. Nonfluent/fluent dichotomy is used in Boston system rather than expressive/receptive diagnosis since both expressive and receptive skills are affected in all aphasias.

7. **Evaluation**

  a. Hearing

  b. Auditory/reading comprehension of single words to paragraph-length material.

  c. Verbal/written expression from single phonemes or words to discourse of paragraph length.

  d. Pragmatics

B. **Developmental language delay**

  a. Delay in acquisition and development of age-appropriate language skills, typically across all domains.

  b. Delay can be due to medical or psychosocial factors.

TABLE 3. Types of Aphasia

Type	Site of Lesion	Associated Characteristics
Fluent aphasias		
Anomic	Temporal-parietal lobes; may extend to angular gyrus	Impaired responsive and confrontational naming; fair to good repetition and comprehension; verbal paraphasias.*
Wernicke's	Posterior, superior temporal gyrus	Impaired comprehension and repetition; neologisms, literal/verbal paraphasias.
Conduction	Arcuate fasciculus	Specific diffulty with repetition; fair to good comprehension; literal paraphasias.
Transcortical sensory	Parietal-occipital lobes	Rare disorder; impaired comprehension and relatively preserved repetition; may be able to recite previously memorized material; paraphasias and neologisms.†
Nonfluent aphasias		
Broca's	Inferior third frontal convolution with extension posteriorly to motor strip	Comprehension is relatively superior to verbal expression; telegraphic output; literal and verbal paraphasias.
Transcortical motor	Anterior and superior to Broca's area	Ability to repeat is nearly intact; fair to good comprehension. Sparse overall output with occasional intact utterances.
Global	Widespread dominant hemisphere	Poor comprehension, repetition, naming with minimal output/mutism.
Subcortical aphasias	Basal ganglia, thalamus	Depends on type of infarct (hemorrhagic vs. nonhemorrhagic) and specific site of lesion within basal ganglia or thalamus. Nonfluent and fluent patterns have been documented.

* Paraphasias include verbal (semantic) and literal (phonemic) errors. Verbal paraphasias are real-word substitutions that generally do not relate to the stimulus. Literal paraphasias are words that include a portion of the target word as well as extraneous phonemes or syllables. Literal paraphasias and, at times, verbal paraphasias may be recognized by the patient, who may attempt self-correction. Similar error patterns may be seen in written output and are labeled as paragraphic errors.
† Neologisms (jargon) are nonwords and are most often associated with fluent aphasia.

C. **Language disorder**
 1. Aberrant or interrupted development, often due to significant medical or psychosocial event.
   a. **Developmental** language disorder is characterized by atypical development of language skills in one or more domains.
   b. **Acquired** language disorder is characterized by language deficits in one or more domains secondary to neurologic insult.
     i. Can and often does result in aberrant development due to interruption in normal course of language acquisition.
     ii. **Causes** of loss or deterioration of language in childhood
       • Aphasias of traumatic origin: head injury, unilateral cerebrovascular lesions, cerebral infections, surgical removal of tumor, cerebral anoxia.
       • Aphasias of convulsive origin: Landau-Kleffner syndrome, others.
       • Other syndromes with loss or deterioration of language: late-onset autism, Rett's syndrome.
     iii. **Acquired childhood aphasia**
       • Language disorder secondary to cerebral dysfunction in childhood after period of normal language development.

- Cerebral dysfunction may result from focal lesion of one of cerebral hemispheres, diffuse lesion of central nervous system above level of brainstem (TBI, cerebral infection), diffuse lesion related to convulsive activity, or unknown etiology.
- Pediatric acquired aphasia tends to be characterized by nonfluency, with primary deficits in verbal expression and parallel deficits in written expression. Auditory comprehension is relatively intact.

2. **Differences in management of pediatric and adult acquired brain injury**
   a. Pediatric brain injury occurs on moving baseline of normal development on which further development is expected.
   b. Assessment tools must be appropriate for developmental age of child; in young children, some functions are not accessible.
   c. Plasticity in developing nervous system may allow preservation of certain functions, particularly those related to language.
   d. Plasticity theoretically may involve relocation of function to opposite hemisphere or elsewhere in same hemisphere.
   e. Normal recovery is dramatic, unexplained phenomenon and should not be confused with plasticity.
   f. Critical periods for development of particular function may exist, which, for most part, cannot be retrieved; for example, development of social communication in young children at relatively high risk for development of autistic features.

3. **Associated medical conditions** specific to children that may result in language delay/disorder:
   a. Chromosomal disorders (e.g., Down syndrome)
   b. Single gene disorders (e.g., clefting, spina bifida, Apert's syndrome)
   c. Sporadic syndromes (e.g., Goldenhar, Moebius, and Prader-Willi syndromes)
   d. Environmental syndromes (e.g., fetal alcohol, failure to thrive, fetal rubella)
   e. Birth-related disorders (e.g., prematurity, asphyxia, cerebral palsy, very low birth weight)
   f. Congenital hearing loss

4. **Importance of relating disorder to developmental stage**
   a. In assessing language disorders in children, it is crucial to understand normal developmental level associated with chronologic age of child.
   b. Determine premorbid developmental levels.
   c. To assess impact of neurologic event or other interruption in typical developmental maturation.

5. **Importance of identifying children at risk:** speech and language delays/disorders in infancy and toddlerhood can result in difficulties in academic learning, social interaction, and development of appropriate peer relationships throughout childhood.

6. **Areas of assessment in pediatric language disorders**
   a. Pragmatics
   b. Play
   c. Cognitive orientation
   d. Attention
   e. Attachment/interaction
   f. Prelinguistic behaviors
   g. Language comprehension
   h. Language production
   i. Hearing

7. **Danger signals of communication problems by age**
   a. **By 6 months**
      i. Does not respond to sound of others talking.
      ii. Does not turn toward speaker out of view.
      iii. Makes only crying sounds.
      iv. Does not maintain eye contact with caregiver.
   b. **By 12 months**
      i. Does not babble.
      ii. Does not discontinue activity when told "no."
      iii. Does not follow gesture commands, such as "want up" or "give me."
   c. **By 24 months**
      i. Does not say any meaningful word.
      ii. Does not refer to self by name.
      iii. Does not follow simple directions.
      iv. Does not talk at all at 2 years.
      v. Vocabulary does not seem to increase.
      vi. Does not have any consonant sounds.
      vii. Does not answer simple yes/no questions.
   d. **By 36 months**
      i. Does not say whole name.
      ii. Does not seem to understand "what" and "where" questions.
      iii. Uses jargon a great deal.
      iv. Answers question by repeating question.
      v. Continues to echo statements made by others.
      vi. Does not use utterances of 2–3 words.
      vii. Points to desired objects rather than naming them.
      viii. Does not name any objects in pictures.
      ix. Leaves off beginning consonants of words.
      x. Cannot be understood even by parents.
      xi. Does not respond when name is called.

IV. Voice Disorders

A. Dysphonia

1. Impairment of voice secondary to cranial nerve involvement, tracheostomy, or laryngeal pathology.
2. May be prominent feature of dysarthria related to cranial nerve involvement.
3. Laryngeal pathologies resulting in dysphonia may include polyps, granulomas, nodules or other lesions affecting vocal fold mucosa.
4. Lesions may necessitate partial or complete laryngectomy with subsequent aphonia.

B. Aphonia

   a. Absence of voice secondary to cranial nerve involvement, tracheostomy, or laryngeal pathology.
   b. Cuffed tracheostomy tube placement may cause aphonia due to obstruction of airflow through larynx.
   c. Patients with tracheostomy tubes may be able to produce voice by following methods:
      i. **Cuff deflation:** partial or complete deflation of cuff may permit enough air leak around tracheostomy tube to achieve voicing, given digital occlusion of tube on exhalation.

ii. **One-way valve:** placement of one-way valve on tracheostomy tube allows airflow into tube on inhalation, closes tube on exhalation to direct air upward through larynx. Cuff must be completely deflated for use.

iii. **Uncuffed tube:** digital occlusion on exhalation or use of plug. If patient requires supplemental oxygen, nasal cannula may be necessary. Plug cannot be used if oxygen via tracheostomy mask is required.

iv. **"Talking" tracheostomy tube:** for use with ventilator-dependent patients who cannot tolerate cuff deflation. Additional line on outer surface of tracheostomy tube attaches to alternate compressed air source. Line allows transmission of air through fenestrations above cuff and upward through larynx for voice production.

v. **Cuff deflation/use of the ventilator cycle:** once they are stable on mechanical ventilation and once positive end-expiratory pressure (PEEP) is no longer required, patients may learn to phonate when cuff is partially to completely deflated. Voice is achieved on inspiratory cycle of ventilator. Adjustments of tidal volume, breath per minute and/or inspiratory to expiratory ratio may help to achieve best voice.

vi. **Electrolarynx/tracheoesophageal puncture:** used after laryngectomy to achieve phonation.

d. **Trouble-shooting**

i. Cuff is deflated, but patient is unable to voice.
- Copious secretions with need for tracheal suctioning.
- Air space around deflated cuff may be too narrow.
- Consider downsizing tracheostomy tube.

ii. When using one-way valve, voice has low volume and is strained.
- Insufficient amount of airflow around deflated cuff: remove valve.
- Consider downsizing tracheostomy tube.

iv. No voice using speaking line of "talking" tracheostomy tube.
- Copious secretions on cuff with need for suctioning of line.
- Angle of tube may cause fenestrations to be occluded by pressure against tracheal wall.
- Consider use of shorter tube or different manufacturer.

v. No speaking voice, but patient has audible cough: patient may need training to reestablish voice.

vi. No voice using inspiratory cycle of ventilator.
- Patient may need position adjustment to align tracheostomy tube vertically within trachea.
- Adjust tidal volume, breaths per minute, and/or inspiratory to expiratory ratio.

V. Fluency Disorders
A. Nonfluency
1. Associated with nonfluent aphasia or apraxia of speech.
2. Short utterances with omission of connecting words such as articles ("the," "a") or verb "to be."
3. Impaired prosody with frequent pausing.
B. Developmental dysfluency (commonly called stuttering)
1. Phoneme/word repetitions, prolongations or arrest of phoneme productions.

2. No adaptation effects.
3. Often includes secondary behaviors such as facial grimacing or other body movements/gestures.
4. Anxiety and concern for difficulty with self-correction are present.

C. **Acquired dysfluency**
1. Motor speech disorder resulting from trauma, vascular injury, or extrapyramidal disease.
2. Phoneme/word repetitions, prolongations or arrest of phoneme productions.
3. Adaptation may occur with ability to improve with repetition of effort.
4. Awareness of errors may be present, but without anxiety.
5. Unilateral lesions are associated with transient dysfluency.
6. Bilateral lesions are associated with chronic/progressive dysfluency.

VI. Communication–Cognition Disorders

A. **Traumatic brain injury** (see Chapter 10, Traumatic Brain Injury)
1. May include impairments of oral motor, speech, voice, fluency, language, verbal reasoning, and executive cognitive functions.
2. Impairments of executive cognitive functions may include impairments in attention (sustained, selective, alternating, divided), awareness of deficits, initiation, impulse control, self-monitoring, self-correction, set-shifting, goal setting, development, and use of strategies.
3. **Site of lesion**
   a. Diffuse axonal injury
   b. Focal cortical/subcortical injury
   c. Contrecoup injury
4. **Evaluation**
   a. Hearing
   b. Oral motor
   c. Motor speech
   d. Language
      i. Auditory comprehension
      ii. Verbal expression
      iii. Reading comprehension
      iv. Written expression
   e. Communicative–cognitive
      i. Orientation
      ii. Attention
      iii. Verbal reasoning
      iv. Verbal/visual memory
      v. Executive cognitive functions
      vi. Pragmatics
      vii. Rancho Los Amigos Levels of Cognitive Functioning Scales

B. **Right hemisphere dysfunction**
1. Impairment of thought processes and executive cognitive skills.
2. Often includes perceptual deficits affecting reading comprehension and written expression secondary to neglect and visual perceptual disorders associated with right parietal function.
3. **Causes**
   a. CVA
   b. Tumor
   c. Aneurysm
   d. TBI
   e. AVM
4. **Site of lesion and associated characteristics**
   a. Right frontal, temporal, parietal, and /or occipital lobes; subcortical structures such as basal ganglia or thalamus
   b. Impairments of executive cognitive functions may include impairments in attention (sustained, selective, alternating, divided), awareness of

deficits (anosagnosia), initiation, impulse control, self-monitoring, self-correction, set shifting, goal setting, development, and use of strategies.

   c. Impairments of visual-perceptual skills such as left neglect or left homonymous hemianopsia affect ability to read text and monitor writing.

5. **Evaluation**

   a. Orientation

   b. Attention

   c. Verbal reasoning

   d. Verbal/visual memory

   e. Executive cognitive functions

   f. Reading/writing

   g. Pragmatics

C. **Language of confusion**

1. Acute change in orientation and attention skills (sustained, selective, alternating, and divided).

2. Acute changes in executive cognitive functions (awareness, insight, self-initiation, impulse control, self-monitoring, set-shifting, goal-setting, and use of strategic behaviors).

3. Degree of impairment often affects focal language skills of auditory/reading comprehension, and verbal/written expression.

4. Status may wax and wane.

5. **Causes**

   a. Encephalopathy

   b. TBI

   c. Aneurysm

   d. CVA

6. **Site of lesion**

   a. Diffuse cortical to subcortical involvement

   b. Focal unilateral or bilateral hemispheric injury

7. **Evaluation**

   a. Orientation

   b. Attention

   c. Comprehension

   d. Expression

   e. Verbal reasoning

   f. Verbal/visual memory

   g. Pragmatics

D. **Language of generalized intellectual impairment**

1. Similar degree of impairment of both language and communicative-cognitive skills.

2. Treatment is generally not recommended because of progressive nature of disease; however, family should be educated about methods to maximize communication skills for activities of daily living.

3. **Causes**

   a. Dementias (e.g., multi-infarct, Alzheimer's disease)

   b. Encephalopathy

4. **Site of lesion**

   a. Bilateral cortex

   b. Bilateral subcortical structures (e.g., hippocampus)

5. **Evaluation**

   a. Hearing

   b. Oral motor

   c. Speech/voice

   d. Language modalities

   e. Communicative-cognitive skills

VII. Verbal/Visual Memory Disorders

A. **Definitions**

1. **Immediate recall:** ability to recall verbal or visual (written/graphic) information immediately after stimulus.

2. **Short-term memory:** ability to recall verbal or visual information for several minutes to several days.
3. **Long-term memory:** ability to recall information from remote past.
4. **Verbal learning impairment:** difficulty in learning new information such as sequence of instructions to complete activity, although comprehension of information is adequate. Impairment of attention adversely affects ability to learn.
5. **Causes**
   a. Developmental seizure disorder   c. TBI
   b. Dementia   d. Encephalopathy
6. **Site of lesion:** bilateral anterior, lateral, or mesial temporal lobes, hippocampus, amygdala
7. **Evaluation**
   a. Attention skills
   b. Recall of related and unrelated words (3–5)
   c. Recall of digit spans
   d. Recall of events within day or previous day
   e. Recall of personal information
   f. Recall of past events

VIII. Swallowing Disorders
A. **Oral dysphagia**
   1. Impairment in oral phase of swallowing.
   2. Involves management of bolus from entry into oral cavity to initiation of pharyngeal swallow at base of tongue.
B. **Pharyngeal dysphagia**
   1. Impairment of the pharyngeal phase of swallowing.
   2. Involves movement of bolus from initiation of swallow at base of tongue through pharynx to level of cricopharyngeus.
C. **Oropharyngeal dysphagia:** impairment of both oral and pharyngeal phases of swallowing.
D. **Causes**
   1. Congenital neurologic disorders
   2. Anatomic or structural abnormalities
   3. Right hemisphere CVA
   4. Large left hemisphere CVA (smaller left lesions often do not cause dysphagia)
   5. TBI
   6. SCI: high cervical lesions
   7. Surgery (e.g., anterior cervical disc fusion, laryngectomy, cardiac)
   8. Degenerative diseases
   9. Neuromuscular diseases
      a. Amyotrophic lateral sclerosis
      b. Myasthenia gravis
   10. Connective tissue disorders
      a. Systemic lupus erythematosus
      b. Scleroderma
   11. Myopathy
      a. Polymyositis   d. Postpoliomyelitis syndrome
      b. Dermatomyositis   e. Muscular dystrophy
      c. Inclusion body myositis

E. **Cranial nerves (CNs) and swallowing**
   1. CN V (trigeminal)
      a. Mastication
      b. Hyoid and tongue elevation
      c. Anterior two-thirds of tongue; cheeks (sensory)
   2. CN VII (facial)
      a. Lower facial muscles
      b. Lips
      c. Hyoid
      d. Base of tongue
      e. Taste for anterior two-thirds of tongue
      f. Salivation
   3. CN XI (glossopharyngeal)
      a. Pharyngeal constrictors
      b. Mucosa in oropharynx (sensory)
      c. Posterior tongue (sensory, taste)
   4. CN X (vagus)
      a. Larynx (sensory from superior and recurrent laryngeal nerves, motor from recurrent laryngeal nerve)
      b. Hypopharynx
      c. Soft palate
      d. Cricopharyngeus
   5. CN XI (spinal accessory)
      a. Elevation and depression of soft palate
      b. Tongue movement
      c. Pharynx
   6. CN XII (hypoglossal)
      a. Tongue
      b. Hyoid
      c. Extrinsic larynx
F. **Conditions associated with swallowing disorders in children**
   1. **Anatomic or structural defects**
      a. Congenital (e.g., tracheoesophageal fistula, choanal atresia, cleft palate)
      b. Acquired (e.g., laryngeal trauma)
   2. **Neurologic deficits**
      a. Cerebral palsy
      b. Traumatic brain injury
      c. Genetic syndromes
      d. Hypoxic/ischemic encephalopathy
      e. Meningitis
      f. Arnold-Chiari malformation
      g. Progressive degenerative neurologic disease
      h. Muscular dystrophy
      i. Guillain-Barré syndrome
   3. **Systemic conditions**
      a. Respiratory diseases (bronchopulmonary dysplasia, reactive airway disease, asthma)
      b. Gastrointestinal (GI) tract disorders (gastroesophageal reflux, esophageal dysmotility)
      c. Connective tissue disorder (scleroderma)
   4. **Complex medical conditions**
      a. Prematurity
      b. Medically fragile

G. **Clinical presentation**
  1. **Pulmonary signs and symptoms**
     a. Chronic: recurrent pneumonia, bronchitis, asthma, upper respiratory infections.
     b. Acute: cough, choke, or gag with eating; changes in voice during/after eating; changes in breathing/respiratory rate; build-up of secretions; fever of unknown origin; decrease in oxygen saturation, decline in alertness/activity during feeding (pediatric).
  2. **GI tract signs and symptoms**
     a. Poor nutritional status
     b. Weight/growth compromise/failure to thrive (pediatric)
     c. Emesis, regurgitation, or gastroesophageal reflux
  3. **Oral motor dysfunction**
     a. Prolonged mealtimes
     b. Excessive drooling
     c. Excessive gagging on oral secretions or during feeds
     d. Delayed or difficult initiation of swallow
     e. Food in mouth after swallow
     f. Multiple swallows to clear oral cavity
  4. **Unusual or inappropriate feeding patterns** (pediatric)
     a. Selective food refusal or resistance
     b. Limited oral intake
     c. Failure to accept age-appropriate foods
     d. Excessive adaptations required to encourage feeding
H. **Clinical swallowing evaluation: adults**
  1. **Complete history** based on medical chart and patient or family interview. (*Note:* Many adults do not associate presence of cough during meals with swallowing disorder).
     a. History of swallowing disorder
     b. Recent upper respiratory infection
     c. Unexplained weight loss and duration of meals
     d. Coughing or choking while eating
  2. **Oral motor/motor speech evaluation**
     a. Strength, speed, range, and accuracy of movement of labial, mandibular, lingual, and palatal musculature.
     b. Oral agility assessed via diadochokinetic rates for repetition of /pa/, /ta/, /ka/, and sequential movement rates and accuracy of /pataka/. This test indicates agility for bilabial, lingua-alveolar, and velar consonants.
     c. Perceptual speech analysis
        i. Respiratory support for speech, including sustained phonation
        ii. Phonation
        iii. Articulation
        iv. Resonance
        v. Prosody
  3. **Swallowing trial**
     a. Use of ice, water (thin liquid), puree (apple sauce or pudding), soft solid (diced fruit) and solid (cookie) food depends on oral motor examination, overall level of arousal, and medical status.
     b. Patients with tracheostomy: liquids/foods tinted blue.
     c. Observe
        i. Tolerance for upright position
        ii. Ability to move oral structures for bolus formation/transit

        iii. Ability to clear oral cavity, number of swallows required to clear

        iv. Onset of laryngeal elevation (should be approximately 1 second after transit begins)

        v. Fatigue over time

        vi. Delayed cough

        vii. Complaint of solids in pharynx after swallow or pain during swallow

  d. Assess

        i. Vocal quality after swallow (wet quality may indicate laryngeal penetration)

        ii. Presence of cough or throat clear

        iii. Strength of volitional cough or throat clearing

I. Clinical swallowing evaluation: infants/toddlers

  1. **History**

  2. **Prefeeding assessment**

    a. Parent-child interaction

    b. Posture and movement patterns

    c. Respiratory patterns

    d. Affect, temperament, and overall responsiveness

    e. Level of alertness/sustained attention

    f. Response to sensory stimulation

    g. Ability to calm/regulate self

  3. **Oral motor exam**

    a. Lip and jaw position

    b. Palatal shape and height

    c. Tongue shape and movement patterns

    d. Oral reflexes

    e. Laryngeal function

    f. Nonnutritive suck (infants)

  4. **Feeding assessment**

    a. Observe infants at least 15–20 minutes; necessary volume per feed in this amount of time indicates functional oral feeder.

    b. Observe older infants and children with familiar feeder

    c. Observe typical positioning.

    d. Observe lip, tongue, and jaw actions with spoon or finger feeding.

J. Instrumental examination

  1. Videofluoroscopic swallow study (VFSS)/fiberoptic endoscopic evaluation of swallowing (FEES): performed when questions about swallowing function remain after bedside/clinical assessment.

  2. **Components assessed**

    a. Oral preparatory phase/oral phase (VFSS)

        i. Ability to take food or liquid into mouth from spoon or cup/straw.

        ii. Efficiency of lingual and mandibular movements needed for mastication.

        iii. Efficiency of bolus formation on the tongue surface.

        iv. Maintenance of bolus within oral cavity without spillage to pharynx before swallow.

        v. Coordination and timing of anterior to posterior bolus propulsion.

        vi. Velar elevation to close nasopharynx.

    b. Pharyngeal phase (VFSS or FEES)

        i. Onset of pharyngeal swallow response.

      ii. Hyoid elevation (superiorly and anteriorly).

      iii. Epiglottic excursion (downward over aryepiglottic folds).

      iv. Passage of bolus (around entrance to airway, posterior to epiglottis).

      v. Pharyngeal motility (pharyngeal constrictors propel bolus toward cricopharyngeus).

      vi. Cricopharyngeus opening (relaxation to allow bolus passage into esophagus).

  c. Esophageal phase (structure and motility assessed by radiologist).

3. **Contraindications for VFSS**

  a. Medical instability (respiratory rate, heart rate, oxygen saturation)

  b. Physical limitations (lethargy, oral defensiveness, absent swallow, lack of cooperation)

  c. Radiation exposure

3. **Prerequisites for VFSS**

  a. Ability to swallow (infants of 37+ weeks' gestation)

  b. Alertness

  c. Sufficient amount to define nature of oropharyngeal function ($\frac{1}{2}$ to 1 ounce of fluid within reasonable period)

  d. Oral feeding experience (pediatric)

  e. Medical stability

  f. Ability to tolerate appropriate position

4. **Alternative evaluation procedures**

  a. FEES

  b. Ultrasonography

  c. Pulse oximetry

  d. Cervical auscultation

  e. Blue dye test

  f. Scintigraphy

5. **Dysphagia diets**

  a. **Thin liquids**

      i. Examples: water, juice, coffee, tea, soda, milk, gelatin (changes from solid to liquid form in oral phase).

      ii. Indications: adequate strength and coordination of lip and tongue musculature; may be used when pharyngeal constrictor function is reduced.

  b. **Thick liquids**

      i. Examples: nectars, milk shakes, cream soups, ice cream (changes from solid to liquid form in oral phase), any liquid mixed with thickening agent to approximate nectar consistency or thicker.

      ii. Indications: weakened oral musculature with adequate pharyngeal constrictor function for bolus propulsion to esophagus.

  c. **Mashed solid/puree**

      i. Examples: pureed meats, fruits, or vegetables; yogurt; pudding; cream of wheat; cream of rice.

      ii. Indications: mastication not required. Used in patients with weak tongue/mandibular musculature or reduced mastication range of motion.

  d. **Semisolid**

      i. Examples: minced meat/fish, cottage cheese, scrambled eggs, soft mashed fruits or vegetables, cooked cereals.

    ii. Indications: some mastication necessary. Fair oral motor control, although with some degree of oral weakness.

  e. **Soft chunk foods**

    i. Examples: yogurt with soft fruit, soft cheeses, smooth peanut butter, minced meats, baked or steamed fish, poached or hard-boiled eggs, banana, canned fruit, mashed vegetables, bread, toast, cold cereal, pancakes, French toast, pasta, rice, noodles, cake, pie, plain soft cookies.

    ii. Indications: Mastication is necessary. Appropriate for patients with adequate oral motor control but decreased endurance.

Bibliography

1. Alexander MP, Naeser MA, Palumbo CL: Correlations of subcortical CT lesion sites and aphasia profiles. Brain 110:961–991, 1987.
2. Caruso AJ, Strand EA (eds): Clinical Management of Motor Speech Disorders in Children. New York, Thieme, 1999.
3. Damasio AR, Damasio H, Rizzo M, et al: Aphasia with nonhemorrhagic lesions in the basal ganglia and internal capsule. Arch Neurol 39:15–20, 1982.
4. Darley F, Aronson A, Brown J: Motor Speech Disorders. Philadelphia, W. B. Saunders, 1975.
5. Goodglass H, Kaplan E: The Assessment of Aphasia and Related Disorders, 2nd ed. Philadelphia, Lea & Febiger, 1983.
6. Hagan C, Malkmus D, Durham P: Levels of cognitive functioning. Presented at Head Trauma Rehabilitation Seminar, Rancho Los Amigos Hospital, Los Angeles, 1977.
7. Helm NA, Butler RB, Benson DF: Acquired stuttering. Neurology 28:1159–1165, 1978.
8. Lees JA: Children with Acquired Aphasias. San Diego, Singular Publishing Group, 1993.
9. Tognola G, Vignolo LA: Brain lesions associated with oral apraxia in stroke patients: A clinico-neuroradiological investigation with the CT scan, Neuropsychologia 18:257, 1980.
10. Ylvisaker M, Szekeres SF: Metacognitive and executive impairments in head-injured children and adults. Top Lang Disord 9(2):34–49, 1989.

Chapter 21

MOBILITY AIDS

Lori L. Brinkey, MPT

I. Description of Common Mobility Devices
  A. Ambulation aids
    1. **Straight cane**
      a. Cane with one point of support.
      b. For patients with mild-to-moderate weakness or balance impairment.
      c. Made of various materials.
      d. Used on opposite side of weakness with tripod gait pattern.
      e. Inexpensive
    2. **Quad cane** (Fig. 1)
      a. Cane with four points of support at base.
      b. For patients with moderate weakness or balance impairment.
      c. Small or large base (the larger the base, the more stability provided).
      d. Used on opposite side of weakness with tripod gait pattern.
    3. **Axillary crutch**
      a. Crutch with single base of support.
      b. Top portion extends upward to axillae but should not touch the axillae.
      c. Proper fit and instruction in correct use is important to prevent radial mononeuropathy secondary to leaning onto axillary pad.
      d. Usually used in pairs, one under each arm.
      e. Usually used for patients with temporary limitations in weight-bearing status of lower extremity (LE), as in patients with fracture.

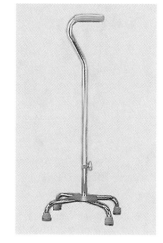

FIGURE 1.   Large-base quad cane.

    f. Occasionally used on permanent basis for patients with mild-to-moderate weakness or balance impairment.

    g. Available in various styles.

    h. When two are used, they can be used in a step-to, step-through, or 4-point gait pattern.

    i. Platform attachment may be added to distribute weight through forearm rather than through wrist or hand.

    j. Inexpensive

4. **Forearm crutch** (Fig. 2)

    a. Crutch with single base of support.

    b. Top portion extends upward to forearm.

    c. Cuffs wrap around forearm, thus freeing hand for other activities, such as grasping door handle.

    d. Frequently used in pairs.

    e. Usually used for patients with permanent moderate-to-severe weakness of LEs.

    f. When two are used, they can be used in a step-to, step-through, or 4-point gait pattern.

5. **Walker** (Fig. 3)

    a. Device that surrounds patient on 3 sides, providing 4 points of support.

    b. For patients with moderate-to-severe weakness, balance impairment, or decreased endurance.

    c. Available in various styles.

    d. May have wheels, wheel brakes, glidebrakes, hand brakes, seat, and back rests.

    e. Light-weight and heavy-duty models are available.

    f. Most models are foldable.

    g. Used without wheels, walker must be lifted to advance it with step-to gait pattern.

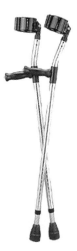 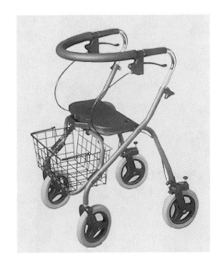

FIGURE 2 *(left).* Forearm crutches.
FIGURE 3 *(right).* Wheeled walker with hand brakes, seat, and back rest.

h. Used with wheels (in front only or on all four points),walker can be pushed forward to advance without having to lift it, encouraging reciprocal gait pattern.

i. Platform attachment may be added to distribute weight through forearm rather than through wrist or hand.

j. May be used in forward or reverse configuration, which promotes trunk extension.

6. **Gait trainer**

a. Wheeled device that provides support at pelvis and trunk.

b. LEs are used to advance patient forward.

c. For patients with severe weakness, motor control problems, or balance impairment.

d. Available in various styles.

e. Used primarily in pediatric setting.

f. Most models provide wide range of support/positioning components, which can be adjusted to patient.

B. **Wheelchairs**

1. **Manual wheelchair**

a. Promotes mobility in seated position.

b. Requires patient to push wheelchair independently or have caregiver push wheelchair.

c. For patients with paralyzed or moderate-to-severe weakness of the LEs, balance impairment, or decreased endurance that limits ambulation; patients who have temporary restrictions limiting ambulation; and patients who are dependent for mobility.

d. Usually patients use upper extremities (UEs) and occasionally LEs to propel wheelchair forward.

2. **Rigid frame** (Fig. 4)

a. Wheelchair that does not fold.

b. Usually used by very active patients who do not need to fold wheelchair for transport.

c. Easier to propel because of less "give" in frame.

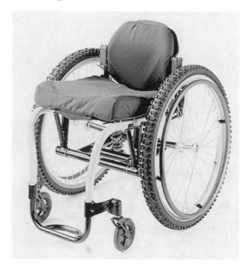

FIGURE 4.   Rigid wheelchair.

    d. Can be very lightweight.

    e. Frequently used in sports activities.

    f. True rigid frames do not allow growth or adjustments, because they are all one piece.

    g. Semirigid frames have removable horizontal cross bar, which can change width of wheelchair.

3. **Folding frame** (Fig. 5)

    a. For patients who need to fold wheelchair for transport or storage.

    b. Removable crossbars allow adjustments in width.

    c. Folding wheelchairs range from light-weight to heavier standard models.

    d. Standard wheelchairs are less expensive and therefore usually used for patients with temporary wheelchair needs.

    e. Growable frame allows adjustments in depth without ordering additional parts.

4. **Tilting frame** (Fig. 6)

    a. Wheelchair that allows seat and back to pivot backward together, maintaining same hip angle throughout tilt.

    b. For patients who are dependent for mobility because of severe motor impairment and patients who are unable to do independent pressure relief or require rests or position changes throughout day.

    c. When wheelchair is tilted, gravity can assist with positioning patient in wheelchair rather than pulling head and trunk forward away from back.

    d. Tilt frame is heavy and relatively long.

    e. Most do not fold.

    f. Caretaker required to tilt wheelchair back.

    g. Since seat-to-back angle remains the same throughout tilt (hips remain flexed), it usually does not trigger spasticity.

5. **Reclining frame** (Fig. 7)

    a. Wheelchair frame that allows back to go down while seat stays in place, thus allowing > 90° of hip extension.

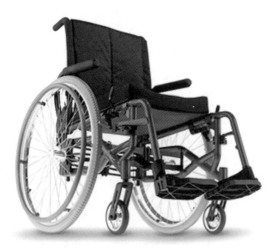

FIGURE 5. Folding wheelchair.

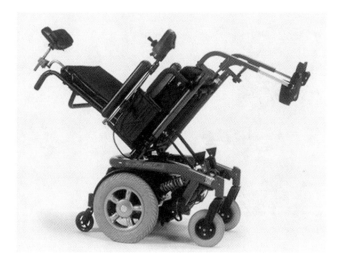

FIGURE 6.   Power tilt in space on a power wheelchair base.

   b. For patients who have limitations in hip flexion and patients who are unable to do independent pressure relief or require rests or position changes throughout day.

   c. When wheelchair is reclined, gravity can assist with positioning patient in wheelchair rather than pulling head and trunk forward away from back.

   d. Reclining frame is heavy and long.

   e. Frequently has elevating leg rests.

   f. Can be folded.

   g. Caretaker required to recline wheelchair back.

   h. Provides excellent pressure relief when fully reclined.

   i. May trigger increased spasticity when moving in and out of reclined positions.

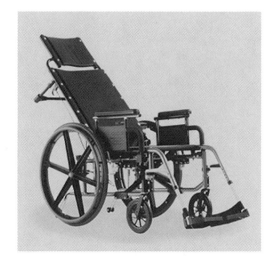

FIGURE 7.   Reclining wheelchair.

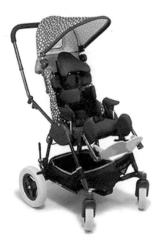

FIGURE 8. Adapted stroller.

6. **Adapted stroller** (Fig. 8)
   a. Stroller that provides additional pads and support to improve positioning.
   b. For infants and toddlers who are too small to fit in or too young to propel manual wheelchair but need more support than what is available in conventional stroller.
   c. Available in many styles; most fold for transport.
   d. Some allow tilt or recline.
   e. Usually has some kind of trunk, head, neck, UE, and LE support.
7. **Power wheelchair** (Fig. 9)
   a. Promotes independent mobility in seated position without requiring caretaker to push wheelchair.
   b. For patients with paralysis or moderate-to-severe weakness of LEs and UEs, balance impairment, or decreased endurance that limits ambulation and patients with UE pain that limits manual wheelchair propulsion.

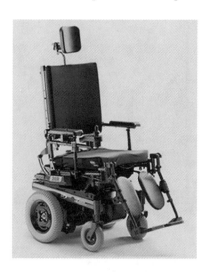

FIGURE 9. Power wheelchair.

    c. Available in front-, mid-, or rear-wheel drive.

    d. Some models can be taken apart and folded for transport.

    e. Power recline and/or tilt systems can be added to some models.

    f. Very heavy because of frame, motors, and batteries.

    g. Various drive options are available, depending on patient's physical abilities (e.g., joystick controlled by UE or chin, switch options controlled by head, extremities, or sip and puff).

    h. Models vary in ability to make adjustments in electronics to accommodate changes in functional status.

    i. Vehicle adaptations may be required for transport (e.g., lift or ramp to get wheelchair into van, tie-down systems to secure wheelchair and rider).

    j. Some can be taken apart for transport in vehicle cargo area.

  8. **Scooter** (Fig. 10)

    a. Promotes independent mobility in seated position on motorized cart, which does not require use of UEs for propulsion.

    b. For patients with mild-to-moderate weakness of LEs and UEs, balance impairment, or decreased endurance that limits ambulation and patients with UE pain that limits manual wheelchair propulsion.

    c. Available in 3- and 4-wheel models.

    d. Limited seating is available on scooters.

    e. Less sophisticated electronics limit amount of adjustment that can be made to accommodate changes in functional status.

    f. Can be taken apart for transport in vehicle cargo area.

    g. For some patients, more esthetically pleasing than power wheelchair.

II. Evaluation for Mobility Device (Fig. 11 at end of chapter)

  A. **Diagnosis**

    1. Current status

    2. Potential for recovery or decline in functional status

  B. **Age:** child, adult, elderly adult

  C. **Physical assessment**

    1. **Range of motion** (ROM)

      a. Spine

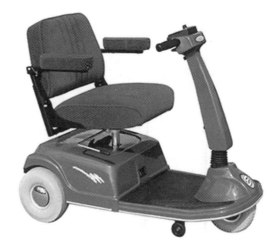

FIGURE 10. Power scooter.

         i. Important for visual orientation.

        ii. Muscle tightness can affect respiratory status.

   b. UEs

        i. Especially important if wheelchair is propelled with UEs.

        ii. Contractures may prohibit grasp of assistive device.

   c. LEs

        i. Hip and knee ROM greatly affect positioning in wheelchair.

        ii. In assessing posture in wheelchair, alignment of hips and pelvis should be addressed first to determine base of support; trunk will respond accordingly.

2. **Strength**

   a. Spine

        i. Weak neck and trunk muscles require more supportive seating on wheelchair.

        ii. For high-level tetraplegia, neck strength and strength of facial muscles should be assessed for power wheelchair mobility.

   b. UEs

        i. Strength determines ability to propel wheelchair or use joystick for power mobility.

        ii. Significant weakness in UEs may require sophisticated electronics for power wheelchair mobility.

       iii. Generally, at least fair UE and LE strength is required to ambulate with assistive device, unless additional support (e.g., orthosis) is provided.

   c. LEs

        i. Occasionally used to propel wheelchair.

        ii. Generally, the greater the weakness, the more support will be needed from assistive device for ambulation.

3. **Endurance**

   a. Affects ability to propel wheelchair.

   b. Ambulation endurance may improve if assistive device is used.

4. **Balance**

   a. History of falls may indicate need for assistive device for safe ambulation.

   b. Severe balance impairment or history of falls while using assistive device may indicate need for wheelchair.

5. **Tone**

   a. Increased tone/spasticity requires support to promote proper alignment and relaxation.

   b. Decreased tone requires support to promote proper alignment.

6. **Posture**

   a. Fixed deformities, such as scoliosis, need to be accommodated in wheelchair seating.

   b. Flexible deformities should be supported appropriately to prevent permanent fixed deformities.

   c. Common postural deformities

        i. Scoliosis with or without trunk rotation.

        ii. Wind-swept LEs (knees oriented in opposite direction of hips, usually with one hip medially rotated and the other laterally rotated).

       iii. Contractures in extremities or neck.

7. **Skin integrity**
   a. Method of pressure relief.
   b. History of pressure areas or skin breakdown.
   c. Common areas of skin breakdown: sacrum, ischial tuberosities, greater trochanters.
   d. Impaired or decreased sensation can lead to pressure ulcers because patient is unable to feel soreness or pain when prolonged pressure is applied to area.

8. **Functional level**
   a. Level of assistance required to complete activities of daily living (e.g., transfers, toileting) helps determine appropriate type of mobility device.
   b. Cognitive status
   c. Activity level
   d. Occupation
   e. Recreational activities

9. **Pain**
   a. Common areas of pain that require use of assistive device for ambulation are back and LEs.
   b. Common areas of pain reported by people using wheelchair: back (which can affect sitting tolerance) and shoulder (which can affect wheelchair propulsion).

10. **Size of patient**
    a. Pediatric devices should be adjustable for growth.
    b. Obese patients may require heavy-duty models.

D. **Home accessibility**
   1. Entrance into home helps determine appropriate type of mobility device: level access, ramp, steps.
   2. House/apartment features
      a. Presence of an elevator
      b. Width of doorways
      c. Over all size of rooms/hallways for maneuvering mobility device

E. **Usual mode of transportation**
   1. Personal vehicle: van, car
   2. Public transportation
   3. School bus

F. **Medical/adaptive equipment used**
   1. Oxygen tank
   2. Ventilator
   3. Feeding pump
   4. Orthoses
   5. Communication device

G. **What equipment has been tried/used before**
   1. What worked well?
   2. What did not work well?
   3. What equipment is currently available?

H. **Patient's goals**

I. **Funding**

III. **Frequently Prescribed Wheelchair and Wheelchair Seating Components**
A. **Manual wheelchair components**
   1. **Anti-tip bars** provide stability to prevent wheelchair from tipping posteriorly or anteriorly.
   2. **Folding frame** mobility base folds for storage or transportation in vehicle.

3. **Grade aids (hill holders)** prevent wheelchair from rolling backward on inclined surfaces.
4. **Handrim with projections (quad knobs)** provide knobby surface area to push against for wheelchair propulsion for patients who are unable to grasp the handrim. They can be oriented in oblique or vertical positions.
5. **Mag wheels** are heavy, durable wheels that increase overall weight of wheelchair.
6. **One-arm drive attachment**, a special axle with two handrims on one wheel, allows patient with only one functional UE to propel manual wheelchair.
7. **Push handles** allow caregivers to push wheelchair and sometimes are used by patient to hook onto in order to complete functional activities such as reaching or pressure relief.
8. **Quick-release axle** allows quick removal of wheels for transportation and maintenance.
9. **Quick-release camber axle** allows quick adjustment of camber for increased stability and maneuverability.
10. **Reverse-configuration rigid frame**, which is low to the ground, allows independent floor-to-floor transfers. Large wheels are in front to allow for easier UE propulsion. Most commonly used with pediatric patients.
11. **Rigid frame**, nonfolding base provides durable and ultralight base for improved propulsion and maneuverability.
12. **Rubber-coated handrim** provides friction surface that allows better grasp for wheelchair propulsion. Used with patients with decreased coordination or fine motor control.
13. **Spoke guards** are coverings that prevent fingers from becoming caught in spokes.
14. **Spoke wheels** are light-weight wheels that decrease overall weight of wheelchair but require high maintenance.

B. **Power wheelchair components**
1. Batteries provide power source for motorized wheelchair. Gel rather than lead acid batteries are recommended for safe transportation and maintenance-free durability.
1. **Chin-control joystick** is operated by chin of patients with decreased UE function.
2. **Midline joystick** is placed toward center of body in patients with restricted UE ROM and limited strength.
3. **Seat elevator** raises and lowers seat height to allow user to complete various activities of daily living, such as transfers at variety of heights, pulling up to high counters and reaching objects normally positioned over their head while seated in wheelchair.
4. **Sip-and-puff switch system** is used to drive the wheelchair. Activated by the user's breathing (variations of sips and puffs) in patients without UE movement and head control.
5. **Swing-away joystick** with mounting hardware allows joystick to be retracted for close access to desk or table.
6. **Tongue-touch switch system** mounted on retainer in user's mouth allows user without UE movement and head control to maneuver wheelchair and operate tilt and recline.

C. **Components common to both power and manual wheelchairs**
1. **Armrests** support UEs. They may be removable or swing away for transfers.

2. **Casters** are small tires in front of wheelchair. They are made of various materials and configurations, depending on user's environment.

3. **Tires** absorb shock and allow safer mobility on uneven terrain. They are made of various materials in various sizes, and treads, depending on user's environment. Flat-free inserts prevent flat tires.

4. **Leg rests** support LEs. They may be removable or swing-away for transfers or transporting wheelchair in a vehicle. They also may elevate to help decrease LE edema.

5. **Footrests** support feet. They may be single platform or individual footplates that swing up out of the way for transfers. They also may be angle-adjustable to accommodate ankle contractures.

6. **Oxygen tank** holder provides secure means of carrying oxygen on wheelchair.

7. **Standing support system** allows user to change from seated position to supported standing either manually or by power.

8. **Suspension shocks** provide smoother, more stable base for heavy patients or those who propel over rough terrain. They reduce fatigue, back and shoulder pain and may be incorporated into the frame or casters.

9. **Recline system** allows back to recline while seat stays in place, thus allowing > 90° of hip extension. It may be operated manually or by power. Power recline provides independent means of position change for medically necessary procedures such as catheterization or pressure relief.

10. **Tilt system** allows seat and back to pivot backward together, maintaining same hip angle throughout tilt. It may be operated manually or by power. Power tilt provides independent means of position change for pressure relief.

11. **Tilt-and-recline system** (combined tilt and recline system) provides optimal pressure relief. It may be operated manually or by power.

12. **Transit option** provides four easy-to-identify securement points on crash-tested frame and seating system. This option allows patient to use wheelchair and seating system as passenger seat during transportation.

13. **Ventilator tray** safely transports ventilator and batteries on wheelchair.

14. **Wheel locks** secure wheelchair in place for safe transfers.

D. **Wheelchair seating components**

1. **Abductor pad positions** medially rotated and adducted hips in more neutral alignment. It may flip down or be removed for safe transfers.

2. **Adductor/knee/thigh/hip guides** position laterally rotated and abducted hips in more neutral alignment.

3. **Adjustable tension back upholstery** consists of Velcro attachments on back of upholstery that allow upholstery to be retightened after it becomes stretched with normal use, promoting trunk extension.

4. **Calf strap wraps** around frame to support LEs and prevent feet from falling posteriorly off footrest.

5. **Custom-molded seat and back** are used to correct flexible deformity or to accommodate fixed deformity by providing full-contact support and lateral stability to trunk, pelvis and LEs. They provide even pressure distribution across seat and back and maximal level of seating control.

6. **Foam in-place molded back** provides full-contact support, lateral stability, and trunk extension for proper postural alignment of trunk. It can accommodate existing deformities and provide even pressure distribution across back.

7. **Headrest** provides support and alignment of head and neck, especially when wheelchair is reclined or tilted. It supports head and neck during transportation and can be flipped down or removed for patients who use headrest for transportation only or to get it out of the way for transfers.

8. **Heel loops and ankle straps** position feet and ankles on footplates to prevent injury to feet.

9. **Lap belt (seat belt)** maintains proper position of hips and pelvis in seat.

10. **Lateral thoracic support** provides lateral trunk control, stability, and proper postural alignment. It may swing-away for transfers.

11. **Lumbar support** is provided by foam back insert that facilitates trunk extension.

12. **Pressure-relieving cushion** distributes seat interface pressures to inhibit decubitus ulcer development. It may be made of contoured foam and gel pads or cells of air.

13. **Shoulder harness** provides anterior support for proper postural alignment and for safety during transportation.

14. **Solid seat** provides solid base of support for seating.

15. **Specialty back** provides firm, padded support to pelvis and trunk to promote erect sitting posture. It may be flat or contoured and is available in various heights, depending on user's level of trunk control. Generally the more trunk control a person has, the lower the back height.

16. **Tray** provides UE support and positioning as well as a support surface for activities such as eating and writing.

WHEELCHAIR EVALUATION

Date:
Patient Name:
UM CPI #:
Diagnosis: spastic quadriplegia/cerebral palsy
Birthdate:
Address:
Telephone:

To Whom It May Concern:
_____ is a ____-year-old male who was evaluated for a wheelchair at _____.
Due to the diagnosis of cerebral palsy, a wheelchair will be required for _____ on a permanent daily basis. The prescription is based on the evaluation and information listed below.

Current physical deficits include but are not limited to the following:
Range of motion: within functional limits for positioning in wheelchair.
Tone/reflexes: increased tone noted in extremities, especially in UE flexor and LE extensor muscles.
Strength/endurance: moves all extremities against gravity. Lacks coordination, strength, and endurance for functional ambulation outside home or classroom.
Posture/alignment: sits with supervision; tends to lean forward with rounded shoulders or to left in sitting; recently received new ankle-foot orthoses.
Functional level: ambulates therapeutic distances at school with reverse walker and contact guard assistance; requires minimal assistance with a stand-pivot transfer; occasionally propels manual wheelchair with UEs.
Skin: no reported problems.
Accessibility/transportation: home is accessible. In family van, he rides in wheelchair secured with docking-type tie-down system. On school bus, 4-point tie-down system is used.
Additional issues: uses a "My Desk" tray with hardware to position his computer at school.

Description of present wheelchair
Wheelchair frame/seating system: Invacare Comet, with large wheels in back; quad knobs on handrims, custom-molded seat and back, flat arm pads.
Reason for replacement: He has outgrown wheelchair and seating.

Wheelchair and seating recommendations
Based on evaluation and functional status, the following wheelchair and seating components are recommended. Please refer to enclosed wheelchair order form for further details about wheelchair specifications.
Wheelchair type: Invacare Allegro. A rigid frame is recommended to provide a durable and lightweight base for improved propulsion and transportation. The added durability of a rigid frame is essential. This particular frame allows for growth in width and depth.
   Width: to be determined at molding.
   Depth: to be determined at molding.
   Frame color: electric blue.
   22" Tires with flat-free inserts to prevent flat tires on wheelchair and to decrease maintenance cost of tubes.
   Plastic-coated handrims with projections to facilitate better grasp and independent wheelchair propulsion for patient with decreased coordination/fine motor control.
   6" Semipneumatic casters to provide durable and low-maintenance casters for wheelchair.
   Contour U-molded back with pans and hardware to provide full-contact support and lateral stability for proper postural alignment of trunk, to accommodate for existing deformity, and to provide maximal level of seating control.
   Contour U-molded seat with pans and hardware to provide full contact, firm base of support for proper postural alignment of the pelvis, LEs and trunk, to accommodate existing deformity, and to provide maximal level of seating control.
   Padded flip-back height adjustable armrests required for proper arm support and to assist with proper alignment and positioning in wheelchair. Flip-back feature allows independence with transfers.
   Arm pads with modular trough pad required to properly position weak UEs and to prevent injury secondary to arms falling off armrest.
   70° removable leg rests required for independent transfers and transporting wheelchair in vehicle.
   Angle-adjustable footrests required to provide LE support and proper postural alignment. Angle adjustability is required due to ankle contractures.

FIGURE 11. Sample therapy evaluation documentation and letter of medical necessity. *(Continued on following page.)*

Body Point Ankle Huggers to properly position and maintain position of feet on footplates.

Otto Bock Small C Headrest with multiaxis hardware to properly position/support head and neck and to prevent neck hyperextension during transportation.

Seat belt (1.5 inch wide with airline-style closure) to properly maintain the position of hips and pelvis in seat and to provide safety during transportation.

Stroller handles required for caregiver to provide assistance with maneuvering over curbs, etc. as needed, and to provide appropriate height for proper body mechanics to prevent caregiver injury.

Padded rear-pull shoulder harness required to provide anterior support of the trunk for proper postural alignment and for safety during transportation.

Equipment recommendations

In addition to the wheelchair, the following equipment is recommended:

Kaye Walker with side bag: due to poor strength, balance, and/or endurance, a walker is required for functional ambulation at home and in the classroom. A reverse walker is required to promote extension of the spine and LEs. Side bag is required to carry school supplies.

Thank you for your time and expedient consideration of _____'s needs. If you have any questions about this equipment please contact _____ at _____.

_____ _____
Physical Therapist Physician

_____
Rehabilitation Technology Supplier

FIGURE 11 *(Continued).*   Sample therapy evaluation documentation and letter of medical necessity.

Bibliography

1. Betz RR, Mulcahey MJ: The Child With a Spinal Cord Injury. Rosemont, IL, American Academy of Orthopedic Surgeons, 1996.
2. Cook AM, Hussey SM: Assistive Technology: Principles and Practice. St. Louis, Mosby, 1995.
3. Cooper D, Dilabio M, Broughton G, Brown D: Dynamic Seating Components for the Reduction of Spastic Activity and Enhancement of Function, Presentation. Seventeenth International Seating Symposium, Feb. 2001.
4. Denison I, Gayton D: Redefining Power Wheelchairs. Presentation, Seventeenth International Seating Symposium, Feb. 2001.
5. Falk Bergen A, Colangelo C: Positioning the Client with Central Nervous System Deficits: The Wheelchair and Other Adapted Equipment. Valhalla, NY, Valhalla Rehabilitation Publications, Ltd., 1985.
6. Ford JR, Duckworth B: Physical Management for the Quadriplegic Patient. Philadelphia, F.A. Davis, 1987.
7. Fraser BA, Hensinger RN, Phelps JA: Physical Management of Multiple Handicaps. Baltimore, Paul H. Brookes Publishing Co, 1987.
8. Minkel JL: Seating and mobility considerations for people with spinal cord injury. Phys Ther 80:701–709, 2000.
9. Paleg G: Made for walking: a comparison of gait trainers. Team Rehabil Rep 41–45, 1997.
10. Pierson FM: Principles and Techniques of Patient Care. Philadelphia, W.B. Saunders, 1999.
11. Tecklin JS: Pediatric Physical Therapy. Philadelphia, JB Lippincott, 1994.

ACKNOWLEDGMENTS

The author would like to thank Invacare Corporation, Leisure-Lift, Inc., and Sunrise Medical for providing the photographs.

Chapter 22

MODALITIES

Jennifer Shifferd, MSPT, and Geeta Peethambaran, B.Sc., P.T.

I. Thermal Modalities
A. Cryotherapy
1. Physiologic effects
a. Knight defines cryotherapy as "the therapeutic application of any substance to the body which results in the withdrawal of heat from the body, thereby lowering tissue temperature."

b. Cryotherapy is broad term that covers a number of specific techniques, including ice packs, cold gel packs, ice massage, ice immersion, cold whirlpool, and vapocoolant spray.

c. Initially, after application of ice pack, patient feels cold, which progresses to burning, warming sensation. Aching, tingling, and finally numbness follow.

d. First response is constriction of arterioles and venules (within 15 minutes or less). Blood flow to area decreases, and body attempts to conserve heat.

e. Vasodilation can be cold-induced after initial period of vasoconstriction when cold is maintained for longer than approximately 15 minutes or when temperature is reduced below $10°$ C.

f. Period of alternating vasodilation and vasoconstriction also may occur, known as "hunting response." This response is most predominant in apical areas where arteriovenous anastomoses are located in skin and has been shown to be absent in deeper tissues. After cold is removed, temperature rises in adjacent body parts.

g. Additional effects of cryotherapy
   i. Decrease in local metabolic rate.
   ii. Decreased conductivity of pain receptors and nerves (when cooled to $\sim 10°$ C).
   iii. Decreased tissue extensibility.
   iv. Spasticity reduction results from decrease in gamma motor neuron activity by excitation of cutaneous afferents. It also acts by decreasing afferent-spindle discharge.
   v. Short applications of cold can be effective adjunct to therapeutic exercise by stimulating muscle function.

2. Application
a. Ice packs
   i. Wrapped in dry or moist toweling.
   ii. Applied for $\sim$ 10–15 minutes for more superficial areas and 15–20 minutes for areas of deeper tissue.

b. **Cold gel packs**
   i. Kept in cooling unit at temperatures of 0–10°F.
   ii. Improper use may cause frostbite.
   iii. They do not lower skin temperature as much as ice; thus, patients may not reach point of anesthesia.

c. **Ice immersion**
   i. Used to treat distal extremities.
   ii. Container big enough to hold extremity is filled with ice and water. Body part is then immersed.
   iii. Temperatures range between 13–18 C for treatment, which may last 10–20 minutes.

d. **Ice massage**
   i. Involves rubbing plastic or foam cup (with edges peeled back) of ice over body part to be treated.
   ii. Used mostly for small areas of inflamed tissue or acute muscle guarding.
   iii. Direction of application should be parallel to muscle fibers.
   iv. Application is continued for 3–10 minutes until anesthesia is reached.

e. **Vapocoolant sprays** (e.g., fluoromethane, ethyl chloride)
   i. Vaporized liquid nitrogen.
   ii. When sprayed on skin, it produces significant cooling through evaporation.
   iii. Container should be held about 2 feet from body part and sprayed in one direction only at rate of 4 inches/second, using 1–2 sweeps while maintaining passive stretch.
   iv. Ethyl chloride is flammable and may freeze skin on contact; therefore, fluoromethane is preferred.
   v. Effective in reducing painful muscle guarding and desensitizing trigger point areas.

3. **Indications**
   a. Michlovitz notes rationale for application of cold 24–48 hours after acute injury.
      i. Decreases fluid filtration into interstitium by vasoconstriction.
      ii. Decreases inflammation.
      iii. Decreases pain and muscle spasm.
      iv. Decreases metabolic rate.
   b. In acute injury cold is used most often in conjunction with compression and elevation.
   c. Cryotherapy is also indicated for treating acute burn. Bloch's extensive review led to conclusion that cooling burns can decrease magnitude of injury by reduction in edema, pain, local fluid loss, tissue injury, and blood volume during the first 48 hours after injury.
   d. Patients with acute spinal cord injury (SCI) also improve with local hypothermia treatments. Bricolo et al. reviewed SCI cases from the literature and noted that complete destruction of spinal cord often may not occur at initial moment of impact but relates to self-destructive process in cord and hypoxic neurologic changes secondary to vascular alterations.
   e. Decreasing spasticity.
   f. Reduction of fever.

    g. Facilitation of muscle contractions by increasing motor neuron excitability.

    h. Especially effective for bursitis and tendinitis.

  4. **Contraindications**

    a. Impaired sensation. Patients cannot report when they become anesthetic from cold. Tissue damage occurs slightly below temperatures that produce numbness.

    b. Impaired circulation: tissue damage may result from vasoconstriction.

    c. Open wounds after 48 hours.

    d. Hypersensitivity to cold, such as Raynaud's phenomenon, cold urticaria, cryoglobulinemia, and paroxysmal cold hemoglobinuria.

    e. Angina pectoris or other severe cardiac disease.

    f. Regenerating peripheral nerves.

  5. **Precautions**

    a. Hypertension

      i. Careful monitoring is needed because of transient increases that can occur in systolic and diastolic blood pressure.

      ii. Treatment should be discontinued if increase in blood pressure is seen.

    b. Elderly patients

      i. Decreased efficiency with vasoconstriction.

      ii. Therefore, they have decreased ability to conserve heat.

    c. Length of treatment

      i. Do not use cold gel packs longer than 15–20 minutes directly on skin, and do not apply any cryotherapy directly to skin for > 1 hour continuously.

      ii. Extended treatment may lead to neurapraxia or axontomesis of superficial peripheral nerves.

B. **Superficial heat modalities**

  1. **Physiologic effects**

    a. Therapeutic heat causes rise in temperature at skin and subcutaneous tissues.

    b. According to Lehmann and DeLateur, tissue temperature must be raised to 40–45°C (104–113°F) to be therapeutic.

    c. Thermal limit for skin tolerance for most people is 113°F.

    d. Greatest degree of heating is at 0.5 cm from the surface and takes 6–8 minutes to reach maximum.

    e. Muscle temperature at 1–2 cm depth increases at lesser degree and takes 15–30 minutes to reach maximum.

    f. Chemical activity in cells and metabolic rate increase 2–3-fold for each 10°C rise in temperature.

    g. Oxygen uptake also increases, making more nutrients available to promote tissue healing.

    h. Vasodilation increases blood flow to area, which can increase edema and hemorrhage.

    i. Decrease in pain results from elevation of pain threshold, alteration of nerve conduction velocity, and decreased firing rate of muscle spindles.

    j. Therapeutic heat has sedative effect that allows relaxation before stretching.

    k. Alterations in viscoelastic properties of connective tissues allow elongation after stretch has been applied.

2. **Application**
   a. **Moist heat**
      i. Moist heat packs
         * Canvas packs filled with silica gel and stored in hot water at 170°F.
         * 6–8 layers of toweling are used before application.
         * Duration of treatment is 10–30 minutes.
      ii. Paraffin wax
         * Melted wax mixed with mineral oil.
         * Kept heated at 125°F.
         * Because of its low specific heat, it heats body part slowly, decreasing risk of burns.
         * Distal body part is dipped 6–10 times and then wrapped with waxed paper or plastic wrap, followed by several layers of toweling.
         * Duration of treatment is up to 20 minutes.
         * Alternative approach is immersing extremity into paraffin wax and allowing wax to solidify. This is followed by repeat immersion for an additional 20–30 minutes.
         * Skin temperatures are maximized to 47°C with both methods.
         * Immersion allows skin temperatures to be maintained at ~47°C, whereas dipping temperatures fall few degrees above baseline at end of 30-minute treatment.
   b. **Dry heat:** fluidotherapy
      i. Warm air is circulated through container holding fine cellulose particles.
      ii. Used for desensitization and application of superficial heat.
      iii. Patients can perform exercises while extremity is in unit.
      iv. Temperature for treatment ranges from 38.8–47.8°C (102–118°F).
      v. Lower temperatures are recommended for patients with predisposition for edema and patients beginning desensitization programs.
      vi. Fluidotherapy is beneficial for treating patients with scar hypersensitivity, later stages of reflex sympathetic dystrophy, and hypersensitivity after amputation of distal extremities.

3. **Indications**
   a. Promotes decrease in musculoskeletal pain (e.g., fibromyalgia, tension myalgia, fibrositis)
   b. Helps decrease joint stiffness and increase range of motion (ROM).
   c. Alleviates muscle spasm and contracture.
   d. Improves tissue healing by increasing blood flow and nutrients to treated area.
   e. Enhances effects of passive stretch by alteration of collagen tissue temperature.
   f. Paraffin treats joint stiffness and contractures in the distal extremities and improves ROM (e.g., rheumatoid arthritis).
   g. Used for burns because mineral oil can lubricate and condition skin.
   h. Used for superficial thrombophlebitis.

4. **Contraindications**
   a. Acute inflammatory conditions (≤ 48 hours), which may be aggravated.
   b. Areas prone to increased bleeding or hemorrhage (i.e., hemophilia) secondary to prolonged bleeding times.
   c. Malignant tumors (heat may contribute to growth and metastasis).

      d. Peripheral vascular disease (patients may have decreased ability to meet metabolic demands of heated tissues).

      e. Cardiac insufficiency (patients may not be able to withstand increased stress from heating).

  5. **Precautions**

      a. Scars with poor vascularization.

      b. Decreased sensation with potential for burns.

  6. **Wet vs. dry heat:** Abramson et al. concluded that dry heat can elevate surface temperatures to greater degree, but moist heat can elevate temperature to slightly deeper tissue level.

C. **Deep heat modalities**

  1. Increases tissue temperatures to depths of 3–5 cm, whereas superficial heating agents can elevate skin and underlying subcutaneous tissues to depth of ~1–2 cm.

  2. Allows heating in deeper structures without causing excessive heating of superficial tissues.

  3. Types

      a. **Ultrasound** (US)

          i. Uses sound waves with frequency > 20,000 Hz (not detectable by human ear).

         ii. Therapeutic US occurs between 0.8 and 3 MHz.

       iii. Piezoelectric crystal produces US waves. Distortions of crystal occur when alternating current is impressed on crystal. This creates vibration and produces mechanical waves identical to sound waves. Size of crystal and frequency of impressed current determine frequencies of waves.

        iv. Sound waves of these frequencies do not travel through air and require coupling medium, such as conductive gel or water, for treatment.

         v. **Physiologic effects**

            • Increased collagen tissue extensibility.

            • Increased local metabolism.

            • Increased blood flow.

            • Increased pain threshold.

            • Increased nerve conduction velocity.

            • Denaturing of scar tissue through mechanical, pulsating, and micromassage effect.

            • Can increase tissue temperature to as much as 43.5°C.

        vi. **Physical properties of continuous (thermal) US**

            • Absorption increases as frequency of US increases.

            • High-frequency (3 MHz) waves are absorbed easily and penetrate to tissue depth of 1–2 cm. High-frequency waves are recommended for treating more superficial areas.

            • Low-frequency (1 MHz) waves have less superficial tissue absorption, allowing absorption of energy at deeper tissue levels, and penetrate to depths of 4–5 cm.

            • Intensity is defined as rate at which energy is delivered per unit area and is expressed as watts per square cm (W/cm^2). For larger quantities of soft tissue, 1.5–3.0 W/cm^2 is recommended; for more superficial tissues, 0.3–1.5 W/cm^2.

   vii. **Types of sound waves**
- Continuous: sound intensity remains constant and produces thermal effect.
- Pulsed: waves are intermittently interrupted, and modes range from 10% and 20% to 50%. Nonthermal effects include cavitation (collapse of bubbles within sound field) and streaming (movements along boundaries of cell membranes as result of US).

  viii. **Duration and technique of treatment**
- May range from 3 to 10 minutes.
- Longer treatment times are recommended for larger areas.
- US gel is used as coupling medium to clean skin.
- US also may be given with distal extremity immersed in water, holding US head parallel to and 0.5–1.0 inches from the skin.

   ix. **Indications**
- US is commonly used to treat soft tissue injuries, joint contractures, scar tissue, bursitis, tendinitis, acute and chronic pain, and muscle spasms/trigger points.
- Also used to allow greater gain in tissue extensibility when followed by passive or active stretching.

   x. **Contraindications**
- Should not be used over eyes, heart, pacemakers, pregnant uterus or low back of pregnant women, testes, malignant tissue, epiphyses in children (continuous US), or spinal cord of patients with laminectomy.
- US makes patients prone to increased bleeding (hemophilia with continuous US)
- Arterial insufficiency (patient may not be able to meet increased metabolic demand).

   xi. **Precautions**
- Care should be taken over anesthetized skin.
- US may be used over metal implants.

b. **Short-wave diathermy**
   i. Converts high-frequency electromagnetic energy to heat energy in patient's tissues through transmission and absorption of nonionizing radiation by body.
   ii. Applied as continuous or pulsed waves that produce heat.
  iii. Radiofrequency most often used is 27.12 MHz.
   iv. Causes increase in ionic motion that in turn causes ions to collide with nearby molecules, which leads to increase in internal kinetic energy and generates heat in tissues.
   v. **Methods of application**
- Condenser field with contraplanar and coplanar methods
- Inductive field

   vi. **Indications** are common to those mentioned for previous thermal modalities.

  vii. **Contraindications**
- Do not use over pregnant uterus, eyes, or pacemaker or on head.
- Acute inflammatory conditions may be aggravated.
- Infections may spread.
- Patients with cardiac disease may not be able to tolerate increased demand placed on heart.

- Metal around treatment site may overheat, causing tissue damage.
- Cancer may spread because of increased blood flow.
- Epiphyses of growing bones (may cause growth disturbances).

  c. **Microwave diathermy**
- i. Produces heat with electromagnetic irradiation.
- ii. Most microwave energy is wasted in heating subcutaneous fat and penetrates muscle only about one-third as deep as short-wave diathermy.
- iii. Primarily used to treat superficial joints and tissues.
- iv. Short-wave diathermy and US have generally replaced this modality.

II. Nonthermal Modalities

A. **Pulsed US** (see under ultrasound section above).

B. **Pulsed short-wave diathermy**
1. Physiologic effects are same as for continuous short-wave diathermy.
2. Power output generally set lower than for continuous short-wave diathermy.
3. Pulse frequency can be 1–7,000 pulses/second.
4. Can be used in thermal or nonthermal modes.
5. Nonthermal effects may heal tissue after injury by repolarizing damaged depolarized cells.
6. Tissues with high electrolyte content, such as muscles, have increased heating, whereas superficial fat has less heating.

C. **Phonophoresis**
1. Uses US energy to deliver topically applied medication by enhancing percutaneous absorption, without direct invasion of the skin.
2. Mechanism is thought to be increase in cell membrane permeability (acoustic streaming).
3. Applied by first rubbing anti-inflammatory medicine (e.g., 10% hydrocortisone ointment) and then coupling gel over the skin to be treated.
4. Used to treat superficial tissues (submuscular and subtendinous levels), because deeper diffusion is not likely.
5. May be considered for patients who will not consider steroid injections for conditions such as bursitis and tendinitis.
6. US contraindications apply to phonophoresis.
7. More extensive research is needed to validate its efficiency.

D. **Hydrotherapy**
1. Good medium for exercise because buoyancy allows gravity-eliminated environment that reduces unnecessary stress on joints.
2. Good for increasing strength because of resistance offered by movement through water.
3. Buoyancy allows patients to move and ambulate with greater ease, thus promoting improved circulation, increased ROM, and patient relaxation.
4. **Forms**
  a. **Whirlpool** (thermal and mechanical effects)
- i. Advocated for treatment of joint stiffness, arthritis, adhesions, and painful scar tissue.
- ii. Water is used to heat or cool body and provides mechanical debridement and massage through agitation.
- iii. Decreased heart rate and lengthened diastole result from immersion of body in cold.
- iv. Enhanced cardiac muscle tone and increased blood pressure result from peripheral vasoconstriction in cold applications.

     v. Heat to entire body in water causes initial increase in blood pressure due to vasodilation.

    vi. Respiratory rate increases with heat and cold application.

   vii. Agitation has analgesic effect due to mechanical stimulation of skin receptors; it also aids in relaxing muscle spasms and blocking pain input by stimulating large sensory afferent nerve fibers.

  viii. Can be comfortable medium for providing assistive or resistive exercises.

b. **Whirlpool baths and Hubbard tanks**

    i. Types
- "Extremity" allows treatment of arms or legs.
- "Lowboy" or "highboy" types are used for lower extremity and trunk immersion.
- Hubbard tanks are designed for full-body immersion and allow patient to perform full-body exercises as therapist assists outside tank.

    ii. Indications
- Acute conditions are treated in cold baths with temperatures of 13–18°C.
- Chronic conditions are treated in hot baths with temperatures of 37–40°C.
- Medium for exercise: tepid temperatures (27–33.5°C).
- Burn treatment:gentle means of debridement to aid in removing necrotic tissue. Mechanical effects also stimulate formation of granulation tissue. Appropriate water temperature helps to soften tissues and increase circulation to affected area.
- Arthritis: Hubbard tanks useful for patients unable to transfer into smaller tank.

   iii. Precautions
- Patients with burns, circulatory disorders, and cardiac conditions should be treated with temperatures of 33–38°C (neutral to warm baths).
- Patients with peripheral vascular disorders should not be treated with whirlpool temperatures > 1 degree above skin temperature.
- Temperatures > 43.5°C are not safe for any whirlpool treatment.
- Monitoring should be continuous.

   iv. Duration of treatment depends on pathology involved.
- Heating: 20 minutes is desired treatment time.
- Debridement: 5–20 minutes, depending on amount of necrotic tissue of affected area.
- Exercising medium: 10–20 minutes.
- Burns: in Hubbard tanks, treatment can be > 20 minutes but should not exceed 30 minutes if no electrolytes have been added to water.

c. **Contrast baths**

    i. Combination of heating and cooling promotes alternating dilation and constriction of blood vessels and helps to stimulate peripheral blood flow and healing.

    ii. Application: body part is dipped into warm water (38–44°C) for 10 minutes; it is then dipped in cold water (10–18°C) for 1 minute, and returned to warm water for 4 minutes. Alternation between warm (4

minutes) and cold (1 minute) occurs for four sets. This cycle continues for 20 minutes.
  ii. Indications
     • Rheumatoid arthritis
     • Reflex sympathetic dystrophy
     • Joint sprains
     • Musculotendinous strains
     • Edema
     • Some peripheral vascular diseases
     • Toughening of amputation stumps
 iii. Contraindications (same as for therapeutic heat and cold, above)
  iv. Precautions
     • Patients with peripheral vascular disease if water temperature > 40°C.
     • Young or elderly patients may have insufficient thermoregulatory systems.

E. **Electrotherapy**
  1. **Transcutaneous electric nerve stimulation** (TENS)
     a. **General principles**
        i. Method of afferent stimulation designed to control pain.
       ii. Gate control theory offers possible explanation of mechanism.
          • TENS is transmitted along large-diameter afferents, which activate inhibitory substantia gelatinosa (SG) interneurons.
          • These interneurons close spinal gate for transmission of nocioceptive information to higher levels in central nervous system; therefore, perception of pain is diminished.
      iii. Skin is cleaned before electrode placement with alcohol preps to ensure good conductivity.
     b. **High-rate conventional TENS**
        i. Used to achieve quick analgesic effect for acute pain.
       ii. Acts by stimulating AC fibers, which conduct faster than C fibers and block pain.
      iii. Adaptation is likely to occur; therefore, increases in amplitude or pulse width may be needed to maintain paresthesia.
       iv. Treatment duration for rapid analgesia is 1–20 minutes; for short-duration analgesia, 30 minutes to 2 hours.
        v. Treatment may be daily or more than once daily, depending on how often it is needed to maintain pain-free state.
     c. **Low-rate TENS**
        i. Used for chronic pain and has slower analgesic effect.
       ii. Treatment time is 30–45 minutes for slower analgesia effect and 2–6 hours for longer duration
      iii. Patients may experience muscle twitch during stimulation.
       iv. Acts by stimulating C fibers and hypothalamus (indirectly). Beta-endorphin is released from pituitary and bonds with opiate receptors in brain to produce analgesic response.
        v. Half-life of beta-endorphin(about 4 hours) suggests long-lasting analgesia.
       vi. Adaptation to this stimulus is minimal.
      vii. Treatment is usually given once daily.

   d. **Pulse width:** generally the opposite of selected rate.

   e. **Modulation modes**

     i. Continuous mode: continuous stimulation at set intensity and rate.

     ii. Burst mode: stimulation for 2.0 seconds, off for 2.0 seconds. It makes low-frequency stimulation more comfortable for patient.

     iii. Modulated mode: intensity remains constant, but there are intermittent rate and/or width changes.

     iv. Multimodulation mode: changes both rate and intensity. As rate decreases, intensity increases and vice versa. Adaptation is decreased with this mode.

   f. **Indications**

     i. For placement on or around painful areas such as trigger points, along meridians, acupuncture, and acupressure points.

     ii. Used for osteoarthritis, rheumatoid arthritis, neurogenic pain, Raynaud's disease, ischemic pain

   g. **Contraindications**

     i. Demand-type cardiac pacemaker.

     ii. No stimulation over carotid sinus, laryngeal or pharyngeal muscles, eyes, or mucosal membranes.

     iii. Not recommended for incompetent patients or patients with myocardial disease or arrhythmias without proper monitoring.

   h. **Precautions**

     i. Can cause skin irritation over site; thus, stimulus area should be rotated.

     ii. Safety of TENS use during pregnancy has not been established.

2. **Neuromuscular electrical stimulation** (NMES)

   a. **General principles**

     i. Used to activate muscular contractions through intact peripheral nervous system or on muscles that are decentralized (SCI). NMES unit sends electrical pulses that cause depolarization of motor endplates and thereby contraction of muscles.

     ii. Some controversial evidence indicates that NMES may have deleterious effects on denervated muscle, causing fiber degeneration and excessive fibrosis as well as retarding reinnervation.

   b. **Indications**

     i. Strengthen and maintain muscle mass during and after periods of immobilization (through improved recruitment of motor neurons).

     ii. Maintain or increase ROM in joints with soft tissue contractures (by taking joints through available ROM several times per day).

     iii. Temporarily reduce effects of spasticity (by interruption of abnormal drive onto motor neuron and antagonist muscle stimulation).

     iv. Increase voluntary motor control (through facilitation and muscle re-education).

     v. Temporarily act as replacement for orthotics or bracing (assist with dorsiflexion in SCI and hemiparetic patients with foot drop and/or shoulder subluxations).

     vi. Conditioning and strengthening muscles for general health benefits in paretic patients.

   c. **Contraindications**

     i. Should not be used over carotid sinuses or demand-type pacemakers.

      ii. Pregnancy

      iii. Cardiac disability

  d. **Precautions**

      i. There is concern about use of NMES for exercise in regard to patient's ability to demonstrate good cardiovascular response with increased demand during electrically induced exercise.

      ii. Safety of extremities during exercise in patients with impaired sensation.

      iii. Monitor patients with arrhythmias, diabetes, and open skin lesions.

      iv. Patients with obesity.

  e. In **functional electrical stimulation** (FES), multiple muscle groups are activated in sequential manner. As technology advances, higher level of coordinated stimulations may help patients (such as those with SCI) to achieve higher functional levels of mobility and activities of daily living.

3. **Alternating current** (AC): interferential stimulation.

  a. **General principles**

      i. Involves mixing two unmodulated sine waves with different frequencies.

      ii. Interferential current (IFC) generators use either fixed frequency of 4,000 Hz or frequency that can be varied from 4,001 to 4,100 Hz.

      iii. Beat frequency can range from 1–100 beats/second. Higher frequencies tend to be more comfortable for patient. Variable frequency helps to prevent adaptation.

      iv. Two methods: quadripolar and bipolar.

      v. Sometimes it is clinically difficult to determine exact site of pain origin. Scanning IFC mode helps to find target tissue areas of pain. Areas of maximal stimulation can be shifted back and forth to help localize area to be treated.

  b. **Indications**

      i. Pain relief, muscle relaxation, and vascular conditions (Raynaud's disease, peripheral vascular disease).

      ii. Urogenital dysfunction: pelvic floor (PF) muscles can become weak in women after childbirth or multiple abdominal surgeries with adherence of scar tissue. This can result in incontinence and/or PF pain.

        • McQuire reports favorable results in women with stress or urge incontinence and pelvic infection (patients were taught PF muscle contractions prior to IFC).

        • Chirarelli et al. noted successful outcomes with IFC in women with partially denervated pudendal nerves, disuse atrophy, damage to sphincter muscles, and deterioration of vaginal mucosal lining.

  c. **Contraindications and precautions**

      i. Similar to those for NMES (see above).

      ii. Should not be used over rib cage in children with small body mass because it may interfere with organ function.

      iii. Patients with arterial or venous thrombosis or thrombophlebitis are at risk for developing pulmonary embolism with IFC treatment.

      iv. IFC can increase metabolism and therefore may exacerbate conditions such as fever, infection, tuberculosis, and neoplasm.

      v. Other contraindications include application of IFC over abdominal, lumbosacral, or pelvic areas of pregnant women and senile or confused patients.

vi. Caution should be used in treating area of decreased sensation (for lower intensities, careful monitoring should be used). Avoid treating areas with extreme edema, and avoid treatment over open wounds.

4. **Direct current** (DC)
   a. **Iontophoresis** (continuous or uninterrupted low-voltage DC)
      i. Method of transdermal administration of ionized drugs that are driven through epidermis by external electrical field.
      ii. Based on principle that electrically charged electrode repels similarly charged ion. Therefore, ions with positive charge can be introduced into tissues from positive electrode and negative ions from negative pole. Path of penetration by ions is primarily through sweat ducts.
      iii. Medications used for iontophoresis must be soluble in water. Commonly used medication is dexamethasone.
      iv. Medicated (active) electrode is saturated with 2.5 ml of chosen agent and placed directly over area to be treated. Dispersive (inactive) electrode is applied over major muscle and should be at least 4 inches from medicated electrode on same side of body.
      v. Before administering iontophoresis, skin must be cleansed with alcohol prep to remove dirt, dry skin, or oil. This reduces skin irritation and helps prevent burns. Allow skin to dry thoroughly.
      vi. After skin has been cleansed, electrodes can be applied. Leads are snapped onto electrodes, with negative lead on medicated electrode and positive on dispersive electrode.
      vii. Patient may receive 3–6 treatments.
      viii. Tissue penetration of medication may reach up to 2 cm.
      ix. Total dosage delivered is 40 mA/min.
      x. Intensity can range from 0.5–4.0 mA.
      xi. **Treatment parameters**

Dose	Current	Minutes
40 mA/min	2 mA	20
40 mA/min	3 mA	13.5
40 mA/min	4 mA	10

      xii. **Indications:** local inflammation such as bursitis, epicondylitis, and tendinitis
      xiii. **Contraindications**
         • Electrodes should not be applied over damaged skin or orbital regions, across thoracic region, or transcranially.
         • Do not use iontophoresis in patients with pacemakers or allergy to corticosteroids.
      xiv. **Precautions**
         • Hot and cold packs should not be applied during treatment.
         • Patient may have redness under one or both electrodes after treatment. It usually disappears after 8 hours.
         • Current settings should never exceed patient's comfort level.
         • Burns and small blisters may occur from skin defects in treated area. These defects create channels of low resistance and tend to carry most of current. If burning or blistering occurs, treatment intensity should be decreased for next application.

  b. **Modulated DC**
    i. Can be reversed, ramped, or interrupted.
    ii. Used to stimulate denervated muscle fiber and to retard atrophy (e.g. Bell's palsy).
    iii. Not commonly used because it may cause skin burns and is uncomfortable to patient.
    iv. Goal with stimulation to denervated muscle is to maintain muscle in healthy state for as long as possible while awaiting reinnervation.
    v. See under NMES for deleterious effects of stimulation to denervated muscle.
  c. **Neuroprobe**
    i. Combined point location and stimulation instrument.
    ii. Referred to as hyperstimulation analgesia and relies on intense stimulation of C fiber for its therapeutic effect.
    iii. Noxious input is used to control pain.
    iv. Small diameter point-probe active electrode is used to deliver non-invasive (surface) pulsed DC stimulation. Small diameter nerve fibers are excited by noxious stimuli that block pain through descending inhibitory pathway at spinal cord level.
    v. Indications: acute and chronic pain conditions.
    vi. Contraindications: see under TENS.
F. **Biofeedback**
  1. Use of instrumentation to transduce motor unit action potentials into auditory or visual feedback.
  2. Can be used as adjunct to therapy for increasing or decreasing voluntary muscle activity, and evaluation of muscle activity. Patient learns how to recognize desired muscular response.
  3. **Indications**
    a. Muscle re-education for volitional movement of muscles with upper motor neuron dysfunction.
    b. Re-education of PF musculature in women with incontinence or pelvic pain.
    c. Functional postural deviations.
    d. Increased motor recruitment of vastus medialis after repair of anterior cruciate ligament.
    e. Recovering peripheral nerve injuries.
    f. To stop unwanted muscular activity (decreased recruitment of upper trapezius with repair of rotator cuff).
    g. To inhibit spasticity.
    h. For muscle relaxation (e.g., women with vulvodynia and vaginismus).
  4. **No contraindications**
  5. **Precautions:** skin irritation with prolonged use and deep relaxation for diabetic patients may adversely affect metabolic level.
III. **Mechanical Modalities**
  A. **Traction**
    1. **General principles**
      a. Force or system of forces applied to body along its length to attempt to:
        i. Elongate or align soft tissue or osseous structures around vertebral joints.
        ii. Separate vertebral segments.

iii. Produce rest by immobilization.
b. Can also improve blood supply to posterior soft tissues and intervertebral discs.
c. Patients with herniated discs may have reduction of bulging nuclear material due to decrease in positive pressure with traction.

2. **Types**
   a. **Cervical traction**
      i. Most often therapist performs trial of manual traction. Tractile force is applied to occiput of patient in supine position.
      ii. Mechanical cervical traction can be done in supine or sitting position.
      iii. For treatment below C2 position, cervical spine is placed in 20–30° of flexion. To treat atlantoaxial segment, patient is placed in neutral.
      iv. Initial pounds of pull should be from 10–15 pounds to overcome weight of head. Treatment weight can range from 10–45 pounds. To achieve separation of vertebral segments, at least 25 pounds should be applied.
      v. Treatment time may range from 5–20 minutes.
      vi. Traction may either be intermittent or static.
         • Intermittent mechanical traction allows periods of rest between traction pulls and usually is well tolerated. Traction is applied for 10–60 seconds; rest periods range from 5–20 seconds.
         • Static or sustained traction applies constant traction force and induces muscle fatigue in paraspinal musculature; in theory, more pull can be transmitted to cervical spine.
      vii. Nonmotorized static mechanical traction
         • Home traction unit with head harness, pulley system, and counterweight (in clinic, weights are used; for home use, bag is filled with water).
         • Patient can be seated (with pulley system attached to door) or supine (pulley system attached to bed). Treatment times may range from 5–25 minutes.
         • Other types of cervical units include inflatable cuffs such as Pronex brand.
      viii. Cervical traction treatment time and cycle may vary according to diagnosis and patient response.
      ix. Indications
         • Decrease muscle spasm and pain.
         • Elongate soft tissue.
         • Reduce pain in spinal disorders (nerve impingement, disc herniation)
         • Treat disc degeneration.
         • Treat foraminal stenosis.
      x. Contraindications
         • Spinal infections/osteomyelitis • Rheumatoid arthritis
         • Osteoporosis   • Unstable fracture
         • Metastatic lesions
   b. **Lumbar traction**
      i. Requires greater amount of force than cervical traction.
      ii. As with cervical traction, manual lumbar traction can be performed as trial before mechanical lumbar traction.

- Patient is in sidelying position for manual traction to specific segment.
- Patient is in supine position for unilateral or bilateral leg pull.

   iii. 30–50% of body weight is used to overcome friction when administering mechanical lumbar traction. Split table is necessary with lumbar traction to diminish effects of friction and restrictive forces.

   iv. Patient lies in supine or prone position. Flexed position increases anterior loading on nuclear material of disc, which results in posterior bulging. When patient is in neutral to extended position, nuclear material is moved anteriorly because of posterior loading.

- Prone positioning is often used for disc herniations with posterior or posterolateral bulging.
- Supine, hook-lying position is most often used for stenosis and facet or intervertebral joint hypomobility.

   v. Pelvic harness is donned with top margin of belt just above iliac crest. Thoracic harness is then donned with straps secured at head end of table. It is best if harnesses are applied against skin to avoid slipping.

   vi. Most therapists use intermittent or static traction.

- Intermittent traction: as with cervical traction, treatment time and cycle may vary according to diagnosis and patient response. Intermittent traction is often used for early treatment of herniated discs to assist in alleviating nerve root compression. Patients tend to tolerate intermittent pulls well.
- Static or sustained traction: discogenic pain is often treated with static lumbar traction after initial period of intermittent traction during early acute stages. As with cervical traction, static lumbar traction can also be used for soft tissue elongation.

B. **Sequential pneumatic pump** (also known as lympha press)

1. Multicompartmental pressure system designed for treatment of lymphedema.
2. Lympha press consists of short-duration and high-pressure cycle, which provides sequential milking effect on limb. It consists of multicompartmental sleeve, which contains 9–12 overlapping cells that can be fitted to limb according to its size.
3. For treatment of lower extremity, additional one-cell boot is used at foot area.
4. Overlapping of air compartments within sleeve guarantees gradient pressure, thus creating milking effect on limb.
5. Sleeve is connected to compressor. Inflation of cell is initiated from most distal cell and progressed proximally. Compressor through distributor powers cells separately so that each successive inflation creates sequential milking mechanism. When entire sleeve is filled with air, it automatically deflates and cycle begins again.
6. Compression period lasts 20 seconds for most distal cell and 2 seconds for most proximal cell.
7. Pressure of compressor can be adjusted; 35–45 mmHg is suggested for treatment of lymphedema.
8. **Advantages**
   a. Easy to use; patient can apply it for home use.

      b. Provides alternative to massage.

      c. Covered by most insurance carriers.

9. **Disadvantages**

      a. Lympha press requires patient to be immobile during treatment.

      b. Lymphatic capillaries may be traumatized if greater pressure is used.

      c. Trunk quadrants are disregarded and may cause genital edema.

10. **Indications**

      a. Primary lymphedema

      b. Secondary lymphedema

      c. Venous disorders

      d. Chronic edema

11. **Contraindications**

      a. Deep venous thrombosis

      b. Acute infection of affected limb

      c. Decompensated heart failure

Bibliography
1. Casely-Smith JR: Modern Treatment for Lymphedema. Adelaide, Australia, Bowden, 1997.
2. Hayes K: Manual for Physical Agents, 4th ed. Norwalk, CT, Appleton & Lange, 1992.
3. Knight K: Cryotherapy Theory: Technique and Physiology. Chattanooga, TN, Chattanooga Corporation, 1985.
4. Michlovitz S: Thermal Agents in Rehabilitation. Philadelphia, F.A. Davis, 1986.
5. Nelson RM, Currier DP: Clinical Electrotherapy, 2nd ed. Norwalk, CT, Appleton & Lange, 1991.
6. Pappas CJ, O'Donnell TF Jr: Long-term results of compression treatment for lymphedema. J Vasc Surg 16:555–564, 1992.

Chapter 23

REHABILITATION PHARMACOLOGY

Jacques Whitecloud, M.D., and M. Catherine Spires, M.D.

Information in this chapter is intended as a general clinical guide to medications commonly used in rehabilitation patients. It should not be considered an official pharmaceutical or therapeutic protocol or document. Information was omitted when a consensus was unavailable in recent medical literature. If available, time to effect and duration are given; if not, half-life is listed.

I. Analgesics

A. Narcotic agonists

1. Opioid agonists exert effects by binding to mu, kappa, and delta receptors in the peripheral and central nervous systems. Mu receptor activation causes analgesia, respiratory depression, and euphoria.

2. **Adverse effects for all narcotic agonists** include nausea and vomiting, constipation, sedation, respiratory depression, and miosis. Adverse effects listed below for each drug are in addition.

3. Care should be taken with **combination agents** (e.g., hydrocortisone/acetaminophen) not to exceed maximum daily doses for each agent.

4. All narcotic agonists have the **potential for abuse and dependence**.

5. **Specific agents** (Table 1 lists doses, equivalencies, peak effect, and duration)

   a. **Codeine**
      i. Additional averse effect: pruritus.
      ii. Also has antitussive effect.
      iii. Doses > 65 mg have no added analgesic effect.

   b. **Fentanyl**
      i. Fever may increase drug release.
      ii. Additional adverse effect: urinary retention.
      iii. 10–14 days are required to reach steady plasma state.

   c. **Hydrocodone:** high abuse potential.

   d. **Hydromorphone:** additional adverse effects include transient hyperglycemia and urinary retention or incontinence.

   e. **Meperidine:** may cause seizures in renally impaired patients.

   f. **Morphine**
      i. Additional adverse effects: pruritus, flushing, sweating.
      ii. Extended-release formulation may be given in bolus dose if crushed.

   g. **Methadone:** additional adverse effects include prolonged ST segment and aseptic hepatitis.

   h. **Oxycodone**
      i. Additional adverse effects: increased serum amylase, pruritus, flushing.
      ii. Extended-release formulation delivered as bolus dose if crushed.

TABLE 1. Narcotic Analgesics

Drug	Dose	Equivalence	Peak	Duration
Codeine	30–65 mg q 4–6 hr	30–200 mg	30–60 min	4 hr
Fentanyl	25–100 µg patch q 3 days	50–100 µg	24–72 hr	72 hr
Hydrocodone	5–7.5 mg PO q 4–6 hr		1.5 hr	4 hr
Hydromorphone	1–4 mg PO, IV, IM q 4–6 hr	1.5 mg IM 7.5 mg PO	1 hr IM 2 hr PO	4 hr IM Up to 6 hr PO
Meperidine	1–1.8 mg up to 150 mg q 4 hr IV, IM, SC, PO	75–100 mg IM 200–300 mg PO	1 hr IM 2 hr PO	3 hr
Morphine	10–15 mg IM 30–60 mg PO	Same	IR: 30 min ER: 1.5 hr	IR: 4 hr ER: 8–12 hr
Methadone	2.5–10 mg IV, PO, SC	10 mg IM 20 mg PO	Onset: 1–4 hr Weeks to peak	48–72 hr
Oxycodone	IR: 5 mg q 4 hr ER: 10–40 mg	15 mg IM 30 mg PO	IR: 1 hr ER: 7 hr	IR: 4 hr ER: 12 hr
Propoxyphene	65 mg PO q 4 hr	32–65 mg		4–6 hr

q = every, PO = orally, IV = intravenously, IM = intramuscularly, SC = subcutaneously, IR = immediate release, ER = extended release.
General rule: scheduled dosing of q 4 hr medications at 8 AM and noon allows better therapy participation than as-needed dosing.

B. **Nonsteroidal anti-inflammatory drugs** (NSAIDs)
  1. All NSAIDs inhibit cyclo-oxygenase (COX) 1 and 2 (except for COX-2-specific NSAIDs, see below) and decrease prostaglandins and platelet thromboxane. COX-1 is present in stomach and kidney; COX-2 is present in inflamed arthritic joints.
  2. **Therapeutic effects** include analgesia, anti-inflammation, anitpyresis, and platelet inhibition.
  3. **Adverse side effects** of all NSAIDs may include renal compromise/failure, interstitial nephritis, gastrointestinal (GI) upset/ulceration, bleeding, edema, rash, pruritus, nausea, and (in elderly patients) confusion and dizziness.
      a. Renal patients may show elevations in creatinine and blood pressure, particularly when NSAIDs are combined with angiotensin-converting enzyme (ACE) inhibitors.
      b. Agent-specific side effects are listed below.
  4. No NSAID has proved superior to another for analgesia. **Choice of agent is based on side-effect profile**.
  5. Clinical experience suggests that peak effect requires days in patients with acute pain. Switching classes may help refractory pain; no studies suggest that different agent in same class will be of additional benefit.
  6. **Classes of NSAIDs and doses for specific agents**
      a. **Acetic acids**
          i. Diclofenac, 75 mg 2 times/day
          ii. Etodolac, 2–400 2 or 4 times/day (COX-2 > COX-1 effects)
          iii. Indomethacin, 25–75 mg every 6 hr (duration: 6–8 hr)
          iv. Ketorolac, 10 mg every 4 hr
          v. Nabumetone, 1000 mg/day (COX-2 > COX-1 effects)
          vi. Sulindac, 150–200 2 times/day (duration: 12 hr)
          vii. Tolmetin, 2–600 3 times/day

    b. **COX-2 inhibitors** (fewer GI effects)
        i. Celecoxib, 200 mg/day (peak effect: 3 hr)
        ii. Rofecoxib, 12.5–50 mg/day (FDA-approved for acute pain)
    c. **Fenamate:** meclofenamate, 500 mg every 6–8 hr (additional side effect: hemolytic anemia)
    d. **Oxicams**
        i. Meloxicam, 7.5 mg/day
        ii. Piroxicam, 20 mg/day (duration: 24 hr; additional side effect: insomnia)
    e. **Propionic acids**
        i. Flurbiprofen, 2–300 mg/day (duration: 4–6 hr)
        ii. Ibuprofen, 2–800 mg 3 or 4 times/day (duration: 4–6 hr)
          • May elevate free phenytoin levels.
          • Probably easiest to use.
        iii. Ketoprofen, 25–75 mg 3 or 4 times/day (duration: 4–6 hr)
        iv. Naproxen, 250–500 mg 2 times/day (duration: 8–12 hr)
        v. Oxaprozin, 1200 mg/day (duration: 4–6 hr)
    f. **Salicylates** (additional side effect: tinnitus; antiplatelet effects last 7–10 days)
        i. Aspirin, 325–1000 mg every 6 hr (duration: 4–6 hr)
        ii. Diflunisal, 2–500 every 12 hr (duration: 12 hr)
        iii. Salsalate, 3000 mg/day total (may have fewer renal effects)
  7. **Special considerations**
    a. Conditions associated with high risk of adverse effects include acute renal failure, renal disease, congestive heart failure (which may cause renal hypoperfusion), hypovolemia, and hypoalbuminemia.
        i. Salsalate *may* be slightly less nephrotoxic than other NSAIDs.
        ii. Monitoring: follow creatinine, electrolytes; digoxin levels affected.
        iii. No NSAID is kidney-sparing, including COX-2 inhibitors.
    b. Patients on oral anticoagulant therapy should avoid NSAIDs (13-fold increase in risk for bleeding). International normalized ratio (INR) should be monitored closely if NSAIDs are used.
    c. Patients with hypertension should adjust doses of thiazide or loop diuretics if they take NSAIDs, which may reduce diuretic efficacy.
    d. Patients with peptic ulcer disease (PUD), advanced age, or on chronic corticosteroid use have 15-fold increase in risk for developing GI ulcer if NSAIDs are used.
        i. Misoprostol helps patients with PUD and elderly patients, but patients taking corticosteroids should avoid NSAIDs when possible.
        ii. Misoprostol is associated with diarrhea.
    e. Prophylactic regimens against adverse NSAID effects
        i. Misoprostol (prostaglandin E_1 analog), 200 mg 3 times/day
        ii. Omeprazole, 20–40 mg/day
        iii. H_2 blockers are inferior to either agent.
C. **Other analgesic agents** (Table 2 summarizes doses, mechanism of action, and pharmacokinetics)
  1. **Acetaminophen**
    a. Analgesic and antipyretic effects; lesser anti-inflammatory and anticoagulant effects.
    b. Adverse effects: hepatotoxicity, nephrotoxicity (in high doses)

TABLE 2. Other Analgesic Agents

Agent	Dose	Mechanism	Pharmacokinetics
Acetaminophen	325–650 mg PO, PR to maximum of 4 gm/day	Inhibits central PG synthesis, less effect in periphery	Hepatic clearance in 0.5–1 hr
Amitriptyline	25–100 mg PO at bedtime; antidepressant effects at 75–300 mg/day	Inhibits postsynaptic reuptake of norepinephrine	Effects may take weeks to appear Hepatic clearance
Capsaicin cream	0.025–0.075% cream 2–5 times/day to affected area	Depletes substance P from C-fiber terminals	Immediate effects
Carisoprodol	350 mg PO 3 or 4 times/day	Inhibits descending reticular formation and spinal cord	Hepatic and renal clearance
Cyclobenzaprine	10 mg PO 3 times/day, maximum of 60 mg/day	May activate locus ceruleus to inhibit motor neurons, producing muscle relaxation	Hepatic and renal clearance
Gabapentin	300–600 mg PO 3 times/day; maximum of 3600 mg/day; titrate every 5 days	May modulate voltage-dependent calcium channels on neurons	Maximum concentration in 3 hr; days to weeks for effects Renal clearance
Metaxalone	800 mg PO 3 or 4 times/day	Centrally acting muscle relaxant	Onset at 1 hr; duration of 4–6 hr Hepatic and renal clearance
Methocarbamol	Acute pain: 1500 mg PO 4 times/day, 1000 mg IV or IM 3 times/day Maintenance dose: 1000 mg PO 4 times/day	Same as metaxalone	Onset in 30 min Hepatic clearance
Mexiletine	400–675 mg PO 3 times/day	Sodium channel blocker	Peak effect at 2–3 hr half-life of 10–12 hr Hepatic clearance
Tramadol	50–100 mg PO every 4–6 hr	Weak mu agonist; inhibits reuptake of norepinephrine and serotonin	Peak concentration at 2–3 hr Hepatic and renal clearance

PO = orally, PR = rectally, IV = intravenously, IM = intramuscularly, PG = prostaglandin.

2. **Amitriptyline**
   a. Used off-label for neuropathic pain; often used as sleep aid.
   b. Adverse effects include sedation, orthostasis, dry mouth/eyes, urinary retention, slow cardiac atrioventricular conduction.
3. **Capsaicin cream**
   a. Adverse effect: burning/stinging sensation on application precedes anesthesia but subsides over time.
   b. More effective for mild-to-moderate neuropathic pain.
4. **Carisoprodol**
   a. Adverse effects: ataxia, sedation, tachycardia, nausea.
   b. No direct effects on muscle; relaxant effects centrally mediated.

5. **Cyclobenzaprine:** adverse effects include sedation, dry mouth, urinary retention, dizziness.
6. **Gabapentin**
   a. Off-label use for pain; primary indication as anticonvulsant for partial complex seizures.
   b. Adverse effects include ataxia, somnolence, dizziness, fatigue, tremor, and diplopia.
7. **Metaxalone:** adverse effects include dizziness, drowsiness, nausea, vomiting, headache.
8. **Methocarbamol:** same adverse effects as metaxalone.
9. **Mexiletine**
   a. Indicated for antiarrhythmic effects; last resort for burning/stabbing pain.
   b. Adverse effects include chest pain, headache, palpitations, sinus node depression in patients with history of cardiac disease.
10. **Tramadol**
    a. Adverse effects include seizures, respiratory depression, mental status changes, headache, constipation, nausea, withdrawal syndrome to that of opioids. Miosis may occur.
    b. Selective serotonin reuptake inhibitors and tricyclic antidepressants may increase plasma levels and therefore seizure risk.
    c. High abuse potential.

II. Anticoagulants
A. **For prophylaxis against deep venous thrombosis** (DVT) (see Chapter 13)
   1. Heparin, low-molecular-weight heparin (LMWH), and warfarin are indicated agents. Table 3 lists specific indications and doses for various forms of heparin.
   2. Heparin inactivates factors IIa (thrombin), Xa, and IXa by potentiating antithrombin III (ATIII).

TABLE 3.   Heparin for DVT Prophylaxis

Form of Heparin	Patient Class	Dose
Low-dose, unfractionated	Standard risk for DVT	5000 units (U) SC every 12 hr
Adjusted dose	Higher risk	3500 ± 500 U SC every 8 hr to achieve high normal PTT values
Low molecular weight	General surgery	40 mg/day SC or 60 mg SC every 12 hr, depending on risk
	Orthopedic surgery	Same as for general surgery; first dose is given 12 hr postoperatively
	Major trauma	30 mg SC every 12 hr
	Acute spinal cord injury	30 mg SC every 12 hr for ASIA class D while in hospital; for ASIA class C, for up to 8 weeks; for ASIA class B or A, for 8 weeks; for ASIA class A with congestive heart failure, fracture, cancer, history of DVT, obesity, or age > 70 year, for 12 weeks or until discharge from rehabilitation.
	Medical conditions	40 mg/day SC

DVT = deep venous thrombosis, U = units, SC = subcutaneously, PTT = partial thromboplastin time, ASIA = American Spinal Cord Injury Association.

3. LMWH has fewer effects on thrombin but more predictable steady state.
4. All forms of heparin are renally cleared.
5. Subcutaneous LMWH is superior to subcutaneous heparin for preventing DVT without increasing bleeding risk. At doses of 1 mg/kg 2 times/day, subcutaneous LMWH is also as effective as IV heparin for DVT treatment.

B. **For treatment of DVT and long-term anticoagulation**
   1. Both **heparin** and **LMWH** are indicated for anticoagulation in patients with DVT until therapeutic INR (2–3) is achieved with **warfarin**. Once INR is therapeutic, heparin or LMWH should be continued for 2–4 days.
      a. Heparin: 80 U/kg bolus, then 18 U/kg/hr
         i. Dose adjusted to achieve partial thromboplastin time (PTT) 2.5 times normal.
         ii. Safe dosing may be difficult with therapies.
      b. LMWH: 1 mg/kg subcutaneously (SC) twice daily; PTT does not need monitoring.
      c. Warfarin: 5 mg/day PO for 3 days; then adjusted to INR.
         i. INR of 2–3 normalizes in 4 days after discontinuance of warfarin; higher INRs require longer time to normalize.
         ii. May have significant interactions in rehabilitation patients.
            • Cephalosporins, sulfonamides, trimethoprim/sulfamethoxazole, and metronidazole potentiate effects of warfarin.
            • Barbiturates and carbamazepine inhibit effects.
   2. Warfarin inhibits synthesis of vitamin K clotting factors II, VII, IX, and X and proteins C and S. **Vitamin K** can be used to reverse supratherapeutic INRs by allowing factor synthesis.
      a. No consensus about dosing of vitamin K.
      b. Recommendations: 1.0–2.5 mg × 1 for INR of 5–9; 5.0 mg × 1 for INR > 9.
      c. For rapid reversal, use slow IV infusion.
      d. For active bleeding, use transfusion of prothrombin concentrate as well as IV vitamin K.
      e. SC vitamin K is less predictable.
   2. **Duration of treatment**
      a. Proximal thrombosis: 3 months
      b. Recurrent thrombosis: 6 months
      c. Symptomatic calf vein thrombosis: 6 weeks to 3 months

III. **Anticonvulsants**
   A. Table 4 summarizes dosage, mechanism of action, and pharmacokinetics of commonly used anticonvulsants.
   B. **Specific agents**
      1. **Carbamazepine**
         a. Adverse effects: aplastic anemia, agranulocytosis, rash, toxic epidermal necrolysis/Stevens-Johnson syndrome.
         b. Therapeutic level: 4–12 μg/ml.
         c. Fewer cognitive effects in patients with traumatic brain injury (TBI).
         d. Check liver function tests (LFTs) every 3 months.
      2. **Gabapentin**
         a. Adverse effects: somnolence, dizziness, ataxia, nystagmus.
         b. Several off-label uses; see analgesics section.

TABLE 4.   Commonly Used Anticonvulsants

Drug	Dose	Mechanism	Pharmacokinetics
Carbamazepine	200–400 mg PO 2–4 times/day	Reduces polysynaptic responses; blocks posttetanic potentiation	Hepatic clearance
Gabapentin	300–600 mg PO 2–3 times/day; maximum: 3600 mg/day	GABA analog; anti-seizure mechanism unknown	Excreted renally
Phenytoin	5 mg/kg or 300 mg/day	Inhibits seizure propagation across motor cortex via efflux of sodium from neurons	PO formulation requires 7–10 days to reach steady state Hepatic clearance
Valproic acid	10–15 mg/kg/day IV/PO up to 60 mg/kg/day	Unknown; may increase GABA concentration in brain	Half-life: 16 hr Hepatic clearance

PO = orally, IV = intravenously, GABA = gamma aminobutyric acid.

3. **Phenytoin**
   a. **Major concern: potentially lethal hypersensitivity syndrome.** First sign is morbilliform rash.
   b. Other adverse effects: nystagmus, ataxia, slurred speech, decreased cognition, sensory peripheral neuropathy (with long-term therapy), nausea, toxic hepatitis, gingival hyperplasia.
   c. Therapeutic level: 10–20 μg/ml.
   d. Off-label uses: mood stabilizer in bipolar disease, migraine headache.
4. **Valproic acid**
   a. **Major concern: potentially lethal hepatotoxicity.**
   b. Other adverse effects: pancreatitis, decreased platelets, headache, nausea, abdominal pain, somnolence, dizziness, tremor.
   c. Check baseline LFTs every 1–3 months in first 3 months, then every 3 months afterward.

IV. **Antidepressants**
   A. **Selective serotonin reuptake inhibitors** (SSRIs)
      1. **Adverse effects of all SSRIs**: anorexia, nausea, vomiting, diarrhea, anxiety, seizures (especially at initiation of treatment), impotence, and anorgasmia. Drug-specific side effects are listed below.
      2. SSRIs may slow metabolism of carbamazepine. Concurrent dosage of SSRIs and carbamazepine may precipitate **serotonin syndrome:** abdominal pain, hyperpyrexia, tachycardia, hypertension, delirium, and seizures.
      3. **Specific agents** (Table 5 summarizes dosage and pharmacokinetics.)
         a. **Citalopram**
            i. Adverse effects: syndrome of inappropriate diuretic hormone (SIADH), somnolence, insomnia.
            ii. Indication: depression.
         b. **Paroxetine**
            i. Adverse effects: impaired platelet activity, sweating, possible potentiation of warfarin, somnolence.
            ii. Indications: depression, panic disorder/phobias, obsessive compulsive disorder (OCD).

TABLE 5.   Selective Serotonin Reuptake Inhibitors

Drug	Dose	Pharmacokinetics
Citalopram	20–40 mg/day	Half-life: 35 hr Hepatic clearance
Paroxetine	10–20 mg/day; titrated to 10–15 mg/day	Half-life: 20 hr (should be tapered if discontinued) Hepatic and renal clearance
Fluoxetine	20–80 mg/day	Half-life: 1–3 days Hepatic clearance
Sertraline	25 mg/day; titrate to 200 mg/day	Half-life: 26 hr (should be tapered if discontinued) Hepatic clearance

   c. **Fluoxetine**
      i. Adverse effects: SIADH, alopecia, sweating, rash (associated with lung, liver, or kidney vasculitis), pulmonary fibrosis, potentiation of warfarin effects)
      ii. Indications: depression, bulimia, OCD, premenstrual dysphoric disorder.
   d. **Sertraline**
      i. Adverse effects: SIADH, insomnia, increased appetite, tinnitus.
      ii. Indications: depression, OCD, panic disorder.
B. **Atypical antidepressants**
  1. **Mechanism of action:** combination of serotonin reuptake inhibition, serotonin receptor antagonism, and/or norepinephrine reuptake inhibition.
  2. **Specific agents** (Table 6 summarizes dosage and pharmacokinetics.)
   a. **Bupropion**
      i. Contraindicated in patients with seizures.
      ii. Adverse effects: agitation, insomnia, hypertension.
      iii. Indications: depression, smoking cessation.
   b. **Nefazodone**
      i. Adverse effects: somnolence; carbamazepine accelerates clearance; carbamazepine levels may be elevated.
      ii. Indication: depression.
   c. **Remeron**
      i. Adverse effects: agranulocytosis, somnolence (significantly higher than placebo).
      ii. Indication: depression.

TABLE 6.   Atypical Antidepressants

Drug	Dose	Pharmacokinetics
Bupropion	100 mg 2 times/day; titrate to maximum of 450 mg/day	Half-life: 14 hr Hepatic clearance
Nefazodone	100 mg 2 times/day; titrate to 300–600 mg 2–3 times/day	Half-life: 2–4 hr Hepatic clearance
Remeron	15–45 mg/day	Half-life: 20–40 hr Hepatic clearance
Venlafaxine	75–375 mg/day divided into 2 or 3 doses; at least 4 days between increases	Half-life: 5–7 hr Renal clearance

d. **Venlafaxine**
   i. Adverse effects: SIADH, somnolence, increased blood pressure; cutaneous/mucus membrane bleeding.
   ii. Indications: depression, generalized anxiety disorder.
V. **Cognitive Enhancers for Traumatic Brain Injury** (see also Chapter 10)
   A. Table 7 summarizes dosage, mechanism of action, and time to effect of drugs used for cognitive enhancement in TBI.
   B. **Specific agents**
      1. **Amantadine**
         a. Adverse effects: nausea, seizures, dizziness, confusion, hallucinations, orthostasis, depression.
         b. Decreases extrapyramidal symptoms in Parkinson's disease.
         c. Antiviral effects against influenza.
      2. **Bromocriptine**
         a. Adverse effects: same as for amantadine plus abdominal cramping and diarrhea.
         b. Decreases release of prolactin and growth hormone.
         c. Decreases extrapyramidal symptoms in Parkinson's disease.
      3. **Dextroamphetamine and racemic amphetamine**
         a. Adverse effects: agitation, tremor, increased blood pressure and heart rate, dry mouth, diarrhea, anorexia.
         b. High abuse potential.
      4. **Methylphenidate**
         a. Adverse effects: same as for dextroamphetamine and racemic amphetamine; also decreases seizure threshold.
         b. High abuse potential.
VI. **Gastrointestinal Medications** (see also Chapter 16)
   A. **Antiemetics**
      1. **Prochlorperazine**
         a. Dose: 5–10 mg intramuscularly, intravenously, or orally; 25 mg rectally.
         b. Mechanism of action: phenothiazine antidopaminergic.
         c. Pharmacokinetics: duration of 3–4 hr; hepatic clearance.
         d. Adverse effects: decreased mental status, decreased blood pressure, parkinsonian signs, neuroleptic malignant syndrome; may increase phenytoin levels.

TABLE 7. Cognitive Enhancers for Traumatic Brain Injury

Drug	Dose	Mechanism	Time to Effect
Amantadine	100–150 mg PO 2 times/day	Increased presynaptic dopamine release	Onset: 4–7 days
Bromocriptine	1.25 mg PO 2 times/ day	Dopamine analog	Onset: 30–90 min Duration: 3–5 hr
Dextroamphetamine/ racemic amphetamine	Titrate from 5 mg/day PO to maximum of 40 mg/day PO	Increases release of dopamine and norepinephrine, decreases their reuptake	Unavailable
Methylphenidate	Titrate from 5 mg to 60 mg/day PO	Unknown; possibly activates reticular activating system	Same as above Peak effect at 2 hr

    2. **Promethazine**
        a. Dose: 12.5–25 mg intramuscularly, orally, or rectally every 4–6 hr.
        b. Mechanism of action: competitive H_1 receptor antagonist.
        c. Pharmacokinetics: onset in 3–4 hr; hepatic clearance.
        d. Adverse effects: decreased mental status, decreased seizure threshold, extra-pyramidal symptoms; potentiates narcotics effects.

B. **Antiulcer medications**
    1. **Famotidine**
        a. Dose: 20 mg 2 times/day orally.
        b. Mechanism of action: H_2 receptor antagonist; decreases gastric secretions.
        c. Pharmacokinetics: onset in 2.5–3.5 hr; renal clearance.
        d. Adverse effects: headache, dizziness, constipation, diarrhea, fatigue.
        e. Rare side effect: negative inotropic effects.
    2. **Ranitidine**
        a. Dose: 150 mg 2 times/day orally.
        b. Mechanism of action: same as for famotidine.
        c. Pharmacokinetics; onset in 2.5–3.0 hr; renal and hepatic clearance.
        d. Adverse effects: same as for famotidine plus increased alanine aminotransferase.

C. **Laxatives**
    1. **Bisacodyl**
        a. Dose: 10–15 mg orally as needed; 10 mg rectally.
        b. Mechanism of action: stimulates colonic parasympathetic activity.
        c. Pharmacokinetics: onset for tablets, 6–12 hr; for suppositories, 15 min to 1 hr.
        d. Adverse effects: electrolyte abnormalities with loose stools.
    2. **Docusate**
        a. Dose: total of 50–400 mg/day, given in 1–4 doses.
        b. Mechanism of action: softens stool by increasing fecal fat and water content.
        c. Pharmacokinetics: maximal effects in 3 days.
        d. Adverse effects: same as for bisacodyl plus nausea and throat irritation.
    3. **Docusate/casanthranol**
        a. Dose: 1–2 capsules orally at bedtime as needed.
        b. Mechanism of action: stool softener, irritant laxative.
        c. Pharmacokinetics: onset in 6–12 hr.
        d. Adverse effects: same as for docusate plus cramping; side effects are rare.
    4. **Lactulose**
        a. Dose: 15–30 ml orally at bedtime.
        b. Mechanism of action: mostly through nonabsorbed disaccharide, which increases GI osmotic pressure.
        c. Pharmacokinetics; onset in 12 hr; effects last up to 48 hr.
        d. Adverse effects: increased blood sugar in diabetics; electrolyte abnormalities, flatulence.
    5. **Magnesium citrate**
        a. Dose: 150–300 ml orally once or twice daily
        b. Mechanism of action: increased GI osmotic pressure, increased release of of cholecystokinin.

    c. Pharmacokinetics: onset in 6–8 hr.

    d. Adverse effects: hypermagnesemia in patients with renal compromise, electrolyte abnormalities.

6. **Magnesium hydroxide**

    a. 30–60 ml orally as needed.

    b. Mechanism of action, pharmacokinetics, and adverse effects same as for magnesium citrate.

7. **Milk and molasses enema**

    a. Remarkably effective home remedy.

    b. Dose: milk and molasses mixed in 1:1 ratio (about 8 oz of each).

    c. Mechanism of action: presumably colonic irritant and osmotic agent.

    d. Pharmacokinetics: effectively evacuates within 1.5 hr.

    e. Adverse effects: presumably electrolyte abnormalities.

8. **Mineral oil**

    a. Dose: 30 ml orally or rectally every 1 hr for impaction.

    b. Mechanism of action: minimally absorbed fecal lubricant.

    c. Pharmacokinetics: onset depends on degree of impaction; cleared by intestines.

    d. Adverse effects: oral route involves aspiration risk in elderly patients; decreased vitamin absorption.

9. **Methylcellulose**

    a. Dose: 1 tablespoon in 8 oz of water 1–3 times/day.

    b. Mechanism of action: increases fecal bulk through water absorption; increased bulk stimulates peristalsis.

    c. Pharmacokinetics: onset in 12 hr; maximal effect in 3 days; cleared by intestines.

    d. Adverse effects: constipation in fluid-restricted patients; flatulence.

    e. Large doses may be used to treat diarrhea.

10. **Polycarbophil** (FiberCon)

    a. Dose: 1 gm/day orally as needed.

    b. Mechanism of action, pharmacokinetics, and adverse reactions: same as for methylcellulose.

11. **Psyllium** (Metamucil)

    a. Dose: 1 teaspoon or 1–2 wafers with water 1–3 times/day.

    b. Mechanism of action and pharmacokinetics: same as for methylcellulose.

    c. Adverse effects: same as for methylcellulose plus hyperkalemia and hyperglycemia secondary to suspensory formulations.

12. **Senna** (Senekot)

    a. Dose: 2 tablets or 10–15 ml orally; 1 rectal suppository.

    b. Mechanism of action: stimulates mesenteric plexus of colonic mucosa, increases water secretion.

    c. Pharmacokinetics: onset in 6–12 hr.

    d. Adverse effects: yellow stools, brown-red urine, cramping, diarrhea; long-term use can impair colonic motility.

13. **Sodium phosphate** (Fleet)

    a. Dose: 1 enema rectally, 20–30 ml oral solution.

    b. Adverse effect: sharp tip can damage rectal mucosa.

14. **TheraVac SB** (docusate 283 mg/glycerin 275 mg)

    a. Dose: 1 mini-enema as needed for bowel movement.

    b. Mechanism: same as for docusate.

     c. Pharmacokinetics: onset in 15 minutes.

     d. Adverse effects: as for docusate; tip can damage rectal mucosa

VII. Sedatives

A. Haloperidol and long-acting benzodiazepines should be **not** be used to treat agitation in patients with TBI.

B. **Adverse effects of all sedatives:** drowsiness, mental status changes, and dizziness, especially in elderly patients. Agent-specific side effects are listed below.

C. **Specific agents** (Table 8 summarizes dosage, mechanism of action, and pharmacokinetics.)

  1. **Chloral hydrate**

    a. Adverse effects: tachyarrhythmia with high doses; nausea and vomiting; dependence is rare.

    b. Tolerance develops over time.

  2. **Diphenhydramine**

    a. Adverse effects: dyskinesia, dystonia (rare), psychosis.

    b. Mild antiparkinson agent.

  3. **Lorazepam**

    a. Adverse effects: **life-threatening withdrawal seizures**.

    b. High abuse potential; poor choice for insomnia.

  4. **Trazodone**

    a. Adverse effects: priapism, decreased blood pressure, arrhythmias with high doses.

    b. Doses as low as 50 mg/day have antidepressant effects.

  5. **Zolpidem**

    a. Adverse effects: nausea, vomiting, diarrhea.

    b. Short half-life leads to less residual drowsiness.

    c. Works better if taken with food.

VIII. Spasticity Management (see also Chapter 19, Spasticity)

A. Table 9 summarizes dosage, mechanism of action, and pharmacokinetics.

B. **Specific agents**

  1. **Baclofen**

    a. Adverse effects: fatigue, muscle weakness, sedation, dizziness, nausea.

TABLE 8. Commonly Used Sedatives

Drug	Dose	Mechanism	Pharmacokinetics
Chloral hydrate	2--50 mg/kg/day 1.5–2.0 gm at bedtime	GABA-a agonist	Onset: 30–60 min Hepatic clearance
Diphenhydramine	25–50 mg PO at bedtime	Antihistamine	Onset: 1 hr Hepatic clearance
Lorazepam	0.5–4 mg IV, PO every 4 hr as needed for agitation	Enhances GABA-a binding GABA	Onset: 20–20 min Duration: 8 hr Hepatic clearance
Trazodone	25–50 mg PO at bedtime	Tricyclic antidepressant- Sedation is side effect	Onset: 1 hr (based on clinical experience) Optimal effects: 2–6 wk Hepatic clearance
Zolpidem	5–10 mg PO at bedtime	Interacts with GABA receptor	Onset: 1 hr Renal clearance

PO = orally, GABA = gamma aminobutyric acid.

   b. **Abrupt cessation is associated with hallucinations and seizures.**
   c. Check LFTs at baseline and every 6 months.
   d. Greater effects in patients with SCI than in patients with stroke.
2. **Clonidine**
   a. Adverse effects: hypotension, bradycardia, dry mouth, drowsiness, constipation, dizziness, depression.
   b. Rarely used as primary agent; may potentiate baclofen and central nervous systems depressants.
3. **Dantrolene**
   a. Adverse effects: weakness, diarrhea, drowsiness, malaise, hepatotoxicity.
   b. Check LFTs at baseline and every 6 months.
   c. Less sedating than other agents, but weakness is more prominent.
4. **Diazepam**
   a. Adverse effects: sedation, cognitive impairment, dependence.
   b. **Abrupt withdrawal is associated with seizures.**
   c. High abuse potential; rarely used as solitary agent.

TABLE 9.   Drugs for Management of Spasticity

Drug	Dose	Mechanism	Pharmacokinetics
Baclofen	Start as low as 5 mg/day titrate upward to 80 mg/day divided into 3 doses	Pre- and postsynaptic inhibition of spinal GABA-b receptors Decreases alpha motor neuron activity, excitatory pathway activity	Half-life: 3.6 hr Hepatic and renal clearance
Clonidine	0.1 mg/day	Centrally acting alpha$_2$ agonist; suspected to decrease sympathetic activity	Peak effect: 3–5 hr Half-life: 12–16 hr Hepatic and renal clearance
Dantrolene	25 mg/day; titrate every 5–7 days to maximum of 400 mg/day in divided doses	Decreases calcium release from SR of skeletal muscle, reducing contractile ability	Maximal plasma concentration: 6 hr Half-life: 6 hr Hepatic clearance
Diazepam	Start at 2 mg; titrate to desired effect and side-effect tolerance	Binds to spinal GABA-a receptors Increased chloride conductance results in presynaptic inhibition	Peak effect: 1 hr Half-life: 20–80 hr Hepatic clearance
Gabapentin	Start at 100 mg PO 3 times/day; titrate to maximum of 3600 mg/day PO in divided doses	GABAnergic effects at hippocampus, neocortex; little interaction at peripheral GABA receptors	Peak effect: 3 hr Renal clearance
Intrathecal baclofen	Start at 25 µg/day; average effects at 4–500 µg/day; maximum of of 1500 µg/day	See under baclofen; action directly at spinal cord	Half-life: 5 hr
Tizanidine	2 mg/day; titrate to maximum of 36 mg/day divided into 3 doses	Centrally acting alpha$_2$ agonist Potentiates glycine Suppresses polysynaptic reflexes	Peak effect: 1–2 hr Half-life: 2.5 hr Hepatic clearance

PO = orally, GABA = gamma aminobutyric acid, SR = sarcoplasmic reticulum.

5. **Gabapentin**
   a. Adverse effect: stomach upset.
   b. Off-label use for spasticity; little evidence suggests that it is effective as first-line agent.

6. **Intrathecal baclofen**
   a. Adverse effects: pump failure, infection, tolerance, drowsiness, headache, nausea, weakness, hypotension.
   b. **Overdose may cause coma; abrupt cessation may cause seizures.**
   c. Allows 4-fold drug concentration at 1% dose; cognitive effects are less.

7. **Tizanidine**
   a. Adverse effects: insomnia, dry mouth, hallucinations, hepatotoxicity.
   b. Check LFTs at baseline and every 3 months.
   c. Strength is relatively spared; possibly better tolerated than baclofen.

IX. **Urologic Agents**
   A. **Choice of agent** determined by pathophysiology of bladder dysfunction.
   B. **Specific agents**
   1. **Bethanechol**
      a. Dose: 5–100 mg orally 4 times/day
      b. Mechanism of action: muscarinic effect; enhances detrusor contraction.
      c. Pharmacokinetics: onset in 1 hr.
      d. Adverse effects: lacrimation, sweating, nausea and vomiting, decreased blood pressure, abdominal cramps
      e. Used with dantrolene for dyssynergia.
   2. **Dantrolene**
      a. Dose: 400 mg/day orally.
      b. For mechanism of action and pharmacokinetics, see Table 9. Also decreases urethral closure pressure.
      c. For adverse effects, see listing under antispasticity drugs.
   3. **Desmopressin**
      a. Dose: 10–40 µg/day intranasally.
      b. Mechanism of action: antidiuretic hormone analog; decreases urine production for 6–8 hr.
      c. Pharmacokinetics: onset at 4–7 hr; duration of 5–24 hr.
      d. Adverse effects: dry mouth, tachycardia, hyponatremia, pruritus, headache.
      e. No effect on endogenous antidiuretic hormone.
   4. **Dicyclomine**
      a. Dose: 10–20 mg orally 3 times/day.
      b. Mechanism of action: antimuscarinic effects; relaxes bladder smooth muscle; increases vesicular capacity.
      c. Pharmacokinetics: peak effect at 1 hr; half-life of 1.8 hr; renal clearance
      d. Adverse effects: dry mouth, blurred vision, hypotension.
      e. Fewer side effects than oxybutynin.
   5. **Ephedrine**
      a. Dose: 25 mg orally 2 or 3 times/day
      b. Mechanism of action: adrenergic agonist; increases urethral tone.
      c. Adverse effects: irritability, insomnia, anorexia.
      d. Also used as decongestant.
   6. **Oxybutynin**
      a. Dose: 2.5 mg/day orally; increased to 5 mg 3 times/day.

   b. Mechanism of action: antimuscarinic effects; decreases detrusor contraction; intravesicular anesthetic.

   c. Pharmacokinetics: onset at 1 hr; hepatic clearance.

   d. Adverse effects (reported in up to one-third of patients): dry mouth, fatigue, blurry vision, increased temperature, hallucinations, nausea, constipation.

  7. **Terbutaline**

   a. Dose: 5 mg orally 3 times/day.

   b. Mechanism of action: beta receptor agonist; decreases urethral pressure.

   c. Pharmacokinetics: duration of 4–8 hr; hepatic clearance.

   d. Adverse effects: palpitation, tremor, tachycardia

  8. **Tolterodine**

   a. Dose: 1–2 mg orally 2 times/day.

   b. Mechanism of action: antimuscarinic effects; decreases detrusor contraction.

   c. Pharmacokinetics: maximal concentration at 2 hr; hepatic clearance.

   d. Adverse effects: dry mouth, blurry vision, fatigue; complaints of dry mouth are less than with oxybutynin.

Bibliography

1. Beydoun A: New Pharmacologic Options for the Management of Neuropathic Pain: A Practical Treatment Guide. Council on Medical Education, 1999.
2. Bonica J: The Management of Pain, 2nd ed. Philadelphia, Lea & Febiger, 1990.
3. Commissiong JW, Karoum F, Reifstein RJ, Neff NH: Cyclobenzaprine: A possible mechanism of action for its muscle relaxant effect. Can J Physiol Pharmacol 59:37–44, 1981.
4. Flitman S: Tranquilizers, stimulants, and enhancers of cognition. Phys Med Rehabil Clin North Am 10:463–472, 1999.
5. Geerts WH, Heit JA, Clagett GP: Prevention of venous thromboembolism. Chest 119(Suppl): 136S, 2001.
6. Gotzsche PC: Non-steroidal anti-inflammatory drugs. BMJ 320:1058–1061, 2000.
7. Hirsh J, Dalen C, Anderson D: Oral anticoagulants: Mechanism of action, clinical effectiveness, and optimal therapeutic range. Chest 114(Suppl):445s–569s, 1998.
8. Hirsh J, Warketin T, Raschke R: Heparin and low-molecular-weight heparin: Mechanisms of action, pharmacokinetics, dosing considerations, monitoring, efficacy, and safety. Chest 114(Suppl):489s–510s, 1998.
9. Kita M, Goodkin DE: Drugs used to treat spasticity. Drugs 59:487–495, 1000.
10. Matthew MT, Nance PW: Analgesics: Opioids, adjuvants, and others. Phys Med Rehabil Clin North Am 10:255–273, 1999.
11. Physicians' Desk Reference, 55th ed. Montvale, NJ, Medical Economics Company, 2001.
12. Schryvers O, Nance P: Urinary and gastrointestinal systems medications. Phys Med Rehabil Clin North Am 10:473–487, 1999.
13. Tannenbaum H, Davis P, Russel A: An evidence-based approach to prescribing NSAIDs in musculoskeletal disease: A Canadian consensus. Can Med Assoc J 155:77–88, 1996.
14. Tasman A (ed): Psychiatry. Philadelphia, W.B. Saunders, 1997.

Chapter 24

PHYSIATRIC PROCEDURES

Donald F. Green, M.D., and Anthony Chiodo, M.D.

I. **Joint, Soft Tissue, and Spinal Injections**
   A. **Purpose**
      1. Injections can serve as a diagnostic and therapeutic tool.
         a. Initial anesthetic effect can localize pain generators.
         b. Corticosteroid effect decreases inflammation.
      2. Injections should be used as part of complete treatment program.
      3. Generally limited to 3 injections into same joint during 1 year.
      4. Tables 1 and 2 compare commonly used anesthetic agents and cortico-
         steroids, respectively.
   B. **Informed consent**
      1. Specify diagnosis to be treated.
      2. Include description of procedure.
      3. Explain risks and complications.
      4. Explain expected benefits.
      5. Explain irreversibility of procedure.
      6. Outline alternative treatments.
      7. Document informed consent (either verbal or written).
   C. **Contraindications**
      1. Local infection over area of injection.
      2. Systemic infections.
      3. Hypersensitivity to injected medications.
      4. Coagulopathy: if patient is taking blood thinners, no intra-articular or spinal
         injections should be performed.
   D. **Complications**
      1. Bleeding.
      2. Infection.
      3. Accidental intravascular injection, potentially leading to seizures, heart ar-
         rhythmias, hypotension, systemic effects of corticosteroids.
      4. Allergic reactions: urticaria, anaphylaxis.
      5. Tendon rupture: more likely in weight-bearing joints.
      6. Nerve injury.
      7. Pneumothorax.
      8. Fat necrosis.
      9. Depigmentation, especially in dark-skinned patients.
      10. Postinjection flare
         a. Joint appears inflamed several hours after injection.
         b. Inflammation subsides in 1–2 days.
      11. Potential systemic effects of corticosteroid injections.

TABLE 1. Comparison of Common Anesthetic Agents

Agent	Brand Name	Potency	Uses	Concentration (%)	Onset	Duration (hr)	Maximal Single Dose (mg)
Lidocaine	Xylocaine	3	Topical application	4	Fast	0.5-1	500
			Infiltration	0.5-1	Fast	1-2	500
			Peripheral nerve block	1-1.5	Fast	1-2	500
			Epidural block	1-2	Fast	0.5-1	500
			Spinal block	5	Fast		100
Prilocaine	Citanest	3	Peripheral nerve block	1-2	Fast	1.5-3	600
			Epidural block	1-3	Fast		600
Mepivacaine	Carbocaine	3	Peripheral nerve block	1-1.5	Fast	2-3	500
			Epidural block	1-2	Fast	1-2.5	500
Bupivacaine	Marcaine	15	Peripheral nerve block	0.25-0.5	Slow	4-12	200
			Epidural block	0.25-0.75	Moderate	2-4	200
			Spinal block	0.5-0.75	Fast	2-4	20
Etidocaine	Duranest	15	Peripheral nerve block	0.5-1	Fast	3-12	300
			Epidural block	1-1.5	Fast	2-4	300
Chloroprocaine			Infiltration	1	Fast	0.5-1	1000
			Peripheral nerve block	2	Fast	0.5-1	1000
			Epidural block	2-3	Fast	0.5-1.5	1000
Procaine	Novocaine	1	Infiltration	1	Fast	0.5-1	1000
			Peripheral nerve block	1-2	Slow	0.5-1	1000
			Spinal block	10	Moderate	0.5-1	200
Tetracaine	Pontocaine	15	Topical application	2	Slow	0.5-1	80
			Spinal block	0.5	Fast	2-4	20

TABLE 2. Comparison of Common Corticosteroids

Agent	Brand Name	Preparations (mg/ml)	Anti-inflammatory Potency	Plasma Half-life (hr)	Onset	Duration	Solubility	Range of Doses for Injection (mg)
Hydrocortisone	Cortisol	25	1	1.5	Fast	Short	Moderate	25–100
Cortisone	Cortone	50	0.8	0.5	Slow	Moderate	Low	10–50
Prednisolone	Hydeltra	20	4	3	Fast	Moderate	Low	10–40
Methylprednisolone	DepoMedrol	20, 40, 80	5	3	Slow	Moderate	Low	10–80
Triamcinolone	Aristocort Kenalog	10, 20, 40	5	5	Moderate	Moderate	Moderate	5–20
Betamethasone	Celestone	6	25	2–5	Fast	Long	High	1.5–6
Dexamethasone	Decadron	4, 8	25	2–5	Fast	Long	Moderate	1.5–4

   a. The more vascular the space, the more pronounced the effects (e.g., increased in intra-articular injections).
   b. More pronounced with more soluble steroids.
   c. Examples
      i. Hyperglycemia
      ii. Glycosuria
      iii. Electrolyte imbalances in diabetic patients
E. **Basic techniques**
   1. Antisepsis
      a. Clean technique: prepare skin with alcohol or betadine; use clean, non-sterile gloves.
      b. Aseptic technique: prepare skin with betadine or chlorhexidine; use sterile gloves and sterile technique.
   2. Local skin anesthesia can be used.
      a. Lidocaine 1% without epinephrine to make small skin wheal (1 ml).
      b. Vapocoolant sprays (dichlorotetrafluoroethane or ethyl chloride).
      c. EMLA cream: place on skin and cover with occlusive dressing for at least 30 minutes.
      d. For joints close to surface, often no local anesthesia is necessary.
   3. Aspirate gently before injection to ensure that needle is not in a vessel.
   4. Do not inject into tendons (some injections are into tendon sheaths).
   5. Introduce injected medications slowly.
   6. Apply gentle pressure to puncture site after injection.
   7. After intra-articular injections, prescribe relative rest for 48 hours.
F. **Aspirated synovial fluid analysis** (Table 3)
   1. Use larger-gauge needle (18–20 gauge).
   2. Use sterile plain tube for Gram stain, culture and sensitivity testing.
   3. Use heparinized tube for cytology and crystals.
   4. Use hematology tube (with EDTA) for cell count and differential.
II. **Specific Injections**
   A. **Upper extremity**
      1. **Glenohumeral joint** (Fig. 1A)
         a. Indications
            i. Osteoarthritis or inflammatory arthritis

TABLE 3.   Interpretation of Synovial Fluid Analysis

	Diseases	Appearance	WBC/m^3	%PMNs
Normal		Clear	< 200	< 25
Noninflammatory	Osteoarthritis Traumatic arthritis Aseptic necrosis Erythema nodosum Osteochondritis dissecans	Clear, yellow	Up to 10,000	< 25
Inflammatory	Rheumatoid arthritis Crystal-induced arthritis Reiter's syndrome Psoriatic arthritis Collagen vascular disease Rheumatic fever	Clear, yellow, turbid	Up to 100,000	40–90
Septic	Bacterial	Turbid	Up to 5,000,000	40–100

WBC = white blood cell, PMNs = polymorphonuclear neutrophils.

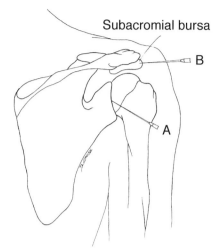

Subacromial bursa

B

A

FIGURE 1. *A*, Injection of the gleno-humeral joint. *B*, injection of the sub-acromial joint.

    ii. Rotator cuff tendinitis or tear
   iii. Adhesive capsulitis
  b. Procedure
      i. Patient sitting, arm relaxed in lap, for posterior approach.
     ii. Aseptic technique with 25-gauge 1.5-inch needle with 6 ml of anes-thetic and steroids (e.g., 4 ml betamethasone and 2 ml lidocaine).
    iii. Palpate posterolateral edge of acromion and coracoid process.
     iv. Insert needle 1 inch below acromion at posterolateral edge.
      v. Direct needle toward coracoid, angled slightly upward, and inject into joint.
  c. **Clinical pearl:** For severe adhesive capsulitis due to chronic immobil-ity, higher volumes (9–12 ml) of saline and anesthetic can be injected into joint to expand capsule.
2. **Subacromial bursa** (Fig. 1B)
  a. Indication: subacromial bursitis.
  b. Procedure
      i. Patient sitting, arm in lap, for posterolateral approach.
     ii. Clean technique with 22-gauge, 1.5-inch needle to deliver 4–6 ml of anesthetic and steroids (e.g., 4 ml 0.25% bupivacaine and 40 mg methylprednisolone).
    iii. Palpate posterolateral edge of acromion.
     iv. Insert needle below edge of acromion.
      v. Direct needle anteriorly and slightly inferiorly and inject into bursa.
  c. **Clinical pearl:** also effective for supraspinatus tendinitis.
3. **Biceps tendon** (Fig. 2)
  a. Indication: bicipital tendinitis.
  b. Procedure
      i. Patient sitting with arm at side, slightly externally rotated.
     ii. Clean technique with 25-gauge, 1.5-inch needle with 2–5 ml of anesthetic and steroids (e.g., 1 ml of bupivacaine and 40 mg methyl-prednisolone).
    iii. Identify bicipital groove and point of maximal tenderness.

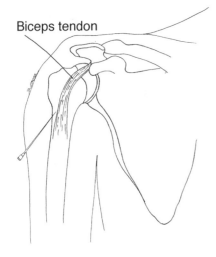

Biceps tendon

FIGURE 2. Injection into the bicipital groove.

    iv. Insert needle into biceps tendon sheath, several inches below acromion, and direct needle slightly upward.

    v. Inject into tendon sheath; little resistance should be felt.

  c. **Clinical pearls**

    i. Restrict heavy lifting for 48 hr after injection.

    ii. Some resistance should be felt; however, if resistance is great, you may be injecting into tendon.

4. **Olecranon bursa** (Fig. 3A)

  a. Indication: olecranon bursitis (common in inflammatory arthritis).

  b. Procedure

    i. Patient lying supine with elbow flexed across chest.

    ii. Clean technique using 18-gauge, 1.5-inch needle with empty syringe.

    iii. Insert needle perpendicular to skin at central swelling.

    iv. Aspirate thick, gelatinous fluid and send for studies.

    v. Change syringes and inject 4 ml of anesthetic and steroids (e.g., 2 ml bupivacaine and 40 mg methylprednisolone).

5. **Lateral epicondyle** (Fig. 3B)

  a. Indication: lateral epicondylitis.

  b. Procedure

    i. Patient sitting with elbow flexed to 90°.

    ii. Clean technique using 22-gauge, 1-inch needle with 2–4 ml of anesthetic and steroids (e.g., 1 ml bupivacaine and 40 mg methylprednisolone).

    iii. Insert needle just below and medial to lateral epicondyle at point of maximal tenderness.

    iv. Insert to bone, then withdraw slightly.

    v. Inject in fanlike pattern with several redirections.

  c. **Clinical pearls**

    i. Consider peritendinous inflammation of nearby muscles (e.g,. extensor digitorum communis, extensor carpi radialis, supinator) in differential diagnosis if injection brings no relief.

    ii. If pain is intractable, consider radial nerve compression.

FIGURE 3. *A*, Injection of the olecranon bursa. *B*, Injection of the lateral epicondyle.

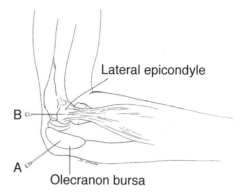

Lateral epicondyle

B

A

Olecranon bursa

6. **Median nerve block at wrist** (Fig. 4)
   a. Indication: carpal tunnel syndrome.
   b. Procedure
      i. Patient's forearm supinated.
      ii. Clean technique using 25-gauge, ⅝-inch needle with 3–5ml of anesthetic and steroids (e.g., 3 ml bupivacaine and 40 mg methylprednisolone).
      iii. Insert needle proximal to wrist crease and on ulnar side of palmaris longus tendon.
      iv. Direct needle toward palm at angle of 30° to depth of ⅝ inch.
      v. Inject into carpal tunnel.
   c. **Clinical pearls**
      i. Severe pain during procedure indicates abnormal needle placement.
      ii. Anesthetic should produce dyesthesia in median nerve distribution after injection.
7. **First dorsal wrist tenosynovitis** (Fig. 5)
   a. Indication: de Quervain's syndrome (stenosing tenosynovitis).
   b. Procedure

FIGURE 4.   Injection of the carpal tunnel.

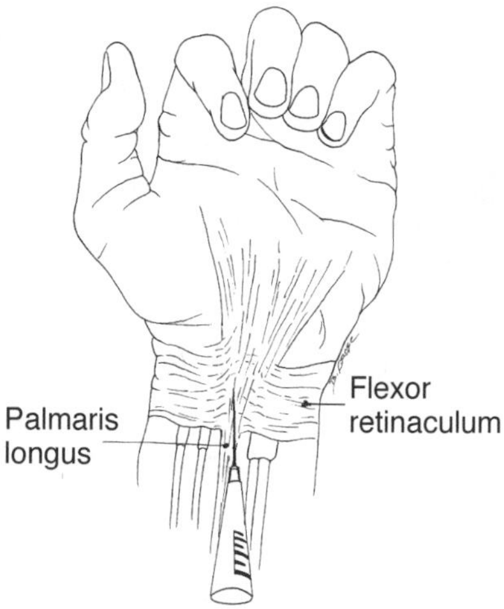

Palmaris longus

Flexor retinaculum

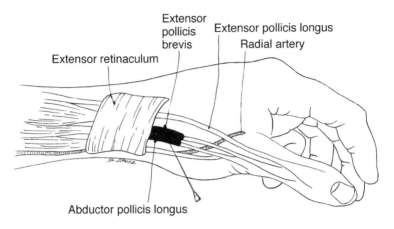

FIGURE 5. Injection of the first dorsal wrist compartment (de Quervain's syndrome).

     i. Patient supine with arm at side, thumb up, wrist relaxed on folded towel.
    ii. Clean technique using 25-gauge, 1-inch needle with 2–4 ml of anesthetic and steroids (e.g., 1 ml bupivacaine and 40 mg methylprednisolone).
   iii. Insert needle just distal to point of maximal tenderness, directed proximally, following line of extensor pollicis longus and abductor pollicis longus tendons.
   iv. Insert needle at 45° angle into tendon sheath and inject.
  c. **Clinical pearl:** Increased resistance indicates that needle is in tendon.
8. **Trigger finger** (Fig. 6)
  a. Indication: trigger finger syndrome.
  b. Procedure
    i. Patient supine with palm upward.

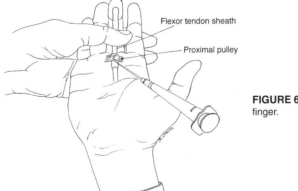

FIGURE 6. Injection of a trigger finger.

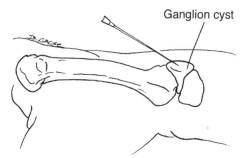

Ganglion cyst

FIGURE 7. Injection of a ganglion cyst.

    ii. Aseptic technique using 25-gauge, 1-inch needle with 1–2 ml of anesthetic and steroids (e.g., 1 ml bupivacaine and 40 mg methyl-prednisolone).

    iii. Hold fingers and insert needle into crease overlying metacarpopha-langeal (MCP) joint at A1 sleeve of tendon.

    iv. Advance needle in distal to proximal direction.

    v. If needle moves greatly with finger flexion, it is in tendon; withdraw slightly and inject into tendon sheath.

  c. **Clinical pearl:** Trigger area can be localized by feeling A1 sleeve near MCP joint of affected finger.

9. **Ganglion cysts** (Fig. 7)

  a. Indication: painful ganglion cyst.

  b. Procedure

    i. Patient with arm ganglion cyst exposed.

    ii. Clean technique with 22-gauge, 1-inch needle with 5-ml empty sy-ringe. Second syringe of 2–3 ml of anesthetic and steroids (e.g., 1.5 ml bupivacaine and 40 mg methylprednisolone) should be prepared.

    iii. Insert needle into cyst and aspirate contents.

    iv. Change syringe and inject anesthetic and steroids.

  c. **Clinical pearls**

    i. If ganglion reappears, surgical excision may be necessary.

    ii. Alternatively, sclerosant may be injected (e.g., sodium tetradecyl).

B. **Lower extremity** (Fig. 8)

  1. **Trochanteric bursa**

    a. Indication: trochanteric bursitis.

    b. Procedure

      i. Patient lying in lateral decubitus position, with involved side up and legs slightly flexed.

      ii. Clean technique using 25-gauge, 3.5-inch needle to deliver 4–6 ml of anesthetic and steroids (e.g., 2 ml bupivacaine and 40 mg methyl-prednisolone).

      iii. Identify greater trochanter and point of maximal tenderness.

      iv. Insert needle over area of maximal tenderness, perpendicular to skin over greater trochanter.

      v. Advance until bone is felt, then withdraw slightly and inject.

    c. **Clinical pearls**

      i. If pain is worse with external rotation, also consider gluteus medius tendinitis.

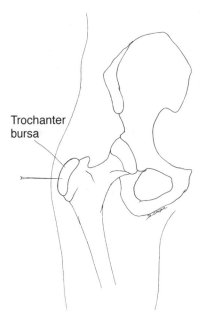

Trochanter
bursa

FIGURE 8. Injection of the greater trochanteric bursa.

   ii. If pain is worse with internal rotation, consider piriformis tendinitis.
2. **Knee** (Fig. 9A)
 a. Indications: osteoarthritis, inflammatory arthritis.
 b. Procedure
   i. Patient supine with knee slightly flexed on a pillow.
   ii. Aseptic technique using 25-gauge, 1.5-inch needle to deliver 6 ml of anesthetic and steroids (e.g., 5 ml bupivacaine and 40 mg methylprednisolone).
   ii. For medial approach, push patella slightly laterally.
   iii. Insert needle even with midpoint of patella between patella and femur.
   iv. Inject after joint space is entered: there should be little resistance.
 c. **Clinical pearl:** Same technique is used to inject intra-articular medications (e.g., hyaluronic acid).
3. **Anserine bursa** (Fig. 9B)
 a. Indication: pes anserine bursitis.
 b. Procedure
   i. Patient supine with knee in full extension.
   ii. Clean technique using 25-gauge, 1.5-inch needle to deliver 4 ml of anesthetic and steroids (e.g., 3 ml bupivacaine and 40 mg methylprednisolone).
   iii. Have patient flex knee against resistance: identify pes anserine bursa distal to joint space at hamstring tendon attachments on tibia.
   iv. Direct needle to point of maximal tenderness, insert to bone, and withdraw slightly.
   v. Inject into bursa: there should be little resistance.
4. **Prepatellar bursa** (Fig. 9C)
 a. Indication: prepatellar bursitis (housemaid's knee).

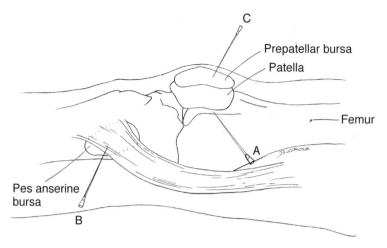

FIGURE 9.   Medial view of the view. *A,* Injection of the knee joint. *B,* Pes anserine bursa injection. *C,* Prepatellar bursa injection.

   b. Procedure
      i. Patient supine with pillow under knee to provide flexion.
      ii. Clean technique using 25-gauge, 1.5-inch needle to deliver 4 ml of anesthetic and steroids (e.g., 2 ml bupivacaine and 40 mg methylprednisolone).
      iii. Identify center of medial aspect of patella.
      iv. Insert needle horizontally into subcutaneous tissue above patella.
      v. Inject into bursa; little resistance should be felt.
5. **Morton's neuroma** (Fig. 10)
   a. Indication: Morton's neuroma.
   b. Procedure
      i. Patient supine with top of foot exposed.

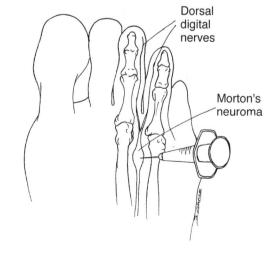

FIGURE 10.   Injection of Morton's neuroma.

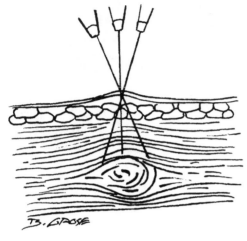

FIGURE 11. Injection of trigger points.

B. GROSE

    ii. Clean technique using 25-gauge, 1.5-inch needle to deliver 4 ml of anesthetic and steroids (e.g., 2 ml bupivacaine and 40 mg methylprednisolone).
    iii. Palpate involved interdigital space.
    iv. Insert needle between metatarsals, advance to mid-depth of foot, and inject.

C. **Trigger points** (Fig. 11)
    a. Indications: trigger points, myofascial pain syndrome.
    b. Procedure
      i. Patient sitting or prone.
      ii. Clean technique using 25-gauge, 1.5-inch needle to deliver 1 ml of anesthetic into each trigger point (e.g., 1 ml bupivacaine).
      iii. Identify trigger points by taut bands and referred pain.
      iv. Insert needle into trigger point, and inject 1 ml in a fanlike pattern with several needle redirections.
    c. **Clinical pearls**
      i. Steroids are generally not used, because they can increase risk for local myopathy.
      ii. Dry needling is also an option.
      iii. Look for muscle spasm or referred pain to be sure that needle is in correct area.

D. **Spinal injection therapy**
    1. **General principles**
      a. Spinal injection is valuable therapeutic and diagnostic tool.
      b. Certainty in needle placement is achieved with fluoroscopic support.
      c. With proper technique, spinal injections can be done quickly and with minimal discomfort.
      d. IV line is recommended for cervical and ablative procedures (cryotherapy, radiofrequency) and can be used to deliver fluid bolus or IV medications, if needed:
        i. Atropine, 0.6 mg IV, for decreased heart rate.
        ii. Diazepam, 5–10 mg IV, for seizures.
        iii. Ephedrine, 12.5–25 mg IV, for decreased blood pressure.

e. Sterile technique makes infection a rare complication.

f. Avoid injection therapy in patients with suspected systemic infection.

g. Injection should not be completed in patients on anticoagulation (e.g., enoxaparin, heparin, warfarin) or with coagulopathy.

h. **Note:** The descriptions that follow should be used only as introduction to these procedures. Complete procedures, contraindications, and complications can be found in several texts listed in bibliography.

2. **Intercostal nerve block**

   a. Indication: radicular pain in thorax.

   b. Procedure

      i. Patient in prone position; with or without fluoroscopic viewing (fluoroscopic view is anteroposterior [AP]).

      ii. Aseptic technique using a 25-gauge, 1.5- or 3-inch needle to deliver 2–3 ml of anesthetic and steroids (e.g., 2 ml bupivacaine and 40 mg methylprednisolone).

      iii. Nerve is located under intercostal vein and artery, just beneath rib of corresponding thoracic nerve segment.

      iv. Insert needle, walk just off bone inferiorly, and advance needle approximately 2 mm.

      v. Injection should be completed after needle aspiration to confirm lack of intravascular injection.

   c. **Clinical pearls**

      i. Same technique is used for chemical neurolysis, cryotherapy, and radiofrequency ablation.

      ii. Pneumothorax is rare but is more likely in patients with chronic obstructive pulmonary disease.

3. **Thoracic and lumbar transforaminal epidural**

   a. Indication: radicular pain from nerve root injury or disease in thorax and lower extremities.

   b. Procedure

      i. Patient in prone position using AP fluoroscopic views.

      ii. Localize injection target with fluoroscope, and mark skin.

      iii. Prepare skin with betadine, and inject skin with local anesthetic wheal.

      iv. Aseptic technique with either 22-gauge, 3.5- or 6-inch spinal needle or 18-gauge introducer with 25-gauge, 6-inch needle to deliver 2–3 ml of anesthetic and steroids (e.g., 2 ml bupivacaine and 80 mg methylprednisolone). Also prepare syringe with 3–5 ml contrast material.

      v. Changing angle of fluoroscope to accommodate lordosis is necessary for adequate visualization in lower lumbar spine.

      vi. Insert needle, checking AP fluoroscopic view as needed, until transverse process is contacted with needle at its caudal aspect.

      vii. Needle is then walked off bone caudally and directed medially and anteriorly to enter neuroforamen at its most cranial (12 o'clock) position.

      viii. Lateral fluoroscopic view assists in positioning needle at correct depth.

      ix. Pop or giving of tissue should be felt as needle advances into epidural space.

      x. Injection of 1–2 ml contrast material highlights nerve root, and epidural flow is seen in AP and lateral views.

      xi. Inject anesthetic and steroids.

c. **Clinical pearls**

    i. This approach allows precise localization of injection at site of suspected pathology based on history, physical examination, and radiologic and electrodiagnostic findings.

    ii. Precise localization and lack of risk of dural injection make this approach preferred procedure in patients with radicular pain from nerve root injury or disease in thorax and lower extremities.

    iii. This approach also can be used for epidural neuroplasty in patients with epidural fibrosis with catheter placement and/or injection of hyaluronidase and hypertonic saline (the latter after IV sedation and adequate epidural local anaesthetic).

    iv. In patients with prior posterior fusion or oblique or hypertrophic facet joint, more lateral injection site or use of curved needle may be necessary.

    v. Injection of larger amounts of contrast allows diagnostic epidurogram and can assist in planning future pain management.

    vi. Oblique view can be used to do this injection as a tunnel-view approach. However, in this circumstance, AP views must be seen to ensure that needle does not advance medial to mid-facet line.

4. **Caudal epidural injection**

a. Indication: leg pain due to lumbar and lumbosacral root disease or trauma.

b. Procedure

    i. Patient in prone position using AP fluoroscopic views.

    ii. Localize injection target with fluoroscope, and mark skin.

    iii. Prepare skin with betadine, and inject skin with local anesthetic wheal.

    iv. Aseptic technique with 25-gauge, 3-inch needle to deliver 9–12 ml of anesthetic and steroids (e.g., 8 ml bupivacaine and 80 mg methylprednisolone). Also prepare syringe with 3–5 ml contrast material.

    v. Insert needle at sacral hiatus, caudal to sacral cornu, using lateral fluoroscopic views to confirm depth.

    vi. Penetration of sacrococcygeal ligament is needed to gain access to epidural space. Pop or giving of tissue should be felt as needle advances into epidural space.

    vii. Injection of 1–2 ml contrast material highlights area and confirms contrast epidural flow.

    viii. High-volume injection is then completed.

c. **Clinical pearl:** Poor selectivity of this block is major limitation, although its relative safety and utility in patients with prior spine surgery have maintained its place in pain intervention armamentarium.

5. **Sacroiliac joint block**

a. Indication: pain mediated by sacroiliac joint.

b. Procedure

    i. Patient in prone position.

    ii. Use oblique fluoroscopic beam, from medial to lateral, which allows tunnel-view approach to well-visualized lower part of joint.

    iii. Localize injection target with fluoroscope, and mark skin.

    iv. Prepare skin with betadine, and inject skin with local anesthetic wheal.

    v. Aseptic technique with 25-gauge, 3-inch needle to deliver 2 ml of anesthetic and steroids (e.g., 1 ml bupivacaine and 80 mg methylprednisolone). Also prepare syringe with 3–5 ml contrast material.

vi. Insert needle, checking fluoroscopic views as needed, until needle is in joint.

vii. Injection of 1–2 ml contrast material creates arthrogram, ensuring proper needle placement.

viii. Inject anesthetic and steroids.

c. **Clinical pearls**

i. Radiographs and nuclear medicine scans are sometimes confirmatory of sacroiliac dysfunction.

ii. Long-acting local anaesthetic is used to assist with diagnostic aspects of block.

Bibliography:

1. Bonica JJ: The Management of Pain, 2nd ed. Philadelphia, Lea & Febiger, 1990.
2. Cyriax J, Coldham M (eds): Textbook of Orthopaedic Medicine, vol. 2: Treatment by Manipulation and Injection. New York, Bailliere Tindall, 1984.
3. Doherty M, et al: Rheumatology Examination and Injection Techniques, 2nd ed. Philadelphia, W.B. Saunders, 1999.
4. Klippel JH, et al (eds): Practical Rheumatology. St. Louis, Mosby, 1997.
5. Lennard TA: Pain Procedures in Clinical Practice, 2nd ed. Philadelphia, Hanley & Belfus, 2000.
6. Moll JMH (ed): Rheumatology in Clinical Practice. Boston, Blackwell Scientific, 1987.
7. Raj PP (ed): Practical Management of Pain, 3rd ed. St Louis, Mosby, 2000.
8. Sliver T: Joint and Soft Tissue Injections. New York, Radcliffe Medical Press, 1996.
9. Waldman SD (ed): Atlas of Pain Management Injection Techniques. Philadelphia, W.B. Saunders, 2000.
10. Walsh NE, et al: Injection procedures. In DeLisa JA, Gans BM (eds): Rehabilitation Medicine: Principles and Practice, 3rd ed. Philadelphia, Lippincott Williams & Wilkins, 1998.

Chapter 25

ORTHOTICS

Sarah Clay Jamieson, M.D., Alicia J. Davis, C.P.O, and M. Catherine Spires, M.D.

I. General Principles
   A. Function of any orthosis is to control, correct, limit, or inhibit motion of extremities or spine
   B. These functions are not mutually exclusive and may be used in concert with one another for patient management.
   C. Orthosis prescription must relate to desired patient outcome.

II. Foot Orthosis and Shoe Modifications
   A. **Purpose:** foot orthoses are means to redistribute contact from heel strike to toe-off to compensate for alterations in foot architecture associated with neuropathies, bony structural changes, and muscle imbalances.
   B. **Composition of orthosis**
      1. Firm base to support or control foot architecture and maintain desired alignment.
      2. Moderate density middle layer for shock absorption.
      3. Soft cover to reduce shear forces against skin.
   C. **Orthotic prescription**
      1. Diagnosis
      2. Activity level and patient's height and weight
      3. Desired biomechanical outcomes
      4. Special considerations: assistive device use, knee/hip problems, gait abnormalities, spasticity
   D. **Pathologies**
      1. **Leg length discrepancy**
         a. Treatment goals
            i. More symmetric posture
            ii. Gait improvement
         b. Shoe modifications
            i. Heel elevation
               • Placed in the shoe if < ½ inch.
               • External placement if > ½ inch.
            ii. Heel and sole elevation if leg length discrepancy is > 1 inch.
            iii. Medial and lateral buttresses for increased stability
      2. **Arthritis, fusion, or instability of subtalar joints**
         a. Treatment goals
            i. Support and limit joint motion.
            ii. Accommodate deformities.

     b. Shoe: high-quarter shoe, reinforced counters, long steel shank, rocker bar, solid ankle cushioned heel.

     c. Orthosis: soft layer for comfort with semirigid layer for support.

3. **Pes planus (valgus)**
     a. Treatment goals
       i. Reduction in eversion
       ii. Support of longitudinal arch
     b. Shoe
       i. Child: high-quarter shoe with broad heel, long medial counter, and medial heel wedge.
       ii. Adult: Thomas heel with medial heel wedge.
     c. Orthosis: medial longitudinal arch support

4. **Pes equinus (fixed)**
     a. Treatment goals
       i. Provide heel strike.
       ii. Contain foot in shoe.
       iii. Reduce pressure on metatarsal heads.
       iv. Equalize leg length.
     b. Shoe: high-quarter shoe with heel elevation, heel and sole elevation on other shoe, modified lace stay for wide opening, possible rocker bar.
     c. Orthosis: medial longitudinal arch support.

5. **Pes varus**
     a. Treatment goals
       i. Flexible deformity: obtain realignment.
       ii. Fixed deformity: accommodate.
       iii. Increase medial and posterior weight-bearing on foot.
     b. Shoe: high-quarter shoe, long lateral counter, reverse Thomas heel, lateral sole and heel wedges for flexible deformity, medial wedges for fixed deformity, and lateral sole and heel flanges.
     c. Orthosis: medial longitudinal arch support.

6. **Pes cavus**
     a. Treatment goals
       i. Distribute weight over entire foot.
       ii. Restore anteroposterior foot.
       iii. Balance and reduce pain on metatarsal heads.
     b. Shoe: high-quarter shoe, high toe box, lateral heel and sole wedges.
     c. Orthosis: metatarsal pads or bars, molded inner sole, medial and lateral longitudinal arch support.

7. **Calcaneal spurs**
     a. Treatment goal: relieve pressure on painful area.
     b. Shoe: inner relief in heel; fill with soft sponge.
     c. Orthosis: heel cushion.

8. **Metatarsalgia**
     a. Treatment goals
       i. Reduce pressure on metatarsal heads.
       ii. Support transverse arch.
     b. Shoe: metatarsal bar or rocker bar, inner sole relief.
     c. Orthosis: metatarsal or sesamoid pad.

9. **Hallux valgus**
     a. Treatment goals

        i. Reduce pressure on first metatarsophalangeal (MTP) joint and great toe by preventing forward foot slide.

        ii. Immobilize first MTP.

        iii. Shift weight laterally.

   b. Shoe: soft vamp with broad ball and toe, relief in vamp with cut-out or balloon patch, low heel, stiff soled shoe with rocker bottom.

   c. Orthosis: metatarsal or sesamoid pad, medial longitudinal arch support.

10. **Hallux rigidus**

   a. Treatment goals

        i. Reduce pressure and motion of first MTP joint.

        ii. Improve push-off.

   b. Shoe: stiff sole shoe or modification to increase rigidity of sole, metatarsal or rocker bar.

   c. Orthosis: sesamoid pad, medial longitudinal arch support.

11. **Hammer toes**

   a. Treatment goals

        i. Relieve pressure on painful areas.

        ii. Support transverse arch.

        iii. Improve push-off.

   b. Shoe: soft upper of shoe, extra depth shoe with high toe box or balloon patch.

   c. Orthosis: metatarsal pad.

12. **Foot shortening (unilateral)**

   a. Treatment goal: fit shoe to foot.

   b. Shoe: extra inner sole and padded tongue for difference < one size.

13. **Foot fractures**

   a. Treatment goal: immobilize fracture.

   b. Shoe: long steel shank to provide rigidity, metatarsal or rocker bar.

   c. Orthosis: longitudinal arch support, metatarsal pad.

14. **Diabetic peripheral neuropathy**

   a. Treatment goal: protect and support associated deformities and problems.

   b. Shoe: extra-depth shoe or custom-molded shoe.

   c. Orthosis: custom orthosis with cover that reduces shear forces.

15. **Charcot changes in foot**

   a. Treatment goal: accommodate fixed deformities, but immobilize foot in active charcot joint.

   b. Shoe

        i. Custom shoes of deer skin with rocker soles.

        ii. Rocker soles can make patient unstable; great care must be used when rocker soles are used.

   c. Orthosis: custom orthosis with appropriate measures to distribute weight-bearing.

III. Ankle-Foot Orthosis (AFO)

  A. **Most often prescribed for lower extremity weakness**

    1. Dorsiflexion weakness

    2. Plantarflexion weakness

    3. Instability in coronal plane

    4. Weakness at knee: ankle plantarflexion encourages knee extension and ankle dorsiflexion encourages knee flexion. AFOs cannot control knee but do influence it.

     5. Also prescribed to reduce axial loading of lower extremity.

B. **Common terms for AFO designs**

    1. Free: allows unrestricted motion in one plane.

    2. Assist: external force applied to increase range, velocity, or force of motion (such as spring).

    3. Resist: external force applied to decrease range, velocity, or force of motion.

    4. Stop: external force to deter undesired motion in one direction.

    5. Variable: adjustment that can be made to degree of motion without causing structural change.

C. **Four primary material designs of AFOs**

    1. **Metal and leather** (also known as double upright AFO)

       a. Not total contact.

       b. Best for patients with edema problems or when total contact is not appropriate.

       c. Attached to stirrup that is permanently attached to shoe.

       d. Most have adjustable ankle joints.

    2. **Metal and plastic**

       a. Best when total contact or cosmesis is important.

       b. Can be placed into different shoes.

       c. Adjustable ankle joints.

    3. **Plastic**

       a. Total contact

       b. Various designs of trim lines afford versatility; rigidity depends on thickness and composition of plastic.

       c. Plastic can be easily modified.

    4. **Laminated**

       a. Total contact

       b. Most rigid material

       c. Best for use with patients who require extremely stable orthosis.

       d. Ankle joints can be incorporated into orthosis.

D. **AFO joint functions** (Table 1)

E. **AFO sagittal control systems**

    1. **Leaf-spring**

       a. Allows dorsiflexion, resists plantarflexion.

       b. Can be made of plastic or metal.

       c. Most common diagnosis: flaccid foot drop.

    2. **Semirigid**

       a. Allows minimal dorsiflexion, resists plantarflexion.

       b. Can be made of plastic or metal.

       c. Plastic model has total contact, and ankle trim lines are at the malleoli.

    3. **Solid ankle**

       a. Does not allow dorsiflexion or plantarflexion.

       b. Can be made of plastic or metal.

       c. Plastic model has total contact, and ankle trim lines are anterior to malleoli.

    4. **Metal and leather:** adjustable stops to allow degrees of dorsiflexion or plantar flexion depending on joint used and patient's progress.

    5. **Floor reaction:** uses ground reaction forces to stabilize both ankle mortise and knee (in extension).

TABLE 1. Ankle-Foot Orthotic Joint Functions

Type of Ankle Joint	Function
Solid ankle	To correct gross medial/lateral instability To manage fused ankle To manage generalized lower leg weakness To relieve ankle pain during ambulation Creates knee flexion moment at heel strike and knee extension moment at midstance through terminal stance.
Limited motion	To provide adjustable plantarflexion and dorsiflexion settings
Free motion	To provide stability in coronal plane Used when dorsiflexor and plantarflexion motion is good
Dorsiflexion assist	To correct weak dorsiflexor muscles without spasticity To correct foot slap or high steppage gait Usually has plantarflexion stop, which creates knee flexion moment at heel strike
Plantarflexion stop	To correct spastic plantarflexor muscles To correct foot slap or high steppage gait To manage knee hyperextension moment Creates knee flexion moment
Dorsiflexion stop	To correct weak plantarflexion muscles To correct weak quadriceps Creates knee extension moment
Floor reaction	Creates knee extension moment by creating posteriorly directed force at knee.

6. **Patellar tendon-bearing type AFO**
   a. Axial unloading
   b. Uses patellar tendon-bearing design to unload ankle.
F. **AFO coronal systems**
   1. **Plastic AFO** uses sustentaculum tali modification (valgus correction) or supramalleolar plastic extension (flange) medially or laterally with long and high medial or lateral distal foot trim line to discourage varus or valgus at ankle.
   2. In **metal or leather AFO**, "T" strap is often used to "pull" ankle into varus or valgus.
   3. In **laminated AFO**, rigidity of lamination and total contact of well-made orthosis control movement.
IV. **Knee Orthoses** (Table 2)
   A. Control various degrees of instability.
   B. Type of instability or motion needed (restricted, free, or partial) dictates type of knee orthoses.
   C. Neoprene orthoses increase warmth, decrease swelling, and help to improve proprioception.
V. **Knee-Ankle-Foot Orthoses (KAFOs)**
   A. **General principles**
      1. Prescribed for knee instability and lower extremity weakness.
      2. Stability achieved through appropriate ankle and knee joint selection.
      3. Composition
         a. Most made with metal knee joint.
         b. Most are hybrids of plastic and metal to achieve stability, comfort, and function.

TABLE 2. Orthotic Knee Joints

Treatment Goal	Appropriate Knee Joint	Advantages	Disadvantages
Medial/lateral stability	Free motion	Light-weight, cosmetic	No flexion or extension control
	Polycentric	Better approximates motion of anatomic knee	Heavy, less cosmetic
Decrease in hyper-extension moment	Posterior offset	Mechanical joint locks before anatomic joint	Heavy, less cosmetic
Maximal stability in standing and ambulation	Drop lock	No upper body involvement to lock joints	Upper body involvement to unlock joints
	Trigger lock	Trigger on proximal thigh section allows release of locking mechanism without bending over	Bulky, needs yearly adjustments
Assist in standing to locked knee position	Step lock	Ratchet action allows flexion stops to complete extension	Bulky, loud (ratchet)
Decrease in knee flexion tightness or contracture	Ultraflex	Constant dynamic stretch Can increase tension over time	Bulky, almost impossible to walk without orthosis on
	Dial lock	Allows static extension adjustments in 6° increments	

    c. Basic design consists of proximal and distal thigh cuffs, calf band, double uprights with mechanical knee joints, and adjustable ankle joint.

B. **Knee joints** (see Table 2)
1. **Free motion**
   a. Knee flexion is unrestricted, but 180° extension stop prevents hyperextension.
   b. Good for patients with medial/lateral instability or tendency to hyperextend knee.
   c. Patient must have good quadriceps strength to control knee in stance and ambulation.
2. **Polycentric joint**
   a. Allows free motion.
   b. Better approximates anatomic knee joint.
3. **Posterior offset**
   a. Extends early in stance because axis of rotation is posterior to knee axis.
   b. Ground reaction forces provide increased stability.
   c. Not intended to be used with knee or hip flexion contracture or with plantarflexion stop at ankle.
4. **Ring or drop lock**
   a. Gravity moves lock into place as patient stands.
   b. Maximal stability: knee is locked in extension.
   c. Difficult gait pattern because locked knee causes vaulting or circumduction.
5. **Lever lock with bail release**
   a. Also called **Cam, Swiss, French, or bail lock**.
   b. Engages when knee is in full extension.
   c. Very stable and easy to unlock.
   d. Bail is engaged when lifted and unlocks knee joint.
   e. Best for patients with compromised upper extremity strength or balance.

6. **Adjustable extension ring lock (dial lock)**
   a. Ring lock as above but is adjustable to differing degrees of extension.
   b. Best for patients with knee flexion tightness or contracture that is improving with treatment.

VI. Hip Orthoses (HOs) and Hip-Knee-Ankle-Foot Orthoses (HKAFOs)

A. **HOs** control hip flexion, extension, abduction, and adduction but **not** rotation.
   1. Used in adult for total hip arthroplasty.
   2. Used in children most often for Legg-Calvé-Perthes disease.
B. **HKAFOs** control hip flexion, extension, abduction, and adduction; rotation is controlled via foot plate.

VII. Cervical Orthoses (COs)

A. **Treatment goals**
   1. Control pain.
   2. Protect from further injury.
   3. Limit or restrict movement.
   4. Support soft tissues.
   5. Assist weak muscles
   6. Control cervical spine position.
   7. Correct abdominal position.
   8. Transfer weight of head to trunk.
B. **Cervical spine characteristics relevant to COs**
   a. Most mobile part of spine
   b. Multiple planes of motion
   c. Small body surface area
   d. Limited amount of external force can be applied.
   e. Achieving adequate purchase on skull and thorax is difficult with external devices.
C. **Occipitoatlantoaxial joint complex**
   1. Occipital–C1 allows significant extension and flexion, lateral flexion, and minimal axial rotation.
   2. Atlantoaxial joint (C1–C2) primarily allows axial rotation (50% of rotation of spine) but also flexion and extension.
   3. Occipitoatlantoaxial joint allows 23° of flexion and 47° of rotation.
   4. C3–C7 allows flexion and extension, lateral bending, and axial rotation.
   5. C2–C3 and C3–C4: lateral bending and axial rotation greater in this area; rotation decreases inferiorly.
   6. C5–C6: site of greatest flexion and extension.
D. **Biomechanical goals** are achieved by
   1. Trunk support
   2. Motion control
   3. Spinal realignment
   4. Weight transfer.
E. **Biomechanical factors determining effectiveness of CO**
   1. Purchase on body
   2. Direction and magnitude of applied forces
   3. How securely device is worn
   4. Force exerted by body against device
   5. Body habitus
F. **Social and economic implications**
   1. Unattractive
   2. Interfere with work and activities of daily living
   3. Psychological and physical dependence on device
   4. Not tolerated well in extremes of temperature and climate
G. **Classification of COs**
   1. Cervical collars
   2. Poster appliances
   3. Cervicothoracic orthoses
   4. Halo devices
H. **Choice of CO** (Table 3)

TABLE 3. Cervical Spine Orthoses

Treatment Goal	Appropriate Orthosis*	Effects†	Advantages	Disadvantages
To treat stable soft tissue injuries: strain, whiplash	Soft cervical collars	Control pain Protect from further injury	Warmth Kinesthetic reminder	Studies have shown that prolonged use increases disability
To limit flexion and extension moments of cervical spine: stable single-column injuries of cervical spine without ligamentous involvement; after surgical stabilization	Philadelphia collar	Control pain Protect from further injury Limit/restrict movement (e.g., after trauma, surgery) Support soft tissues, assist weak muscles	Limits motion in cervical spine Warmth Kinesthetic reminder	Can be hot and decrease tolerance by patients
	Aspen and Miami J collar	Same as above plus control of cervical spine position	More stable than Philadelphia Used to wean patients off more rigid orthoses	Hot Nor for use with moderate-to-severe injuries
	Hard collar	Same as above	Rigid and adjustable	Low patient compliance
	2- or 4-poster cervical collar	Same as above	Increased immobilization of extension and flexion compared with above collars	Does not prevent rotation or lateral side bending Although more stable, does not immobilize and not recommended for unstable injuries
	Philadelphia/Aspen and Miami J with thoracic extension	Same as above	Addition of thoracic extension increases immobilization in both flexion and extension	Do not use for unstable injuries
	Lerman-Minerva	Same as above	Thoracic extension and head band increase immobilization	
To limit flexion moment of cervical spine (e.g., after surgery or injury)	Sternal occipital mandibular immobilization (SOMI)	Same as above	Must be put on in supine position Radiographically translucent Increased patient compliance	*Does not prevent extension*
To immobilize cervical spine in patients with unstable cervical injuries	Halo	Same as above plus correction of abnormal position and transfer of weight of head to trunk	Provides greatest degree of cervical immobilization No contact with neck; thus allows inspection of neck (e.g., after surgery or injury) Increased patient compliance	Invasive (pins) Infection of pin sites Alters center of mass and thus can impair balance *Contraindications:* multiple skull fractures

* Orthoses are listed in order from least to most restrictive. No orthosis completely immobilizes the cervical spine.
† All orthoses are only as good as their fit, the orthotist's recommendation, and patient compliance.

VIII. Thoracic, Lumbar, and Sacral Spinal Orthoses

A. **Treatment goals**
1. Decrease motion.
2. Unload spinal structure.
3. Protect structures.
4. Stabilize or correct thoracolumbo-sacral spine alignment
5. Control musculoskeletal pain.

B. **Classification of spinal orthoses**
1. Trochanteric band
2. Sacral orthosis
3. Lumbosacral orthosis
4. Thoracolumbosacral orthosis (TLSO)

C. **Biomechanical foundation of TLSOs**
1. TLSO used depends on stability of fracture site and ligamentous involvement.
2. Three-point force control system with anterior compression of abdomen.
   a. Control of pelvis, which provides base for spinal alignment.
   b. Abdominal compression reduces longitudinal forces of spine, decreases lordosis and intervertebral joint motion, and can provide axial unloading of intervertebral discs.
   c. Abdominal support typically provided by abdominal apron or modification of semirigid (plastic) orthosis.
   d. Anterior support and abdominal compression are counterbalanced by rigid posterior positioning system.
   e. Provide abdominal support *except* hyperextension orthoses.
3. Pressure over bony prominences must be of sufficient magnitude to remind wearer to maintain or correct position.

D. **Functional impact of TLSOs**
1. Augment gait (e.g., shorten stride length).
   a. Oxygen consumption may increase.
   b. Depending on fit of orthosis, patient may slow cadence to equilibrate for increased energy needs.
   c. Balance may be affected
2. Muscle atrophy may occur with orthosis use; thus, patients will need strengthening programs.
3. Restriction created by orthosis causes increased motion in intervertebral joints caudal and cephalic to orthosis.

E. **Choice of spinal orthosis** (Table 4)

IX. Upper Extremity Orthoses

A. **General concepts**
1. 85% of upper extremity orthoses are interim; 15% are definitive.
2. Prehension (grasp)
   a. Three-point palmar prehension
   b. Tenodesis
      i. Tendency for fingers to flex and thumb to oppose and adduct during wrist extension.
      ii. Most grasp-and-release systems are for definitive use.

B. **Goals**
1. Maintain palmar arch.
2. Keep thumb in opposition.
3. Support web space.
4. Provide means of attachment for other systems (both static and dynamic).

C. **Components**
1. Palmar bar: maintains palmar arch.

TABLE 4. Spinal Orthoses

Treatment Goal	Appropriate Orthosis	Effects*	Advantages	Disadvantages
To support pelvis, control pain	Trochanteric band	Control musculoskeletal pain Decrease motion Protect from further injury	Support after pelvic fractures Supports sacroiliac joint or pubic symphyses diastasis	Must be worn tight to be effective; thus patient compliance may be an issue
	Sacroiliac corset	Same as above	Light-weight support Cosmetic	May press on bladder, exacerbating bladder control problems
To alleviate low back pain	Lumbosacral corset	Same as above plus unload-ing of spinal structure	Increases intra-abdominal pressure, creating axial unloading of lumbar spine Decreases lordosis (with appropriate use of stays) Can be used in pregnancy, but consult obstetrician before prescribing May be used to wean from more rigid orthosis	May complicate respiratory distress May cause trunk muscle deconditioning
To limit lumbar extension (lordosis)	Lumbosacral chairback orthosis	Same as above	Limits extension Allows minimal flexion Some have lateral bars that inhibit lateral side-bending Reduces lordosis	Does not control higher or lower lumbar fractures Not indicated for compression fractures Not for complete immobilization No total contact
	Lumbosacral polymer orthosis	Same as above	Total contact: custom or prefabricated Provides lateral control	Increases intra-abdominal pressure Hot
To limit flexion	Thoracolumbar corset	Same as above	Soft, cosmetic Moderate control	Axillary straps decrease patient compliance
	Thoracolumbar orthosis	Same as above	More rigid Provides intra-abdominal pressure May provide lateral control by addition of lateral bars to orthosis	Axillary straps decrease patient compliance Anterior extension on sternum or in deltopectoral groove not well tolerated
To limit flexion, extension, and rotation	Thoracolumbosacral (hypertension) orthosis	Same as above plus stabilization or correction of thoracolumbosacral spine alignment	Controls least stable injuries Increases intra-abdominal pressure (for axial unloading) Provides triplanar control Maintains spinal alignment through total contact	Does not control for T7 or higher Total contact may lead to skin problems

* Orthosis success depends on patient compliance and fit and appropriateness of orthosis.

2. Opponens bar: maintains thumb in opposition, gives medially directed force to thumb for appropriate positioning, and is often used with thumb adduction stop.

3. Radial and ulnar extensions: oppose one another and increase total contact.

4. Wrist piece: should not interfere with flexion and extension of the wrist.

D. **Types of upper extremity orthoses**

1. **Static:** no motion or hinge; holds joint in fixed position; resting orthoses.

2. **Dynamic:** incorporate flexible (spring or elastic) component; exert constant force; allow joint position change under tension.

3. **Static progressive:** static orthosis that incorporates range of motion (ROM) joint that may be changed over time as patient progresses in function.

E. **Pathologies and treatment options**

1. **Thumb instability**

   a. Thumb adduction stop: "C" bar used to increase ROM in first web space.
      i. Static orthosis: both advantage and disadvantage
      ii. Adjustable over time
   b. Rigid thumb orthosis: stabilizes thumb for prehension
      i. Advantage: patient can grasp without dislocation of thumb.
      ii. Disadvantage: static orthosis that allows only one position.

2. **Digits**

   a. **Mallet finger**
      i. Distal phalynx fracture or extensor tendon rupture to distal interphalangeal (DIP) joint.
      ii. Goal: to prevent flexion.
      iii. Treatment: hold DIP joint in extension with DIP extension assist.
         • Advantage: static, removable orthosis.
         • Disadvantage: removable orthosis may affect patient compliance.

   b. **Boutonnière deformities**
      i. Flexion deformity of proximal interphalangeal (PIP) joint with hyperextension of DIP joint.
      ii. Goal: prevent flexion of PIP and hyperextension of DIP joint.
      iii. Treatment: extension assist at PIP with extension resist and flexion at DIP.

   c. **Swan neck deformities**
      i. Hyperextension deformity of PIP and flexion deformity of DIP.
      ii. Goal: decrease hyperextension of PIP and flexion of DIP.
      iii. Treatment: extend DIP and flex PIP (assist opposite positioning).

3. **Metacarpophalangeal (MCP) joints** (ulnar and/or median nerve damage)

   a. **Extension contractures of MCP joints**
      i. Flexion assist is needed (dynamic: rubber bands/springs)
      ii. Hand orthosis (HO)
         • Rubber bands or springs for increase in ROM; line of pull should be perpendicular to shaft of bone
         • Stops are just proximal to joint that requires stabilization.
         • MCP joints determine IP joint positioning; can use MCP stops and IP extension assists
         • Advantage: tension on system can be increased or decreased by adding rubber bands.
         • Disadvantage: removable.

    b. **Rheumatoid deformities** (volar subluxation and ulnar deviation)

        i. Goal: decrease ulnar deviation and subluxation.

        ii. Treatment: static wrist-hand orthosis (WHO) during acute phase.

          • Advantage: medial and lateral trims at hand and digits may be modified to prevent ulnar deviation.

          • Disadvantage: static orthosis that only holds position.

4. **Wrist instability**

    a. Treatment: WHO.

    b. Dynamic systems for ROM and balancing

    c. Static systems for positioning and stabilization

5. **Prehension (grasp)**

    a. Treatment: tenodesis-type HO

    b. Wrist-driven HO uses available motion to increase prehension.

        i Uses parallelogram linkage and creates three-point palmar prehension.

        ii. Advantages: uses body power and increases fine motor skills.

        iii. Disadvantage: patient may not have enough body power to create prehension.

    c. External power HO uses battery or pneumatic system.

        i. Advantages: does not fade over time; may be used for long duration.

        ii. Disadvantages: can be bulky; decreased cosmesis may decrease acceptance.

6. **Elbow positioning**

    a. Elbow extension contracture

        i. Static treatment: turnbuckle orthosis for positioning and stabilization.

        ii. Dynamic treatment: flexion assist orthosis for increase in ROM and balancing.

          • Usually uses ratchet-type hinge with locking mechanism.

          • May use external power (either contralateral arm or myoelectric control)

    b. Elbow flexion contracture

        i. Static treatment: turnbuckle orthosis for positioning and stabilization.

        ii. Dynamic treatment: extension assist orthosis for increase in ROM and balancing.

7. **Proximal stability of extremity and placement of hand in space**

    a. Shoulder-elbow-wrist-hand Orthosis (SEWHO).

    b. Very difficult to achieve stability and function at this level.

    c. Increased hardware gains only limited function.

    d. Low-functional outcome and labor-intensive treatment.

8. **Peripheral neuropathies**

    a. Ulnar nerve at wrist (claw hand)

        i. Goals: decrease hyperextension of MCP and flexion of PIP and DIP joints.

        ii. Treatment: MCP extension stop with palmar orthosis.

          • Static for nighttime

          • Dynamic for therapy

    b. Median nerve palsy at wrist

        i. Goal: thumb opposition with assist in wrist extension and MCP extension.

        ii. Treatment: HO with an opponens bar and MCP stop.

    c. Radial nerve palsy
- i. Goals: extend wrist and MCP joints, prevent contracture.
- ii. Treatment: WHO (dynamic or static) to assist in wrist extension and assist for MCP extension.

    d. Combined median and ulnar nerve paralysis
- i. Goals: MCP flexion, thumb opposition for prehension.
- ii. Treatment: HO with opponens bar and MCP stop (or MCP flexion assist with thumb stabilized in opposition).

9. **Spinal cord injuries and upper extremity orthoses**
    a. **C1–C3**
- i. Goals: upper extremity (UE) positioning and prevention of contracture from spasticity
- ii. Treatment: WHO for positioning (long opponens)

    b. **C4**
- i. Goals: place hand in space for functional use, prehension, positioning.
- ii. Treatment: mobile arm support (balanced forearm orthosis [BFO]), power tenodesis, long opponens.

    c. **C5**
- i. Goals: UE positioning, prevention of contracture from spasticity, and positioning UE in space for functional use, prehension.
- ii. Treatment: WHO for positioning, BFO to place hand in space, externally powered tenodesis for prehension (initially), ratchet tenodesis.
- iii. Disadvantages
  - BFO: bulky, difficult to maneuver.
  - Power tenodesis: bulky, relies on external power.
  - Ratchet tenodesis: depends on manually controlled prehension.

    d. **C6**
- i. Goals: place thumb in opposition for functional prehension and assist wrist extension to gain functional prehension; improve strength of grasp and dynamic grasp.
- ii. Treatment: opponens orthosis for thumb opposition, wrist-driven tenodesis (may use ratchet type for ease in prehension for extended periods).
  - Advantage: grasp size (leverage) can be varied.
  - Disadvantage: requires fair wrist extension strength.

    e. **C7**
- i. Goal: functional prehension.
- ii. Treatment: initially, possibly wrist-driven tenodesis; later, thumb opponens HO and adduction bar for functional positioning for prehension (MCP flexion/extension).

    f. **C8**
- i. Goal: maintain functional thumb position for opposition.
- ii. Treatment: short opponens HO (small and noncumbersome).

10. **Fracture management**
    a. **Humeral fracture**
- i. Goals: full circumferential compression of soft tissue to maintain pseudohydrostatic environment for stability and alignment.
- ii. Treatment: humeral fracture orthosis (Sarmiento).

- Advantage: allows adjustment as edema decreases.
- Disadvantage: removable.

b. **Humeral fracture, distal third**

i. Goals: same as for humerus plus forearm extension to maintain alignment.

ii. Treatment: humeral fracture orthosis with forearm extension.
- Advantage: reduces pronation and supination.
- Disadvantage: removable.

c. **Ulnar fractures**

i. Goals: same as for humeral fracture.

ii. Treatment: ulnar fracture orthosis (Sarmiento)
- Advantage: soft tissue pressure in interosseous space maintains stability and alignment.
- Disadvantage: not indicated for > 10° of angulation or for proximal fracture.

d. **Radial fractures** do not respond well to fracture orthoses.

Bibliography
1. Alexander IJ: The Foot: Examination and Diagnosis, 2nd ed. New York, Churchhill Livingstone, 1997.
2. Bunch WH, et al (eds): Atlas of Orthotics. American Academy of Orthopedic Surgeons, 2nd ed. St. Louis, Mosby, 1985.
3. Bussell MH, Femwick L: Lower-limb orthotics. In Gabois M, et al (eds): Physical Medicine and Rehabilitation: The Complete Approach. Malden, MA, Blackwell Science, 2000, pp 544–548.
4. Cailliet R: Foot and Ankle Pain, 3rd ed. Philadelphia, F.A. Davis, 1997.
5. Goldberg B, Hsu JD: Atlas of Orthoses and Assistive Devices, 3rd ed. St. Louis, Mosby, 1997.
6. Inman VT, et al: Human Walking. Baltimore, Williams & Wilkins, 1994.
7. Levy C, Waite S, Davis AJ. Spinal orthoses in rehabilitation medicine. In Grabois M, et al (eds): Physical Medicine and Rehabilitation: The Complete Approach. Malden, MA, Blackwell Science, 2000.
8. Lusardi MM, Nielsen CC: Orthotics and Prosthetics in Rehabilitation. Boston, Butterworth Heinemann, 2000.
9. Malick MH, Meyer C: Manual on Management of the Quadriplegic Upper Extremity, 2nd ed. Pittsburgh, PA, Harmorville Rehabilitation Center, 1987.
10. Molnar GE, Alexander MA (eds): Pediatric Rehabilitation, 3rd ed. Philadelphia, Hanley & Belfus, 1999.
11. Perry J: Gait Analysis: Normal and Pathological Function. New York, McGraw-Hill, 1992.
12. Redford JB: Orthotics Etcetera, 2nd ed. Baltimore, Williams & Wilkins, 1980.
13. Wu KK: Foot Orthoses: Principles and Clinical Application. Baltimore, Williams & Wilkins, 1990.

Chapter 26

PROSTHETICS

Sarah Clay Jamieson, M.D., and Alicia J. Davis, C.P.O.

I. Lower Extremity Amputations (also see Chapter 1, Amputation Rehabilitation)
  A. **Incidence, biomechanical concerns, and prosthetic intervention by level**
    1. **Toes:** ~ 56,000 amputations in 1994, according to U.S. National Center for Health Care Statistics (NCHCS).
      a. **Great toe**
        i. Loss of great toe decreases balance through loss of tripod effect: (1) great toe, (2) digits 2–5, (3) calcaneus.
        ii. Loss of push-off with loss of insertion of flexor hallucis longus (FHL) and flexor hallucis brevis (FHB).
        iii. Types of prosthesis
          • Toe filler   • Rocker sole to aid in roll-over
          • Spring steel shank
      b. **Digits 2–5**
        i. Loss of push-off.
        ii. Loss of stability.
        iii. Deficit depends on number of digits amputated.
        iv. Types of prosthesis: same as for great toe.
    2. **Foot:** ~ 11,000 amputations in 1994, according to NCHCS.
      a. **Transmetatarsal**
        i. Loss of anterior lever arm (two-thirds of tripod).
        ii. Types of prosthesis: same as for great toe.
      b. **Total ray**
        i. Loss of width of base of support of foot.
        ii. If fifth ray is amputated, loss of insertion of both peroneus brevis and peroneus tertius.
        iii. Types of prosthesis
          • Toe filler
          • Look for adducted forefoot and treat orthotically.
      c. **Partial foot**
        i. Possible loss of tibialis anterior, extensor digitorum longus (EDL), flexor digitorum longus (FDL), extensor hallucis longus (EHL), FHL, and peroneus tertius.
        ii. Plantarflexors act unopposed, leading to equinovarus foot.
        iii. No loss of overall length of limb.
        iv. Type of prosthesis: total-contact ankle-foot orthosis (AFO) with toe filler.
    3. **Syme amputation**
      a. Good end-bearing.

   b. Heel pad migration (posterior migration is most common).
   c. Prosthetic components become a concern because of minimal space between distal end of residuum and floor.
   d. Types of prosthesis
      i. Symes prosthesis with low-profile foot.
      ii. Prosthesis may of variable design to accommodate residuum.
4. **Transtibial amputation**
   a. ~ 33,000 in 1994, according to NCHCS.
   b. Loss of residuum is a major concern.
   c. Most appropriate technique for prosthetic components and ambulation is to leave at least one-third of overall length of tibia intact.
   d. Longer lever arm increases ambulation stability.
   e. Tibia that is too long (> two-thirds) reduces choice of prosthetic components.
   f. Type of prosthesis: transtibial prosthesis appropriate to patient's activity level, residual limb integrity, and medical, social, and functional history.
5. **Knee disarticulation**
   a. Good end-bearing.
   b. Long lever arm.
   c. No anatomic knee joint; therefore, prosthetic knee joint required.
   d. Discrepancy in height due to ratio of prosthetic knee to anatomic knee.
   e. Type of prosthesis: knee disarticulation prosthesis appropriate to patient's activity level, residual limb integrity, and medical, social, and functional history.
6. **Transfemoral amputation**
   a. ~ 32,000 in 1994, according to NCHCS.
   b. Loss of knee increases energy expenditure.
   c. The longer the residual limb, the less energy is expended to ambulate.
   d. Type of prosthesis: transfemoral prosthesis appropriate to patient's activity level, residual limb integrity, and medical, social, and functional history.
7. **Hip disarticulation**
   a. < 1% of all amputations in 1994, according to NCHCS.
   b. Loss of hip and knee joints.
   c. Increase in energy expenditure.
   d. Decrease in velocity.
   e. Decrease in ability to dissipate heat from body.
   f. Type of prosthesis: hip disarticulation prosthesis with very stable knee joint, appropriate to patient's activity level, residual limb integrity, and medical, social, and functional history.
B. **Factors affecting prosthetic prescription**
   1. Diagnosis
   2. Patient's weight
   3. Activity level
   4. Socket design
   5. Socket-skin interface
   6. Suspension
   7. Joints (if any)
   8. Foot type
   9. Endoskeletal vs. exoskeletal
   10. Special considerations
   11. Contractures, weakness, impaired sensation, poor balance, underlying bony deficits, pressure-intolerant areas (scars, grafts, burns, or bypass grafts)
C. **Prosthetics for specific amputation levels**
   1. **Hip disarticulation/hemipelvectomy socket**
      a. For hip disarticulation or residual femur < 5 cm.

b. Rigid frame.
c. Contains tissues of amputated side, buttocks, and contralateral ilium with flexible anterior shell that opens for donning of prosthesis.
d. Weight-bearing for hip disarticulation occurs over ipsilateral ischial tuberosity and gluteal tissues.
e. Weight-bearing for hemipelvectomy occurs over contralateral ischial tuberosity, sacrum, and ipsilateral remaining tissue.
f. Proximal portion of socket is contoured to fit between iliac crest and rib cage for control and to help suspend the prosthesis.

2. **Transfemoral (above-knee) amputation**
   a. **Transfemoral socket**
      i. **Rigid socket**
         • Securely holds ischium on shelf (either contained or noncontained).
         • Can be made of laminate material or plastic.
      ii. **Flexible socket**
         • Hard, windowed outer frame with semiflexible plastic or silicon polymer socket inside.
         • Fabricated using ischial containment, quadrilateral, or hybrid socket design.
         • Inner liner can become more flexible as it warms to body heat.
      iii. **Ischial-containment, normal shape, normal alignment, and contoured adducted trochanteric-controlled alignment method (CAT-CAM)**
         • Wide anteroposterior and narrow mediolateral dimensions provide compression of soft tissues and limits lateral shift of femur within socket during stance phase.
         • Maintains more anatomic alignment of residual femur.
         • Posterior brim has a high posteromedial wall that cups ischial tuberosity, creating bony lock of socket to ischium during stance phase and limiting lateral socket shift.
      iv. **Quadrilateral hard socket** (most commonly used between 1940 and 1980; use now declining).
         • Narrow anteroposterior and wide mediolateral dimensions.
         • Anterior wall provides counterpressure against limb to ensure proper placement of ischium on posterior shelf.
         • Posterior brim has broad, flat seat for weight-bearing of ischial tuberosity but does not contain ischial tuberosity.
         • Medial wall provides pressure against adductor longus muscle to help control socket.
         • Lateral wall provides surface pressure against shaft of femur and pressure relief for distal cut femur; aids in pelvic stability and overall control of prosthesis; and provides counterpressure for medial wall.
   b. **Transfemoral standard bench alignment**
      i. Bench alignment is variable because of differences in knee manufacturer specifications.
      ii. Stability of knee is generally achieved through trochanter-knee-ankle (TKA) alignment
         • Alignment depends on both knee and prosthetic foot choice.
         • With single-axis or dynamic foot, weight line moves anterior to knee more quickly, thus achieving greater stability.

  iii. Most common gait deviations
- Circumduction: prosthesis too long or knee will not bend.
- Vaulting: same as above.
- Whip (foot swings either medially or laterally in swing phase): knee is internally or externally rotated.
- Lateral trunk bending: medial wall too proximal.
- Knee does not bend: TKA is incorrect, knee is too far posterior.

 c. **Transfemoral prosthetic suspension systems** (Table 1)
 d. **Transfemoral prosthetic knee systems** (Table 2)
 e. **Prosthetic feet** (Table 3)

3. **Knee disarticulation**
 a. **Knee disarticulation socket**
  i. Must accommodate for femoral condyles.
  ii. Can be made self-suspending, depending on shape of residual limb.
  iii. Problems
- Femoral condyles: difficult socket fit.
- May not have adequate room distal to socket for prosthetic knee unit; therefore, knee center will not be anatomically correct

 b. **Knee disarticulation standard bench alignment**
  i. TKA
  ii. Four-bar knee unit is often used because its axis of rotation is more proximal and allows distal aspect of prosthesis to swing under proximal section.

TABLE 1. Transfemoral Prosthetic Suspension Systems

System	Advantages	Disadvantages
Suction	Light-weight Excellent suspension Good proprioception	Unsuitable for elderly or people with heart conditions (because of stress in donning) Not recommended for people with poor blood flow Not recommended for people with volume fluctuation
Lanyard	Easy to don with good hand function and strength Can be used when patient has fluctuating volume (managed with limb socks) Aids in proprioception	Possibility of skin problems Can be difficult to don Expensive
Silesian belt	Axillary suspension Used when suction is not an option Aids in rotational control Adjustable Ease in donning	Chafing Can be particularly uncomfortable in obese patients (cuts into soft tissue)
Hip joint and pelvic band	Controls rotation Maximal mediolateral stability Provides good swing-phase control Used for weak hip adductors or short residuum	Heavy, bulky, and cumbersome Inherent pistoning
Suspenders	Last resort suspension Used if forces around pelvis are an issue (e.g., colostomy)	Patient discomfort Cosmetic issues

TABLE 2. Prosthetic Knee Systems

Knee	Stance-Phase Stability	Swing Phase	Indications	Advantages	Disadvantages	Cost
Outside hinges	Achieved through TKA alignment	Pendulum effect	Good hip extensors Knee disarticulations	Knee center most closely approximates anatomic alignment	Cosmesis Bulky Can ruin clothes	$
Single axis	Achieved through TKA alignment Possible extension assist	Friction	Good strength Long residual limb	Durable Light-weight	Little inherent knee stability	$
Weight-activated stance control	TKA Achieved through "brake" mechanism, which is weight-activated—even in flexion up to 35°	Friction Extension assist	Short residual limb Poor balance New amputee Weak hip extensors Hip flexion contracture	Excellent stability Durable	Cannot descend stairs one after another (brake activates) Expensive Maintenance	$
Polycentric four-bar	Mechanically engineered TKA	Extension assist	Knee disarticulations Short residuum	Excellent stability Durable Knee center approximates anatomic alignment Swing clearance	Increased weight Maintenance	$$$
Manual locking	Manual locking mechanism	Locked	Very weak	Totally stable	Swing phase is impaired	$
Hydraulic	TKA Each knee unit has its own mechanism for stability	All fluid is resistant to flow Viscosity and density determine flow rate	Active strong patients Patients who vary their cadence	Swing changes with cadence	Weight Cost	$$$
Electronic	TKA	Electrically engineered microprocessor	Patients who need assistance with phases of gait	Electronicallly accommodates changes in patient cadence	Extremely high cost Very high maintenance	$$$$$

TKA = trochanter-knee-ankle.

TABLE 3.   Prosthetic Feet

Type	Indications	Contraindications	Action	Advantages	Disadvantages	Cost
Solid ankle cushioned heel (SACH)	New amputees Limited ambulators	Active patient Patients with need for stability on uneven terrain	Plantarflexion simulated by compression of heel wedge No dorsiflexion	Moderate weight Durable Rigid forefoot provides anterior lever arm and proprioception Minimal maintenance Minimal cost	Limited plantarflexion and no dorsiflexion Heel cushion deteriorates over time Rigid forefoot provides poor shock absorption	Low
Single-axis	When foot flat is needed to move weight line anterior to ankle at heel strike	Plantarflexion may cause knee hyperextension at heel strike Weight of foot	Plantarflexion is simulated by compression of heel bumper and joint	Plantarflexion of foot reduces knee flexion moment at heel strike Plantarflexion resistance is adjustable	Maintenance Noise Increased weight No transverse rotation motion	Low, Medium
Multiaxis	When patient needs to ambulate on uneven terrain To reduce transverse rotation on residuum	Patient cannot tolerate added weight Patient does not have access to maintenance	Provides motion in all three planes, including transverse rotation	Reduces torque on residuum Adjustable Shock-absorbing	Increased weight Increased maintenance Increased noise Cost	Medium, High
Dynamic response	Highly active patient When energy storage helps to off-load contralateral limb	Patients who require ambulation aids (e.g., cane, walker)	Heel of foot acts like spring, compressing in stance phase, "storing energy," and rebounding at toe-off to "push-off."	Reduces force at heel strike on contralateral side Some designs are quite light-weight	High cost Some require regular maintenance	High, Very high

4. **Transtibial (below-knee) amputation**
    a. **Transtibial socket** (Table 4)
        i. **Patellar-tendon bearing (PTB):** designed to place greater force over pressure tolerant areas.
            - Pressure-tolerant areas: patella tendon, medial flare and shaft of tibia, soft tissues of anterior compartment between tibia and fibula, lateral shaft of fibula, distal end of residual limb, and posterior compartment.
            - Pressure-sensitive regions: tibial crest, anterior distal end of tibia, fibular head, cut end of fibula, peroneal nerve, and lateral tibial condyle.
        ii. **Variations of PTB**
            - Supracondylar PTB: used for short residual limbs and lax ligaments; no sleeve necessary.
            - Supracondylar/suprapatellar PTB: for very short residual limb; gives anteroposterior stability because it provides rigid hyperextension stop.
            - PTB with joint and corset: prevents hyperextension; good for ligament laxity and heavy duty use (e.g., construction workers, firemen). Corset can cause thigh atrophy.

TABLE 4.   Transtibial Prosthetic Sockets

Socket Design	Indications	Advantages	Disadvantages
PTB	Most common Good ligamentous structure	Total contact in weight-tolerant areas Does not bear weight on intolerant areas (tibial crest, fibular head, distal cut tibia, fibula)	Residual limb bears all weight of patient Requires auxiliary suspension
Total-surface bearing	Most patients Good ligamentous structure	Total contact increases proprioception Minimizes distal edema	Must use interface material (silicone is most common)
PTBSC	Mediolateral instability Very short residual limbs Need for less suspension	Increases mediolateral stability Self-suspending on thin patients	Will not self-suspend on limbs with excessive adipose tissue or very muscular thighs
PTBSCSP	Same as for PTBSC	Same as PTBSC Provides extension stop (SP portion)	Same as PTBSC Enclosing patella can inhibit kneeling and other activities
Joint and corset	Increased weight-bearing surface Mediolateral instability at knee Very short residual limbs Need for rigid extension stop	Off-loads residual limb by bearing weight through thigh Increases mediolateral stability Provides rigid knee extension stop	Bulky and heavy Requires auxiliary suspension (fork strap and waist belt) Patient's limb will piston within socket
Plug fit	When distal residual limb contact is not desired	No contact on distal residual limb	Lack of distal end contact may lead to choke syndrome

PTB = patellar-tendon bearing, PTBSC = patellar-tendon bearing supraconylar, PTBSCSP = patellar-tendon bearing supracondylar/suprapatellar).

  iii. **Total-surface bearing**
- Captures all regions for weight-bearing and distributes pressure equally to all areas of residual limb.
- Incorporates silicone suspension methods.
- Total contact increases proprioception, minimizes distal edema, and increases overall surface bearing on limb.

 b. **Transtibial suspension systems** (Table 5)

 c. **Prosthetic feet** (see Table 3).

 d. **Standard bench alignment**
  i. Center of mass of socket is located 25 mm anterior to ankle center when viewed in sagittal plane.
  ii. Center of foot is located 12 mm medial to midline of socket as viewed posteriorly in coronal plane, producing narrower base of support and therefore requiring less energy to walk or run. This also produces varus moment at midstance to load pressure-tolerant regions of limb.
  iii. Most common gait deviations
- Excessive valgus (loads pressure sensitive areas)
- Excessive varus (causes inefficient gait and requires more energy to ambulate)
- Lateral trunk bending (results if prosthesis is too short or too tall)
- Drop-off (if socket weight line is forward to foot, causing knee to break too quickly)
- Hyperextension at knee (socket is too posterior in coronal plane)

5. **Syme amputation**: ankle disarticulation with reattachment of heel pad.

TABLE 5.   Transtibial Suspension Systems

System	Advantages	Disadvantages
Sleeve	Ease in donning Hides proximal prosthesis trim lines	Wears out Some pistoning Increased perspiration Can cause skin problems May not be indicated for vascular patients
Supracondylar cuff	Ease in donning Provides good suspension over patella	Not indicated for people with excessive adipose tissue
Supracondylar	No auxiliary suspension needed	Same as above
Bony lock	No auxiliary suspensions needed Cosmetic benefit	Can be difficult in all planes of motion to maintain suspension
Silicone suspension	One of most reliable suspension methods Cosmetic benefit Eliminates pistoning Provides cushioning to residuum as well as some shear absorbency	Can be difficult to don Possibility of skin problems Hot—problematic in warm climate
Suction	No auxiliary suspension needed Cosmetic benefit Light-weight	Patient cannot have volume changes

      a. Narrow internally just proximal to bulbous flair of malleoli, allowing it to be self-suspending; use of compressible liners or expandable air bladders make this possible.

      b. Low-profile foot is used because of limited space between distal end of socket and ground.

  6. **Partial foot amputation**

      a. In great-toe and transmetatarsal amputations, goal is to normalize gait mechanics and provide energy return during toe-off.

        i. Add spring steel shank.

        ii. Add foam toe filler.

        iii. Add rocker sole to create smooth transition from foot flat to toe-off.

      b. Midfoot amputations may use self-suspending split socket and custom prosthetic foot.

II. Upper Extremity Amputations (also see Chapter 1, Amputation Rehabilitation)

  A. **General principles**

    1. Goal is to preserve function, which is usually accomplished by preserving length.

    2. Skin traction is used for open amputations.

    3. Skin grafting may be necessary.

    4. Disarticulation in children prevents bony overgrowth and preserves growth plate.

    5. Supination and pronation of the forearm decrease as the site of amputation becomes more proximal.

  B. **Amputation levels**

    1. **Transphalangeal** (finger)

      a. Biomechanical concerns: prehension, cosmesis.

      b. Type of prosthesis: passive.

    2. **Ray**

      a. Biomechanical concerns: prehension, grasp, cosmesis.

      b. Type of prosthesis: passive glove.

    3. **Transmetacarpal/transcarpal**

      a. Biomechanical concerns: prehension, grasp, cosmesis.

      b. Type of prosthesis: passive glove.

    4. **Wrist disarticulation**

      a. Biomechancial concerns: preservation of forearm supination/pronation, prehension, grasp, cosmesis.

      b. Type of prosthesis: conventional prosthesis, figure-of-eight harness, single control for terminal device (TD), flexible hinges, wrist and TD appropriate to patient's needs. Length of prosthesis may be longer than contralateral limb, depending on components.

    5. **Below elbow** (BE)

      a. Types

        i. Long

          • Biomechanical concerns: prehension, grasp, cosmesis.

          • Types of prosthesis: same as for wrist disarticulation; myoelectric TD, if appropriate.

        ii. Medium: same concerns and types of prosthesis as long.

        iii. Short/very short

          • Biomechanical concerns: same as for long plus ability to flex elbow to move hand in space for activities of daily living (ADLs).

- Types of prosthesis: same as for long, but socket must be pre-flexed.
  b. Minimum of 10 cm below lateral epicondyle is preferred (provides better lever am and therefore greater forearm strength).
  c. Save elbow joint whenever feasible to preserve natural flexion/extension; in addition, one less prosthetic joint is needed.
  d. 2 cm proximal to wrist allows 70–80% of pronation/supination and room for prosthetic components.
  e. Short forearm length (60% of length or less) requires method of rotating forearm in prosthesis.
6. **Elbow disarticulation**
  a. Biomechanical concerns: prehension, grasp, cosmesis, locked elbow for ADLs.
  b. Types of prosthesis: same as for BE; outside locking hinges at elbow.
  c. Allows effective humeral rotation.
  d. Disadvantages: distal end of prosthesis is bulky and requires outside locking hinges.
7. **Above elbow** (AE)
  a. Types
    i. Long (standard)
      - Biomechanical concerns: prehension, grasp, cosmesis, locked elbow for ADLs.
      - Types of prosthesis: same as for elbow disarticulation. TDs include conventional type (dual control or nudge control) and myoelectric.
    ii. Short: same concerns and types of prosthesis as long.
    iii. Very short: same concerns and types of prosthesis as long; however, socket design includes shoulder cap and chest strap.
  b. Residual limb 10 cm long (measured from axillary fold) is preferred to preserve humeral rotation.
8. **Shoulder disarticulation**
  a. Same concerns and types of prosthesis as for AEs.
  b. Retention of surgical neck of humerus helps maintain shoulder fullness.
9. **Forequarter**
  a. Same concerns and types of prosthesis as for AEs.
  b. Includes amputation of arm, scapula, and part of clavicle.
C. **Upper extremity prosthetic management**
  1. **Time frame**
    a. Immediate: in operating room or recovery room.
    b. Early: 7–30 days ("Malone's golden period"); has shown greatest prosthetic success and use.
    c. Late: > 30 days; poor results.
    d. Children: "sit to fit" (6–9 months); passive vs. functional.
  2. **Prosthetic prescription/upper extremity components**
    a. **Type**
      i. Provisional: first prosthesis, not intended for long-term use.
      ii. Definitive: intended for long-term use.
    b. **Control system**
      i. Endoskeletal vs. exoskeletal
      ii. Conventional (body-powered)
      iii. Single cable

    iv. Dual cable

    v. External power

    vi. Myoelectric

    vii. Switch/nudge control

    vii. Hybrid of myoelectric and switch/nudge control

  c. **Socket**

    i. Double wall

    ii. Silicone liner: used as growth liner (to be discarded as patient grows).

    iii. Split wall: used to gain range of motion.

  d. **Suspension system**

    i. Harness

    ii. Figure-of-eight system

    iii. Chest strap

    iv. Shoulder saddle

    v. Self–suspending system

    vi. Body-suspending system

    vii. Silicone suction-suspending system

  e. **Shoulder**

    i. Four-way hinge

    ii. Shoulder cap

  f. **Elbow**

    i. Internal locking/turntable

    ii. Forearm lift assist

    iii. External locking

    iv. Externally powered

    v. BE hinges

      • Flexible   • Cuff attached to socket

      • Rigid   • Step-up

  g. **Wrist**

    i. Friction: for patients who do not routinely change TDs.

    ii. Quick disconnect: for patients who routinely change TDs.

    iii. Power rotator: for patients who need rotation capabilities (using external power).

    iv. Flexion wrist: for bilateral amputees so that activities at midline of body can be performed.

  h. **Terminal device**

    i. Mechanical hand: more cosmetic, but not as functional as hook.

    ii. External power hand: can generate up to 35 pounds of pinch force.

    iii. Hook

      • Voluntary opening: opened by voluntary coordinated muscle contraction (glenohumeral flexion and biscapular abduction).

      • Voluntary closing: hook remains open until coordinated muscle contraction closes TD.

      • Increased sensory feedback; increase in muscle contraction = increased pinch force.

      • Rubber bands on hooks: 1 rubber band = 1 pound of pinch force.

      • Most common types of hooks: (1) 5XA (aluminum with neoprene lining on hook to prevent grasp slipping), (2) 7 (farmer's hook; good for grasping tools, and (3) 8 (for children).

   i. **Accessories**
      i. Compression socks   v. Electrodes
      ii. Limb socks   vi. Batteries
      iii. Rubber bands   vii. Battery charger
      iv. Band applicator

D. **Problems of upper extremity prostheses**
  1. Function is usually less than patients expect or need.
  2. Changes in residual limb volume create problems with socket fit.
  3. Skin can develop folliculitis, and excessive perspiration can cause other dermatologic problems.
  4. Changes in residual limb volume may create choke syndrome acutely or chronically (verrucous hyperplasia).

Bibliography

1. Ayyappa E: Normal human locomotion. Part 1: Basic concepts and terminology. J Prosthet Orthot 9:10–17, 1997.
2. Bowker JH, Michael JW (eds): Atlas of Limb Prosthetics: Surgical, Prosthetic, and Rehabilitation Principles. St. Louis: Mosby, 1992.
3. Bowker JH: Kinesiology and functional characteristics of the lower limb. In Bowker JH (ed): Atlas of Limb Prosthetics. St. Louis, Mosby, 1981, pp 261–271.
4. Colwell MO, Spires MC, Wontorcik L, et al: Lower extremity prosthetics and rehabilitation. In Grabois M, et al (eds): Physical Medicine and Rehabilitation: The Complete Approach. Malden, MA, Blackwell Science, 2000, pp 583–607.
5. Gard SA, Childress DS, Uellendahl JE: The influence of four-bar linkage knees on prosthetic swing-phase floor clearance. J Prosthet Orthot 8:34–40, 1996.
6. Greene MP: Four-bar linkage knee analysis. Orthot Prosthet Int 37:15–24, 1983.
7. Harris M: Diabetes in America: Epidemiology and scope of the problem. Diabetes Care 21(Suppl 3):C11–C14. 1998.
8. Inman VT, et al: Human Walking. Baltimore, Williams & Wilkins, 1994.
9. Leonard JA, Meier RH: Upper and lower extremity prosthetics. In DeLisa JA, et al (eds): Rehabilitation Medicine: Principles and Practice, 3rd ed. Philadelphia, J.B. Lippincott, 1998, pp 669–696.
10. Lusardi MM, Nielsen CC: Orthotics and Prosthetics in Rehabilitation. Boston, Butterworth Heinemann, 2000.
11. Michael JW: Prosthetic knee mechanisms. Phys Med Rehabil State Art Rev 8:147–164, 1994.
12. Moore WS, Malone JM: Lower Extremity Amputation. Philadelphia, W.B. Saunders, 1989.
13. Nader M, Nader HG: Otto Bock Prosthetic Compendium: Lower Extremity Prostheses. Berlin, Schiele & Schon, 1994.
14. New York University Postgraduate Medical School: Lower Limb Prosthetics. New York, Prosthetic Orthotic Publications, 1993.
15. Perry J: Gait Analysis: Normal and Pathological Function. New York, McGraw-Hill, 1992.
16. Spires MC, Leonard JA: Prosthetic pearls. Phys Med Rehabil Clin North Am 7:3:509–526. 1996.
17. Spires MC, Miner L: Upper extremity prosthetics and rehabilitation principles. In Grabois M, et al (eds): Physical Medicine and Rehabilitation: The Complete Approach. Malden, MA, Blackwell Science, 2000, pp 549–582.
18. Wagner FW: Partial-foot amputations. In Bowker JH, Michael JW (eds): Atlas of Limb Prosthetics: Surgical, Prosthetic, and Rehabilitation Principles, 2nd ed. St. Louis, Mosby. 1992, pp 389–401.

EMERGENCY GUIDELINES

Cardiac Arrest

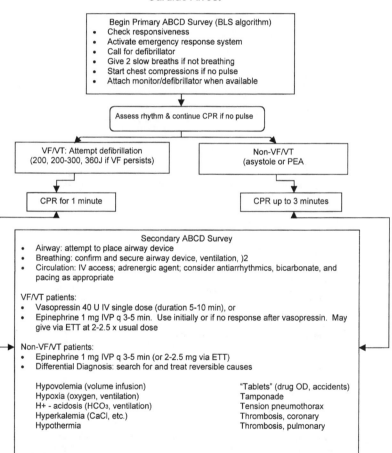

Begin Primary ABCD Survey (BLS algorithm)
- Check responsiveness
- Activate emergency response system
- Call for defibrillator
- Give 2 slow breaths if not breathing
- Start chest compressions if no pulse
- Attach monitor/defibrillator when available

Assess rhythm & continue CPR if no pulse

VF/VT: Attempt defibrillation (200, 200-300, 360J if VF persists)

Non-VF/VT (asystole or PEA

CPR for 1 minute

CPR up to 3 minutes

Secondary ABCD Survey
- Airway: attempt to place airway device
- Breathing: confirm and secure airway device, ventilation,)2
- Circulation: IV access; adrenergic agent; consider antiarrhythmics, bicarbonate, and pacing as appropriate

VF/VT patients:
- Vasopressin 40 U IV single dose (duration 5-10 min), or
- Epinephrine 1 mg IVP q 3-5 min. Use initially or if no response after vasopressin. May give via ETT at 2-2.5 x usual dose

Non-VF/VT patients:
- Epinephrine 1 mg IVP q 3-5 min (or 2-2.5 mg via ETT)
- Differential Diagnosis: search for and treat reversible causes

Hypovolemia (volume infusion)	"Tablets" (drug OD, accidents)
Hypoxia (oxygen, ventilation)	Tamponade
H+ - acidosis (HCO3, ventilation)	Tension pneumothorax
Hyperkalemia (CaCl, etc.)	Thrombosis, coronary
Hypothermia	Thrombosis, pulmonary

Adapted from Guidelines 2000 for cardiopulmonary resuscitation and emergency cardiovascular care. Circulation 102(Suppl 1), 2000, with permission.

Ventricular Fibrillation & Pulseless VT

```
┌──────────────────────────────────────────────────────────────┐
│       Primary ABCD Survey: basic CPR and defibrillation        │
│   •  Check responsiveness                                      │
│   •  Activate emergency response system                        │
│   •  Call for defibrillator                                    │
│   Airway: open the airway                                      │
│   Breathing: provide positive-pressure ventilation             │
│   Circulation: chest compressions                              │
│   Defibrillation: assess for and shock VF & pulseless VT, up to 3 times │
│   (200J, 200-300J, 360J, or equivalent biphasic) if necessary  │
└──────────────────────────────────────────────────────────────┘
                              │
                              ▼
              ┌──────────────────────────────────┐
              │     Persistent or recurrent VF/VT │
              └──────────────────────────────────┘
                              │
                              ▼
┌──────────────────────────────────────────────────────────────┐
│     Secondary ABCD Survey: more advanced assessment & rx       │
│   Airway: place airway device as soon as possible              │
│   Breathing: confirm airway device placement by exam & confirmatory test │
│   Breathing: secure airway device; purpose-made tube holders preferred │
│   Breathing: confirm effective oxygenation and ventilation     │
│   Circulation: IV access                                       │
│   Circulation: Identify rhythm → monitor                       │
│   Circulation: administer drugs appropriate for rhythm and condition │
│   Differential diagnosis: search for and treat identified reversible causes │
└──────────────────────────────────────────────────────────────┘
                              │
                              ▼
┌──────────────────────────────────────────────────────────────┐
│   •  Epinephrine 1 mg IV push (or 2-2.5 mg via ETT), q 3-5 minutes, or │
│   •  Vasopressin 40 U IV x 1; may switch to epinephrine after 5-10 min. │
└──────────────────────────────────────────────────────────────┘
                              │
                              ▼
          ┌──────────────────────────────────────────┐
          │   Resume attempts to defibrillate          │
          │   1 x 360 J (or equivalent biphasic) within 30-60 seconds │
          └──────────────────────────────────────────┘
                              │
                              ▼
┌──────────────────────────────────────────────────────────────┐
│   Consider antiarrhythmics:                               A    │
│   •  Amiodarone ( IIb) 300 mg IVP (may give repeat doses of 150 mg IVP) │
│   •  Lidocaine (recommendation indeterminate) 1-1.5 mg/kg IVP or 2-4 │
│      mg/kg via ETT (may repeat 0.5-0.75 mg/kg bolus q 3-5 min to max 3 │
│      mg/kg)                                                     │
│   •  Magnesium ( IIb if hypomagnesemic or polymorphic VT) 1-2 g IV │
│   •  Procainamide ( IIb for intermittent/recurrent VF/VT) 20-50 mg/min to │
│      total 17 mg/kg                                            │
└──────────────────────────────────────────────────────────────┘
                              │
                              ▼
          ┌──────────────────────────────────────────┐
          │   Resume attempts to defibrillate          │
          │   360J after each med or each minute of CPR │
          └──────────────────────────────────────────┘
```

A. Levels of evidence: Class I – interventions always acceptable, proven safe, and definitely useful. Class IIa – acceptable, safe and useful; standard of care of intervention of choice: IIb – acceptable, safe and useful; within standard of care, but considered optional or alternative intervention: Class III – not useful, potentially harmful.

Adapted from Guidelines 2000 for cardiopulmonary resuscitation and emergency cardiovascular care. Circulation 102(Suppl 1), 2000, with permission.

Pulseless Electrical Activity
(Rhythm on ECG monitor without detectable pulse)

Primary ABCD Survey: basic CPR and defibrillation
- Check responsiveness
- Activate emergency response system
- Call for defibrillator

Airway: open the airway
Breathing: provide positive-pressure ventilation
Circulation: give chest compression
Defibrillation: assess for VF & pulseless VT; shock if indicated

---

Secondary ABCD survey: more advanced assessment and treatment
Airway: place airway device as soon as possible
Breathing: confirm airway device placement by exam & confirmatory test
Breathing: secure airway device; purpose-made tube holders preferred
Breathing: confirm effective oxygenation and ventilation
Circulation: establish IV access
Circulation: identify rhythm → monitor
Circulation: administer drugs appropriate for rhythm and condition
Circulation: assess for occult blood flow ("pseudo-PEA")
Differential diagnosis: search for and treat identified reversible causes

---

Review for most frequent causes   **A**

- Hypovolemia (volume infusion)
- Hypoxia (oxygen, ventilation)
- H+ - acidosis (HCO_3, ventilation)
- Hyperkalemia (CaCl, *etc.*)
- Hypothermia

- "Tablets" (drug OD, accidents)
- Tamponade
- Tension pneumothorax
- Thrombosis, coronary
- Thromboembolism, pulmonary

Epinephrine 1 mg IVP, repeat every 3 to 5 minutes   **B**

Atropine 1 mg IV push (if PEA rate is slow), repeat every 3 to 5 minutes as needed, to a total dose of 0.04 mg/kg   **C**

A. Sodium bicarbonate 1mEq/kg indications: Class I: pre-existing hyperkalemia. Class IIa: known pre-existing bicarbonate-responsive acidosis; tricyclic antidepressant overdose: to alkalinize urine in salicylate or other drug overdose. Class IIb: in intubated and ventilated patients with long arrest interval: on return of circulation after long arrest interval. Class III (may be harmful) in hypercarbic acidosis.
B. Epinephrine 1 mg IVP q 3-5 minutes (Class indeterminate). If this approach fails, higher doses up to 0.2mg/kg may be used but are not recommended. Evidence does not yet support routine use of vasopressin in PEA or asystole.
C. Atropine with shorter dosing interval (q 3-5 min) is possibly helpful in cardiac arrest.

Adapted from Guidelines 2000 for cardiopulmonary resuscitation and emergency cardiovascular care. Circulation 102(Suppl 1), 2000, with permission.

Asystole

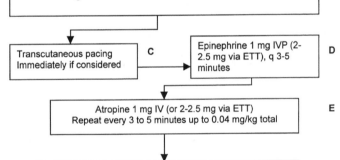

Primary ABCD Survey: basic CPR and defibrillation   **A**
- Check responsiveness
- Activate emergency response system
- Call for defibrillator

Airway: open the airway
Breathing: provide positive-pressure ventilation
Circulation: give chest compression
Confirm: true asystole
Defibrillation: assess for VF & pulseless VT; shock if indicated
Rapid scene survey: any evidence team should not attempt resuscitation?

⬇

Secondary ABCD Survey: more advanced assessment and rx
Airway: place airway device as soon as possible
Breathing: confirm airway device placement by exam & confirmatory test
Breathing: secure airway device; purpose-made tube holders preferred
Breathing: confirm effective oxygenation and ventilation
Confirm asystole: check lead & cable connections; monitor power on? monitor gain up? Verify asystole in another ECG lead.
Circulation: establish IV access
Circulation: identify rhythm → monitor
Circulation: administer drugs appropriate for rhythm and condition   **B**
Differential diagnosis: search for and treat identified reversible causes

⬇

| Transcutaneous pacing Immediately if considered   **C** | Epinephrine 1 mg IVP (2-2.5 mg via ETT), q 3-5 minutes   **D** |

⬇

Atropine 1 mg IV (or 2-2.5 mg via ETT)   **E**
Repeat every 3 to 5 minutes up to 0.04 mg/kg total

⬇

If asystole persists consider terminating resuscitation effort
- Consider quality of resuscitation effort
- Atypical clinical features absent? Not a victim of drowning or hypothermia? No reversible therapeutic or illicit drug OD?
- Support for cease-efforts protocols in place?

A. Assess clinical indicators that resuscitation not indicated, i.e. signs of death.
B. Sodium bicarbonate 1mEq/kg indicated for TCA overdose, urine alkalinization in overdose, tracheal intubation plus long arrest intervals, or upon return of circulation if there is a long arrest interval. Ineffective or harmful in hypercarbic acidosis.
C. Transcutaneous pacing must be performed early, combined with drug therapy. Not routinely indicated for asystole.
D. Epinephrine 1 mg IVP q 3-5 min. If this fails, higher doses (up to 0.2mg/kg) may be used but not recommended. Insufficient evidence supports vasopressin for asystole.
E. Atropine: shorter dosing interval q 3-5 min in asystolic arrest

Adapted from Guidelines 2000 for cardiopulmonary resuscitation and emergency cardiovascular care. Circulation 102(Suppl 1), 2000, with permission.

Bradycardia

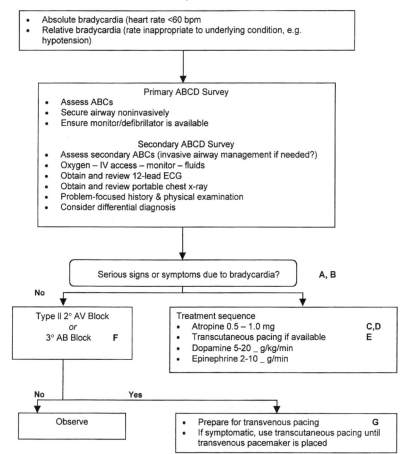

- Absolute bradycardia (heart rate <60 bpm
- Relative bradycardia (rate inappropriate to underlying condition, e.g. hypotension)

Primary ABCD Survey
- Assess ABCs
- Secure airway noninvasively
- Ensure monitor/defibrillator is available

Secondary ABCD Survey
- Assess secondary ABCs (invasive airway management if needed?)
- Oxygen – IV access – monitor – fluids
- Obtain and review 12-lead ECG
- Obtain and review portable chest x-ray
- Problem-focused history & physical examination
- Consider differential diagnosis

Serious signs or symptoms due to bradycardia?   **A, B**

No

Type II 2° AV Block
or
3° AB Block   **F**

Treatment sequence
- Atropine 0.5 – 1.0 mg   **C,D**
- Transcutaneous pacing if available   **E**
- Dopamine 5-20 _ g/kg/min
- Epinephrine 2-10 _ g/min

No   **Yes**

Observe

- Prepare for transvenous pacing   **G**
- If symptomatic, use transcutaneous pacing until transvenous pacemaker is placed

A. If the patient has serious signs or symptoms make sure they are related to bradycardia.
B. Symptoms: chest pain, shortness of breath, decreased level of consciousness; Signs: low blood pressure, shock, pulmonary congestion, congestive heart failure.
C. Denervated transplanted hearts will not respond to atropine. Go at once to pacing.
D. Atropine should be given in repeat doses every 3 to 5 minutes up to a total of 0.03 to 0.04 mg/kg. Use a shorter dosing interval (q 3 min.) in severe clinical situations.
E. If the patient is symptomatic, do not delay transcutaneous pacing while awaiting IV access or for atropine to take effect.
F. Never treat the combination of 3° heart block and ventricular escape beats with lidocaine (or any agent that suppresses ventricular escape rhythms).
G. Verify mechanical capture and patient tolerance. Use analgesia and sedation prn.

Adapted from Guidelines 2000 for cardiopulmonary resuscitation and emergency
cardiovascular care. Circulation 102(Suppl 1), 2000, with permission.

Stable Ventricular Tachycardia

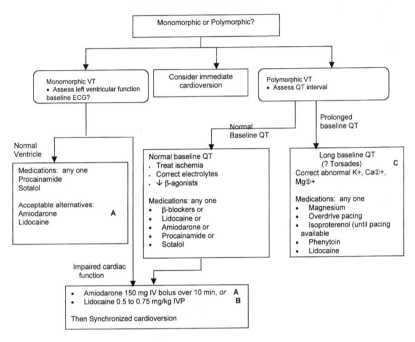

A.   Amiodarone dosing: 150 mg IV bolus over 10 minutes. Repeat 150 mg IV every 10-15 minutes prn. Alternative
infusion 360 mg over 6 hours (1 mg/min) then 540 mg over 18 hours (0.5 mg/min). Maximum total dose 2.2g in 24
hours including all resuscitation doses.
B.   Lidocaine dosing in impaired cardiac function: 0.5-0.75 mg/kg IV push. Repeat q 5-10 min then infuse 1-4 mg/min.
Maximum total dose 3 mg/kg over one hour.
C.   If rhythm suggests *torsades de pointes*: stop/avoid all treatments that prolong QT. Identify and treat abnormal
electrolytes.

**Adapted from Guidelines 2000 for cardiopulmonary resuscitation and emergency
cardiovascular care. Circulation 102(Suppl 1), 2000, with permission.**

Tachycardia

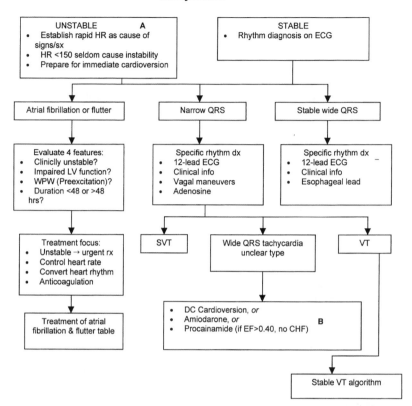

A. Cardioversion:
   - 02 sat monitor, suction, IV access, intubation equipment
   - Pre-medicate when possible (with benzo or barbiturate + narcotic)
   - Synchronized shocks in following sequence: 100, 200-300, 360J or equivalent biphasic

B. Give amiodarone (150 mg IV over 10 minutes, then 1 mg/kg x 6 hrs., then 0.5 mg/min) or
   procainamide (20 mg/min to total 17 mg/kg, or development of hypotension or QRS widening)

**Adapted from Guidelines 2000 for cardiopulmonary resuscitation and emergency
cardiovascular care. Circulation 102(Suppl 1), 2000, with permission.**

Management of Acute Seizures

0–5 minutes
Airway, breathing, circulation
Vital sign monitoring with pulse oximetry
    Management of fever
    Supplemental oxygen as required
Neurologic examination
Glucose testing
Start IV fluids
Draw blood for basic electrolytes, including magnesium, calcium, complete blood count, renal/liver function, and serum drug levels
Thiamine 100 g IV prior to dextrose
Consider EEG monitoring
Lorazepam 0.1mg/kg IV at 2 mg/min

5–25 minutes
If seizures continue:
    Phenytoin 20 mg/kg IV at 50 mg/min
                or
    Fosphenytoin 20 mg/kg PE IV at 150 mg/min
Continued vital signs monitoring

25–30 minutes
If seizures continue:
    Additional **phenytoin 5–10 mg/kg IV at 50 mg/min**
                or
    Additional **fosphenytoin 5–10 mg/kg PE IV at 150 mg/min**

35–50 minutes
If seizures continue:
    Phenobarbital 20 mg/kg IV at 50–75 mg/min
Consider midazolam or propofol anesthesia if in the ICU, hyperthermia, or continued seizing more than 60 minutes

50–60 minutes
If seizures continue:
    Additional **phenobarbital 5–10 mg/kg at 50–75 mg/min**

> 60 minutes
ICU admission with general anesthesia:
    Midazolam 0.2 mg/kg IV followed by 75–100 micrograms/kg/hr
                or
    Propafol 1-2 mg/kg IV followed by 2–10 mg/kg/hr

PE= phenytoin equivalents.
Adapted from Lowenstein DH, Alldredge BK: Status Epilepticus. N Engl J Med 338:970–976, 1998.

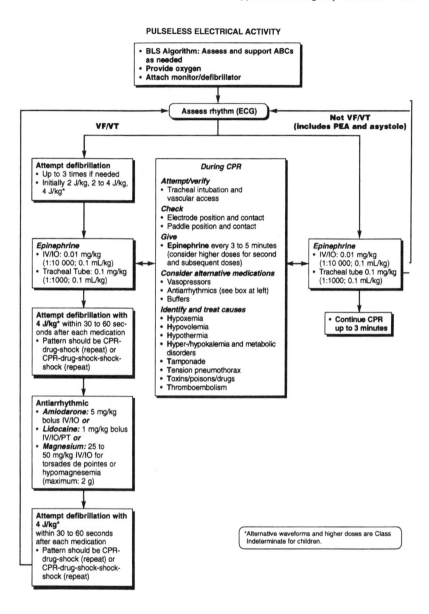

Pediatric Advanced Life Support (PALS) pulseless arrest algorithm. From Guidelines 2000 for cardiopulmonary resuscitation and emergency care. Circulation 102(Suppl 1), 2000, with permission.

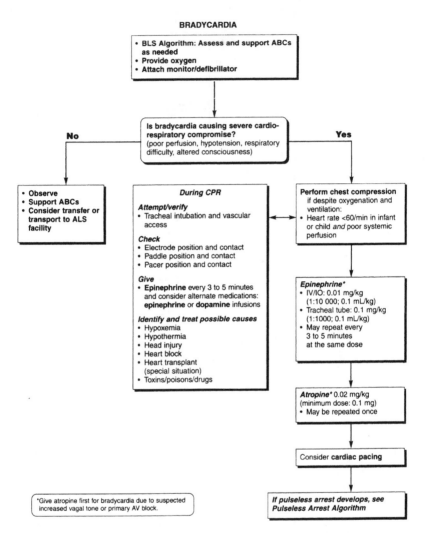

BRADYCARDIA

- BLS Algorithm: Assess and support ABCs as needed
- Provide oxygen
- Attach monitor/defibrillator

Is bradycardia causing severe cardio-respiratory compromise?
(poor perfusion, hypotension, respiratory difficulty, altered consciousness)

No

- Observe
- Support ABCs
- Consider transfer or transport to ALS facility

Yes

During CPR

Attempt/verify
- Tracheal intubation and vascular access

Check
- Electrode position and contact
- Paddle position and contact
- Pacer position and contact

Give
- **Epinephrine** every 3 to 5 minutes and consider alternate medications: **epinephrine** or **dopamine** infusions

Identify and treat possible causes
- Hypoxemia
- Hypothermia
- Head injury
- Heart block
- Heart transplant (special situation)
- Toxins/poisons/drugs

Perform chest compression
if despite oxygenation and ventilation:
- Heart rate <60/min in infant or child *and* poor systemic perfusion

Epinephrine*
- IV/IO: 0.01 mg/kg (1:10 000; 0.1 mL/kg)
- Tracheal tube: 0.1 mg/kg (1:1000; 0.1 mL/kg)
- May repeat every 3 to 5 minutes at the same dose

Atropine* 0.02 mg/kg (minimum dose: 0.1 mg)
- May be repeated once

Consider **cardiac pacing**

*Give atropine first for bradycardia due to suspected increased vagal tone or primary AV block.

If pulseless arrest develops, see Pulseless Arrest Algorithm

PALS bradycardia algorithm, From Guidelines 2000 for cardiopulmonary resuscitation and emergency care. Circulation 102(Suppl 1), 2000, with permission.

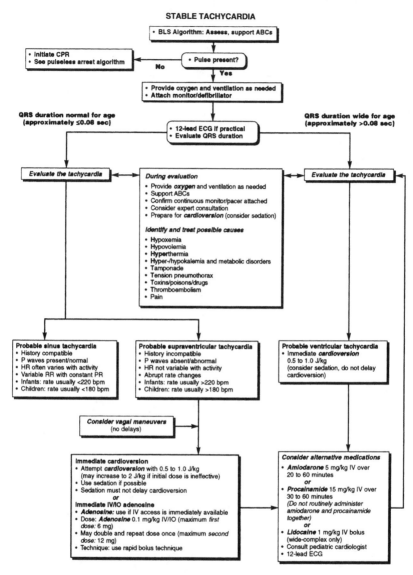

PALS tachycardia algorithm for infants and children with rapid rhythm and adequate perfusion. From Guidelines 2000 for cardiopulmonary resuscitation and emergency care. Circulation 102(Suppl 1), 2000, with permission.

ELECTROMYOGRAPHY

Henry Tong, M.D.

This appendix is designed to be a reference tool for the beginning electromyographer. It is not intended to include all possible methods of care of different clinical problems. Normative data are not included because they depend on the specific technique used and the patient population. Several textbooks describe specific study techniques and provide reference values. Sources are listed because data from one source may conflict with data from another source.

Reduction of Stimulus Artifact with Nerve Conduction Studies

- Remove perspiration from skin between stimulator and recording electrodes.
- Use only a small amount of electrolyte cream beneath all electrodes.
- Place ground electrode next to active recording electrode, between the stimulator and the active recording electrode.
- Use only enough current strength and duration to achieve a supramaximal response.
- Reduce the impedance between the skin and all electrodes.
- Elevate the low-frequency filter (use sparingly, if it all, because it tends to distort the waveform).
- Rotate the anode about the cathode.
- Use a needle cathode/ (anode).

From Dumitru D, Amato A, Zwarts MJ (eds): Electrodiagnostic Medicine, 2nd ed. Philadelphia, Hanley & Belfus, 2002, with permission.

Reducing Motor Artifact in Antidromic Ulnar Sensory Studies to Fifth Digit

1. Place the active ring electrode over the middle phalanx and the reference ring electrode over the distal phalanges of digit 5; the space between electrodes should be at least 3–4 cm.
2. Extend/straighten and abduct fingers; gauze may be used to separate the fifth digit from the fourth.

From Rutkove SB: Reduction of motor artifact in antidromic ulnar sensory studies. Muscle Nerve 22:520–522, 1999.

Reducing 60 Cycle per Second interference in Needle EMG Study

I. Reduce existing 60 cycle per second interference around patient/electrodes.
  • Unplug unused equipment (e.g., lamps, radios). Plugged power cords, even with the equipment turned off, are a source of interference.
  • Keep plugged power cords as far away from the patient as possible.
  • Keep EMG machine as far away from patient/preamplifier as reasonable (usually limited by cable or preamplifier holder).
  • Try rotating preamplifier.
2. If you are using a monopolar needle, decrease (and hopefully match) impedance of active/reference electrode.
  • Keep surface reference electrode near needle.
  • If surface reference electrode moved several times, reapply electrode cream and use new tape. Ensure that surface electrodes are well attached.
  • In ICU setting or electrically hostile environment, consider using 3-cm ground electrode or subcutaneous needle electrode for reference electrode.

From Gitter A: Instrumentation lecture for 1996 Review Course in Physical Medicine and Rehabilitation. Sponsored by the University of Washington School of Medicine [videocassette]. Mt. Laurel, NJ, CME video program, 1995.

Insertional Activity

Type	Duration	Shape	Cause
Normal	< 300 msec	Spikes	Muscle depolarization
Increased	> 300–500 msec	Spikes Positive waves	Normal variant Normal variant Denervation Myopathy
Decreased	Absent or < 300 msec	Absent/spikes	Fat/not in muscle Fibrosis Periodic paralysis Compartment syndrome/ischemia

From Dumitru D, Amato A, Zwarts MJ (eds): Electrodiagnostic Medicine, 2nd ed. Philadelphia, Hanley & Belfus, 2002, with permission.

Grading of Fibrillation Potentials

0	=	absence
±	=	equivocal
+	=	persist over 1–2 areas, present in ≥ 2 areas
2+	=	moderate number present in ≥ 3 areas
3+	=	large numbers in all areas
4+	=	profuse, widespread, pesistent; fill baseline

From Daube JA: AAEM Minimonograph No. 11: Needle Examination in Electromyography. Rochester, MN, American Association of Electrodiagnostic Medicine, 1979.

Recommended Initial Mache Settings*

	Filter Setting		Starting Stimulus		Initial Motor Settings	
	Low Frequency (High Pass)	High Frequency (Low Pass)	Druation (msec)	Intensity	Sweep (msec/division)	Gain/Sensitivity (µV/division)
Nerve conduction velocity (sensory)	20 Hz	2 kHz	0.05	Start at 0 mA, then 25, 50, and 75 mA...	2	10–20
Nerve conduciton velocity (motor)	2 Hz	10 kHz	0.1	Same as sensory	2	2000–5000
Repetitive nerve stimulation	Same as motor NCV			Motor supramaximal settings, but stimulate 2–3 Hz × 4–10 responses		
F wave	Same as motor NCV			Motor supramaximal settings	Arm: 5; leg: 10	100–500
H reflex	Same as motor NCV		0.7–1	Start 0 mA and slowly increase every 2–3 sec	Leg: 10	200–500
Blink reflex	20 Hz	10 kHz	0.05		5–10	200
Sympthetic skin response	0.5 Hz	2 kHz	0.2		500	200
EMG: routine	20 Hz	10 kHz			10	Insertion: 50–100 MUAP: 200
EMG: quantative	2–5 Hz	10 kHz			0.2–05	200
SFEMG	500–1000 Hz	10–20 kHz				
SEP†	5–30 Hz	3 kHz	0.1–05 msec	2.5–3 times sensory threshold or see muscle contraction	Arm: 40 Leg: 80	1–5

EMG =electromyography, SFEMG = single-fiber electromyography, SEP = somatosensory evoked potential, MUAP = motor unit action potential.

* There are no universally accepted guidelines for filter settings, only recommendations.

† Goldberg G, Lagatutta FP, Kraft GH: Somatosensory Evoked Potentials: Basics. An AAEM Workshop. Rochester, MN, Johnson Printing, 1993.

From Sethi RK, Thompson LL: The Electromyographer's Handbook. Boston, Little, Brown, 1989, p 179, and TD20 MK1 Version, number 27, 10 EMG/EP System Operating Notes. Pleasantville, NY, TECA Corporation, 1987.

Voluntary Motor Unit Action Potential (MUAP) Parameters

I. **Recruitment**
  A. Recruitment principles
    1. Henneman size principle: initially smaller motor units are activated. With more force generation, there is an orderly recruitment of sequentially larger motor units.
    2. Rule of fives
      • Motor units begin firing at stable rates at ~ 5 Hz. Minimum onset frequency of motor unit: ~ 3–4 Hz.
      • When first motor unit fires ~ 10 Hz, second motor unit is activated at 5 Hz.
  B. Recruitment frequency: the firing frequency of a MUAP when the next MUAP just begins to fire regularly.
    1. Normal recruitment frequency: 5–10.
    2. Decreased recruitment frequency: >10.
    3. Increased recruitment: many motor units are seen for the amount of force generated by muscle.
  C. Recruitment ratio: firing frequency of fastest MUAP/number of different MUAPs.
    1. Normal: ~5-10 (rough guide).
    2. Decreased recruitment: ratio > 10.
    3. Ratio < 5 is consistent with increased recruitment.
II. **Amplitude:** height between the sequential most positive peak to most negative peak.
  A. Highest when needle tip is in region of motor unit; fast rise time is seen (e.g., < 0.5 msec for concentric needle).
  B. Amplitude with monopolar needle is 5–30% higher than with concentric needle.
III. **Duration:** time between point of initial departure from baseline and final return to baseline.
  A Normal duration: about 7–10 msec.
  B. For more details, see table below by Kelly and Stolov.
IV. **Phases:** number of baseline crossing plus one.
  A. Polyphasia: five or more phases.
  B. In muscle, 20% polyphasic motor units is upper limit of normal.

From Ball RD: Basics of Needle Electromyography: An AAEM Workshop. Rochester, MN, American Academy of Electrodiagnostic Medicine, 1985, and Dumitru D: Needle electromyography. In Dumitru D (ed): Electrodiagnostic Medicine. Philadelphia, Hanley & Belfus, 1995, pp 211–248.

Mean MUAP Duration for Selected Muscles

Age	Temporalis	Masseter	Sternocleidomastoid		
0–10	6.7	6.2	7.1		
13–20	8.4	7.9	8.2		
25–50	8.7	8.2	9.2		
55–80	8.9	8.4	10.3		
Age	Deltoid	Bicep	Tricep	EDC	BR	FDI
0–10	8.6	8.5	9.9	7.8	8.1	8.5
13–20	9.9	9.7	11.3	8.9	9.2	9.7
25–50	11.1	10.9	12.2	10.1	10.4	10.9
55–80	12.5	12.3	12.7	11.3	11.7	12.3
Age	Glut. Max	Biceps Fem.	Vast. Med.	Tibial Ant.	Gastroc.
0–10	10.2	9.4	8.7	10.5	8.0
13–20	11.7	10.8	9.9	11.9	9.1
25–50	13.1	12.1	11.1	13.4	10.3
55–80	14.7	13.6	12.5	15.1	11.5

Data obtained with concentric needle electrode and reported in ms but may be used with monopolar needle electrodes if the MUAP's rise time is less than 1.0 ms. EDC = extensor digitorum communis, BR = brachioradialis, FDI: = first dorsal interosseous, Glut. Max. = gluteus maximus, Biceps Fem. = biceps femoris, Vast. Med. = vastus medialis, Tibial Ant. = tibialis anterior, Gastroc. = gastrocnemius. Values 20% greater than those listed are considered abnormal. From Dumitru D, Amato A, Zwarts MJ (eds): Electrodiagnostic Medicine, 2nd ed. Philadelphia, Hanley & Belfus, 2002, with permission.

Electrodiagnostic Findings in Peripheral Neuropathies

Parameter	Early Demyelinating	Chronic Demyelinating	Acute Axonal	Chronic Axonal
Distal latency	Increased	Increased	Normal or slightly increased	Normal or slightly increased
NCV	Decreased	Decreased	Normal or slightly decreased	Normal or slightly decreased
F latency	Increased or absent	Increased or absent	Normal or absent	Normal or absent
H-reflex latency	Increased or absent	Increased or absent	Absent	Absent
SNAP amplitude	Decreased or absent	Decreased or absent	Decreased or absent	Decreased or absent
CMAP amplitude	Normal or decreased	Normal or decreased	Decreased	Decreased
MUAP duration	Normal	Normal (hereditary) Increasd (acquired)	Normal	Increased
MUAP amplitude	Normal	Normal or increased	Normal	Increased
Polyphasics	Normal	Increased	Normal	Increased
Recruitment	Normal or decreased	Decreased, rapid	Decreased, rapid	Decreased, rapid
Abnormal spontaneous activity	None	None or fibrillations, PSWs, CRDs	Fibrillations, PSWs, CRDs	None, or fibrillations, PSWs, CRDs

NCV = nerve conduction velocity, SNAP = sensory nerve action potential, CMAP = compound motor action potential, MUAP = motor unit action potential, PSWs = positive sharp waves, CRDs = complex repetitive discharges.
From Krivikas L: Electrodiagnosis in neuromuscular diseases. Phys Med Rehabil Clin North Am 9:83–114, 1998, with permission.

Suggested Electrodiagnostic Testing for Specific Disorders*

Suspected Condition	Sensory Testing	Motor Testing	Electromyography	Proximal Conductions	Other Special Tests
Myopathy	One sensory NCS in clinically involved limb	One or two motor NCS in clinically involved limb	Two muscles (proximal and distal) in two limbs, one of which is symptomatic		Consider RNS studies
NMJ disorders	One sensory NCS in clinically involved limb	One motor NCS in clinically involved limb	One proximal and one distal muscle in clinically involved limb		RNS at 2–3 Hz in clinically weak muscle and, if normal, another weak muscle SFEMG with high suspicion and negative RNS; can be first test in ocular MG
Polyneuropathy	Sensory NCS in at least two extremities If abnormalities in one limb, contralateral limb should be studied. Four or more may be necessary to classify polyneuropathy	Motor NCS in at least two extremities If abnormalities in one limb, contralateral limb should be studied. Four or more may be necessary o classify polyneuropathy	One distal muscle in both legs and distal muscle in one arm	Consider proximal nerve conduction studies (H reflexes, F waves, and blink reflexes)	
Motor neuron disease	One sensory NCS in at least two clinically involved limbs	One motor NCS in at least two clinically involved limbs Proximal stimulation sites to exclude multi-focal motor neuropathy	Several muscles in three extremities, or two extremities and cranial nerve-innervated muscles as well as lumbar or cervical paraspinal muscles. Thoracic paraspinal muscles may be considered as an extremity. Sample distal and proximal muscles.	Consider F waves	Consider RNS

NCS = nerve conduction study, RNS = repetitive nerve stimulation, NMJ = neuromuscular junction, SFEMG = single-fiber EMG, MG = myasthenia gravis.

* These recommendations represent a minimum study for addressing the target disorder. Expanding the study to exclude other conditions is often necessary. These guidelines not only acknowledge but also recommend expansion of testing.

From Dillingham T: Electrodiagnostic approach to patients with suspected generalized neuromuscular disorders. Phys Med Rehabil Clin North Am 12:253, 2001, with permission.

Electrodiagnostic Findings in Neuromuscular Junction Transmission Disorders

Parameter	Myasthenia Gravis	Lambert-Eaton Myasthenic Syndrome	Botulism
Distal latency	Normal	Normal	Normal
NCV	Normal	Normal	Normal
SNAP amplitude	Normal	Normal	Normal
CMAP amplitude	Usually normal	Decreased	Normal or decreased
Slow repetitive stimulation	Decrement	Decrement	± Decrement
Fast repetitive stimulation or brief exercise	± Mild increment	Large increment (lasting 20–30 sec)	Intermediate increment (lasting up to 4 min)
Postactivation exhaustion	Yes	Yes	No
MUAP configuration	MMAV (weak muscles) ± decreased amplitude and duration	MMAV (all muscles), decreased amplitude and duration, increased polyphasics	MMAV (weak muscles) decreased amplitude and duration, increased polyphasics
Recruitment	Normal or increased	Increased	Increased
Spontaneous activity	Fibrillations in severe disease	None	Fibrillations in severe disease
SFEMG	Increased jitter and blocking (increases with increased firing rate)	Increased jitter and blocking (decreases with increased firing rate)	Increased jitter and blocking (decreases with increasesd firing rate)

NCV = nerve conduction velocity, SNAP = sensory nerve action potential, CMAP = compound motor action potential, MUAP = motor unit action potential, SEFMG = single-fiber EMG, MMAV = moment-to-moment amplitude variation.

From Krivikas L: Electrodiagnosis in neuromuscular diseases. Phys Med Rehabil Clin North Am 9:83–114, 1998, with permission.

Electrodiagnostic Findings in Myopathies

Parameter	Muscular Dystrophy	Congenital	Mitochondrial	Metabolic	Inflammatory	Chanellopathy
Distal latency	Normal	Normal	Normal	Normal	Normal	Normal
NCV	Normal	Normal	Normal	Normal	Normal	Normal
H-reflex latency	Normal or absent	Normal or absent	Normal	Normal	Normal or absent	Normal
SNAP amplitude	Normal	Normal	Normal	Normal	Normal	Normal
CMAP amplitude	Normal or decreased	Normal or decreased	Normal or decreased	Normal or decreased	Normal or decreased	Normal
MUAP duration	Decreased and/or increased	Decreased or normal	Decreased or normal	Decreased or normal	Decreased and/or normal (IBM)	Decreased or normal
MUAP amplitude	Decreased and/or increased	Decreased or normal	Decreased or normal	Decreased or normal	Decreased and/or normal (IBM)	Decreased or normal
Polyphasics	Increased	Increased or normal	Increased or normal	Increased or normal	Increased	Increased or normal
Recruitment	Increased	Increased or normal	Increased or normal	Increased or normal	Increased	Increased or normal
Fibrillations and PSWs	Yes	Centronuclear myopathy	No	Yes	Yes	Occasionally
CRDs	Yes	Centronuclear myopathy	No	Yes	Yes	Occasionally
Myotonic potentials	Myotonic dystrophy	Centronuclear myopathy	No	Acid maltase deficiency	No	Yes
Electrical silence	No	No	No	Contractures in McArdle's disease	No	During attacks of paralysis

NCV = nerve conduction velocity, SNAP = sensory nerve action potential, CMAP = compound motor action potential, MUAP = motor unit action potential, PSWs = positive sharp waves, CRDs = complex repetitive discharges, IBM = inclusion body myositis.
From Krivikas L: Electrodiagnosis in neuromuscular disease. Phys Med Rehabil Clin North Am 9:83–114, 1998, with permission.

Normal Spontaneous Activity in Needle Electromyography

	MEPPs	Endplate Spikes
Sounds like	Sea shell murmur	Grease in pan
Morphology	Monophasic negative	Biphasic negative/positive
Rhythm	Irregular	Irregular
Amplitude	10–50 µV	100–200 µV
Duration	0.5–2 msec	3.0–4.0 msec
Origin site	Endplate	Single muscle fiber
Comments	Disappear	Disappear

MEPP = miniature endplate potential.
Modified from Dumitru D, Amato A, Zwarts MJ (eds): Electrodiagnostic Medicine, 2nd ed. Philadelphia, Hanley & Belfus, 2002, with permission.

Muscle Generators of Abnormal Spontaneous Activity

	Fibrillation Potentials	Positive Sharp Waves	Complex Repetitive Discharge	Myotonic Discharges
Sounds like	Rain falling on tin roof	Dull thud	Heavy machinery; idling motorcycle	Dive bomber
Morphology	Biphasic spike with initial positive deflection	Positive wave with negative phase	Any form, but is constant	Brief spikes/positive waveforms
Rhythm	0.5–20 Hz	Regular but can be irregular	10–100 Hz, regular	20–100 Hz, wax and wane
Amplitude	20–1000 µV	20–200 µV	50–1000 µV	20–1000 µV
Duration	< 5.0 msec	10–30 msec	Varies	Varies
Origin site	Single muscle fiber	Controversial	Ephaptic conduction between muscle fibers	Uncertain; may originate in muscle membrane
Comments			Abrupt onset and cessation	Frequency and amplitude waxes and wanes

Modified from Dumitru D, Amato A, Zwarts MJ (eds): Electrodiagnostic Medicine, 2nd ed. Philadelphia, Hanley & Belfus, 2002, with permission.

Neural Generators of Abnormal Spontaneous Activity

	Fasciculation	Myokymic Discharges	Neuromyotonic Discharges
Sounds like		Marching soldier	
Morphology	Simple or polyphasic MUAP	*Bursts* of 2–10 normal motor unit potentials	Burst of MUAPs; amplitude typically wanes
Rhythm	0.1–10 Hz; irregular spontaneous firing	20–250 Hz trains firing every 0.1–10 Hz	15–300 Hz for a few seconds; starts and stops abruptly
Amplitude	> 300 *m*V	Varies	Varies
Duration	~ MUAP	Varies	Varies
Origin site	Single motor unit	Group of motor units firing	Motor axons
Comments		Electrical silence between bursts	

MUAP = motor unit action potential.
Modified from Dumitru D, Amato A, Zwarts MJ (eds): Electrodiagnostic Medicine, 2nd ed. Philadelphia, Hanley & Belfus, 2002, with permission.

Simple Schematic of Brachial Plexus

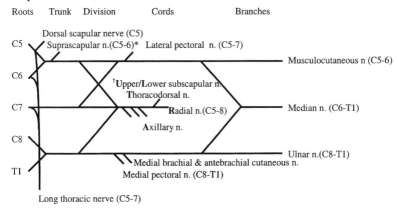

Roots   Trunk   Division   Cords   Branches

Dorsal scapular nerve (C5)

C5   Suprascapular n.(C5-6)*   Lateral pectoral n. (C5-7)

Musculocutaneous n (C5-6)

C6

†Upper/Lower subscapular n.
Thoracodorsal n.

C7   Radial n.(C5-8)   Median n. (C6-T1)

Axillary n.

C8

Ulnar n.(C8-T1)

Medial brachial & antebrachial cutaneous n.

T1   Medial pectoral n. (C8-T1)

Long thoracic nerve (C5-7)

* Nerve to subclavius muscle also originates around here

†Posterior cord: the nerves do not branch off in this order and are listed in this order for mnemonic reasons (ULTRA- personal communication from John Lekas, M.D.)

Root/Plexus Tract for Sensory Nerves Used for Sensory Nerve Conduction Studies

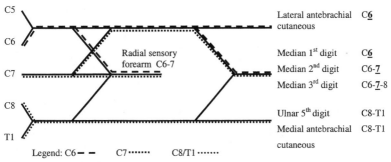

C5

Lateral antebrachial   C**6**
cutaneous

C6

Radial sensory
forearm   C6-7

Median 1ˢᵗ digit   C**6**

C7   Median 2ⁿᵈ digit   C6-**7**

Median 3ʳᵈ digit   C6-**7**-8

C8

Ulnar 5ᵗʰ digit   C8-T1

Medial antebrachial   C8-T1

T1   cutaneous

Legend: C6 ‒ ‒   C7 ∙∙∙∙∙∙∙   C8/T1 ∙∙∙∙∙∙∙

Sensory data reference: Ferrante MA. Wilbourn AJ. The utility of various sensory nerve conduction responses in assessing brachial plexopathies. Muscle&Nerve. 1995;18:879-89.

Muscles, Root Levels, and Innervation, Organized by Nerve

Muscle/Arm	Root†	Nerve	Comments
Sternocleidomastoid*	CN XI, C2–C3	CN XI	
Trapezius*	CN XI, C3–C4	CN XI	
Diaphragm*	C3, <u>C4</u>, C5	Phrenic	
Serratus anterior*	C5, C6, C7	Long thoracic	
Levator scapulae*	C3, <u>C4</u>, C5	Dorsal scapular	
Rhomboideus major*	C5	Dorsal scapular	
Rhomboideus minor*	C5	Dorsal scapular	
Supraspinatus*	<u>C5</u>, C6	Suprascapular	
Infraspinatus*	<u>C5</u>, C6	Suprascapular	
Pectoralis major (clavicular)*	C5–C7	Lateral pectoral	
Pectoralis major (sternal)*	C8–T1	Medial pectoral	
Pectoralis minor*	C8–T1	Medial pectoral	
Subscapularis	C5–C7	Upper/lower subscapularis	
Teres major*	<u>C5</u>–C6	Lower subscapularis	
Latissimus dorsi*	C6, <u>C7</u>, C8	Thoracodorsal	
Teres minor*	<u>C5</u>–C6	Axillary	
Deltoid*	<u>C5</u>–C6	Axillary	Nerve runs from posterior to anterior
Triceps long*, lateral*, medial	<u>C7</u>–C8	Radial	Medial head is lowest of three muscles before they enter spinal groove, first muscle after they leave spinal groove
Anconeus*	<u>C7</u>–C8	Radial	Last muscle before nerve enters spinal groove
Brachioradialis*	C5–C6	Radial	Last muscle before nerve exits spinal groove
Extensor carpi radialis longus*	<u>C6</u>–C7	Radial	
Extensor carpi radialis brevis*	<u>C6</u>–C7	Radial	
Supinator*	C5–<u>C6</u>	Posterior interosseus	
Extensor carpi ulnaris*	C7–<u>C8</u>	Posterior interosseus	
Extensor digitorum communis*	<u>C7</u>–C8	Posterior interosseus	First muscle innervated by posterior interosseus nerve after it leaves the supinator
Extensor digiti minimi	C7–C8	Posterior interosseus	
Abudctor pollicis longus*	C7–<u>C8</u>	Posterior interosseus	
Extensor pollicic longus*	C7–<u>C8</u>	Posterior interosseus	
Extensor pollicis brevis*	C7–<u>C8</u>	Posterior interosseus	
Extensor indicis*	C7–<u>C8</u>	Posterior interosseus	Last radial-innervated muscle
Coracobrachialis	C6–C7	Musculocutaneous	
Biceps brachii*	C5–C6	Musculocutaneous	
Brachialis*	C5–C6	Musculocutaneous	
Pronator teres*	C6–C7	Median	
Flexor carpi radialis*	C6–<u>C7</u>	Median	First muscle innervated after nerve leaves pronator
Palmaris longus	C7–T1	Median	
Flexor digitorum superficialis* (splits to form anterior interosseus n.)	<u>C7</u>–<u>C8</u>–T1	Median	

Table continued on following page

Muscles, Root Levels, and Innervation, Organized by Nerve *(Continued)*

Muscle/Arm	Root†	Nerve	Comments
Flexor pollicis brevis (superficial head)	C8–T1	Median	Do not stick since one-half innervated by ulnar nerve
Abductor pollicis brevis*	C8–T1	Median	Check abductor pollicis brevis or opponens for distal median-innervated muscle
Opponens pollicis*	C8–<u>T1</u>	Median	
Lumbricals 1–2	C8–T1	Median	
Flexor digitorum profundus 1–2	C7–C8	Anterior interosseus	
Flexor pollicis longus*	C7–<u>C8</u>	Anterior interosseus	
Pronator quadratus*	C7–<u>C8</u>–T1	Anterior interosseus	
Flexor carpi ulnaris*	<u>C8</u>–T1	Ulnar	Can come before or after cubital tunnel
Flexor digitorum profundus 3–4*	<u>C8</u>–T1	Ulnar	Always after cubital tunnel
Abductor digiti minimi (quinti hand)*	C8–T1	Ulnar	
Opponens digiti minimi	C8–T1	Ulnar	
Flexor digiti minimi	C8–T1	Ulnar	
Volar interossei	C8–T1	Ulnar	
Dorsal interossei–first dorsal interosseus*	C8–T1	Ulnar	Last ulnar-innervated muscle
Lumbricals 3–4	C8–T1	Ulnar	
Flexor pollicis brevis (deep head)	C8–T1	Ulnar	
Abductor pollicis*	C8–T1	Ulnar	

Muscle/Leg	Root†	Nerve	Comments
Iliopsoas*	L2–L3	Femoral	
Pectineus	L2–L4	Femoral	
Sartorius	L2–L4	Femoral	
Rectus femoris*	L2–L3–L4	Femoral	
Vastus medialis*	L2–L3–L4	Femoral	
Vastus intermedius	L2–L4	Femoral	
Vastus lateralis*	L2–L3–L4	Femoral	
Obturator externus	L2–L5	Obturator	
Adductor longus and brevis*	L2–<u>L3–L4</u>	Obturator	
Gracilis*	L2–L4	Obturator	
Adductor magnus (one-half tibial sciatic)*	L2–<u>L3–L4</u>	Obturator	
Obturator internus	L4–S2	Sacral plexus	
Inferior gemelli	L4–S2	Sacral plexus	
Piriformis	L4–S2	Sacral plexus	
Gluteus medius*	L4–<u>L5</u>–S1	Superior gluteal	
Gluteus minimus	L5–S1	Superior gluteal	
Tensor fascia lata	L5–S1	Superior gluteal	
Gluteus maximus*	L5–<u>S1</u>–S2	Inferior gluteal	
Quadratus femoris	L4–S1	Sciatic, tibial division	
Semitendinosus (internal hamstring)*	L4–<u>L5</u>-S1–S2	Sciatic, tibial division	
Semimembranosus*	L4–<u>L5</u>–S1–S2	Sciatic, tibial division	
Biceps femoris long head*	L5–<u>S1</u>–S2	Sciatic, tibial division	External hamstrings/tibial

Table continued on following page

Muscles, Root Levels, and Innervation, Organized by Nerve *(Continued)*

Muscle/Leg	Root[†]	Nerve	Comments
Adductor magnus (one-half obturator)	L2–L4	Sciatic, tibial division	
Biceps femoris short head*	L5–<u>S1</u>–S2	Sciatic, peroneal division	External hamstrings/ peroneal
Tibialis posterior*	<u>L5</u>–S1	Tibial	
Popliteus	L5–S1	Tibial	
Soleus*	<u>S1</u>–S2	Tibial	
Gastrocnemius—medial*	L5–<u>S1</u>–S2	Tibial	
Gastrocnemius—lateral*	<u>S1</u>–S2	Tibial	
Flexor digitorum longus	L5–S1	Tibial	
Flexor hallucis longus	L5–S2	Tibial	
Flexor digitorum brevis	S1–S2	Medial plantar	
Flexor hallucis brevis	S1–S2	Medial plantar	
Abductor hallucis*	<u>S1</u>–S2	Medial plantar	Distal tibial muscle
Lumbrical 1	S1–S2	Medial plantar	
Abductor digiti minimi (pedis)*	S1–S2	Lateral plantar	
Abductor hallucis	S1–S2	Lateral plantar	
Flexor digiti minimi	S1–S2	Lateral plantar	
Interossei (first dorsal inter-osseus of foot)	S1–S2	Lateral plantar	Other distal tibial muscle
Quadratus plantae	S1–S2	Lateral plantar	
Lumbricals 2–4	S1–S2	Lateral plantar	
Peroneus longus*	<u>L5</u>–S1	Superficial peroneal	Use needle to look at superficial peroneal n.
Peroneus brevis	L5–S1	Superficial peroneal	
Tibialis anterior*	L4–<u>L5</u>	Deep peroneal	
Extensor digitorum longus*	<u>L5</u>–S1	Deep peroneal	
Extensor hallucis longus*	<u>L5</u>–S1	Deep peroneal	
Peroneus tertius	L5–S1	Deep peroneal	
Extensor digitorum brevis	L5–S1	Deep peroneal	Last deep peroneal muscle

For muscles with asterisk (*), root levels were taken from Geiringer SR: Anatomic Localization for Needle Electromyography, 2nd ed. Philadelphia, Hanley & Belfus, 1999.

For muscles without asterisk (*), root levels were taken from Kimura J: Electrodiagnosis in Disease of Nerve and Muscle: Principles and Practice, 2nd ed. Philadelphia, F.A. Davis, 1989.

[†] Underlined root levels indicate that the root level is believed to innervate the majority of muscle fibers in the muscle (according to Geiringer, above).

Upper Limb Nerves and Entrapment Sites

n.b. Entrapment sites in italics

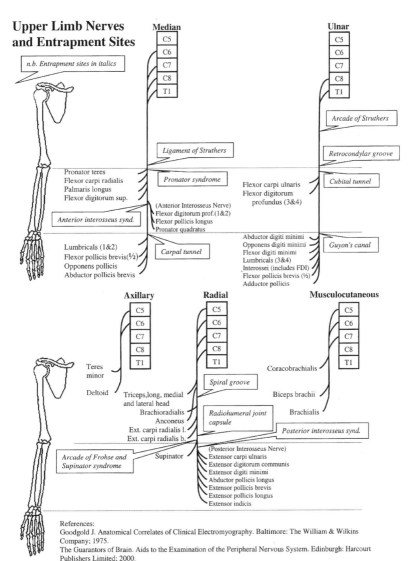

Median

C5
C6
C7
C8
T1

Ligament of Struthers

Pronator teres
Flexor carpi radialis
Palmaris longus
Flexor digitorum sup.

Pronator syndrome

Anterior interosseus synd.

(Anterior Interosseus Nerve)
Flexor digitorum prof.(1&2)
Flexor pollicis longus
Pronator quadratus

Lumbricals (1&2)
Flexor pollicis brevis(½)
Opponens pollicis
Abductor pollicis brevis

Carpal tunnel

Ulnar

C5
C6
C7
C8
T1

Arcade of Struthers

Retrocondylar groove

Flexor carpi ulnaris
Flexor digitorum
profundus (3&4)

Cubital tunnel

Abductor digiti minimi
Opponens digiti minimi
Flexor digiti minimi
Lumbricals (3&4)
Interossei (includes FDI)
Flexor pollicis brevis (½)
Adductor pollicis

Guyon's canal

Axillary

C5
C6
C7
C8
T1

Teres minor

Deltoid

Radial

C5
C6
C7
C8
T1

Spiral groove

Triceps,long, medial
and lateral head
Brachioradialis
Anconeus
Ext. carpi radialis l.
Ext. carpi radialis b.

*Radiohumeral joint
capsule*

*Arcade of Frohse and
Supinator syndrome*

Supinator

Posterior interosseus synd.

(Posterior Interosseus Nerve)
Extensor carpi ulnaris
Extensor digitorum communis
Extensor digiti minimi
Abductor pollicis longus
Extensor pollicis brevis
Extensor pollicis longus
Extensor indicis

Musculocutaneous

C5
C6
C7
C8
T1

Coracobrachialis

Biceps brachii

Brachialis

References:
Goodgold J. Anatomical Correlates of Clinical Electromyography. Baltimore: The William & Wilkins Company; 1975.
The Guarantors of Brain. Aids to the Examination of the Peripheral Nervous System. Edinburgh: Harcourt Publishers Limited; 2000.
Wertsch JJ, Oswald TA, Kincaid JC. Ulnar Techniques: An AAEM workshop. AAEM; September 1994.

Lower Limb Nerves and Entrapment Sites

n.b. Entrapment sites in italics

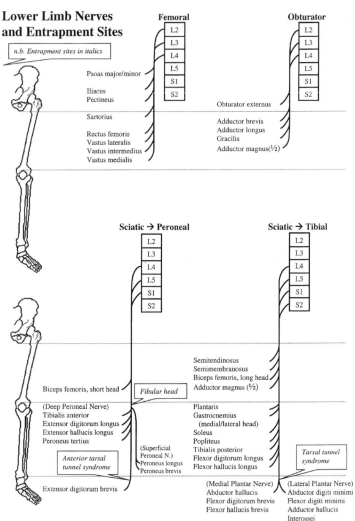

Femoral

L2
L3
L4
L5
S1
S2

Psoas major/minor

Iliacus
Pectineus

Sartorius

Rectus femoris
Vastus lateralis
Vastus intermedius
Vastus medialis

Obturator

L2
L3
L4
L5
S1
S2

Obturator externus

Adductor brevis
Adductor longus
Gracilis
Adductor magnus(½)

Sciatic → Peroneal

L2
L3
L4
L5
S1
S2

Biceps femoris, short head *Fibular head*

(Deep Peroneal Nerve)
Tibialis anterior
Extensor digitorum longus
Extensor hallucis longus
Peroneus tertius

Anterior tarsal tunnel syndrome

(Superficial Peroneal N.)
Peroneus longus
Peroneus brevis

Extensor digitorum brevis

Sciatic → Tibial

L2
L3
L4
L5
S1
S2

Semitendinosus
Semimembranosus
Biceps femoris, long head
Adductor magnus (½)

Plantaris
Gastrocnemius
   (medial/lateral head)
Soleus
Popliteus
Tibialis posterior
Flexor digitorum longus
Flexor hallucis longus

Tarsal tunnel syndrome

(Medial Plantar Nerve)
Abductor hallucis
Flexor digitorum brevis
Flexor hallucis brevis

(Lateral Plantar Nerve)
Abductor digiti minimi
Flexor digiti minimi
Adductor hallucis
Interossei

References:
Goodgold J. Anatomical Correlates of Clinical Electromyography. Baltimore: The William & Wilkins Company; 1975.
The Guarantors of Brain. Aids to the Examination of the Peripheral Nervous System. Edinburgh: Harcourt Publishers Limited; 2000.

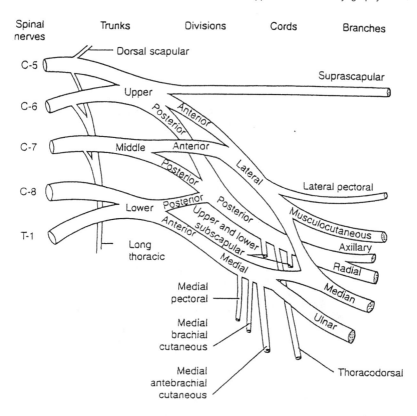

Diagram of the brachial plexus. The small nerve to the subclavius, from the upper trunk, is omitted. (From Jenkins DB (ed): Hollinshead's Functional Anatomy of the Limbs and Back, 7th ed. Philadelphia, W.B. Saunders, 1998, p 71, with permission.)

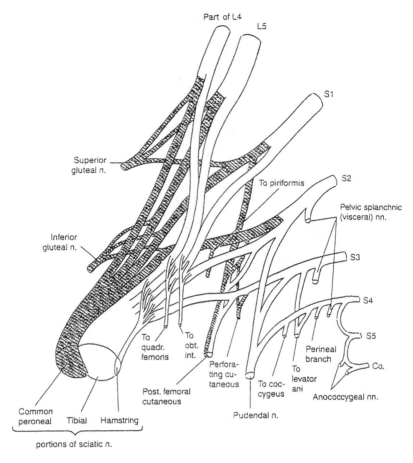

Diagram of the sacral plexus. The posterior parts of the plexus are shaded. (From Jenkins DB (ed): Hollinshead's Functional Anatomy of the Limbs and Back, 7th ed. Philadelphia, W.B. Saunders, 1998, p 272, with permission.)

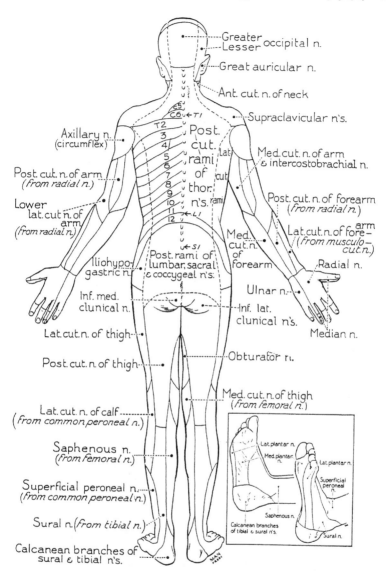

The cutaneous fields of peripheral nerves from the posterior aspect. The boundaries of cutaneous supply of the posterior primary rami are indicated by broken lines. The designation, *Post. cut. rami of thor. n's.*, refers to the cutaneous branches of the posterior primary rami; *Lat. cut. rami* indicates the distribution from the lateral branches of the anterior primary rami. For purposes of orientation, the spinous processes of the first thoracic (T1), the first lumbar (L1), and the first sacral (S1) vertebrae are indicated by arrows. (From Haymaker S, Woodhall B: Peripheral Nerve Injuries: Principles of Diagnosis, 2nd ed. Philadelphia, W.B. Saunders, 1953, p 40, with permission.)

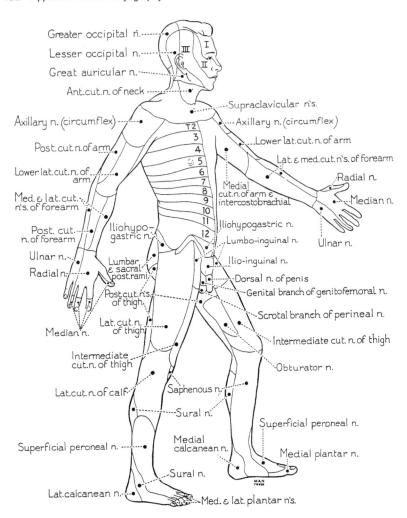

Side view of the cutaneous fields of peripheral nerves. The face and anterior half of the head are innervated by the three divisions of the trigeminal: I, ophthalmic; II, maxillary; III, mandibular. The fields of the intercostal nerves are indicated by numerals. the unlabeled cutaneous field between the great and second toes is supplied by the deep peroneal nerve. (From Haymaker S, Woodhall B: Peripheral Nerve Injuries: Principles of Diagnosis, 2nd ed. Philadelphia, W.B. Saunders, 1953, p 40, with permission.)

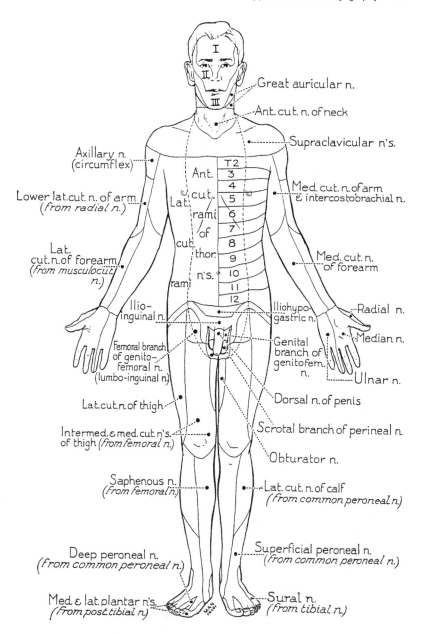

The cutaneous fields of peripheral nerves from the anterior aspect. the numbers on the left side of the trunk refer to the intercostal nerves. On the right side are shown the cutaneous fields of the lateral and medial branches of the anterior primary rami. The asterisk just beneath the scrotum is in the field of the posterior cutaneous nerve of the thigh. (From Haymaker S, Woodhall B: Peripheral Nerve Injuries: Principles of Diagnosis, 2nd ed. Philadelphia, W.B. Saunders, 1953, p 43, with permission.)

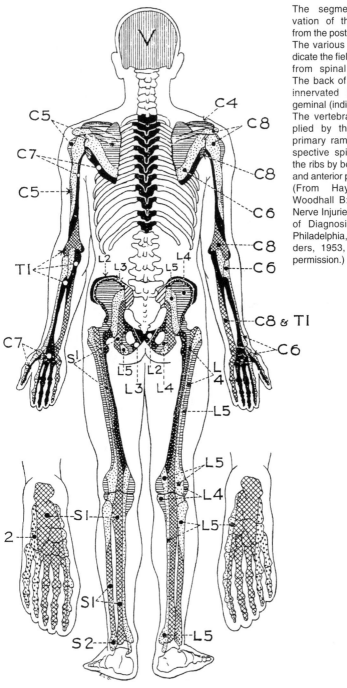

The segmental innervation of the skeleton from the posterior aspect. The various patterns indicate the fields of supply from spinal segments. The back of the skull is innervated by the trigeminal (indicated by V). The vertebrae are supplied by the posterior primary rami of the respective spinal nerves, the ribs by both posterior and anterior primary rami. (From Haymaker S, Woodhall B: Peripheral Nerve Injuries: Principles of Diagnosis, 2nd ed. Philadelphia, W.B. Saunders, 1953, p 48, with permission.)

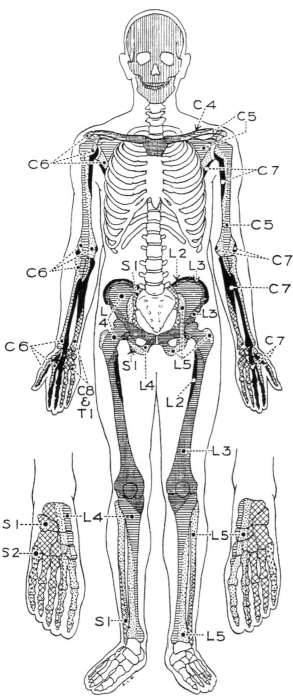

The innervation of the skeleton by spinal segments from the anterior aspect. The various sclerotomes are indicated by the different styles of shading. The insets show sclerotomes of the dorsal aspect of the feet. (From Haymaker S, Woodhall B: Peripheral Nerve Injuries: Principles of Diagnosis, 2nd ed. Philadelphia, W.B. Saunders, 1953, p 49, with permission.)

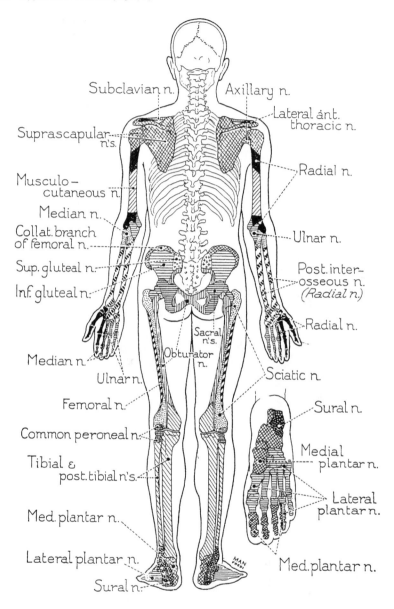

The peripheral nerve supply to the skeleton from the posterior aspect. The various fields are indicated by different patterns. (From Haymaker S, Woodhall B: Peripheral Nerve Injuries: Principles of Diagnosis, 2nd ed. Philadelphia, W.B. Saunders, 1953, p 50, with permission.)

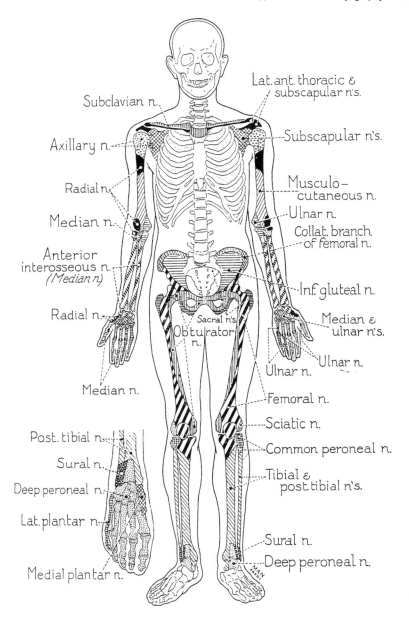

The peripheral nerve supply to the skeleton from the anterior aspect. The various peripheral nerve fields are indicated by different types of shading. (From Haymaker S, Woodhall B: Peripheral Nerve Injuries: Principles of Diagnosis, 2nd ed. Philadelphia, W.B. Saunders, 1953, p 51, with permission.)

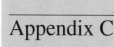

Appendix C

NUTRITION

Determining Energy Requirements Based on Weight and Activity

Estimated Maintenance Energy Requirements at Ideal Body Weight (IBW)

Activity Level	Kcal/lb IBW	Kcal/kg IBW
Basal metabolism	10	22
Sedentary, very light activity	13	29
Moderate, equivalent to 4 hours of walking/day	15	33
Strenuous, heavy manual labor, athletes in training	16–20	35–44

Estimated Maintenance Energy Requirements at Actual Body Weight (ABW)

Maintenance of excessive weight requires 4 kcal/lb excessive weight.

Maintenance enegy needs for ABW = maintenance energy needs at IBW + (excessive weight in lb × 4 kcal/lb)

Determining Daily Maintenance Fluid Requirements

Estimation: 100 ml/kg for the first 10 kg of body weight
50 ml for the second 10 kg of body weight
20 ml/kg for each kg of body weight over 20 kg

For every degree increase in body temperature above 38°C, approximately 10% more fluid above maintenance should be given unless otherwise contraindicated.

Determining Daily Protein Requirements

General requirements: 1.25–15.gm/lg	Dialysis: 1.0–1.5 gm/kg
Uremia (not dialyzed): 0.8 gm/kg	Hepatic encephalopathy: 0.5 gm/kg
Burns: 2.0–2.5 gm/kg	

Nitrogen Balance

Nitrogen balance = (total protein intake in gm/6.25) – (UUN + 4 gm), where UUN = urinary urine nitrogen in gm/24 hr.

0 = normal health
Negative = continuing deficit
Positive = growth and repair

4 = factor for skin and gastrointestinal nitrogen loss.

Calculations are not accurate in patients with burns, draining wounds, fistulas, or renal failure.

Basic Principles of Enteral Feeding

Gastric feeding: start at full strength at 30 ml/hr; advance 20 ml/hr every 8 hr to goal; check residual volumes every 4 hr; hold feedings 1 hr if residuals > 150 ml.

Jejunostomy feeding: start with full strength at 20 ml/hr; advance 20 ml/hr every 8 hr to goal; follow clinically to assess feeding; no need to check residuals.

Bolus feeding: start with full strength at 120 ml every 4 hr; advance 60 ml every 2–3 boluses to goal.

From University of Michigan Diet Manual.

Food and Nutrition Services Adult Enteral Formulary

	Non-stressed	Moderate Protein	Fiber Formula	High Protein	1.5 Kcal/ml Moderate Protein	2 Kcal/ml Moderate Protein	Renal Low Protein	Renal Moderate Protein	High Protein CAPD	Chemically Defined	Encephalopathy Formula
Trade name	Isocal	Isocal HN	Ultracal	Replete	Nutren 1.5	Deliver 2.0	Suplena	Magnacal Renal	Isotein HN	Pro-peptide	Nutrihep
Description	Isotonic tube feeding formula	Isotonic tube feeding formula	Isotonic tube feeding formula with fiber	Stress/trauma tube feeding-oral supplement	High-calorie, moderate-osmolality tube feeding	Hypertonic concentrated oral and tube feeding	Renal disease oral supplement-tube feeding	Renal disease oral supplement tube feeding	Renal disease oral supplement tube feeding	Elemental tube feeding maldigestion or malabsorption	Hepatic disease branched chain amino acids (BCAAs)
Kcal/ml	1.06	1.06	1.06	1.0	1.5	2.0	2.0	2.0	1.2	1.0	1.5
Protein source mg/L	34 Soy protein, calcium and sodium caseinate	44 Soy protein, calcium and sodium caseinate	44 Calcium and sodium caseinate	62.5 Calcium potassium caseinate	60 Calcium potassium caseinate	75 Calcium and sodium caseinate	30 Sodium and calcium caseinate	75 Calcium and sodium caseinate	68 Delactosed lactalbumin	40 Hydrolyzed whey protein	40 L-amino acids, whey protein 50% BCAAs
Fat source gm/L	44 MCT oil Soy oil	45 MCT oil Soy oil	45 Canola oil MCT oil	34 Soy lecithin Canola oil MCT oil	67.6 MCT oil Canola oil Corn oil Soy lecithin	102 MCT oil Soy oil	95.6 High-oleic sunflower oil Soy oil	101 Canola oil High-oleic sunflower oil MCT oil Corn oil	34 Partially hydrogenated soybean oil MCT oil	39.2 MCT oil Sunflower oil	21.2 MCT oil Canola oil Lecithin Corn oil
Carbohydrate source gm/L	135 Maltodextrin	123 Maltodextrin	123 Maltodextrin	113 Maltodextrin Corn syrup	42 Maltodextrin	200 Corn syrup	255.2 Maltodextrin Sucrose	200 Maltodextrin Sugar	158 Maltodextrin Fructose	127.2 Maltodextrin Starch	290 Maltodextrin Modified corn starch

Table continued on following page

Food and Nutrition Services Adult Enteral Formulary *(Continued)*

	Non-stressed	Moderate Protein	Fiber Formula	High Protein	1.5 Kcal/ml Moderate Protein	2 Kcal/ml Moderate Protein	Renal Low Protein	Renal Moderate Protein	High Protein CAPD	Chemically Defined	Encephalopathy Formula
Sodium mg (mEq/L)	530 (23)	930 (40)	930 (40)	876 (38.1)	1170 (50.8)	800 (35)	790 (34)	800 (35)	620 (27)	500 (21.7)	320 (13.9)
Potassium mg (mEq/L)	1320 (34)	1610 (41)	1610 (41)	1560 (40)	1872 (48)	1700 (43)	1120 (28.6)	1270 (33)	1074 (28)	1252 (32.1)	1320 (33.8)
Nonprotein kcal/gm nitrogen	168:1	125:1	128:1	75:1	131:1	144:1	393:1	144:1	86:1	131:1	209:1
Volume to meet 100% RDA (ml)	1890	1180	1180	1500	1000	1000	947	1000	1770	1500	1000
mOsm/kg water	300	270	310	300	430	640	600	570	300	270	690
Free water (ml/L)	840	840	850	840	780	710	713	710	854	880	760
Phosphorus (mg/L)	530	850	850	1000	1000	1000	730	800	566	700	1000
Comments	Lactose-free gastric and small bowel feeding	Lactose-free gastric and small bowel feeding	Lactose-free gastric and small bowel feeding, 14.4 gm/L dietary fiber	Lactose-free oral, gastric, and small bowel feeding	Unflavored Lactose-free Gluten-free	Lactose-free oral or gastric feeding	Lactose-free oral supplement Gastric feeding Low protein Low electro-lyte	Lactose-free oral supplement Gastric feeding for dialysis patients	Lactose-free oral supplement Gastric and small bowel feeding for patients on CAPD	Lactose-free isotonic peptide-based elemental formula	Lactose-free Not palatable

CAPD = continuous ambulatory peritoneal dialysis.

Premixed Oral Supplements

	Carnation Instant Breakfast 8 oz–240 ml	Resource per 6 oz–180 ml
Description	Low-fat oral supplement (vanilla/chocolate)	Clear liquid oral supplement
Kcal	228 with 2% milk	190
Protein gm	11	6
Carbohydrate gm	35	41.5
Fat gm	4 with 2% milk	0
Sodium mg	197	100
Potassium mg	568	50
Comments	Contains lactose	Lactose-free

Pediatric Oral and Tube Feeding Formulas and Canned Oral Supplements

	PediaSure	PediaSure with Fiber	Boost	Boost Plus
Description	Pediatric oral supplement tube feeding	Pediatric oral supplement tube feeding	Oral food supplement 1.0 k/cal/ml	Oral food supplement 1.5 kcal/ml
Kcal/ml	1	1	1.06	1.5
Protein source gm/L	30 Whey protein and sodium caseinate	30 Whey protein and sodium caseinate	43 Milk protein concentrate	60 Sodium and calcium caseinate
Fat source gm/L	50 Soy oil Safflower oil, fractionated	50 Soy Oil Safflower oil, fractionated	18 Corn oil Canola oil Sunflower oil	57 Corn oil
Carbohydrate source gm/L	110 Hydrolyzed corn starch Sucrose	110 Hydrolyzed corn starch Sucrose	170 Corn syrup Sucrose	188 Corn syrup
Sodium mg/L (mEq)	380 (16.5)	380 (16.5)	541 (24)	833 (36)
Potassium mg/L (mEq)	1310 (33.5)	1310 (33.5)	1667 (43)	1458 (37)
Nonprotein kcal/gm nitrogen	185:1	185:1	125:1	134:1
Volume to meet 100% RDA (ml)	1000 (ages 1–6) 1300 (ages 7–10)	1000 (ages 1–6) 1300 (ages 7–10)	1200	1180
mOsm/kg water	365	365	610	670
Free water ml/L	840	840	833	770
Comments	Lactose-free Gluten-free	Lactose-free Gluten-free Dietary fiber 5 gm/L	Lactose-free Oral or gastric feeding	Lactose-free Oral or gastric feeding

Food and Nutrition Services Infant Formulas

	Enfamil 20*	Similac 20*	Prosobee 20	Isomil 20	Pregestimil	Nutramigen	Neocate	Portagen	Enfamil 24 Premature	Similac Special Care†	Neosure 22 kcal/oz
Description	Milk-based infant formula	Milk-based infant formula	Soy protein infant formula	Soy protein infant formula	Protein hydrolysate formula	Protein hydrolysate formula	Elemental	For use in fat malabsorption	For low-birth-weight infants	For growing, low-birth-weight infants	Prematurity
Kcal/ml	0.67	0.67	0.67	0.67	0.67	0.67	0.67	0.67	0.8	0.8	0.73
Protein source gm/L	14 Reduced mineral whey and nonfat milk taurine	14 Nonfat milk Whey Protein concentrate	20 Soy protein isolate L-methionine Taurine L-carnitine	16.3 Soy protein isolate Methionine	19 Casein hydrolysate L-cystine L-tyrosine L-tryptophan Taurine L-carnitine	19 Casein hydrolysate L-cystine L-tyrosine L-tryptophan	20.6 (protein equivalent) Aminos acids	23.3 Sodium caseinate Taurine L-carnitine	24 Whey Nonfat milk Taurine L-carnitine	22 Nonfat milk Whey Protein concentrate	19 Nonfat milk Whey Protein concentrate
Fat source gm/L	35.3 Palm, soy, coconut, sunflower oils	36 Soy, coconut oils, High oleic	35 Palm, soy, coconut, sunflower oils	37 Soy, coconut oils	38 MCT, safflower oil, soy oil	33 Palm, soy, coconut, sunflower oils	30 Safflower, coconut, soy, MCT oils	32 MCT oil, corn oil	40.4 MCT oil, soy oil	44 MCT oil, soy oil, coconut oil	40.1 Soy, safflower, MCT, coconut oils
Carbohydrate source gm/L	73 Lactose	72 Lactose	67 Corn syrup solids	69 Corn syrup and sucrose	69 Corn syrup solids Glucose Modified corn starch	73 Corn syrup solids Modified corn starch	78 Corn syrup	77 Corn syrup solids Sucrose	88 Corn syrup solids Lactose	85 Lactose Hydrolyzed corn starch	75 Corn syrup Lactose
Sodium mg/L (mEq)	180 (8)	160 (7)	240 (10.4)	293 (12.7)	260 (11.3)	313 (13.6)	248.6 (10.8)	367 (16)	310 (13.4)	347 (15)	241 (10.4)
Potassium mg/ml (mEq)	720 (18.4)	700 (18)	800 (20.5)	720 (18.4)	727 (18.6)	733 (19)	1034 (25.5)	833 (21.3)	817 (20.9)	1040 (27)	1036 (26.5)

Table continued on following page

Food and Nutrition Services Infant Formulas *(Continued)*

	Enfamil 20*	Similac 20*	Prosobee 20	Isomil 20	Pregestimil	Nutramigen	Neocate	Portagen	Enfamil 24 Premature	Similac Special Care†	Neosure 22 kcal/oz
mOsm/kg water	300	300	200	230	320	320	342	230	310	280	290
Free water ml/L	910	899	910	899	910	910	875 gm/L	910	880	879 gm/L	896 gm/L
Comments	Contains lactose	Contains lactose	Lactose-free	Lactose-free	Lactose-free	Lactose-free	Lactose-free	Lactose-free	Lactose-free	Contains lactose	Contains lactose

* Also stocked in 24 kcal/oz. Ready to feed with or without iron.
† Similac Special Care is stocked only in 24 kcal/oz without iron.
Note: This list is not all-inclusive; additional formulas are available.
Chart adapted from the University of Michigan Food and Nutrition Services.

Pediatric Elemental Formula

	Peptamen Jr.	L-Emental
Description	Elemental tube feeding	Elemental tube feeding
Kcal/ml	1	0.8
Protein source gm/L	30 Hydrolyzed whey	24 Free amino acids
Fat source gm/L	MCT oil, soybean, canola oil, soy	MCT oil
Carbohydrate source gm/L	137.5 Maltodextrin, corn starch	130 Maltodextrin, modified starch
Sodium mg/L (mEq)	460 (20)	400 (17)
Potassium mg/L (mEq)	1320 (33.8)	1200 (31)
Volume to meet 100% RDA (ml)	1000	1000 (1–6 yr) 1170 (7–10 yr)
mOsm/kg water	260	360
Free water ml/L	850	893
Comments	Unflavored liquid, 1–10 yr	Powder

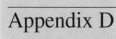

Appendix D

PEDIATRIC REHABILITATION

Growth from Birth to Maturity

Head Circumference		Weight	
Birth	35 cm	Birth (full-term)	3400 gm
4 months	41 cm	5 months	Double
12 months	47 cm	12 months	Triple
Maturity	57 cm	Until adolescent growth spurt	2 kg annually

Height/Stature		Sitting Height		
			Girls	Boys
Birth	50 cm	Newborn	34 cm	35 cm
12 months	75 cm	5 years	61 cm	62 cm
4 years	100 cm	10 years	73 c m	74 cm
Early school age	5 cm/yr	18 years	88 cm	92 cm
Prepubescence/adolescence	5–8 cm/yr			

Physiologic Postural Reflex Responses*

Postural Reflex	Stimulus	Response	Age of Emergence	Clinical Significance
Head righting	Visual and vestibular	Align face/head vertical, mouth horizontal	Prone: 2 mo Supine: 3–4 mo	Delayed or absent in CNS immaturity or damage
Head and body righting	Tactile, vestibular proprioceptive	Align body parts in anatomic position relative to each other and gravity	4–6 mo	As above
Protective extension or parachute reactions	Displacement of center of gravity outside supporting base in sitting position	Extension/abduction of lateral extremity toward displacement to prevent falling	Sitting anterior: 5–7 mo Lateral: 6–8 mo Posterior: 7–8 mo Standing: 12–14 mo	As above
Equilibrium or tilting	Displacement of center of gravity	Adjustment of tone and posture of trunk to maintain balance	Sitting: 6–8 mo Standing: 12–14 mo	As above

* Emerge with central nervous system (CNS) maturation, present through life, modulated by volition, used in gross motor activities.
From Molnar GE, Alexander MA (eds): Pediatric Rehabilitation, 3rd ed. Philadelphia, Hanley & Belfus, 1999, with permission.

Reflex Development*

Reflex	Stimulus	Response	Age of Suppression	Clinical Significance
Moro	Sudden neck extension	Shoulder abduction, shoulder, elbow, and finger extension, followed by arm flexion adduction	4–6 mo	Persists in CNS pathology, static encephalopathy
Startle	Sudden noise, clapping	Same as Moro reflex	4–6 mo	Persists in CNS pathology, static encephalopathy
Rooting	Stroking lips or around mouth	Moving mouth, head toward stimulus in search of nipple	4 mo	Diminished in CNS pathology, but may persist
Positive supporting	Light pressure or weight-bearing on plantar surface	Legs extend for partial support of body weight	3–5 mo; replaced by volitional weight-bearing with support	Obligatory or hyperactive abnormal at any age, early sign of extremity spasticity, may be associated with scissoring
Asymmetric tonic neck	Head turning to one side	Extremities extend on face side, flex on occiput side	6–7 mo	Obligatory response abnormal at any age, persists in static encephalopathy
Symmetric tonic neck	Neck flexion Neck extension	Arms flex, legs extend, Arms extend, legs flex	6–7 mo	Same as asymmetric tonic neck
Palmar grasp	Touch or pressure on palm or stretching finger flexors	Flexion of all fingers, hand fisting	5–6 mo	Diminished in CNS suppression, absent in LMN paralysis; persists/hyperactive in spasticity
Plantar grasp	Pressure on sole distal to metatarsal heads	Flexion of all toes	12–14 mo when walking is achieved	Same as palmar grasp
Automatic neonatal walking	On vertical support plantar contact and passive tilting of body forward and side to side	Alternating automatic steps with support	3–4 mo	Variable activity in normal infants; absent in LMN paralysis
Placement or placing	Tactile contact on dorsum of foot or hand	Extremity flexion to place hand or foot over an obstacle	Before end of first year	Absent in LMN paralysis or with lower extremity spasticity
Neck righting or body derotational	Neck rotation in supine	Sequential body rotation from shoulder to pelvis toward direction of face	4 mo; replaced by volitional rolling	Nonsequential leg rolling suggests increased tone
Tonic labyrinthine	Head position in space, strongest at 45° from horizontal		4–6 mo	Hyperactivity/obligatory abnormal at any age; persists in CNS damage/static encephalopathy
	Supine Prone	Predominant extensor tone Predominant flexor tone		

* Primitive reflexes: present at birth, suppressed at certain ages in normal development.
CNS = central nervous system, LMN = lower motor neuron.
From Molnar GE, Alexander MA (eds): Pediatric Rehabilitation, 3rd ed. Philadelphia, Hanley & Belfus, 1999, with permission.

AGE MOS.	GROSS MOTOR	FINE MOTOR	SELF-HELP	PROBLEM SOLVING	SOCIAL EMOTIONAL	RECEPTIVE LANGUAGE	EXPRESSIVE LANGUAGE
1	Chin up in prone	Hands fisted near face		Fixes on ring / Follows face	Discriminates mother voice / Cries out of distress	Alerts to voice / sound	Throaty noises
2	Chest up in prone / Head bobs when held in sitting	Hands unfisted 50% / Retains rattle if placed in hand / Holds hands together		Visual threat present / Follows ring / Recognizes mother	Reciprocal smiling - responds to adult voice & smile		Coos / Social smile (6 wks) / Vowel like noises
3	Props on forearms in prone / Suspended in prone-head above body	Hands unfisted 50% / Inspects fingers / Bats at objects		Reaches for face / Follows ring in circle (in supine) / Regards cube	Expression of disgust (sour taste, loud sound) / Understands relationship between speaker and voice	Regards speaker	Chuckles / Vocalizes when talked to
4	Sit w/ trunk support / No head lag -pull to sit / Props on wrists / Rolls front to back	Clutches at clothes / Hands to mouth / Reaches persistently / Plays with rattle		Mouths objects / Aware of strange situation / Shakes rattle / Reaches for ring/rattle	Smiles spontaneously at pleasurable sight/sound / Stops crying at parent voice / To & fro alternating vocalizations	Orients to voice / Stops crying to soothing voice	Laughs out loud / Vocalizes when alone
5	Sits w/ pelvic support / Rolls back to front / Anterior protection - parachute	Palmar grasp/cube / Transfers object: hand-mouth-hand / Holds hands together / Attains dangling ring	Gums/mouth pureed food	Attains dangling ring / Turns head--look for dropped spoon / Regards pellet	Recognizes caregiver visually / Forms attachment relationship to caregiver	Orients: Bell I / Begins to respond to name	"Ah-goo" / Razz, squeal / Expresses anger other than crying
6	Sits momentarily propped on hands / Pivots in prone / Prone--bears weight on 1 hand	Transfers hand-hand / Rakes pellet / Takes second cube - holds on to 1*	Feeds self crackers / Places hands on bottle	Touches reflection and vocalizes / Removes cloth on face / Bangs & shakes toys	Stranger anxiety (familiar vs. unfamiliar - people)	Orients to Bell-II / Attends to music	Reduplicative babble w/ consonants / Listens then vocalizes when adult stops / Smiles/Vocalizes to mirror
7	Bounces when held / Sits w/o support-- Steady / Lateral protection	Radial-palmar grasp		Inspects ring / Observes cube in each hand / Finds partially hidden object			
8	Gets into sitting / Commando crawls / Pulls to sitting/kneeling	Bangs spoon w/ demo / Scissor grasp of pellet / Takes cube out of cup / Pulls large peg out	Holds own bottle / Finger feeds Cheerios or string beans	Seeks object after it falls silently to the floor	Lets parents know when happy vs. upset / Engages in gaze monitoring: adult looks away and child follows adult glance with own eyes	Responds to "come here" / Looks for family members "Where's mama?....etc"	"Dada" inappropriate / Echolalia (8-30 mos.) / Shakes head for no
9	Gets to 4-pt. / Begins creeping / Pulls to stand / Bear walks	Scissor grasp of pellet / Radial-digital grasp of cube / Bangs 2 cubes together	Bites, chews cookie	Inspects bell / Rings bell / Pulls string to obtain ring	Uses sounds to get attention / Follows a point "Oh look at.. / Recognizes familiar people visually	Enjoys gesture games / Orients to name well / Orients: Bell III	"Mama" inappropriate / Non-reduplicative babble / Imitates sounds
10	Creeps well / Cruises around furniture- 2 hands / Stands-1 hand held / Walks-2 hands held	Clumsy release of cube / Immature pincer grasp of pellet / Isolates index finger and pokes	Drinks from cup held for him	Uncovers toy under cloth / Pokes at pellet in bottle / Tries to put cube in cup, but may not be able to let go	Experiences fear / Looks preferentially when name is called	Enjoys Peek-A-Boo / Waves bye-bye back	"Dada" appropriate / Waves bye-bye
11	Walks--1 hand held / Pivots in sitting / Cruises - 1 hand / Stands few seconds	Throws objects / Stirs with spoon		Finds toy under cup / Looks at pictures in book	Gives objects to adult for action after demonstration (lets adult know he needs help)	Stops activity when told "no" / Bounces to music	1st word / Vocalizes to songs

AGE MOS.	GROSS MOTOR	FINE MOTOR	SELF-HELP	PROBLEM SOLVING	SOCIAL EMOTIONAL	RECEPTIVE LANGUAGE	EXPRESSIVE LANGUAGE
12	Stands well Posterior protection Independent steps	Marks after demo Fine pincer grasp of pellet Holds crayon Attempts tower of 2	Finger feeds part of meal Takes hat off	Rattles spoon in cup Lifts box lid to find toy	Shows objects to parent to share interest Proto-imperative pointing to indicate wants	1-step command w/ gesture Recognizes names of two objects-looks when named	Proto-imperative pointing to get desired object
13	Throws ball-sitting Walks w/ high guard	Attempts to release pellet in bottle	Drinks from cup w/ spilling	Dangles ring by string Solves glass frustration test Unwraps toy in cloth	Shows desire to please care giver Solitary play Functional play	Looks appropriately "Where's ball?"	3° word Immature jargoning - Inflection without real words
14	Stands w/o pulling up Falls by collapse Walks well	Imitates back-forth scribble Attains 3rd cube by combining 2 2 cube tower One round peg in & out	Removes socks/shoes Chews well Spoon to mouth – turns over	Dumps pellet out of bottle after demo	Proto-declarative pointing to indicate interest Purposeful exploration of toys through trial and error	1-step command without gesture	Names one object Proto-declarative pointing
15	Stoops to pick up toy Creeps up stairs Runs stiff-legged Walks carrying toy Climbs on furniture	3-4 cube tower Place 10 cubes in cup Releases pellet into bottle	Uses spoon–some spill Attempts to brush own hair Fusses to be changed	Turns pages in book Places circle in single shape puzzle	Shows empathy (someone else cries child looks sad) Hugs adult in reciprocation Hands toy to adult if can't operate (no demo - see 11 month above)	Points to 1 body part Points to 1 object of 3 Gets object from another room upon demand	3-5 words Mature jargoning w/ real words
16	Stands on 1 foot w/slight support Walks backwards Walks up stairs - 1 hand held	All round pegs in with urging Scribbles spontaneously	Picks up & drinks from cup Fetches & carries objects (same room)	Dumps pellet out w/o demo Places circle in form board Finds toy under layered Covers	Kisses by touching lips to skin Periodically visually relocates caregiver Self-conscience, embarrassed when aware of people observing them	Understands simple commands "Bring to mommy" Points to 1 picture	5-10 words
18	Creeps down stairs Runs well Seats self in small chair Throws ball—standing	4 cube tower Crudely imitates vertical stroke	Removes garment Gets onto adult chair unaided Moves about house without adult	Matches pairs of objects Circle reversed after searching	Passes CHAT Engages in pretend play (e.g. tea party, birthday party - with other people) Begins to show shame (when does wrong) & possessiveness	Points to 2 of 3 objects Body parts: 3 Points to self Understands "mine"	10-25 words Giant words (all gone, stop that) Imitates environmental sounds Names one picture on demand
20	Squats in play Carries large object Up stairs holding onto one hand	Completes round peg board w/o urging 5-6 cube tower Completes square peg board	Places only edibles in mouth Feeds self w/spoon entire meal	Deduces location of hidden object Places square	Begins to have thoughts about feelings Engages in tea party with stuffed animals Kisses with pucker	Points to pictures: 3 Begins to understand her / him / me	Holophrases ("Mommy?" and points keys "These are Mommy's keys") 2-word combinations Answers requests w/ "no"
22	Up stairs with rail, marking time Kicks ball w/ demo Walks w/one foot on walking board	Closes box with lid Imitates vertical line Imitates circular scribble	Uses spoon well Drinks from cup well Unzips zippers Puts shoes on partway	Adapts to FB reversal within 4 trials Completes form board		Pictures: 4-5 Body parts 5-6 Clothing: 4 pieces	25-50 words Asks for more Adds 1-2 words/week

Charts on pp 469–471 from Children's Association for Maximum Potential. San Antonio, with permission.

Age	Gross Motor	Fine Motor / Adaptive	Self-Help	Cognitive	Social / Play	Receptive Language	Expressive Language
24	Down stairs with rail, marking time Jumps in place Kicks ball w/o demo Throws overhand	Train of cubes w/o stack Imitates single circle Imitates horizontal line	Opens door using knob Sucks through straw Takes off clothes w/o buttons Pulls off pants	Sorts objects Matches objects to pictures Shows use of familiar objs	Parallel play Begins to mask emotions for social etiquette	Follows 2-step command Understands me / you Points to 5-10 pictures	2 word sentence (N+V) Telegraphic speech 50 + words 50% intelligibility Refers to self by name Names 3 pictures
28	Jumps from bottom step—1 foot leading Walks on toes after demo Walks backward 10 ft	Strings beads awkwardly Unscrews jar lid	Holds self/ verbalizes toilet needs Pulls pants up with assistance	Matches shapes Matches colors		Understands "just one"	Repeats 2 digits Begins to use pronouns (I, me, you) Names 10-15 pictures
30	Up stairs with rail, alternating feet Jumps in place Stands w/ both feet on balance beam Walks w/ one foot on balance beam	8 cube tower Train of cubes with stack	Washes hands Puts things away Brush teeth w/assistance	Reverses form board spontaneously Points to small details in pictures	Pretend play - advanced	Follows 2 prepositions: "Put block in ... on box" Understands action words: "playing...washing...blowing"	Echolalia & jargoning gone Names objects by use Refers to self w/correct pronoun
33		9-10 cube tower 6 square pegs in pegboard Imitates cross	Toilet trained Puts on coat unassisted	Points to self in photos Points to body parts acc'd to function ("what do you hear with?")		Understands 3 prepositions Understands dirty, wet Points to objects by use: ride in ... put on feet. ... write with	Gives first & last name Counts to 3 Begins to use past tense
3yr	Balances 1 ft - 3 sec Upstairs, alternating feet, without rail Pedals tricycle Heel to toe walk Catches ball—arms stiff	Copies circle Cuts w/ scissors: side to side (awkwardly) Imitates bridge Strings small beads well	Independent eating Pours liquid from one container to another Puts on shoes w/o lace Spreads w/ knife Unbuttons	Adds 2 parts to DAP Understands long/short "big/small, more/less" ws own gender ws own age	Starts to share with/without prompt Fears imaginary things Imaginative play Uses words to describe what someone else is thinking (Mom thought I was asleep)	Points to parts of pictures (nose of cow, door of car) Understands long / short Names body parts w/ funct Understands negatives Groups objects (foods, toys)	200+ words 3 word sentences Uses pronouns correctly 75% intelligibility Uses plurals Names body parts by use
4yr	Balances 1 ft 4-8 sec Hops 1 ft 2-3 times Standing broad jump:1-2 ft Galops Throws ball overhand 10 ft Catches bounced ball (4½ yrs)	Copies square Imitates gate Ties single knot Cuts 5 inch circle Uses tongs to transfer	Goes to toilet alone Wipes after BM Washes lace / hands Brushes teeth alone Buttons Uses fork well	P = 4-6 parts Number concepts to 2 Simple analogies: • dad / boy: mother / ??? • ice / cold: fire / ??? • Ceiling / up: floor / ??? Points to 4 colors	Passes Sally & Anne test Deception – interested in "tricking" others, & concerned about being tricked by others Has a preferred friend Labels happiness, sadness, fear & anger in self Group play	Follows 3 step commands Points to 4 colors Understands action words- II (swims in water, cut with, is read, sit at, tells time..) Understands adjectives: busry, long, thin, pointed	Digits: 3 forward 300-1000 words Tells stories Counts to 4 Names 4 colors 100% intelligibility Uses "feeling" words
5yr	Down stairs, alternate feet, w/ rail Balances 1 ft >8 sec Hops 1 foot 15 feet Skips Running broad jump: 2-3 ft Walks backward heel-toe Jumps backward	Copies triangle Builds stairs from model Puts paper clip on paper Can use clothespins to transfer small objects	Spreads with knife Independent dressing Bathes independently	DAP = 8-10 parts Number concepts to 3 Identifies coins Standardized IQ test needed	Has a group of friends Apologizes for mistakes Responds verbally to good fortune of others	R & L on self (5-7 yrs) Points to different one in a series Understands "er" endings (batter, skater).	Digits: 4 forward Counts to 10 Colors: 4-6 Defines simple words 2000 words Knows telephone number Responds to why questions
6yr	Tandem walks	Builds stairs from memory Draws diamond Copies flag	Ties shoes Combs hair Looks both ways at street	DAP = 12-14 parts Number concepts to 10 Simple addition Understands seasons	Has best friend of same sex Plays board games	Reads at first grade level Use PPVT	Days of the week 10,000 words when enters first grade

WeeFIM® instrument

L E V E L S	7 Complete Independence (Timely, Safely) 6 Modified Independence (Device)	**No Assistance**
	Modified Dependence 5 Supervision (Subject = 100%) 4 Minimal Assist (Subject = 75%+) 3 Moderate Assist (Subject = 50%+) **Complete Dependence** 2 Maximal Assist (Subject =25%+) 1 Total Assist (Subject = less than 25%)	**Assistance**

ASSESSMENT   **GOAL**

Self-Care
1.   Eating
2.   Grooming
3.   Bathing
4.   Dressing - Upper
5.   Dressing - Lower
6.   Toileting
7.   Bladder
8.   Bowel
Self-Care Total   *Quotient*

Mobility
9.   Chair, Wheelchair
10.   Toilet
11.   Tub, Shower
12.   Walk/Wheelchair
13.   Stairs
Mobility Total   *Quotient*

W Walk
C wheelChair
L crawL
B comBination

Cognition
14.   Comprehension
15.   Expression
16.   Social Interaction
17.   Problem Solving
18.   Memory
Cognitive Total   *Quotient*

A Auditory
V Visual
B Both

V Vocal
N Nonvocal
B Both

WeeFIM Total   *Quotient*

NOTE: Leave no blanks. Enter 1 if patient not testable due to risk

Michigan Special Education – Varies State to State

SPECIAL EDUCATION ACRONYMS

AI	autistic impaired
DD	developmental disability
EI	emotionally impaired
EMI	educable mentally impaired
EP	epilepsy
HH	homebound and hospitalized
HI	hearing impaired
IE	independent evaluation
IEP	Individualized Education Program
IEPC	Individualized Education Planning Committee
ISD	intermediate school district
LD	learning disability
LEA	local educational agency
LRE	least restrictive environment
OT	occupational therapy
P&A	Michigan Protection and Adocacy Service
PAC	Parent Advisory Committee
POHI	physically or otherwise health impaired
PPI	pre-primary impaired
PT	physical therapy
SLI	speech and language impaired
SMI	severely mentally impaired
SSI	Supplemental Security Income
SXI	severely multiply impaired
TBI	traumatic brain injury
TC	teacher consultant
TMI	trainable mentally impaired
VI	visually impaired
504	Section 504 of the Rehabilitation Act of 1973 (federal)

FLOW CHART FOR REFERRAL TO PLACEMENT OR APPEAL

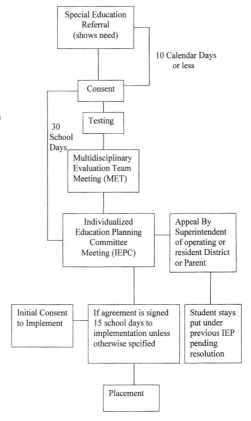

Children's Orientation and Amnesia Test (COAT)

General Orientation

1. What is your name? First (2) _____   (5) _____
    Last (3) _____

2. How old are you? (3) _____ When is your birthday?
    Month (1) _____ Day (1) _____   (5) _____

3. Where do you live? City (3) _____
    State (2) _____   (5) _____

4. What is your father's name? (5) _____
    What is your mother's name? (5) _____   (10) _____

5. What school do you go to? (3) _____
    What grade are you in? (2) _____   (5) _____

6. Where are you now (5) _____   (5) _____
    (Question may be rephrased: Are you at home now? Are you in
    the hospital? If rephrased, the child must correctly answer both
    questions to receive credit.)

7. Is it daytime or night-time? (5) _____   (5) _____

                 General Orientation Total   _____

Temporal Orientation (administer to children ages 8–15 years)

8. What time is it now? (5) _____   (5) _____
    (correct = 5; < hr off = 4; 1 hr off = 3; > 1 hr off = 2; 2 hr off = 1)

9. What day of the week is it? (5) _____   (5) _____
    (correct = 5; 1 off = 4; 2 off = 3; 3 off = 1; 4 off = 1)

10. What day of the month is it? (5) _____   (5) _____
    (correct = 5; 1 off = 4; 2 off = 3; 3 off = 2; 4 off = 1)

11. What is the month? (10) _____   (10) _____
    (correct = 10; 1 off = 7; 2 off = 3; 3 off = 1)

12. What is the year? (15) _____   (15) _____
    (correct = 15; 1 off = 10; 2 off = 5; 3 off = 1)

                 Temporal Orientation Total   _____

Memory

13. Say these numbers after me in the same order. (Discontinue when the child fails both
    series of digits at any length. Score 2 points if both digit series are correctly repeated.
    Score one point if only 1 is correct.)

3	5	35296	81493
58	42	539418	724856
643	926	3129365	4739128
7216	3279		

14. How many fingers am I holding up? Two fingers (2) _____   (10) _____
    Three fingers (3) _____ Ten fingers (5) _____

15. Who is on Sesame Street (10) _____   (10) _____
    (Other major television show may be substituted)

16. What is my name? (10) _____   (10) _____

                        Memory Total   _____

                        OVERALL TOTAL   _____

Normative Data for Children's Orientation and Amnesia Test

Age (yr)	Total Score		
	n	*Mean*	*Standard Deviation*
3	16	46.8	12.6
4	26	59.4	8.5
5	25	61.6	6.3
6	12	64.1	8.5
7	10	58.3	6.1
8	17	114.8	5.6
9	8	113.3	7.4
10	14	117.6	5.7
11	10	116.4	4.1
12–15	8	119.8	1.5

For ages 3–7 years the total score is based on the general orientation (questions 1–7) and memory (questions 13–16) items. The total score for children aged 8–15 is based on questions 1–16.

From Ewing-Cobbs L, Levin HS, Miner ME, Eisenberg HM: The Children's Orientation and Amnesia Test: Relationship to severity of acute head injury and to recovery of memory. Neurosurgery 27:683–691, 1990, with permission.

Appendix E

STROKE

Central Nervous System Ischemic Vascular Syndromes

Vessel	Major Structure Supplied	Major Clinical Findings (Syndromes)
Brachiocephalic trunk	Right side of head, arm	Lower blood pressure in ipsilateral arm, other findings as for ICA syndrome
Common carotid artery	Each side of head	Findings as for ICA syndrome; poorly conducted heart sound along ICA, absence of superficial temporal artery pulse
Internal carotid artery (ICA)	All structures of frontal, parietal, and temporal lobes, medial surfaces of both hemispheres	Contralateral hemiparesis, hemianesthesia, hemianopia, aphasia; global aphasia (DH) or denial or neglect (NDH)
Ophthalmic artery	Orbit, forehead, dura of anterior fossa	Ipsilateral monocular blindness or amaurosis fugax
Anterior choroidal artery	Medial aspects of cerebrum, superior border of frontal and parietal lobes	Weakness, clumsiness, and sensory loss affecting mainly distal contralateral leg
Small branches	Rostrum of corpus callosum, septum pellucidum, and lamina terminalis	Tactile anomia or ideomotor apraxia of limbs
Huebner's artery	Anterior limb of internal capsule, anterior portion of putamen, globus pallidum	Contralateral weakness of arm and face with or without rigidity or dystonia
Cortical branches	Major portion of medial aspects of hemisphere, paracentral lobe	Contralateral weakness and sensory loss in leg; if bilateral, behavior disturbances
Middle cerebral artery	Most of lateral surface of each hemisphere and deep structures of frontal and parietal lobe	Hemiplegia (face, arm, leg equally affected), hemianesthesia or hemianopia, aphasia (DH), hemineglect or dressing apraxia (NDH)
Upper division	Internal capsule (superior portion of anteroposterior limb), corona radiata, external capsule, putamen, caudate nuclei (body)	Hemiplegia (face, arm more affected than leg), hemianesthesia or hemianopia, Broca's aphasia (DH) or spatial disorientation
Lower division	Lateral surface of cerebral hemisphere at insula of lateral sulcus	Hemianopia or pure Wernicke's aphasia (DH) or other intellectual deficits (NDH)
Penetrating cortical branches	Anterior limb of internal capsule, basal ganglia	Pure contralateral hemiplegia or hemiparesis
	Temporal, parietal or frontal opercular surface of hemisphere	Monoparesis, discriminative and proprioceptive sensory loss, quadrantanopia, Broca's aphasia or Gerstmann's syndrome (DH), other intellectual deficits (NDH)
Vertebral artery	Midbrain, pons, medulla, and cerebellum	Various combinations of signs: ataxia, diplopia, vertigo, bulbar syndrome, facial weakness

Table continued on following page

Central Nervous System Ischemic Vascular Syndromes *(Continued)*

Vessel	Major Structure Supplied	Major Clinical Findings (Syndromes)
Posteroinferior cerebellar artery	Lateral medulla, cerebellum (posteroinferior aspect), cranial nerves V, IX, and X, vestibular nuclei, solitary nucleus/tract	Wallenberg's syndrome (alternating hemianesthesia, pharyngeal and laryngeal paralysis, dysphagia, hoarseness, decreased gag reflex, gait and ipsilateral limb ataxia) or Derjine's syndrome
Anterior spinal artery	Caudal medulla (paramedian area), cranial nerve VII, solitary nucleus and tract, spinal cord (dorsolateral quadrants)	Radicular pain, loss of pain or temperature sensation, spastic weakness in legs with (cervical level) or without (below cervical level) focal atrophy and weakness of arms
Posterior spinal artery	Spinal cord (dorsal funiculus), dorsal gray horns	Loss of deep tendon reflexes and joint position sense, astereogenesis at level involved
Basilar artery	Pons, midbrain, cerebellum, occipital lobe, part of temporal lobe	Diplopia, coma, bilateral motor and sensory signs, cerebellar and cranial nerve signs
Short paramedian arteries	Medial basal pons (pontine nuclei, corticospinal fibers, medial lemniscus)	Paraparesis, quadriparesis, dysarthria, dysphagia, tongue hemiparesis and atrophy, gaze paralysis, cranial nerve VI palsy, contralateral hemiparesis; Milard-Gruber-Foville, Raymond-Cestan, Marie-Foix syndromes
Internal auditory artery	Auditory and facial cranial nerves	Vertigo, nausea, vomiting, nystagmus
Anteroinferior cerebellar artery	Lateral aspect of pons and anteroinferior cerebellum	Ipsilateral facial paralysis, taste loss on half of tongue, deafness or tinnitus, limb ataxia, contralateral sensory loss over body
Superior cerebellar artery	Lateral midbrain, superior surface of cerebellum	Ipsilateral cranial VI and VII palsy, gait and limb ataxia, cerebellar signs, contralateral hemiparesis
Posterior cerebellar artery	Entire occipital lobe, inferior and medial portion of temporal lobe	Hemianopia, quadrantanopia (macular vision spared), Gerstmann's syndrome, or cortical blindness
Small perforating arteries	Midbrain, posterior thalamus	Midbrain (Weber's, Benedict's) or thalamic (Dejerine-Roussy) syndromes
Pial spinal arteries	Nerve roots and spinal cord	Anterior or posterior spinal artery syndromes

DH = dominant hemisphere, NDH = nondominant hemisphere.
From Wiebers DO, Feigin VL, Brown RD: Handbook of Stroke. Philadelphia, LIppincott Williams & Wilkins, 1997, pp 342–344, with permission.

Symptoms of Unruptured Intracranial Aneurysms

Artery Affected and Most Common Location	Major Structure(s) Involved (Compressed)	Clinical Findings
Internal carotid artery (infraclinoid-intracavernous part)	Cranial nerves III, IV, V, VI and pituitary fossa	Ipsilateral total ophthalmoplegia with small, poorly reactive pupil often associated with cranial nerve IV, V, VI palsy, facial pain or paresthesias or partial sensory loss, hypopituitarism, pulsatile noise in head
Internal carotid artery (supraclinoid part)	Cranial nerves II, III, optic chiasm	Visual field defects associated with ipsilateral cranial nerve II palsy, decreased visual acuity, scotoma, optic atrophy or blindness; partial ophthalmoplegia due to cranial nerve III palsy
Middle cranial fossa, near petrous apex	Trigeminal ganglion, cranial nerves IV, V	Raeder's paratrigeminal syndrome (unilateral oculosympathetic paresis—miosis and ptosis—associated with ipsilateral head, facial, or retroorbital pain and cranial nerve IV and VI palsy)
Ophthalmic artery	Cranial nerve II, optic foramen, pituitary fossa	Ipsilateral painless loss of vision, optic nerve atrophy, x-ray enlargement of optic foramen, hypopituitarism]
Anterior cerebral artery (at junction with anterior communicating artery)	Olfactory tract, optic chiasm, frontal lobes	Ipsilateral anosmia, bitemporal hemianopia (may begin with lower bitemporal quadrants); large aneurysm can produce intellectual deficits
Middle cerebral artery (at level of lateral fissure)	Lateral surface of cerebral hemisphere, surface between frontal and temporal lobes	Ipsilateral pain in or behind eye and in low temple associated with contralateral focal motor seizures, hemiparesis, dysphasia (DH involvement), homonymous hemianopia or upper quadrantanopia
Posterior communicating artery (at junction with internal carotid artery)	Cranial nerves III, IV	Painful palsy of cranial nerve III (pain typically occurs above brow and radiates back to ear) with or without ipsilateral nerve VI palsy (cranial nerve III paresis usually incomplete)
Vertebral artery (on surface of medulla)	Cranial nerves IX, X, XI, XII	Ipsilateral Collet-Sicard, Villaret, Schmidt, Jackson, or Tapia syndromes and occasionally paralysis of cranial nerve VII
Basilar artery (upper border of pons)	Cranial nerve V	Ipsilateral facial pain with or without tic douloureux
Anteroinferior cerebellar artery	Cranial nerve VII and brainstem structures	Ipsilateral paralysis of all facial muscles, loss of taste, occasionally signs of hydrocephalus
Superior cerebellar artery (at vertebrobasilar junction)	Cranial nerve III and brainstem structures	Homolateral focal headache, occipital or posterior cervical location, associated with ipsilateral ptosis, divergent strabismus, horizontal-vertical diplopia, pupil dilation, ataxia
Posterior cerebral artery (proximal portion)	Midbrain structures	Focal ipsilateral headache (occipital or posterior cervical region), pseudobulbar signs, decreased level of consciousness

DH = dominant hemisphere.
From Wiebers DO, Feigin VL, Brown RD: Handbook of Stroke. Philadelphia, LIppincott Williams & Wilkins, 1997, pp 345–346, with permission.

National Institutes of Health Stroke Scale

Item	Points	Function
Level of consciousness	[ ] 0 points	Fully alert
	[ ] 1 point	Drowsiness, with consciousness slightly impaired
	[ ] 2 points	Stuporous when not stimulated; difficult to arouse
	[ ] 3 points	Comatose; unresponsive to all stimuli
Orientation		
Two questions	[ ] 0 points	Answers both questions correctly
	[ ] 1 point	Answers one question correctly
	[ ] 2 points	Answers both questions incorrectly or cannot answer
Two commands	[ ] 0 points	Follows both commands correctly
	[ ] 1 point	Follows one command correctly
	[ ] 2 points	Follows no command or cannot respond
Eye movements (gaze)	[ ] 0 points	Normal
	[ ] 1 point	Partial gaze problem in one or both eyes
	[ ] 2 points	Forced deviation or total paresis cannot be overcome
Visual fields	[ ] 0 points	Normal
	[ ] 1 point	Partial hemianopia
	[ ] 2 points	Complete hemianopia
	[ ] 3 points	Bilateral hemianopia
Facial motor activity	[ ] 0 points	Normal
	[ ] 1 point	Minor asymmetry, but good movement
	[ ] 2 points	Definite weakness with partial movement
	[ ] 3 points	Complete paralysis of half of face
Upper extremity motor		
Right	[ ] 0 points	Normal
	[ ] 1 point	Drift is present
	[ ] 2 points	Cannot resist gravity
	[ ] 3 points	No movement
Left	[ ] 0 points	Normal
	[ ] 1 point	Drift is present
	[ ] 2 points	Cannot resist gravity
	[ ] 3 points	No movement
Limb ataxia	[ ] 0 points	Absent
	[ ] 1 point	Present in upper or lower limb
	[ ] 2 points	Present in both upper and lower limbs
Sensory status	[ ] 0 points	Normal; no sensory loss
	[ ] 1 point	Mid-to-moderate loss to pin prick
	[ ] 2 points	Profound loss of sensation
Neglect	[ ] 0 points	None
	[ ] 1 point	Partial visual, tactile, or auditory
	[ ] 2 points	Severe neglect to more than one modality
Articulation	[ ] 0 points	Normal speech
	[ ] 1 point	Mild-to-moderate slurring present
	[ ] 2 points	Near unintelligible speech out of proportion to any present aphasia
Language	[ ] 0 points	Normal with no aphasia
	[ ] 1 point	Mild-to-moderate aphasia
	[ ] 2 points	Severe aphasia
	[ ] 3 points	Mute or global aphasia

Adapted from Goldstein LB, Bertels C, Davis JN: Interrater reliability of the stroke scale. Arch Neurol 46:660–662, 1989; and Brott T, et al: Measurements of acute cerebral infarction. Stroke 20:864–870, 1989.

Hunt and Hess Classification for Subarachnoid Hemorrhage

Grade	Clinical Presentation
1	Asymptomatic
2	Severe headache or nuchal rigidity; no neurologic deficit
3	Drowsy; minimal neurologic deficit
4	Stuporous; moderate-to-severe hemiparesis
5	Deep coma; decerebrate posturing

Adapted from Hunt WE, Hess RM: Surgical risk as related to time of intervention in the repair of intracranial aneurysms J Neurosurg 28:14–20, 1968.

Mini-Mental State Examination

Points	Domain
	Orientation
5	What is the (year) (season) (day) (month)?
5	Where are we (state) (country) (town) (hospital) (floor)?
	Registration
3	Name 3 unrelated objects. Allow one second to say each. Then ask the patient to repeat them after you have said them. Give one point for each correct answer. Repeat until he or she learns all three.
	Attention and calculation
5	Ask the patient to count backward from 100 by sevens. Give one point for each correct answer. Stop after five answers. Alternatively, spell the word "world" backward.
	Recall
3	Ask the patient to recall the three objects previously stated. Give one point for each correct answer.
	Language
9	Show the patient a wristwatch; ask the patient what it is. Repeat for a pencil. (2 points) Ask the patient to repeat the following: "No ifs, ands, or buts." (1 point) Ask the patient to follow a three-step command: "Take a paper in your right hand, fold it in half,and put it on the floor." (3 points) Ask the patient to read and obey the following sentence, which you have written on a piece of paper: "Close your eyes." (1 point) Ask the patient to write a sentence. (1 point) Ask the patient to copy a design. (1 point)

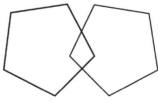

___/30 points

Adapted from Folstein MF, Folstein FE, McHugh PR: Mini-Mental State: A practical method of grading the cognitive state of patients for the clinician. J Psychol Rev 12:196–198, 1975.

Barthel Index

Activity	Score	Function
1. Feeding	[ ] 10 points	Independent; feeds self from tray or table; can put on assistive device if needed; accomplishes feeding in reasonable time.
	[ ] 5 points	Assistance needed with meal preparation.
	[ ] 0 points	Cannot meet criteria.
2. Moving (transfers)	[ ] 15 points	Independent in all phases of the activity.
	[ ] 10 points	Minimal help needed or patient needs to be reminded or supervised for safety of one or more parts of the activity.
	[ ] 5 points	Patient can come to a sitting position without the help of a second person but needs to be lifted out of bed and assisted with transfers.
	[ ] 0 points	Cannot meet criteria.
3. Personal toileting	[ ] 5 points	Can wash hands, face; combs hair, cleans teeth. Can shave (males) or apply makeup (females) without assistance; females need not be able to style hair.
	[ ] 0 points	Cannot meet criteria.
4. Getting on and off the toilet	[ ] 10 points	Able to get on and off the toilet, fastens/unfastens clothes, can use toilet paper without assistance. May use wall bar or other support if needed; if bedpan is necessary, patient can place it on chair, empty, and clean it.
	[ ] 5 points	Needs help because of imbalance or other problems with clothes or toilet paper.
	[ ] 0 points	Cannot meet criteria.
5. Bathing self	[ ] 5 points	May use bath tub, shower, or sponge bath. Patient must be able to all functions without another person being present.
	[ ] 0 points	Cannot meet criteria.
6. Walking on level surface	[ ] 15 points	Patient can walk at least 50 yards without assistance or supervision; may use braces, prostheses, crutches, canes, or walkers, but not a rolling walker. Must be able to lock/unlock braces, assume standing or seated position, get mechanical aids into position for use, and dispose of them when seated.
	[ ] 10 points	Assistance needed to perform above activities, but can walk 50 yards with little help.
	[ ] 0 points	Cannot meet criteria.
7. Propelling a wheelchair	*Do not score if patient gets a score for walking.*	
	[ ] 5 points	Patient cannot ambulate but can propel a wheelchair independently; can go around corners, turn around, and maneuver chair to table, bed, or toilet; must be able to push chair 50 yards.
	[ ] 0 points	Cannot meet criteria.
8. Ascending/ descending stairs	[ ] 10 points	Patient is able to go up and down a flight of stairs without supervision using canes, handrails, or crutches when needed and can carry these items as ascending or descending.
9. Dressing and undressing	[ ] 10 points	Patient is able to put on, fasten, and remove all clothing; ties shoelaces unless necessary adaptations are used. Activities include fastening braces and corsets when prescribed; suspenders, loafer shoes, and dresses opening in the front may be used when necessary.
	[ ] 5 points	Patient needs help putting on, fastening, or removing clothing; must accomplish at least half of the task alone within reasonable time; women need not be scored on use of brassiere or girdle unless prescribed.
	[ ] 0 points	Cannot meet criteria.

Table continued on following page

Barthel Index *(Continued)*

Activity	Score	Function
10. Continence of bowels	[ ] 10 points	Patient can control bowels and has no accidents. Can use a suppository or take an enema as necessary (as used in patients with spinal injury). device if needed; accomplishes feeding in reasonable time.
	[ ] 5 points	Patient needs in using a suppository or taking an enema or has occasional accidents.
	[ ] 0 points	Cannot meet criteria.
11. Control of bladder	[ ] 10 points	Patient is able to control bladder day and night. Patients with spinal injury must be able to put on external devices and leg bags independently, clean and empty bag, and must stay dry day and night.
	[ ] 5 points	Occasional accidents occur; patient cannot wait for bed pan, does not get to toilet in time, or needs help with external device.
	[ ] 0 points	Cannot meet criteria.

Full credit is not given for an activity if the patient needs even minimal help or supervision. A score of 0 is given when the patient cannot meet criteria as defined.
Adapted from Mahoney FL, Barthel DW: Functional evaluation: The Barthel Index. Md State Med J 14:61–65, 1965.

Modified Rankin Scale

Score	Description
0	No symptoms.
1	No significant disability despite symptoms; able to carry out all usual duties and activities.
2	Slight disability; unable to carry out all previous activities but able to look after own affairs without assistance.
3	Moderate disability requiring some help but able to walk without assistance.
4	Moderate severe disability; unable to walk without assistance and unable to attend to own bodily needs without assistance.
5	Severe disability; bedridden, incontinent, and requiring constant nursing care and attention.

Adapted from Rankin J: Cerebral vascular accidents in patients over the age of 60. II: Prognosis. Scott Med J 2:200–215, 1957.

	7 Complete Independence (Timely, Safely) 6 Modified Independence (Device)	NO HELPER
L **E** **V** **E** **L** **S**	Modified Dependence 5 Supervision 4 Minimal Assist (Subject = 75% +) 3 Moderate Assist (Subject = 50% +) Complete Dependence 2 Maximal Assist (Subject = 25% +) 1 Total Assist (Subject = 0% +)	HELPER

	ADMIT	DISCHG	FOL-UP
Self-Care			
A. Eating			
B. Grooming			
C. Bathing			
D. Dressing - Upper Body			
E. Dressing - Lower Body			
F. Toileting			
Sphincter Control			
G. Bladder Management			
H. Bowel Management			
Transfers			
I. Bed, Chair, Wheelchair			
J. Toilet			
K. Tub, Shower			
Locomotion	Walk / Wheelchair / Both	Walk / Wheelchair / Both	Walk / Wheelchair / Both
L. Walk/Wheelchair			
M. Stairs			
Motor Subtotal Score			
Communication	Auditory / Visual / Both	Auditory / Visual / Both	Auditory / Visual / Both
N. Comprehension			
O. Expression	Vocal / Non-vocal / Both	Vocal / Non-vocal / Both	Vocal / Non-vocal / Both
Social Cognition			
P. Social Interaction			
Q. Problem Solving			
R. Memory			
Cognitive Subtotal Score			
Total FIM			

NOTE: Leave no blanks; enter 1 if patient not testable due to risk

From Uniform Data System for Medical Rehabilitation: Guide for the Uniform Data Set for Medical Rehabilitation (Adult FIM), version 4.0. Buffalo, NY, State University of New York, 1993, with permission.

TRAUMATIC BRAIN INJURY

Glasgow Coma Scale (GCS)	
Domain	**Score**
Eyes	
Open spontaneously	4
Open to verbal command	3
Open to pain	2
No response	1
Best motor response	
Follows simple commands	6
To painful stimulus	
Localizes pain (pulls examiner's hand away)	5
Flexion–withdrawal (pulls limb away)	4
Flexion–abnormal (decorticate)	3
Extension (decerebrate)	2
No response	1
Best verbal response	
Oriented and converses	5
Disoriented and converses	4
Inappropriate words	3
Incomprehensible sounds	2
No response	1
GCS total	**3–15**

Galveston Orientation and Amnesia Test (GOAT)

No.	Question to Ask	Credit	Error Points
1A	What is your name?	For first and last name	2
1B	When were you born?	For entire date of birth	4
1C	Where do you live?	For correct city (address not needed)	4
2A	Where are you now?	For correct city	5
2B		For "hospital" (hospital name not needed)	5
3A	On what date were you admitted to this hospital?	For exact date	5
3B	How did you get here?	For correct mode of transportation	5
4	What is the first event you can remember *after* the injury? Can you describe in detail the first event you recall? (e.g., date, time, friends)	For no recall	10
		For description of plausible event after injury but no recall of detail	5
		For clear recall of emergency department or waking up in hospital with detail	0
5	Can you describe the last event you can recall before the injury? Can you describe in detail the last event before the injury? (e.g., date, time, friends)	(same as above)	
		For no recall	10
		For plausible, vague recall	5
		For recall of details	0
6	What time is it now?	Deduct 1 point for every half hour up to 5 points	5
7	What day of the week is it?	Deduct 1 point for every day removed up to 3	5
		Deduct 5 for inability to answer	
8	What day of the month is it?	Deduct 1 for every day removed up to 3	5
		Deduct 5 for inability to answer	
9	What month is it?	Deduct 5 for each month off up to 15	15
10	What is the year?	Deduct 10 for each year off up to 30	30

Add up deductions and subtract from 100 (100 − total error points = GOAT score).

Norms:
 Median = 95
 Below 65 = posttraumatic amnesia
 66–75 = borderline
General rule: Score > 75 for 2 consecutive days indicates that the patient is out of posttraumatic amnesia.

Adapted from Levin HS, O'Donnell VM, Grossman RG: The Galveston Orientation and Amnesia Test: A practical scale to assess cognition after head injury. J Nerve Ment Dis 167(11):675–684, 1979.

Rancho Los Amigos Scale for Level of Cognitive Functioning

Level	Response
I	No response. Patient does not respond to external stimuli and appears asleep.
II	Generalized response. Patient reacts to external stimuli in nonspecific, inconsistent, and nonpurposeful manner with stereotypic and limited responses.
III	Localized response. Patient responds specifically and consistently with delays to stimuli but may follow simple commands for motor action.
IV	Confused, agitated response. Patient exhibits bizarre, nonpurposeful, incoherent, or inappropriate behaviors; has no short-term recall; attention is short and nonselective.
V	Confused, inappropriate, nonagitated response. Patient gives random, fragmented, and nonpurposeful responses to complex or unstructured stimuli. Simple commands are followed consistently, memory and selective attention are impaired, and new information is not retained.
VI	Confused, appropriate response. Patient gives context-appropriate, goal-directed responses, dependent on external input for direction. There is carry-over for relearned, but not for new tasks, and recent memory problems persist.
VII	Automatic, appropriate response. Patient behaves appropriately in familiar settings; performs daily routines automatically, and shows carry-over for new learning at lower than normal rates. Patient initiates social interactions, but judgment remains impaired.
VIII	Purposeful, appropriate response. Patient is oriented and responds to the environment, but abstract reasoning abilities are decreased relative to premorbid levels.

Adapted from Hagen C, Malkmus D, Durham P: Levels of cognitive functioning. In Rehabilitation of the Head Injured Athlete: Comprehensive Physical Management. Downey, CA, Professional Staff Association of Rancho Los Amigos Hospital, 1979.

Consultation for Loss of Consciousness

1. Regular physical exam including neurologic exam covering mental status, cranial nerves, motor abilities, reflexes, sensory status, cerebellar functions, gait, and cognition.
2. Brief but sensitive mental status exam (supplementing Mini-Mental Status Exam) to address five areas:

1. Attention	Observe patient's attention	
	____ Count backward from 20	
	____ Say the months backward	
2. Language	Describe spontaneous speech	
	____ Speech is fluent	Nonfluent ____
	____ Names objects	
	____ Repeats sentences	
	____ Comprehends yes/no questions	
	____ Points to objects	
	____ Reads and writes a sentence	
	____ (?) Apraxia: show me how you brush your teeth, comb your hair	
3. Visuospatial	____ Line bisection	
	____ Copy geometric design	
	____ Draw clock	
4. Memory	____ Five-word recall and recognition	
	____ If able to do 3–5 words, try Hopkins Recall/Recognition Test	
	____ Digit span (more difficult)	
	____ Long-term recall: birthdates, recent public events	
5. Executive function	____ Name as many animals as possible in 1 minute (norm = 20)	
	____ Oral trail-making test (a-1, b-2, c-3, etc.)	
	____ Luria three-step test: alternate hand pattern and see if patient can mimic	

In summary and recommendations, comment on need for supervision, impulsivity, medications to avoid, and how to handle agitation without using sedating medications. Encourage team to treat pain appropriately because pain may contribute to agitation. Make recommendations for follow-up in your clinic or appropriate disposition options if TBI is more severe. Above all, *communicate with the primary team.*

Index

Entries in **boldface type** indicate complete chapters.

Pneumonia
  aspiration, in stroke patients, 151
  nosocomial, bed rest-related, 222
Poliomyelitis, heterotopic ossification associated
    with, 242
Polycarbophil (FiberCon), 266, 373
Polydactyly, 115
Polyethylene glycol (GoLytely), 267
Polymeric dressings, 291, 292, 293
Polyneuropathy, electrodiagnosis of, 438, 439
Polysporin, as pressure ulcer treatment, 288, 289
Ponstel. *See* Mefenamic acid
Pontine, upper, injuries to, 176
Pontine micturition center, 247
Pontocaine, 380
Popliteus muscle, innervation of, 446
Positioning, of burn patients, 25
Positive supporting reflex, 468
Positron emission tomography (PET), for traumatic
    brain injury evaluation, 172, 176
Postconcussive syndromes, 195–198
Postoperative pain, 207
Posttraumatic pain, 207
Posttraumatic stress disorder, 217
  in burn patients, 30, 32
  in traumatic brain injury patients, 178
Postural instability, Parkinson's disease-related, 74,
    75
Postural reflexes, physiologic, 467
Povidone-iodine preparations, 290
Pramipexole, as Parkinson's disease treatment, 77
Prazosin, as neurogenic bladder treatment, 254
Precocious puberty
  neural tube defects-related, 93
  traumatic brain injury-related, 101
Prednisolone, 381
Prednisone, as juvenile rheumatoid arthritis
    treatment, 108
Prehension grasp, 406
Prenatal diagnosis, of neural tube defects, 91
Pressure therapy, for burn-related scar prevention,
    27, 28, 29
Pressure ulcers. *See* Ulcers, pressure
Prilocaine, 380
Primitive reflexes, in cerebral palsy, 84
Proantheline, as neurogenic bladder treatment, 255
Problem-solving ability, development of, 469–471
Procaine, 380
Progressive supranuclear palsy, traumatic brain
    injury-related, 193
Promethazine, 372
Pronator quadratus muscle, innervation of, 445
Pronator teres muscle, innervation of, 444
Propionic acids, 365
Propoxyphene, pharmacokinetics of, 364
Propranolol, use in traumatic brain injury patients
  as aggression treatment, 199
  as disinhibition/emotional lability treatment, 200
  as motor restlessness treatment, 200
  as tremor treatment, 199
Prostate cancer, treatment side effects in, 40
Prostheses, 12, **409–420**
  for cancer patients, 42
  lower-extremity, 9, 409–417
  pediatric, 11
  transtibial immediate postoperative, 5
  upper-extremity, 10, 417–420

Prosthetic training, of amputees, 9–10
Protective extension reactions, 467
Protein, dietary
  daily requirements for, 459
    in pediatric patients, 82
  enteral formula content of, 460–461
Protein C resistance, as deep venous thrombosis risk
    factor, 231
Pruritus, burn-related, 28
Pseudoaneurysm, pressure ulcer-related, 286
Psoriasis, arthritis-associated, in pediatric patients,
    110–111
Psychological adjustment, by burn patients, 30–31,
    32
Psychology, rehabilitation, **271–279**
  referrals in, 275–276
  team resources and treatment in, 276–279
Psychosis
  dopaminergic drugs-related, 75
  Parkinson's disease-related, 79
Psychosocial impairments, traumatic brain injury-
    related, 179
Psyllium (Metamucil), 266, 373
Pulmonary disorders, cerebral palsy-related, 89
Pulseless electrical activity, emergency care in, 423
Pupils, examination of, in traumatic brain injury,
    170, 171
Pyelogram, intravenous, 251
Pyelonephritis, 259

Q
Quadratus femoris muscle, innervation of, 445
Quadratus plantae muscle, innervation of, 446
Quadriplegia
  incidence of, 120
  respiratory muscle dysfunction in, 129–130
  spastic, cerebral palsy-related, 85, 88, 90, 117

R
Radiation, as burn cause, 14
Radiation therapy
  for heterotopic ossification, 244
  side effects of, 39–40
Radiculopathy, electrodiagnosis of, 438
Radioiodine [^{125}I]-labeled fibrinogen uptake test, 237
Radius
  distal, resection of, in limb-sparing procedures, 42
  fractures of, orthotic treatment for, 407
Raloxifene, as osteoporosis prophylaxis and
    treatment, 225, 226
Rancho Los Amigos Scale for Level of Cognitive
    Functioning, 100, 200, 201, 202, 487
Range-of-motion exercises, for spasticity
    management, 301
Ranitidine, 372
Rankin Scale, Modified, 483
Raschischisis, 116
Rash, in traumatic brain injury patients, 182
Ray amputations, prosthetic interventions for, 417
Raynaud's phenomenon, 113
Rectal digital examination, in neurogenic bowel
    evaluation, 264
Rectum
  bleeding from, 268, 269
  examination of, in neurogenic bowel evaluation,
    264
  prolapse of, 269